TRANSITION SERIES
TOPICS FOR THE PARAMEDIC

TRANSITION SERIES
TOPICS FOR THE PARAMEDIC

DANIEL A. BATSIE, BA, NREMT-P
EDUCATION DIRECTOR
ATLANTIC PARTNERS EMS
BANGOR, MAINE

JOSEPH J. MISTOVICH, MED, NREMT-P
CHAIRPERSON, DEPARTMENT OF HEALTH PROFESSIONS
PROFESSOR OF HEALTH PROFESSIONS, YOUNGSTOWN STATE UNIVERSITY, YOUNGSTOWN, OHIO

DANIEL LIMMER, AS, EMT-P
EMS EDUCATOR, KENNEBUNKPORT, MAINE
PARAMEDIC, KENNEBUNKPORT EMS, KENNEBUNKPORT, MAINE

MEDICAL EDITOR

HOWARD A. WERMAN, MD, FACEP
PROFESSOR OF CLINICAL EMERGENCY MEDICINE, THE OHIO STATE UNIVERSITY
COLLEGE OF MEDICINE, COLUMBUS, OHIO

Brady
is an imprint of

PEARSON

Boston   Columbus   Indianapolis   New York   San Francisco   Upper Saddle River
Amsterdam   Cape Town   Dubai   London   Madrid   Milan Munich   Paris   Montreal   Toronto
Delhi   Mexico City   São Paulo   Sydney   Hong Kong   Seoul   Singapore   Taipei   Tokyo

Library of Congress Cataloging-in-Publication Data

Batsie, Dan.
  Topics for the paramedic / Dan Batsie, Joseph J. Mistovich, Daniel Limmer ; medical editor,
Howard A. Werman.
      p. ; cm. — (Transition series)
  Includes bibliographical references and index.
  ISBN-13: 978-0-13-708245-2
  ISBN-10: 0-13-708245-2
  I. Mistovich, Joseph J.   II. Limmer, Daniel.   III. Title.   IV. Series: Transitions series (Pearson
Education, Inc.)
  [DNLM: 1. Emergency Treatment.   2. Allied Health Personnel.   3. Emergency Medical Services. WB 105]
  LC Classification not assigned
  362.18—dc23   2012016372

Publisher: Julie Levin Alexander
Publisher's Assistant: Regina Bruno
Editor-in-Chief: Marlene McHugh Pratt
Acquisitions Editor: Sladjana Repic
Senior Managing Editor for Development:
   Lois Berlowitz
Project Manager: Deborah Wenger
Assistant Editor: Jonathan Cheung
Director of Marketing: David Gesell
Executive Marketing Manager: Derril Trakalo
Marketing Manager: Brian Hoehl
Marketing Specialist: Michael Sirinides
Marketing Assistant: Crystal Gonzalez
Managing Editor for Production: Patrick Walsh
Production Project Manager: Debbie Ryan

Production Liaison: Patricia Gutierrez
Production Editor: Debbie Ryan
Manufacturing Manager: Alan Fischer
Editorial Media Manager: Amy Peltier
Media Project Manager: Lorena Cerisano
Art Director: Jayne Conte
Cover Designer: Karen Salzbach
Cover Image: Daniel Limmer
Interior Design: Ilze Lemesis
Composition/Full Service Project Management:
   Niraj Bhatt/Aptara®, Inc.
Printer/Binder: Courier/Kendallville
Cover Printer: Courier/Kendallville
Text Font: Avenir LT Std

Many of the designations by manufacturers and sellers to distinguish their products are claimed as trademarks. Where those designations appear in this book, and the publisher was aware of a trademark claim, the symbols ® or ™ will appear at the first mention of the product.

Notice on Care Procedures: The author and the publisher of this book have taken care to make certain that the information given is correct and compatible with the standards generally accepted at the time of publication. Nevertheless, as new information becomes available, changes in treatment and in the use of equipment and procedures become necessary. The reader is advised to carefully consult the instruction and information material included with each piece of equipment or device before administration. Students are warned that the use of any techniques must be authorized by their medical adviser, where appropriate, in accord with local laws and regulations. The publisher disclaims any liability, loss, injury, or damage incurred as a consequence, directly or indirectly, of the use and application of any of the contents of this book.

Notice on Gender Usage: The English language has historically given preference to the male gender. Among many words, the pronouns "he" and "his" are commonly used to describe both genders. Society evolves faster than language, and the male pronouns still predominate in our speech. The authors have made great effort to treat the two genders equally, recognizing that a significant percentage of EMTs are female. However, in some instances, male pronouns may be used to describe both males and females solely for the purpose of brevity. This is not intended to offend any readers of the female gender.

10 9 8 7 6 5 4 3 2 1

PEARSON

ISBN 13: 978-0-13-708245-2
ISBN 10:   0-13-708245-2

DEDICATION

To my beautiful family, Margo, Mary, and Grace. Thank you for sharing me with all my projects while still reminding me of what is important in life. I cannot imagine a better inspiration.

DB

To my best friend and beautiful wife, Andrea, for her unconditional love and inspiration to pursue my dreams. To my daughters Katie, Kristyn, Chelsea, Morgan, and Kara, who are my never-ending sources of love, laughter, and adventure and remind me why life is so precious. I love you all!

In memory of my father, Paul, who was a continuous source of encouragement and the epitome of perseverance. I have come to realize that he is my hero.

JJM

To Stephanie, Sarah, and Margo. A man is truly fortunate to be surrounded by such beauty, intelligence, and love. You are each amazing and wonderful—the foundation for all that I am.

DL

CONTENTS

ACKNOWLEDGMENTS

Contributors

Thanks to the following people for their contributions to *Transition Series: Topics for the Paramedic.*

Scott Smith
Critical Care Nurse Practitioner
Baltimore Shock Trauma
Baltimore, MD

Kelsi A. Bean, BA, AAS, NREMT-P
Paramedic Mayo EMS
Hampden, ME

Nicole M. Beehler, BSAS, RN, CEN, EMT-P
Adjunct Faculty, Emergency Medical Technology Program
Department of Health Professions
Bitonte College of Health and Human Services
Youngstown State University
Youngstown, OH

Randall W. Benner, MEd, NREMT-P
Program Director, CFD
University of Cincinnati College of Medicine
Department of Emergency Medicine
Cincinnati, OH

Tom Brazelton, MD, MPH, FAAP
Associate Professor
Division of Critical Care Medicine
Department of Pediatrics
University of Wisconsin School of Medicine & Public Health
Madison, WI

Cornelia A. Bryan, MHHS, NREMT-P
Adjunct Faculty
Youngstown State University
Youngstown, OH

Keisha T. Robinson, DrPH, MPH
Assistant Professor/Director of Public Health Program/YSU MPH
    Program Coordinator
Department of Health Professions
Youngstown State University
Youngstown, OH

Reviewers

Thanks to the following reviewers for providing invaluable feedback, insight, and suggestions in the preparation of *Transition Series: Topics for the Paramedic.*

John L. Beckman, AA, BS, FF/EMT-P
EMS Instructor
Addison Fire Protection District
Fire Science Instructor, Technology
    Center of DuPage Addison, IL

Richard Belle, BS, NREMT-P
Continuing Education Manager
Acadian Ambulance/National EMS
    Academy
Lafayette, LA

George Blankinship, FP I/C
Moraine Park Technical College
Fond du Lac WI

Major Raymond W. Burton
Plymouth Regional Police/Corrections
    Academy
Plymouth, MA

Jerry Chaney, EMT-P/EMD
EMS Instructor
Onslow County Emergency Services
Jacksonville, NC

Helen T. Compton
Paramedic
Mecklenburg County Rescue Squad
Clarksville, VA

Jesse N. Davis, NREMT-P, I/C
EMS Instructor/Chaves County Training
    Coordinator
Eastern New Mexico University—Roswell
Roswell, NM

Chuck Fedak, EMT-P, BS
EMT Program Director
Baldy View ROP–EMT Program
Ontario, CA

Robert Ferris
EMS Specialist, FF/EMT-P
Memorial Health System EMS
Colorado Springs, CO

D. Randy Kuykendall, MLS, NREMT-P
Chief, Emergency Medical and Trauma
    Services Section
State of Colorado Department of
    Public Health and Environment
Denver, CO

Peggy Lahren, BS, NREMT-P
EMS Regional Coordinator
Arizona Department of Health, Bureau of
    EMS & Trauma
Phoenix, AZ

Alan Lambert, NREMT-P
Deputy Director
Louisiana Bureau of Emergency
    Medical Services
Baton Rouge, LA

James Massie, BS, NREMT-P
Assistant Professor of EMS Program
College of Southern Idaho
Twin Falls, ID

Christopher Matthews, AGS, NREMT-P
EMS Instructor
Truckee Meadows Community College
    EMS Programs
Reno, NV

Gregory S. Neiman, BA, NREMTP,
    CEMA (VA)
BLS Training Specialist
Virginia Office of EMS
Richmond, VA

Joel Perkins, EMT-P
Instructor
Westfield State University
Westfield, MA

Michael S. Vastano, AAS, NREMT-P
EMT Program Director
Captain James A. Lovell Federal Heath
    Care Center
North Chicago, IL

ABOUT THE AUTHORS

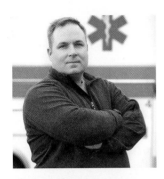

DANIEL A. BATSIE

Daniel A. Batsie has been involved in EMS for more than 20 years and has been an EMS educator since 1994. He is currently the Education Director for Atlantic Partners EMS in Bangor, Maine. In this capacity, he oversees licensure education for two regions of Maine EMS. He is department chair for EMS at Eastern Maine Community College and an adjunct faculty member for the Kennebec Valley Community College paramedic program.

Mr. Batsie graduated from Hobart College in 1993 and served in the United States Marine Corps. He has worked as a paramedic in Syracuse, New York, and Portland, Maine. He is a contributing author for numerous EMS books and journal articles.

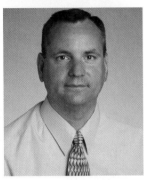

JOSEPH J. MISTOVICH

Joseph J. Mistovich is Chairperson of the Department of Health Professions and a Professor at Youngstown State University in Youngstown, Ohio. He has more than 25 years of experience as an educator in emergency medical services.

Mr. Mistovich received his Master of Education degree in Community Health Education from Kent State University in 1988. He completed a Bachelor of Science in Applied Science degree with a major in Allied Health in 1985 and an Associate in Applied Science degree in Emergency Medical Technology in 1982 from Youngstown State University.

Mr. Mistovich is an author or co-author of numerous EMS books and journal articles and is a frequent presenter at national and state EMS conferences.

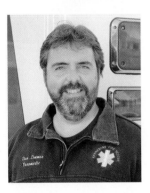

DANIEL LIMMER

Daniel Limmer has been involved in EMS for 31 years. He is active as a paramedic with Kennebunkport EMS in Kennebunkport, Maine. A passionate educator, he teaches basic, advanced, and continuing education EMS courses throughout Maine. He previously taught at George Washington University in Washington, D.C., where he coordinated international EMS education programs, and at the Hudson Valley Community College in Troy, New York. He is a charter member of the National Association of EMS Educators.

Mr. Limmer has also been involved in law enforcement, serving both as a dispatcher and police officer in Colonie, New York. He has received several awards and honors in law enforcement, including the distinguished service award (officer of the year), lifesaving award, and three command recognition awards. He also has served in the police department communications, patrol, juvenile, narcotics, and training units. Mr. Limmer retired from police work in New York but remains active as a police officer in Maine on a part-time basis.

In addition to authoring many EMS journal articles, Mr. Limmer has co-authored numerous EMS texts, including *Emergency Care*; *First Responder: A Skills Approach*; *EMT Complete: A Basic Worktext*; *Advanced Medical Life Support*; and *Active Learning Manual for EMTs*.

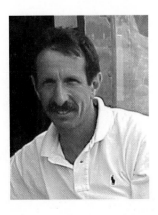

HOWARD A. WERMAN (MEDICAL EDITOR)

Howard Werman is Professor of Clinical Emergency Medicine at The Ohio State University. He is an active teacher of medical students in the College of Medicine and the residency training program in Emergency Medicine at The Ohio State University Medical Center. He has been a member of the faculty at Ohio State since 1984 and has been a contributing author to several prehospital and emergency medicine texts. He is past Chairman of the Board of the National Registry of Emergency Medical Technicians.

Dr. Werman has been active in medical direction of several emergency medical services and is currently Medical Director of MedFlight of Ohio, a critical care transport service that offers helicopter and mobile ICU services.

TRANSITION TO THE NATIONAL EMS EDUCATION STANDARDS

The National Highway Traffic Safety Administration (NHTSA) published the *National EMS Education Standards* in 2009 in response to the *EMS Education Agenda for the Future: A Systems Approach*. The National EMS Core Content and National EMS Scope of Practice Model served as the foundation for the development of the new Education Standards. The Education Standards replaced the 1985 Department of Transportation (DOT) Emergency Medical Technician–Intermediate Curriculum (I-85) and the 1999 EMT-Intermediate National Standard Curriculum (I-99). Unlike the old prescriptive DOT NSC, the Education Standards allow for much greater flexibility, adaptability, and creativity. Four levels of provider are given in the National EMS Education Standards: Emergency Medical Responder (EMR), Emergency Medical Technician (EMT—note "basic" has been deleted from the level), Advanced EMT (AEMT), and Paramedic. Although the paramedic level itself did not change, the content of the education standards was altered, giving more depth and breadth to the highest EMS level.

The Education Standards define the competencies, clinical behaviors, and judgments necessary for entry-level AEMTs to practice in the prehospital environment. For the Education Standards to be fully implemented, it is necessary for the education program and instructors or EMS service to work closely with the state EMS office to ensure that the National Scope of Practice Model has been adopted. Regardless of the adoption of the Education Standards, however, paramedic educators are obligated to present the most updated and current information to students. Likewise, practicing paramedics have a responsibility to stay current with the latest medical information relevant to their respective level of prehospital practice through continuing education.

Transition Series: Topics for the Paramedic provides both an overview of new information contained within the Education Standards at the paramedic level and a source of continuing education for practicing paramedics. If your initial paramedic training was under the old National Standard Curriculum, you will note new "topics" that were not contained in the prior curricula and previous "topics" that are presented at a much greater depth and breadth than what was contained previously. Paramedics educated and trained under the new Education Standards will be provided with a much greater foundation of knowledge for practicing prehospital care.

The National Association of State EMS Officials (NASEMSO) published a Gap Analysis Template in 2009 comparing the EMS knowledge and skills of the new National EMS Education Standards to the old Department of Transportation (DOT) National Standard Curricula (NSC). These changes, reflected as deletions, additions, and expansion from the previous NSC curriculum, identified by the Gap Analysis Template at the paramedic level, are as follows:

SKILLS NO LONGER TAUGHT TO PARAMEDICS

- Pressure points and elevation for hemorrhage control
- Umbilical vein access
- Urinary catheterization
- Forceful restraint in a prone position, with wrists and ankles tightly tied together ("hobbled") behind the back.

SKILLS FOR THE PARAMEDIC TRANSITIONING TO A 2009 PARAMEDIC

- Use of BiPAP/CPAP
- Waveform capnography
- Monitoring and management of a chest tube
- Assist in the insertion of a chest tube
- Performing a percutaneous cricothyrotomy
- Accessing indwelling catheters and implanted central IV ports
- Central line monitoring
- Initiation of intraosseous infusion in all patients (previously used IOs on children only)
- Intranasal medication administration
- Eye irrigation with the Morgan® lens
- Initiation and monitoring of thrombolytic medication
- Blood chemistry analysis (includes psychomotor skills involved with collection of blood for analysis [point-of-care testing] and the cognitive material necessary to understand implications of results)

NEW EMT EDUCATION CONTENT

- Preparatory—EMS System
  - More detailed discussion on patient safety issues.
  - Strategies to decrease medical errors.
- Preparatory—Research
  - The section is focused primarily on evidence-based decisions and how to interpret research; the section on conducting research is gone.
- Preparatory—Workforce Safety and Wellness
  - Emphasizes the difference between body substance isolation and personal protective equipment; brief discussion on bariatric issues, neonatal isolettes, and medical restraint.
  - The 1998 EMT-P National Standard Curriculum mentioned CISM; the new standards does not use that term, focusing more instead on stress management issues.

- Preparatory—Documentation
  - The Health Insurance Portability and Accountability Act (HIPAA) did not exist when the 1998 EMT-P National Standard Curriculum was authored.
- Preparatory—Therapeutic Communications
  - Increased depth of cultural competence issues.
- Preparatory—Medical/Legal Ethics
  - Health Insurance Portability and Accountability Act (HIPAA) did not exist when the 1998 EMT-P National Standard Curriculum was authored; increased depth of discussion regarding advance directives; the term "end-of-life" was not previously used; increased emphasis on end-of-life issues; increased depth and breadth on ethics.
- Anatomy and Physiology (A&P)
  - The current recommendation calls for more comprehensive coverage of A&P than provided in the previous 1998 EMT-P National Standard Curriculum. Programs should evaluate their current A&P program to see how much upgrade they need to reach a comprehensive and complex understanding, especially in the cardiovascular, respiratory, and neurologic systems.
- Medical Terminology
  - Although not detailed, this content is new to this level.
- Pathophysiology
  - The current recommendation calls for more comprehensive coverage of pathophysiology than provided in the previous 1998 EMT-P National Standard Curriculum. Programs should evaluate their current pathophysiology program to see how much upgrade they need to reach a comprehensive and complex understanding, especially in the cardiovascular, respiratory, and neurologic systems.
- Public Health
  - Consistent with *the EMS Agenda for the Future*, there is a greater emphasis on public health issues.
- Pharmacology—Principles of Pharmacology
  - Programs should evaluate their current pharmacology program to see how much upgrade they need to reach a comprehensive and complex understanding.
- Pharmacology—Medication Administration
  - Programs should evaluate their current pharmacology program to see how much upgrade they need to reach a comprehensive and complex understanding.
- Pharmacology—Emergency Medications
  - In the 1998 EMT-P National Standard Curriculum, there was no list of medications; the list in the IGs represents medications commonly used in numerous EMS systems and is a minimum list that all paramedics should know. States and programs are encouraged to add to the list, but should not delete. This list may become dated quickly.
- Airway Management, Respiration, and Artificial Ventilation—Anatomy and Physiology
  - Confusion exists about the differences among oxygenation, ventilation, and respiration. The *Education Standards* were organized to attempt to highlight the differences among the concepts. There is a greater emphasis on

ventilation and respirations and the importance of artificial ventilation. Research suggests that EMS can make a difference in this area.
- Airway Management, Respiration, and Artificial Ventilation—Airway Management
  - Confusion exists about the differences among oxygenation, ventilation, and respiration. The *Education Standards* were organized to attempt to highlight the differences among the concepts. There is a greater emphasis on ventilation and respirations and the importance of artificial ventilation. Research suggests that EMS can make a difference in this area.
- Airway Management, Respiration, and Artificial Ventilation—Respiration
  - Confusion exists about the differences among oxygenation, ventilation, and respiration. The *Education Standards* were organized to attempt to highlight the differences among the concepts. There is a greater emphasis on ventilation and respirations and the importance of artificial ventilation. Research suggests that EMS can make a difference in this area.
- Airway Management, Respiration, and Artificial Ventilation—Artificial Ventilation
  - Confusion exists about the differences among oxygenation, ventilation, and respiration. The *Education Standards* were organized to attempt to highlight the differences among the concepts. There is a greater emphasis on ventilation and respirations and the importance of artificial ventilation. Research suggests that EMS can make a difference in this area.
- Patient Assessment—Scene Size-Up
  - No new information here, but a re-emphasis on the need for scene safety for everyone present.
- Patient Assessment—Primary Assessment
  - New terminology that more closely mimics that of other health care professionals.
- Patient Assessment—History Taking
  - New terminology that more closely mimics that of other health care professionals.
- Patient Assessment—Secondary Assessment
  - New terminology that more closely mimics that of other health care professionals; more thorough than in the previous curriculum.
- Patient Assessment—Monitoring Devices
  - Includes capnography, chemistry analysis, arterial blood gas interpretation.
- Patient Assessment—Reassessment
  - New terminology that more closely mimics that of other health care professionals; more thorough than in the previous curriculum.
- Medicine—Medical Overview
  - Reuse of the new assessment terminology; emphasis on pathophysiologic basis; updated destination decisions for some medical conditions, such as stroke and acute coronary syndrome.

- Medicine—Neurology
  - The term "demyelinating" was not used in the 1998 EMT-P National Standard Curriculum; more detailed information on stroke assessment and management.
- Medicine—Abdominal and Gastrointestinal Disorders
  - In the 1998 EMT-P National Standard Curriculum, the topic was gastroenterology; new section on mesenteric ischemia, rectal foreign body obstructions, and rectal abscess.
- Medicine—Immunology
  - The term "anaphylactoid" is used here; that term was not used in the 1998 EMT-P National Standard Curriculum; transplant-related problems and collagen vascular disease added.
- Medicine—Infectious Disease
  - This section includes updated infectious disease information—for example, methicillin-resistant *Staphylococcus aureus*, hepatitis, and acquired immunodeficiency syndrome update; discussion on cleaning and sterilizing equipment and decontaminating the ambulance.
- Medicine—Endocrine Disorders
  - Added long-term effects of diabetes and how the disease affects other conditions.
- Medicine—Psychiatric
  - Includes new material on excited delirium; other psychiatric conditions are recategorized, with an increase in depth and breadth.
- Medicine—Cardiovascular
  - Increased emphasis on anatomy, physiology, and pathophysiology; acute coronary syndrome, 12-lead interpretation; updated information on heart failure.
- Medicine—Toxicology
  - Includes section on over-the-counter medication toxicology.
- Medicine—Respiratory
  - More in-depth evaluation of a patient with respiratory problems.
- Medicine—Hematology
  - Reorganized with added section on blood transfusion reactions.
- Medicine—Genitourinary/Renal
  - More detailed discussion of this organ system; urinary catheter management (not insertion).
- Medicine—Gynecology
  - Includes brief discussion of sexually transmitted diseases and pelvic inflammatory disease.
- Medicine—Nontraumatic Musculoskeletal Disorders
  - Added section on disorders of the spine, joint abnormalities, muscle abnormalities, and overuse syndromes.
- Medicine—Diseases of the Ears, Eyes, Nose, and Throat
  - New section emphasizing major eye, ear, nose, and throat disease.
- Shock and Resuscitation
  - Reorganized for emphasis, more pathophysiology.

- Trauma—Trauma Overview
  - Discussion on the Centers for Disease Control and Prevention (CDC) Field Triage Decision Scheme: The National Trauma Triage Protocol and trauma scoring.
- Trauma—Bleeding
  - More detailed discussion.
- Trauma—Chest Trauma
  - More detailed discussion—programs should evaluate their current trauma program to see how much upgrade they need to reach a comprehensive and complex understanding.
- Trauma—Abdominal and Genitourinary Trauma
  - More detailed discussion—programs should evaluate their current trauma program to see how much upgrade they need to reach a comprehensive and complex understanding.
- Trauma – Orthopedic Trauma
  - More detailed discussion—programs should evaluate their current trauma program to see how much upgrade they need to reach a comprehensive and complex understanding.
- Trauma—Soft Tissue Trauma
  - More detailed discussion—programs should evaluate their current trauma program to see how much upgrade they need to reach a comprehensive and complex understanding.
- Trauma—Head, Facial, Neck, and Spine Trauma
  - More detail about neck, eye, oral, and brain injuries; emphasizes the harm of overventilation in most situations.
- Trauma—Nervous System Trauma
  - More detail on brain anatomy; emphasizes the harm of hyperventilation; references the Brain Trauma Foundation; increased emphasis on neurologic assessment.
- Trauma—Special Considerations in Trauma
  - All sections with new or increased emphasis.
- Trauma—Multisystem Trauma
  - New material at this level; critical thinking skills emphasized, includes discussion of kinematics and blast injury.
- Special Patient Populations—Obstetrics
  - Added section on hyperemesis gravidarum.
- Special Patient Populations—Neonatal Care
  - This section is much more detailed than in the previous version.
- Special Patient Populations—Pediatrics
  - This section is much more detailed than in the previous version.
- Special Patient Populations—Geriatrics
  - Added section on herpes zoster.
- Special Patient Populations—Patients with Special Challenges
  - Added section on bariatrics.

Section (* = Education Standards Content Not Specifically Identified in the NASEMSO Essential Content: EMT Gap Analysis)	Transition Topics: EMT Topic Number	Transition Topics: EMT Topic Title
Preparatory: EMS Systems	1	Workforce Safety and Wellness
	2	Patient Safety
Preparatory: Research	5	Research: Evidence-Based Decision Making in EMS
Preparatory: Therapeutic Communication	4	Therapeutic Communication
Preparatory: Medical, Legal, Ethics	3	Legal Issues in EMS
Anatomy and Physiology; Pathophysiology	6	The Cellular Environment and Metabolism
	7	Anatomy and Physiology: The Blood
	8	The Nervous System
	10	Cellular Adaptation and Injury
	11	Self-Defense Mechanisms and Inflammation
	12	The Cardiovascular System
Medical Terminology*	9	Medical Terminology
Life Span Development*	13	Life Span Development
Public Health*	14	Public Health and EMS
Pharmacology	15	Medication Administration
	16	Paramedic Medications
Airway Management, Respiration and Oxygenation	17	Airway Assessment and Decision Making
	18	Noninvasive Airway Intervention
	19	Invasive Airway Management
Patient Assessment	20	Critical Thinking
	21	Patient Assessment
	22	Patient Monitoring Devices
Medicine: Neurology	32	Neurology: Stroke
Medicine: Abdominal and Gastrointestinal Disorders	33	Abdominal Emergencies and Gastrointestinal Bleeding
Medicine: Infectious Disease	Appendix A	Infectious Disease
Medicine: Immunology*	34	Immunology: Anaphylactic and Anaphylactoid Reactions
Medicine: Endocrine Disorders	35	Endocrine Emergencies: Hypoglycemia
	36	Endocrine Emergencies: Hyperglycemic Disorders
Medicine: Psychiatric	37	Psychiatric Disorders
Medicine: Cardiovascular	26	Cardiovascular Emergencies: Acute Coronary Syndrome
	27	Acute Coronary Syndrome and the Multilead ECG
	28	Cardiovascular Emergencies: Heart Failure
Medicine: Toxicology*	Appendix B	Toxicology
Medicine: Respiratory	29	Respiratory Emergencies: Airway Resistance Disorders
	30	Respiratory Emergencies: Lung and Gas Exchange Disorders
	31	Respiratory Emergencies: Infectious Disorders
Medicine: Hematology	38	Hematology
Medicine: Genitourinary/Renal	39	Genitourinary and Renal Disorders
Medicine: Gynecologic Emergencies*	40	Gynecologic Emergencies
Medicine: Emergencies Involving the Eyes, Ears, Nose, and Throat*	41	Emergencies Involving the Eyes, Ears, Nose, and Throat
Shock and Resuscitation	23	Cardiac Arrest and Resuscitation
	24	Shock
Trauma: Overview	Appendix C	Multisystem Trauma
Trauma: Bleeding*	42	Bleeding and Bleeding Control
Trauma: Chest Trauma	43	Chest Trauma
Trauma: Abdominal and Genitourinary Trauma	44	Abdominal Trauma

(Continued)

Section (* = Education Standards Content Not Specifically Identified in the NASEMSO Essential Content: EMT Gap Analysis)	Transition Topics: EMT Topic Number	Transition Topics: EMT Topic Title
Trauma: Soft-tissue Trauma*	45	Soft-Tissue Injuries: Crush Injury and Compartment Syndrome
Trauma: Orthopedic Trauma*	46	Orthopedic Trauma
Trauma: Head, Facial, Neck, and Spine Trauma	47 48	Head and Neck Trauma Traumatic Brain Injury
Trauma: Nervous System Trauma	47 48 49	Head and Neck Trauma Traumatic Brain Injury Complete and Incomplete Spine and Spinal Cord Injuries
Trauma: Special Considerations in Trauma	50 51 52	Trauma in Special Populations: Pediatrics Trauma in Special Populations: Geriatrics Trauma in Special Populations: Pregnancy
Trauma: Environmental Emergencies*	53 54	Diving Emergencies: Decompression Sickness and Arterial Embolism Lightning Strike Injuries
Special Patient Populations: Obstetrics	55	Obstetrics (Antepartum Complications)
Special Patient Populations: Newborn Care*	56	Neonatology
Special Patient Populations: Pediatrics*	57	Pediatrics
Special Patient Populations: Geriatrics*	58	Geriatrics
Special Patient Populations: Patients with Special Challenges*	59	Patients with Special Challenges
EMS Operations: Principles of Safely Operating a Ground Ambulance	60	Operating an Ambulance Safely
EMS Operations: Incident Management	61	Multiple Casualty Incident and Incident Management
EMS Operations: Hazardous Materials Awareness	n/a	Note: NASEMSO recommends Hazardous Waste Operations and Emergency Response (HAZWOPER) First Responder Awareness Level training. Hazardous material awareness training is handled as stand-alone course/material.
EMS Operations: Mass Casualty Incidents Due to Terrorism and Disaster	61	Multiple-Casualty Incident and Incident Management

INSTRUCTOR RESOURCES

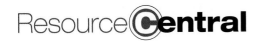

This *new* Web site contains all your instructor resources in one location! It provides all your teaching resources: PowerPoint program with instructor's notes and teaching tips, answer key to end-of-chapter questions, sample syllabi, and multiple-choice questions. To access Resource Central, go to **www.bradybooks.com** and select Resource Central. You can also find three appendices at Resource Central: Appendix A, Infectious Diseases; Appendix B, Toxicology: Street Drugs; and Appendix C, Multisystem Trauma.

Learning Management System

A dynamic and interactive online learning management system is available with this text. You can easily create a course and customize it with your own materials. All instructor resources for this edition are already loaded to enable you to run your online course with ease.

Standard Preparatory

Competency Integrates comprehensive knowledge of EMS systems, safety/well-being of the paramedic, and medical/legal and ethical issues, which are intended to improve the health of EMS personnel, patients, and the community.

TOPIC

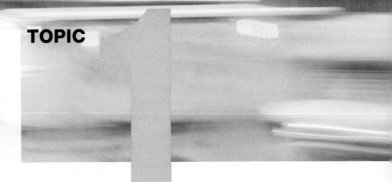

WORKFORCE SAFETY AND WELLNESS

INTRODUCTION

The number-one rule for all EMS providers is "Go home safely at the end of your shift." For all the formulas, algorithms, and skills you must learn, there is no more important theory to embrace than this rule. Often when we think of scene safety, angry patients wielding knives come to mind; in actuality, though, different, less dramatic threats are far more prevalent and even more dangerous to our well-being. Although responding to violence is certainly an important skill, often our safety education falls short on other topics that are equally as threatening.

In this topic, we take a realistic look at the causes of injury and death to EMS providers. We concentrate our efforts on preventive measures rather than reactive steps. Rather than discussing defensive tactics to ward off violent attackers, we describe preventive strategies to stop the spread of infectious diseases, to prevent back injuries, and to control potentially career-ending stress reactions. Furthermore, as advanced providers, we must discuss the role of leadership in workplace safety. It is not enough to simply protect yourself. As a paramedic, you must also consider your role in protecting the EMS team. Your role may include safety engineering, system design, and, at a minimum, serving as an example for others to follow.

All providers, from emergency responder to paramedic, should commit themselves to providing a safe work environment. "Go home safely at the end of your shift!" Safety must be an everyday, ongoing strategy and not one considered only in the case of an acute threat. Well-being rarely occurs by accident.

ACTUAL SAFETY THREATS

According to the National Highway Traffic Safety Administration (NHTSA) Fatality Analysis Reporting System, EMS providers are nearly six times more likely to be killed in a vehicle crash than to be killed by a murderous assailant. These numbers also show that as paramedics, you are as likely to die of a heart attack as you are to be murdered.

EMS workplace injury numbers follow a similar pattern. A 2007 article in the *American Journal of Industrial Medicine* and

several other related smaller studies show that back injuries and exposure to bloodborne pathogens are the leading causes of missed work among EMS professionals. Although violence remains a threat and contributes to workplace injuries, other more subtle threats debilitate hundreds of providers each day. Given this information, we must take a realistic look at scene safety threats and respond accordingly.

RESPONDING TO THE ACTUAL THREATS—WELLNESS AND INJURY PREVENTION

The core principles of injury prevention and wellness should reflect all the threats EMS providers face, not just the dramatic threats that play well on television. Although data collection in this area is quite immature, prevention strategies should be prioritized to address the most common concerns, and measures should be designed to actually protect providers from the most likely causes of injury.

Data collection is an important component in this process. Our capabilities must be improved. With regard to injury prevention, the more information we have, the better we can design our systems to protect providers. In the following sections, we discuss some of the most common safety threats to EMS providers and successful strategies to address them.

Motor Vehicle Crashes

According to the NHTSA, vehicle crashes account for nearly 80 percent of EMS line-of-duty deaths. Given this statistic, shouldn't our first safety and wellness concern be to operate emergency vehicles safely? Safe ambulance operation is discussed in greater detail in Topic 60, but as a basic injury prevention principle, seatbelt use must be of the highest priority. The fact that seatbelts prevent injuries is, at this point, a redundant statement. We all know this is true, yet each year EMS providers die unnecessarily when they are unrestrained in motor vehicle crashes. If the number one rule for paramedics is "come home safely," the number one strategy to achieve this goal should be "wear a seatbelt."

> **Vehicle crashes account for nearly 80 percent of EMS line-of-duty deaths.**

Back Injuries

Research conducted through the *American Journal of Industrial Medicine* in 2007 demonstrated that back injuries are among the most common causes of lost work and long-term disability among EMS providers. Although these injuries lack the dramatic flair and media attention of violent attacks, far more people end their careers as a result of back injuries than because of injuries from assaults.

Back injuries rarely are a singular event; they occur over the course of an often too-short career in EMS. Progressive poor lifting technique creates ongoing stress on the back; as time goes by, injuries multiply and worsen. Proper lifting and moving habits minimize stress; they should be reinforced from the beginning and used during every patient move. Although there are strategies to treat and recover from a back injury, it is far better to prevent one.

KEY ELEMENTS OF PROPER LIFTING Well-being through proper lifting technique encompasses many separate strategies revolving around the single goal of protecting your back. Key concepts of lifting and moving include the following:

1. **Anticipate a career of lifting.** It is difficult to imagine spending time as an EMS provider and not being tasked with lifting patients. In many ways, that is the nature of our profession. As such, EMS providers must consider the ongoing impact of our vocation on their backs. The risk of injury is high by default. Steps should be taken to minimize the risk of injury, including using proper lifting technique and maintaining physical fitness, core strength, and flexibility. Proper health also helps prevent injury by controlling weight gain. Remember that excessive personal weight gain adds stress to your back and can compound progressive injuries.

2. **Know your limitations.** Paramedics are faced with many lifting challenges each day. Most lifts can be accomplished with the predesignated crew, but some cannot. Unfortunately, many EMS systems have a culture that frowns on asking for help. This can be due to crew availability, budget cuts, or even ego, but regardless of the cause, attempting a lift beyond your capabilities is a recipe for disaster. Morbidly obese, or *bariatric*, patients present specific challenges. In this subset of patients, not only are our lifting capabilities overwhelmed, but the capacities of our patient carrying equipment are also often challenged.

Thankfully, advances in technology are improving our capabilities. Today's stretchers are capable of carrying heavier loads, and many of them use pneumatic or electronic technology to raise and lower the patient. This technology relieves the crew from having to deadlift a heavy stretcher loaded with a patient. Remember, though, that new technology brings with it new requirements for ongoing maintenance and upkeep. Always follow manufacturers' recommendations for use and maintenance.

Even with nonbariatric patients, every EMS provider should know when to call for help. As a paramedic, you must set the example and help build a culture in which lift assistance is the norm, rather than the exception. There should be no shame in recognizing that your capabilities are outmatched by the weight of your patient and that attempting a lift without the proper capabilities is unsafe both to you and to your patient.

Just as decision making is important in treatment strategies, it plays an important role in lifting and moving tactics. Often, as the advanced provider, you will be tasked with making important judgments on when to lift the patient or when to seek assistance in completing that lift. You must use good judgment to know not only your own capabilities, but also the capabilities of your team. When making decisions, remember that it is best not to lift if it can be avoided. Although this is not always possible, technology can frequently replace the need for old-fashioned power lifting. Use stair chairs to negotiate stairs. Use power stretchers to take the place of back stress, and when a lift is necessary, plan, ensure proper resources, and communicate. Specialized equipment is also available to assist with bariatric patients. Bariatric stretchers that are rated for much heavier loads, as well as specialized patient lifts, are sometimes available to assist with the unusually heavy patient. You should know the resources that are available in your system and use them to your advantage.

Overall, the key is to lift only when necessary and only when fully prepared with the necessary resources. Consider these concerns as just another part of your scene safety assessment.

3. **Lift using the proper power-lift technique.** Set up on a firm, level surface and position your feet shoulder-width apart. Lift with only your legs. Try not to lift with your back. Never turn or twist during a lift and avoid leaning to either side. Keep your back straight and locked and keep the weight as close to your body as you can. The farther the weight is from your body, the greater your chance of injury.

4. **Pay attention to minor injuries.** Seek medical attention for injuries that occur as a result of lifting or that arise in the line of duty. Remember that these injuries add up over time and may be the root cause of more serious injuries later. Proper initial treatment and therapy often can prevent minor injuries from developing into major injuries.

Infection Control

Exposure to potentially infectious materials is also an extremely common reason that EMS providers seek medical attention. For a paramedic, avoiding potentially infectious patients is likely impossible; however, many exposures (especially high-risk exposures) are preventable by using simple preventive strategies and appropriate personal protective equipment. Consider the following prevention strategies:

1. **Wash your hands.** The single most effective strategy to prevent the transmission of disease is basic hand washing. Effective washing must include the following key elements:
   a. Use warm flowing water with soap.
   b. Scrub all surfaces, including between the fingers and the thumbs, for at least 15 seconds.
   c. Rinse thoroughly.
   Remember to also avoid reexposure through touching faucet handles and doorknobs. Consider using paper towels as a barrier to minimize this type of contamination. Alcohol-based hand sanitizers can be used when hand washing is not available; remember, though, that not all microorganisms are destroyed by these products. Specifically, *Clostridium difficile* (C-Dif) is not destroyed by alcohol-based gels and foams.

2. **Handle sharps safely.** Although the incidence of needle sticks has declined in recent years, this route of exposure still poses a very high risk of bloodborne transmission. Safety engineering is a key practice in preventing sharps exposures. System design should minimize a paramedic's necessity to handle sharps. For example, alternative systems have eliminated the need for needles in most medication administration situations. Here, needles are only used when absolutely necessary.

   Consideration should be given to the availability of specialized sharps containers before using needles. When using sharps, be conscious of safe handling and disposal. Never recap needles and use only approved disposal receptacles. Remember that, as the paramedic, you will be setting the example.

3. **Use Standard Precautions.** Standard Precautions are the protective steps you take with every patient to guard against the potential of infectious exposure. Although risk can often be stratified by considering the circumstances (e.g., a patient with spurting blood would be a higher risk than a patient who is not bleeding), it is impossible to rule out infectious disease simply by looking at a patient. With that in mind, we should protect ourselves from potential hazards when in contact with any patient, not just high-risk patients.

   Standard Precautions include, at a minimum, gloves and probably eye protection, but can include other elements as well, depending on the level of risk. As a paramedic you must evaluate the situation and choose the appropriate level of personal protective equipment accordingly. For example, spurting blood or body fluids would definitely require eye protection and could include the need for a gown or full face protection. As an advanced provider, you may not be making this decision only for yourself, but you will likely also make the decision (or at least set the example) for others.

Infection control also requires proper post-exposure response. A plan must be in place and discussed *before* an exposure occurs. As a paramedic, you may have a role in planning or implementing such procedures. At a minimum, you may play a role in ensuring that an exposure is dealt with properly. Most postexposure plans include extensive documentation and follow-up with a medical provider. Always follow your service's specific plan. It may be your role as a paramedic to ensure that a team member completes each step of the plan. Although the exposure may be minor or low risk, consider the consequences of an infectious disease acquired on the job. Documentation is important for even the most trivial of exposures.

WELLNESS

About 10 percent of workplace deaths each year in EMS are attributed to cardiovascular disease. Although not all these deaths can be prevented, we do know that leading a healthy lifestyle can decrease the risk of heart attack and stroke. Although this may seem like a simple concept, the life of a paramedic often runs counter to this goal. EMS workers are challenged by long shifts, quick meals (that often are obtained at fast food establishments), and ongoing stress. However, when you consider that cardiovascular health poses a very high risk to our personal well-being, proactive steps must be taken. As paramedics, we must help establish a cultural shift away from the unhealthy patterns of yesterday and toward a future culture of fitness and health. The following are some important concepts to consider:

> The single most effective strategy to prevent the transmission of disease is basic hand washing.

- **Regular exercise.** A well-planned workout regimen will help you control your weight, improve flexibility, and reduce the risk of cardiovascular disease. Remember that regular exercise will also improve muscle strength and flexibility, and therefore lower the risk of back injury as well.

- **Healthy diet.** Minimizing your intake of high-calorie foods and foods high in saturated fat will improve your cardiovascular health. A proper diet will also help control your weight. Often EMS providers must be proactive and plan for healthy meals. If healthy options are not available on the job, consider bringing meals to work with you.

- **Rest.** Sleep patterns are important to any healthy lifestyle. Long and unusual EMS shifts often can interfere with getting enough sleep. Recognize that proper sleep is not just a luxury, but also an important part of healing and well-being. Choose shifts appropriately, and take active steps to maintain normal sleep patterns.

  Remember that fatigue is also a scene safety hazard. As an advanced provider, you will be making decisions that affect both your patient and your team. Fatigue can rob you of essential cognitive ability. Although caffeine and energy drinks can often relieve the pressure of fatigue, a sleep debt must eventually be repaid. Excessive caffeine and stimulant use can also increase the risk of cardiovascular disease.

- **Routine and regular medical care.** Many diseases can be successfully treated if not prevented with proper routine physicals and diagnostic testing. Consider how frustrating it is when a patient waits too long to call EMS. Avoiding routine preventive care is the same type of poor decision making.

Stress Management

The stimulus for stress is different in every individual—and the world of EMS is filled with potential stressors. From the effects of dramatic and tragic calls to those of long hours and low pay, the effects of stress can be seen throughout our industry. It is important to remember that stress has a physiologic impact, and stress management must be an important element in any wellness plan.

STRESS REACTIONS Paramedics face three types of stress reactions: acute stress reactions, delayed stress reactions, and cumulative stress reactions. The physiologic impact of stress can range from immediate to ongoing issues that build up over time. Sometimes stress occurs as the result of a dramatic or tragic call (critical incident), but often it can result from the ongoing pressure of many separate stressors that need not be dramatic in nature. Prolonged stress that leads to a cumulative stress reaction is a common reason for EMS providers to leave their field of employment.

- **Acute stress reaction.** Acute stress reactions most commonly occur immediately. A stressor elicits an immediate reaction that can include behavioral, cognitive, or even physical changes. Typically, these changes occur in response to an unusual or extra ordinary event, but again, different people have different stressors. It is reasonable to expect physiologic and behavioral changes in response to a critical incident. Shaking, crying, and increased sympathetic tone are all normal responses. However, if any of these changes impair the performance of routine duties or have an impact on a normal lifestyle, then a mental health provider should be contacted (and, in some cases, a medical professional as well). It is

exceptionally important to deal with this type of stress immediately to prevent cumulative effects from harming you later.

- **Delayed stress reaction.** Sometimes a stressor can trigger a response days, months, or even years later. A delayed stress reaction, also known as *post-traumatic stress disorder* (PTSD), can be difficult to deal with because often the signs and symptoms of stress are not recognized as being associated with a specific event. This type of stress reaction is no less harmful, however, and requires the intervention of a mental health professional to treat appropriately. Flashbacks, nightmares, irritability, and difficulty sleeping are all common signs of a delayed stress reaction.

- **Cumulative stress reaction.** Ongoing stress or stressors can also lead to cumulative stress reactions (also known as *burnout*). This type of reaction often develops over the course of years and is the result of many different stressful situations. Burnout is often difficult to diagnose, as it is usually a combination of many subtle signs. Anxiety, sleep disturbance, exhaustion, headaches, and gastrointestinal (GI) disorders are all common findings associated with cumulative stress reactions.

  Over time and without the appropriate treatment, these symptoms will grow worse and be a real threat to health and the ability to continue in a career as a paramedic. Cumulative stress reactions are not simple to deal with and frequently require the aid of a mental health professional to treat successfully.

Regardless of the type of stress reaction, the physiologic changes of stress can seriously damage your health and well-being. As part of your wellness strategy, you

must learn to recognize and minimize the effects of stress.

MINIMIZING STRESS Although it would be simple to manage stress if we could easily rid ourselves of all the things that cause difficulty in our lives, short of winning the lottery, that is not a likely answer for most EMS providers. However, you can employ strategies to minimize the impact of stress. The following are considered successful stress mitigation strategies:

- **Exercise regularly.** A regular and frequent workout regimen will reduce the effects of stress in your life, as well as improving your cardiovascular health.
- **Relax.** Find time to relax each day. Many different relaxation strategies are possible and can range from simple hobbies to quiet meditation. Find a strategy that works for you, and the effects of stress will be reduced.
- **Sleep.** Regular sleep cycles reduce the effects of stress.
- **Eat right.** Avoid excessive caffeine and energy drinks, and eat a balanced diet.
- **Seek medical attention when necessary.** Not all stress can be successfully treated by yourself. Recognize when your own strategies are unsuccessful, and seek the advice of a medical professional.

CONCLUSIONS

Very real threats face EMS providers every day. Self-protection must be the most important decision a paramedic makes. Providers should constantly be vigilant against ever-present threats, but must also recognize the ongoing, subtle threats to their well-being. Not every threat is secondary to violence. Injury prevention and wellness strategies must be considered an important strategy in staying safe.

TRANSITIONING

REVIEW ITEMS

1. According to the NHTSA, what is the most common cause for line-of-duty death in EMS?
   a. violent attack
   b. motor vehicle crashes
   c. infectious disease
   d. heart attack

2. According to the report completed in the *American Journal of Industrial Medicine*, what is the most common cause of lost work among EMS workers?
   a. back injury
   b. infectious disease
   c. cardiovascular disease
   d. violent attacks

3. Which of the following would be considered a bariatric patient?
   a. a pathologically obese person
   b. a patient with a diving injury
   c. a patient over the age of 65
   d. a potentially violent patient

4. Which of the following describes the proper technique used to conduct a power lift?
   a. shift the weight to one side when lifting
   b. lift with your back only
   c. bend at the waist when lifting
   d. lift with your legs only

5. Nightmares about a specific call that occur two months after the call would be considered a(n) _____.
   a. delayed stress reaction
   b. acute stress reaction
   c. cumulative stress reaction
   d. preemptive stress reaction

APPLIED KNOWLEDGE

1. List three important elements of hand washing.

2. List four techniques for mitigating stress.

3. List three important concepts in a wellness plan.

4. Describe the proper technique used to complete a power lift.

CLINICAL DECISION MAKING

You are assessing a 65-year-old female patient with chronic obstructive pulmonary disease (COPD). She is morbidly obese and weighs roughly 400 pounds. She is complaining of difficulty breathing and reports a three-day history of fever and coughing. She is actively coughing now.

1. What personal protective equipment would be appropriate to put on before assisting this patient?

You have determined the need to transport this patient to the hospital, and you now must move her from her bedroom to the ambulance. At this point, your team consists of yourself and your partner.

2. Would you be capable of moving this patient with the current team?

3. What additional resources would you require (if any)?

4. Would your standard lifting and moving equipment be capable of handling this patient?

5. What resources (if any) would be necessary on your arrival at the hospital?

RESOURCES

Maguire, B. J., K. L. Hunting, G. S. Smith, and N. R. Levick. "Occupational Fatalities in Emergency Medical Services: A Hidden Crisis." *Annals of Emergency Medicine* 40 (2002):625–632.

National Highway Traffic Safety Administration, Fatality Analysis Reporting System Encyclopedia, 2010.

Studnek, J. R., A. Ferketich, and J. M. Crawford. "On the Job Illness and Injury Resulting in Lost Work Time among a National Cohort of Emergency Medical Services Professionals." *American Journal of Industrial Medicine* 50 (2007):921–931.

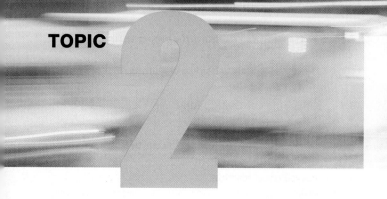

Standard Preparatory

Competency Integrates comprehensive knowledge of EMS systems, safety/well-being of the paramedic, and medical/legal and ethical issues, which is intended to improve the health of EMS personnel, patients, and the community.

PATIENT SAFETY

TRANSITION *highlights*

- Recognition of areas of patient safety risk.
- Strategies to minimize patient risk.
- Analysis of how errors occur.
- Error prevention strategies.

INTRODUCTION

According to a November 1999 Institute of Medicine (IoM) report, as many as 98,000 patients die in hospitals each year because of preventable medical errors. As every medical provider strives first to do no harm, this statistic should be considered completely unacceptable. As a paramedic, you have been entrusted with a wider array of tools and medications to more skillfully treat your patients; however, with these added capabilities your responsibilities have increased significantly. Your medications and skills could harm or even kill your patient if not used correctly.

Paramedics, as the highest level of provider in EMS, shoulder the heaviest weight of risk as they make patient care decisions. In light of the high potential to do harm and the (at least alleged) poor track record of medical errors in health care, it is essential for today's advanced life support provider to embrace the key principles of patient safety and error reduction. This topic discusses high-risk situations common to paramedics and describes strategies designed to reduce the risk of error.

> **Patient handoff is the single largest situation associated with patient errors.**

AREAS OF RISK

As an advanced provider, you face many situations that place you and your patient at risk. Paramedic-level care makes avoiding these situations altogether impossible; however, recognizing high-risk situations can help raise awareness and lead to a more cautious approach. This cautious approach is the key to keeping your patient safe.

Think of the scene assessment you conduct as you arrive at a call. There are certainly situations that you recognize as high risk for scene safety concerns. Dangerous conditions, violent patients, and bad neighborhoods all elicit a higher level of awareness than other more routine situations. High-risk patient safety situations should be dealt with in the same way. Some situations simply pose a higher risk than others. Just as going into a bad neighborhood does not automatically ensure a violent outcome, negotiating a high-risk patient safety situation does not automatically mean that an error will be made.

Situational awareness in both cases recognizes increased risk and helps you take appropriate steps to avoid problems. This awareness protects both you and your patient. The following are examples of patient situations that are considered high risk. Statistically speaking, these situations are considered the greatest concern with regard to patient safety.

Patient Transfer and Handoff

According to the IoM report, patient handoff was the single largest situation associated with patient errors. This certainly makes logical sense. As hospitals become busier and busier and staffs are cut more and more, the transfer of patients becomes increasingly difficult. EMS is by no means exempt from this risk.

Consider the following example: You arrive at a busy emergency department (ED) at a time when your shift has three priority 1 calls holding. Your suspected stroke patient seems stable enough, but you are obviously concerned about the overall outcome. En route you give a radio report; on arrival, you recognize the triage nurse as the person with the voice you spoke to on the radio. She says, "Go ahead and put him in the hall bed; we will be right there." In the meantime, dispatch radios you for the fourth time and asks if you are available. Having been acknowledged by the nurse, you and your partner transfer the patient and leave for the next call. Although this situation seems simple enough, there are a few problems:

- What if the patient's mental status changes in the next few minutes?
- Have you given enough information over the radio for that patient to receive appropriate care at the ED?
- Have you communicated the patient's medication list or allergies?
- What if there is a potentially dangerous contraindication to therapies that are about to be performed at the ED?
- Have you communicated all the therapies you completed en route?
- Is there a danger in the ED accidentally repeating those therapies?

The dangers go on and on. Instead of assigning blame, we need to recognize patient transfer as a dangerous situation. Although the situation outlined above is extreme, we are far too often faced with similar problems. Indeed, many challenges face busy EMS systems; however, we should look on patient transfer and the documentation required in that setting as just another part of patient care. You would not withhold a necessary treatment from a patient just because the system is busy, and you should not withhold the appropriate transfer of information during patient handoff.

Communication Issues

Communication (or miscommunication) certainly plays a role in many high-risk patient situations and can lead to patient errors. Patient handoff is a good example of a situation in which communication problems can raise the level of risk for your patient, but communication issues do not end there.

In many other areas, communication difficulty might put your patient at risk. Perhaps on-line medical direction has given you an order to administer a medication. Are you sure you heard the correct dose? Are you sure you heard the correct concentration? Every year hundreds of medications are administered incorrectly as a result of communication errors.

Communication issues occur even in the back of an ambulance. Are you sure your partner heard you? Are you sure you asked about allergies? Any of these situations can expose your patient to tremendous risk.

Communications must be treated with the utmost seriousness. Orders should be repeated back (this is called *closed-loop communication*); even better, they should be written down when possible. Although you may be facing time constraints and a challenging work environment, you should slow down and focus on important communication.

Medication Issues

Incorrect medication administration can potentially result in disastrous consequences. As a paramedic, you are faced with an increasing and ever-changing list of medications that can benefit your patient in the right circumstances, but can be deadly when given incorrectly. Moreover, many medications either sound or look similar to each other. For instance, epinephrine 1:1,000 is a very different drug from epinephrine 1:10,000. Atropine is very different from adenosine.

Consider packaging as well. Many EMS systems use preloaded syringes; these often are very difficult to discern at first glance. Care must be taken to ensure that the proper medication in the proper dose is given. Think back to basic pharmacology and recall the five rights of medication administration: right medication, right dose, right time, right route, and right patient. Take the time to address each of these separate questions before administering a medication. Just as with a bullet, you cannot take a medication back.

Airway Issues

Airway issues—particularly misplaced endotracheal intubations—continue to be a serious problem in the world of EMS. Unfortunately, mishandled airways have proven to be both prevalent and disastrous. Two powerful forces converge in airway management to cause tragic results. The first force is the flawed theory that intubation is the best way to manage an airway and the second is the stress associated with such a situation. Airway management will be discussed in greater detail in Topics 18 and 19, but in general we need to approach this type of decision making with an entirely different frame of reference.

Intubation is only one of many tools in the airway toolbox. It can be very appropriate, but may not always be the best choice. In light of the risk of killing your patient by placing the breathing tube into the esophagus, the decision to use endotracheal intubation should be reserved for only those situations in which its benefit truly outweighs its risk.

We also now know that stress leads to poor decision making. With regard to airway management, we need to bypass human frailties and rely on technology. In the moment, everyone thinks their tube has been placed in the trachea, but many studies have demonstrated that this initial judgment is not significantly reliable. In too many cases, this assumption is dangerously incorrect. Endotracheal tubes *must* be confirmed using technology. The risk is just too great otherwise. Waveform capnography removes the human element and replaces it with objective findings. Even simple qualitative devices such as end-tidal carbon dioxide ($ETCO_2$) detectors have the capability to identify a misplaced tube. These are inexpensive and readily available but must be used if we wish to prevent deadly airway mistakes.

Patient Movement

Patients are at risk whenever we are moving them. Dropping a patient can run the risk of both injuring the patient and exposing yourself to serious legal and civil liability. Care must be taken to move patients safely. In Topic 1, we discussed the importance of making good decisions about lifting capabilities. Lifting beyond your capacity not only puts you at risk for injury, but also exposes your patient to tremendous risk. Always know your limitations and seek help when necessary.

As Topic 1 described, you should always use technology to avoid patient lifts. Lifting a patient on a powered stretcher should always be considered preferable to lifting the stretcher yourself. Remember to utilize resources when the need of the lift outweighs your crew's capabilities. It is far better to await extra hands than to drop and injure a patient. Consider also the following helpful tips on moving patients:

- **Lift only when necessary.** Use technology when possible. Be sure you have enough personnel to effect the lift.
- **Communicate.** Patient movement almost always requires teamwork. Poor communication is frequently the cause of dropped patients.

Patient movement almost always requires teamwork.

- **When using a stretcher, move only in a head or toe direction, and never move laterally.** Consider also lowering the stretcher to reduce the top-heavy profile when traversing long or uneven distances. Consider the load capabilities of your stretcher. Patients who exceed that capacity pose a risk for equipment failure.

Ambulance Crashes

Ambulance crashes remain the single largest cause of lawsuits against EMS providers and are the source of the majority of iatrogenic injuries caused to patients by providers. Because of the high risk, we must approach this environment with an increased level of awareness and caution. Topic 60 discusses safe ambulance operation in greater detail, but some key points are worth the risk of redundancy:

- **Lights and sirens.** Is this priority transfer really necessary? We know that the risk of collision increases exponentially when lights and sirens are used. Before "lighting it up," you must seriously consider the benefits against the very high risk.
- **Securing the patient.** In the event of a crash, an unsecured patient is at an extremely high risk for injury. Have you used the appropriate restraint systems? Has the long board been properly secured to the stretcher?
- **Securing equipment.** Gear projected through the patient compartment in a crash can be deadly. Have you secured all equipment in the back?

Spinal Immobilization

Spinal immobilization is not so much a prevalent risk as it is a potentially disastrous risk. Although the data are very unclear as to the true benefit of spinal immobilization, it is an important standard of care designed to prevent secondary injuries. With patients at high risk and/or with a positive mechanism of injury, it is important to care appropriately for a potentially devastating injury. Spinal immobilization is no time to be complacent, as no provider wishes to experience the terrible consequence of a secondary injury as a result of EMS care.

HOW ERRORS HAPPEN

In the previous section, we described a number of situations in which patients were at high risk. Problems occur in many other situations as well. It is important to consider not only high-risk situations, but also behaviors that increase the risk to patients.

Errors involving patients can generally be categorized into one of three types: skill-based errors, knowledge errors, or rule-based failures. Each category results in potentially dangerous consequences and should be examined to understand how to prevent similar situations in your own practice.

Skill-Based Errors

Skill-based errors occur when technology fails or a technical skill is completed incorrectly. These types of errors can occur as a result of equipment failure or user incompetence. EMS is at high risk for these types of errors.

We have already discussed endotracheal intubation. This is a high-risk skill that is increasingly difficult to properly train providers to do. As operating rooms have more and more students and rely more and more on alternative airways for simple procedures, primary training for new providers is difficult to come by. As with any other skill, proficiency is gained through repetitive training; without appropriate training opportunities, many providers find themselves unprepared in serious situations. Frankly, it is no wonder that errors occur. The simplest way to prevent such errors is to maintain high standards of both initial and ongoing training, especially with regard to high-risk skills.

Other skill-based errors occur as a result of equipment failure. These issues underscore the need for regular equipment checks and ongoing preventive maintenance.

Knowledge-Based Errors

Knowledge-based errors occur when a wrong decision is made as a result of either incomplete or incorrect information. In many cases, these errors are due to poor initial training or a lack of ongoing education. The world of medicine is dynamic, and excellent providers recognize the need to continue their education. Even new providers should undergo field training to ensure competency.

Not every knowledge-based error is the result of incompetency, however. In many cases, these errors occur because of incomplete information. The smartest, best-educated provider may make an error if he or she has incorrect or incomplete information regarding the patient being treated. Topic 4 discusses the importance of therapeutic communication and a complete patient interview. Often, errors can be avoided by simply being thorough in your assessment.

Rule-Based Failures

A rule-based failure occurs when a provider fails to follow prescribed rules, regulations, or protocols. Generally, rules are created for a purpose and often represent the most appropriate method of accomplishing a skill or solving a problem. When providers ignore rules, errors frequently occur. The most dangerous situations are those in which safety precautions are ignored. For example, protocols are designed based on recommended treatment strategies and commonly reflect the most accepted therapies. When a paramedic ignores protocols, he likely exposes his patient to potentially hazardous treatment. Simply put, patients would be much safer if all providers followed the rules and protocols.

PREVENTING ERRORS

The two main approaches to preventing errors are systemic strategies and individual tactics. System approaches engineer safety into rules, regulations, and procedures. These strategies are designed to be used by all providers and are often the result of universal or common errors.

A good example of a systemic approach in EMS would be the design of clear protocols. These guidelines provide direction in situations that are often complex and otherwise difficult to manage. Other systemic strategies include safety engineering, such as the use of needleless systems, and could even include smaller tactics, such as improved lighting in the back of an ambulance or more distinct packaging of medications. Paramedics, as leaders of the EMS community, are frequently involved in systemic changes.

Individual tactics include situational awareness, reflection, and an understanding of personal limitations. Most individual errors occur as a result of stress and/or distraction. Therefore, the best way to prevent these errors is to slow down and pay attention. Of course, that is easier said than done. It is essential, however, especially when faced with high-risk situations.

Reflection is a different challenge and includes simply being thoughtful, but also recognizing that you are not perfect. Excellent providers constantly evaluate their own performance and recognize errors that they have made. To accomplish a high level of performance, you must learn from every mistake and consider each time how you could do it better. Embrace quality improvement and continuing education.

Finally, to prevent errors you must know your own limitations. Consider your own capabilities and seek help when you are overwhelmed. Never push a bad situation. If you have a hard time remembering doses or other numbers, for example, create and carry memory aids. If you are bad at lifting, work to improve, but recognize when the lift outweighs your own capabilities.

Ideally, systemic strategies will be combined with self-aware providers who take steps to personally prevent errors.

When these two approaches combine, patient safety is improved by far.

CONCLUSIONS

There is no single approach that will be successful in improving patient safety. Rather, patient safety is improved by weaving any number of strategies together. Recognizing high-risk situations and behaviors and adding systemic and personal strategies to reduce errors are the ways to ensure safe patient encounters.

TRANSITIONING

REVIEW ITEMS

1. Which of the following conditions associated with patient handoff would create the highest risk for patient safety?
   a. destination errors
   b. medical record transfer
   c. transfer of patient belongings
   d. communication issues

2. Which of the following would be considered closed-loop communication?
   a. speaking to a coworker in private
   b. writing down specific orders
   c. answering a specific question
   d. repeating an order back after receiving it

3. With regard to airway management, which of the following would be considered the highest-risk patient situation?

   a. bag-valve-mask ventilation
   b. misplaced endotracheal tubes
   c. poor suction use
   d. improperly sized airway adjuncts

4. Which of the following would be considered a skill-based failure?
   a. ignoring protocols
   b. ignoring a standard operating procedure
   c. administering an incorrect drug dose
   d. applying a Kendrick extrication device (KED) incorrectly

5. True or false: Using lights and sirens increases the risk of a motor vehicle crash.
   a. True   b. False

APPLIED KNOWLEDGE

1. Describe three techniques for minimizing the risk involved with patient movement.

2. Describe how patient transfer can cause an increased risk to the patient.

3. Discuss how airway management risk can be reduced.

4. Discuss why spinal immobilization is associated with increased risk to the patient.

5. Discuss how skill-based errors are different from rule-based errors.

CLINICAL DECISION MAKING

You are treating a 77-year-old female patient in cardiogenic shock. You believe that her low blood pressure requires a dopamine infusion, so you call on-line medical direction to obtain such an order.

1. Based on the points discussed in the communication section, describe the steps you would take to improve patient safety while communicating with on-line medical direction.

On-line medical direction approves an order for 5 mcg/kg/min of dopamine to be infused.

2. What individual tactics might you employ to improve patient safety while administering this medication?

3. How might systems engineering improve patient safety with regard to the administration of this particular medication?

While administering the dopamine, your reassessment determines the need for more aggressive airway management, and you elect to intubate this patient.

4. What are the patient safety risks associated with this procedure?

5. What steps can you take to minimize these risks?

Standard Preparatory

Competency Applies fundamental knowledge of the EMS system, safety/well-being of the paramedic, and medical/legal and ethical issues to the provision of emergency care.

TOPIC

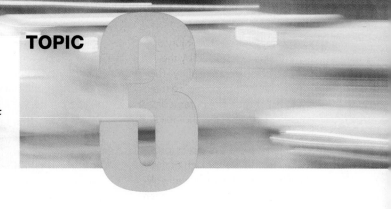

LEGAL ISSUES IN EMS

INTRODUCTION

Compassionate, professional care in the best interest of our patients should always be the guiding principle of paramedic-level treatment. As a medical professional, though, you must also operate within a system of laws, rules, and protocols designed to protect the public and to ensure the integrity of the system. Practicing in a professional manner implies an understanding of these rules and obligations.

As a paramedic, not only must you be familiar with your specific treatment guidelines, but you should also understand the regulations and requirements that specifically apply to your level of care. Decisions at the advanced level are more challenging and have more dangerous consequences in the event of an error. Legal guidelines are designed not only to provide you with specific treatment pathways, but also to protect you from liability when working within these frameworks.

Today's society is a litigious one. Lawsuits are prevalent. Being familiar with the legal concepts that are important to EMS will help ensure that you are protected from liability while doing the right thing for your patient. This topic discusses the key legal concepts that are important to every EMS provider.

LEGAL TERMS

Terminology is important when discussing legal concepts. In many ways, the medical legal world has a language of its own. As a paramedic, you should be familiar with the following concepts.

Scope of practice. The scope of practice refers to the actions and care that are legally allowed to be performed by the state in which the paramedic is providing emergency medical care. It defines the extent to which a paramedic may provide care and limits what the paramedic may do in response to an emergency. The scope of practice of the paramedic is greater than that of other levels and contains advanced modalities that come with greater legal risks and ramifications.

In most states, a medical practice act defines who may provide medical care. It is typically within this law that a paramedic's role and skill set are defined. Commonly, paramedic care is considered an extension of the capabilities of

TRANSITION *highlights*

- *Legal terms commonly associated with pertinent EMS laws and regulations.*
- *Patients' rights as applied to emergency and health care.*
- *The paramedic's role in organ donation and other special reporting situations.*

a medical direction physician. This implies specific involvement of doctors and mid-level providers within the EMS system. For example, some skills may require on-line medical direction approval. In other cases, physicians play a significant role in run review and quality assurance.

This medical practice act may also define the breadth of liability assumed by the paramedic while he is operating within the rules of the system. That does not mean paramedics cannot be sued; rather it means they may enjoy certain protections from litigation based on their appropriate actions. The laws pertaining to EMS vary from state to state; you should be familiar with the regulations guiding your own practice.

Standard of care. The standard of care is the care that is expected to be provided by a paramedic with similar training managing a patient in a similar situation. It is what a "reasonable person" with the same training in the same area would do for a similar patient. Unlike the scope of practice, which states *what* a paramedic can do, the standard of care focuses on *how* the paramedic does it.

Negligence. Negligence is a tort, or wrongful act, in which the paramedic had no intent to do any harm to the patient but in which there was a breach in the duty to act, and harm occurred. The plaintiff must prove the following four elements, or the suit will fail:

- The paramedic had a duty to act.
- The paramedic breached that duty to act.

- The patient suffered an injury or harm that is recognized by the law as a compensable injury. This means that by not providing the standard of care, the paramedic caused physical or psychological harm to the patient.
- The injuries were the direct (proximate) result of the breach of the duty. If a patient who files a negligence suit contributed in any manner to his own injury or illness, then the patient may be found guilty of contributory negligence.

Intentional torts. An intentional tort is an action knowingly committed by an individual that is considered to be civilly wrong according to the law. Common intentional torts in EMS include the following:

- *Abandonment* occurs when the treatment of a patient is stopped prior to transferring the care to another competent health care professional of an equal or higher level of training and certification or licensure.
- *Assault* is a willful threat to inflict harm on a patient.
- *Battery* is the act of physically touching a patient unlawfully without the patient's consent.
- *False imprisonment* or *kidnapping* is the intentional loading and transporting of a competent patient without the patient's consent.
- *Defamation* results when damaging information to a person's character or reputation is released to the public. The spoken form of defamation is slander; the written form is libel.

> **Medical direction should be contacted whenever a question arises about the scope of practice or the direction of the emergency care.**

Duty to act. The concept known as duty to act refers to the paramedic's legal obligation to provide emergency care to a patient. A paramedic who is on duty and comes across an emergency is generally required to stop and provide care. An off-duty paramedic usually does not have the same legal duty to act. Always be sure you are familiar with the laws of your state. If a paramedic responds to an emergency scene and stops to provide emergency care, a duty to act will be created.

Good Samaritan laws. Good Samaritan laws have been developed in all states to provide immunity to individuals trying to help people in emergencies. Most of these laws will grant immunity from liability if the rescuer acts in good faith to provide care unless the actions taken constitute gross negligence. The laws governing private and public providers vary.

Sovereign immunity. Sovereign immunity, or governmental immunity, prevents patients who receive care from governmentally operated EMS services from suing the government for civil liability. Sovereign immunity does not apply to private EMS agencies, and it may not apply to EMS providers as individuals (only to the government agency itself).

Statute of limitations. Statute of limitations refers to the period of time during which an individual may file a negligence claim. The time begins when the injury or illness was caused or when it was first discovered that the problem existed.

Medical direction. Medical direction provides active physician interaction and oversight of the emergency care provided to patients within an EMS system. Because the paramedic acts as an extension of the physician in the field, it is necessary for the paramedic to communicate appropriately and follow the orders and protocols established by medical direction. Medical direction should be contacted whenever a question arises about the scope of practice or the direction of the emergency care.

ETHICS AND ETHICAL DECISION MAKING

Advanced providers are faced with difficult decisions every day. Decisions regarding safety, transport, and treatment all must be weighed in the best interest of the patient. As a maker of such decisions, paramedics should rely heavily on ethics not only to guide appropriate treatment choices, but also to provide direction when choices are not clear. Unfortunately, advanced care is rarely "black and white"; when faced with a "gray area," ethics can help direct the most appropriate outcome.

Ethics is a branch of philosophy specifically directed toward the study of morals or concepts such as what is right and wrong. All illegal actions are considered unethical. The National Association of Emergency Medical Technicians has issued a Code of Ethics for paramedics. Ethical responsibilities of all EMS personnel include the following:

- Providing competent and professional emergency care to every patient
- Respecting all persons and their rights
- Maintaining professional knowledge and skill mastery
- Participating in research and improving patient care outcomes
- Upholding all professional standards and conduct
- Reporting events thoroughly and honestly
- Working harmoniously with other health care professionals

Sometimes, decision making is easy. Frequently, our choices are predetermined by protocol or rule. However, when the situation is unclear, ethics should guide our choices. What is the right thing to do? Paramedics should always remember the Latin phrase *Primum non nocere*—First, do no harm. As a rule, choices should always be guided by the patient's best interest. Decision making will be discussed in greater detail in Topic 20, "Critical Thinking," but ethics should always be on the forefront of any choice you make.

PATIENTS' RIGHTS
Privacy and Confidentiality

As a paramedic, it is your responsibility to maintain the privacy and confidentiality of the patient's medical status, history, and records. The Health Insurance Portability and Accountability Act (HIPAA) of 1996 is a federal law that protects the privacy of patient health care information and gives the patient control over how the information is distributed and used. Releasing confidential information requires a written release form signed by the patient or a legal guardian.

By law, you are allowed to release confidential patient information without the permission of the patient or the patient's guardian if:

- Another health care provider needs to know the information in order to continue medical care.
- An official public health or other governmental agency requires mandatory reporting of information related to your contact with the patient.
- You are requested by the police to provide the information as part of a potential criminal investigation.
- A third-party billing form requires the information.
- You are required by legal subpoena to provide the information in court (▶ Figure 3-1).

Access to Emergency Care

The Consolidated Omnibus Budget Reconciliation Act (COBRA) of 1985 and the Emergency Medical Treatment and Active Labor Act (EMTALA) of 1985 are federal regulations that ensure the public's access to emergency health care regardless of one's ability to pay. The regulations were intended to prevent "patient dumping," in which a patient requiring medical care is turned away or is transferred to a public hospital because of his inability to pay for the services.

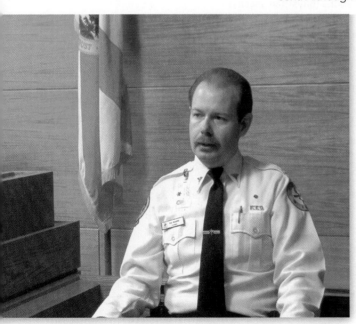

Figure 3-1 A paramedic may be required to testify in court in a variety of legal settings.

Consent

The conscious, competent, and rational patient has the right to accept or refuse emergency medical care. The patient must be informed of the care to be provided and the associated risks and consequences of receiving or refusing the care. This is referred to as *informed consent*. In addition, expressed consent from the patient must be obtained prior to initiating any care.

In a true emergency when a patient is unresponsive or is not competent, the law assumes that the patient would give consent for the treatment if able to do so. This is referred to as *implied consent*.

Some patients, such as those who are mentally incompetent or incarcerated, may not have the legal right to determine their own medical care. In these cases, it is necessary to gain consent for treatment from the legal authority that makes decisions on the patient's behalf. Minors, unless emancipated, are not considered legally competent to make their own medical decisions. Parental or legal guardian consent is needed before treating minors. If the parent or guardian is not present and cannot be reached, the concept of implied consent is used to initiate care.

With a greater skill set and assessment skills, the paramedic also has additional responsibility when it comes to patient consent and obtaining true informed consent. Although many would agree that the benefits of advanced modalities are significant, there are also greater risks. It is up to you to get the appropriate consent before beginning any care.

Refusing Care

Competent adult patients have the right to refuse emergency care and treatment even if this may result in death. A patient who displays an altered mental status, is mentally ill (although a history of mental illness alone does not automatically preclude an individual from refusing), or is under the influence of drugs or alcohol may be considered incompetent or incapacitated. Before leaving the scene of a patient refusing care, you must do the following:

- Ensure that the patient is legally competent and is capable of making an informed decision.
- If you are unsure of the patient's competency, contact medical direction.
- If you are required to contact medical direction by protocol, do so.
- Inform the patient of the risks, including the possibility of death, associated with refusing emergency care and transport to a hospital.
- Ask the patient again to accept emergency care or transport.
- If the patient is competent and still refuses, ask him to sign a refusal form. If possible, get a neutral third party to witness the refusal.
- Encourage the patient to call back if he changes his mind or if other symptoms develop.
- Completely, accurately, and thoroughly document all aspects of the call.

Transport

In an emergency, it is important to transport the patient to the closest appropriate medical facility. As a paramedic, you should not bypass a medical facility that is able to treat the patient, unless you are instructed to do so by medical direction or the patient or by predetermined protocol. If you bypass a facility, you should document the reason you did so. There are sometimes legitimate reasons to bypass a facility (e.g., if it is not a trauma hospital or stroke center) to provide the patient with appropriate care.

If you are transporting a patient from one facility to another, you should obtain informed consent, receive an accurate patient report, and receive proper documentation from the transferring facility before you place the patient on your cot. You should provide care only within your scope of practice and contact medical direction if any problems occur.

End-of-Life Issues

Some of the most important patients' rights involve end-of-life decision making. Much consideration is now given to the choices made before and during end-of-life circumstances. As an advanced provider, you should be familiar with the laws and regulations pertaining to end-of-life issues not only to be in compliance with the law, but also to respect these solemn wishes and protect the dignity of patients whose lives are coming to a close.

ADVANCE DIRECTIVES Patients are entitled to express their wishes about the events surrounding their end-of-life treatment and care. *Advance directives* are legal documents that state the patient's preferences about future medical and end-of-life care prior to serious injury or illness. Become familiar with the laws regarding living wills, do not resuscitate (DNR) orders, and health care proxies for your region or state and the laws and rules governing their implementation.

- *Living wills* are written legal documents that indicate the patient's decision about the use of long-term life support and comfort measures, such as respirators and pain medications.
- *Medical power of attorney* (POA) is a legal document that designates a person, known as a *health care proxy*, to make medical decisions for a patient when the patient is unable to do so.
- A *do not resuscitate* (DNR) *order* is a written and signed request for health care providers to withhold resuscitative measures (▶ Figure 3-2). A DNR order may indicate a variety of detailed instructions for the paramedic to perform or omit, so it should be obtained and considered before beginning any resuscitative efforts. If the DNR order cannot be located immediately, it is

---

PREHOSPITAL DO NOT RESUSCITATE ORDER

ATTENDING PHYSICIAN

In completing this prehospital DNR form, please check part A if no intervention by prehospital personnel is indicated. Please check Part A and options from Part B if specific interventions by prehospital personnel are indicated. To give a valid prehospital DNR order, this form must be completed by the patient's attending physician and must be provided to prehospital personnel.

A) _____ **Do Not Resuscitate (DNR):**
No Cardiopulmonary Resuscitation or Advanced Cardiac Life Support be performed by prehospital personnel

B) _____ **Modified Support:**
Prehospital personnel administer the following checked options:
_____ Oxygen administration
_____ Full airway support: intubation, airways, bag/valve/mask
_____ Venipuncture: IV crystalloids and/or blood draw
_____ External cardiac pacing
_____ Cardiopulmonary resuscitation
_____ Cardiac defibrillator
_____ Pneumatic anti-shock garment
_____ Ventilator
_____ ACLS meds
_____ Other interventions/medications (physician specify)
_____

Prehospital personnel are informed that (print patient name)_____
should receive no resuscitation (DNR) or should receive Modified Support as indicated. This directive is medically appropriate and is further documented by a physician's order and a progress note on the patient's permanent medical record. Informed consent from the capacitated patient or the incapacitated patient's legitimate surrogate is documented on the patient's permanent medical record. The DNR order is in full force and effect as of the date indicated below.

_____   _____
Attending Physician's Signature

_____   _____
Print Attending Physician's Name   Print Patient's Name and Location
                                          (Home Address or Health Care Facility)

_____
Attending Physician's Telephone

_____   _____
Date   Expiration Date (6 Mos from Signature)

Figure 3-2 Example of a do not resuscitate (DNR) order.

best to err on the side of patient care and perform all resuscitative measures, and then contact medical direction.

You may also hear the term *surrogate decision maker*. This is another term for someone who is allowed to make health care decisions for another individual. This is often done through a *health care proxy* or *durable POA*, which names someone to make decisions when the patient is incapacitated or incompetent.

ORGAN DONATION Patients may donate their organs if they sign a document giving permission to have their organs harvested. If the patient is a potential organ donor, medical direction should be contacted. A patient who is an organ donor should not be treated differently from any other patient requiring emergency care.

SPECIAL REPORTING SITUATIONS

Paramedics and other health care professionals are required to report certain types of incidents. Know the requirements in your state. Some special reporting situations include the following:

- **Suspected abuse or neglect.** Be careful to report and document the call objectively. Do not make accusations. Provide the proper emergency care to those involved and follow local protocol. Safe haven laws allow a person who is unwilling or unable to care for a child to drop the child off at any police, fire, or EMS station. Some areas have also expanded this program to include elderly individuals.
- **Potential crime scenes.** The primary purpose for paramedics at a crime scene is to assess and provide emergency care to the patient. They should attempt not to disturb evidence and should cooperate with other professionals on the scene.
- **Suspected infectious disease exposure.** Certain diseases are tracked by health authorities. You will also be required to report exposures to your employer to receive workers' compensation benefits.
- **Treatment or transport of incapacitated patients or those who are patients against their will.** You will likely be transporting these patients in conjunction with law enforcement or mental health authorities.
- **Dog bites.** Because of the potential for rabies and required isolation periods, many states require reports of dog bites to the appropriate authorities.

TRANSITIONING · · · · · · · ·

REVIEW ITEMS

1. An alert and oriented adult patient initially refuses care and transport. He becomes unconscious before you leave. What type of consent will you have to obtain before emergency care may be provided in his current mental state?
   - a. expressed consent
   - b. implied consent
   - c. informed consent
   - d. false imprisonment

2. An alert and oriented adult patient is complaining of severe abdominal pain. What must be obtained prior to providing emergency care?
   - a. expressed and informed consent
   - b. expressed and implied consent
   - c. informed and implied consent
   - d. implied consent only

3. Which of the following must be proven for negligence?
   - a. There was not a requirement for the paramedic to provide care.
   - b. The paramedic caused the injury.
   - c. The paramedic followed his protocols.
   - d. There was not a breach of duty.

4. Your alert and oriented patient has stated he has a severe phobia of stethoscopes and has asked you and your partner not to use one during your assessment. Immediately following the conversation, your partner removes a stethoscope from the bag and states he is going to auscultate the patient's breath sounds. Which of the following charges could result from this action?
   - a. abandonment
   - b. negligence
   - c. assault
   - d. battery

5. Following the administration of nitroglycerin to an alert and oriented patient complaining of chest pain, you place the patient on the cot to transport her to the hospital. Prior to leaving, the patient states she has changed her mind and does not wish to go to the hospital. If you continue to take her to the hospital, it may result in which of the following charges?
   - a. abandonment
   - b. slander
   - c. kidnapping
   - d. defamation

6. You left your patient in the hallway of the hospital with the nursing assistant. You are guilty of _____.
   - a. assault
   - b. abandonment
   - c. battery
   - d. libel

APPLIED KNOWLEDGE

1. List the four elements necessary to prove negligence.

2. Explain the difference between implied and expressed consent.

3. Explain why it is important for a paramedic to always behave ethically.

4. What determines a paramedic's standard of care?

5. What can a paramedic do to reduce the chance of being sued?

CLINICAL DECISION MAKING

Your supervisor calls you into her office as soon as you clock in for your morning shift at the station. She introduces you to the company's lawyer and informs you that you have been named in a lawsuit. She states that the plaintiff, Mrs. Smith, was a patient you treated more than three years ago and is now claiming that you were negligent.

1. Based on the scenario, what questions do you have?

2. On how many emergency calls have you been dispatched since that date?

3. Could you recall the specifics of that call based on this information?

4. What would you like to have to refresh your memory?

The lawyer hands you a copy of your run report of the call. As you read over your report, you are still unable to recall any specific details of the call. You look at the document and notice that you left a couple of blanks and misspelled several words on your report.

5. What concerns do you have now?

According to your prehospital care report, your patient was a 68-year-old woman whose daughter called 911 after her mother said she did not feel good. On your arrival, the patient was alert and oriented with no suspected injuries or impairments and refused any assessment or treatment.

6. At this point, what should you have done?

You and your partner attempted to persuade the patient to receive care, informed her of any risks associated with refusal, and contacted medical direction per your protocol. You advised the patient to call back if the symptoms progressed or if she changed her mind. You had her sign a refusal form.

7. What else should have been done?

8. What type of consent was rendered by the patient?

9. If you or your partner treated her at this time, of what would you be guilty?

As you were about to leave, the patient had a syncopal episode.

10. What should you have done next?

11. What type of consent was used? Why?

According to your protocol, you responded appropriately and performed emergency treatments that met the standard of care for your area. You loaded the patient into the ambulance and transported her to the closest hospital. You documented the call thoroughly.

12. Do you believe the plaintiff can prove negligence or kidnapping? Why?

13. Are you concerned about the lawsuit now? Why or why not?

Standard Preparatory

Competency Integrates comprehensive knowledge of EMS systems, safety/well-being of the paramedic, and medical/legal and ethical issues, which are intended to improve the health of EMS personnel, patients, and the community.

TOPIC

4

THERAPEUTIC COMMUNICATION

INTRODUCTION

For all the diagnostic tools and devices at the disposal of today's paramedic, the most important capability is the ability to communicate. At no other level of prehospital care is communication so important. As an advanced provider, you will be faced with difficult and complex decisions. You must make these decisions based not only on physical findings but also on a thorough medical history and examination of the patient's chief complaint. Failed communication leads to underinformed decision making and errors. Excelling at communication is a key skill to develop as a paramedic; this skill should be constantly nurtured and improved.

Communication is an active process that incorporates verbal and nonverbal expressions into messages that are received by others. Many factors—such as age, gender, culture, and experiences—can influence how these messages are sent and interpreted. As a paramedic, you must incorporate all these elements in order to maximize the amount of information available to you as you make critical decisions. To do this, you must be competent, confident, and compassionate.

THE PROCESS OF COMMUNICATION

The process of communication begins when the sender creates and encodes a message based on the information he wants to convey to the receiver. For the receiver to understand the message, it must be decoded (▶ **Figure 4-1**). The process of decoding can be influenced by the receiver's beliefs, thoughts, perceptions, and values. It is important that the message be decoded accurately to ensure effective communication. The receiver

TRANSITION *highlights*

- *Review of communication from a process perspective.*
- *Techniques to facilitate communication between individuals.*
- *Insight into communicating with patients from other cultural backgrounds.*
- *Strategies on how to communicate best with difficult patients.*

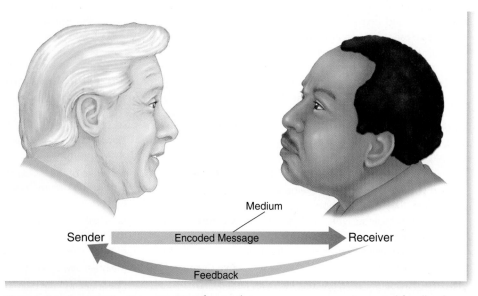

Sender — Encoded Message → Receiver

Medium

Feedback

Figure 4-1 Communication consists of a sender, a message, a receiver, and feedback.

TABLE 4-1	Techniques That May Facilitate Communication
Clarification	Ask more questions to clarify the patient's meaning.
Summary	Rephrase the response and ask whether this is what the patient meant.
Explanation	Present the information in a way the patient can understand.
Silence	Give the patient time to form an appropriate response.
Reflection	Redirect the patient's statements back to him empathetically.
Empathy	Try to understand how the patient feels and has been affected.
Confrontation	Avoid confrontation unless absolutely necessary. Always be respectful and act in the patient's best interest.
Facilitation	Help the patient express himself with the aid of communication devices.

should provide feedback by encoding a message back to the sender about the information that was received. In turn, the feedback should be decoded and interpreted. This exchange of messages and feedback is repeated continually during communication. If there is difficulty in interpreting the messages, communication will be impaired.

You should understand that both you and your patient will bring personal values, perceptions, and experiences to your communication efforts. Some techniques that may help you facilitate communication with your patient are listed in Table 4-1.

GUIDELINES FOR INITIAL PATIENT CONTACT

The paramedic is often the team leader. Assuming this role and providing a focal point for contact with the patient is an important element of communication. Confidence and poise often can restore order to an otherwise disorganized scene. Sometimes disorder comes from the patient, the patient's family, or bystanders, but often disorder is a side of effect of poor team dynamics among the EMS crews. Proper leadership can frequently improve these situations.

As a paramedic, the first impression you give to a patient when you arrive on the scene provides a foundation for the rapport you will continue to develop with the patient. The rapport should be positive and help facilitate your understanding and care for the patient. Some guidelines involving the initial patient contact include the following:

- Dress and behave professionally.
- Introduce yourself and your team.

- Ask the patient how he would like to be addressed.
- Gain consent from the patient for everything you do.
- Be aware of defense mechanisms the patient may use.
- Speak clearly, calmly, and slowly, using a professional tone of voice.
- Respect the patient's privacy.
- Limit interruptions unless they are necessary for emergency care.
- Try to control the environment surrounding the patient.
- Be courteous, compassionate, respectful, and a good listener.

CONDUCTING THE PATIENT INTERVIEW

The patient interview is an incredibly valuable component of the patient assessment. No other element of assessment will gain as much information as can be achieved through talking to the patient. As such, paramedics must look at this interaction with respect for the opportunity that it is. When the patient interview is performed effectively, valuable information is gained that will help determine the best choices in the interest of the patient.

The interview is used to gain valuable data about the patient's current problem and helps the paramedic determine an appropriate course of action. Although much of the interview is verbal, it is important for the paramedic not to overlook the nonverbal elements used throughout this process.

Nonverbal Communications

Nonverbal communications can convey valuable information between you and your patient. Nonverbal communication can include your posture, distance, gestures, use of eye contact, facial expressions, and touch. Suggested actions for using nonverbal communication appear in Table 4-2.

Each type of nonverbal communication technique conveys messages to your patient. It is important that you be aware of your patient's responses to nonverbal communications and that you react to them appropriately. Remember that what you *do not* say may be perceived by a patient as more important than what you *do* say.

Interviewing the Patient

When conducting the patient interview, you should use the following guidelines:

- Consider the patient's age and stage of development when asking a question. Use language the patient can understand.

TABLE 4-2	Nonverbal Communications	
Type of Communication	Suggested Actions
Posture	Approach the patient with open arms, open hands, and relaxed shoulders. Remain at eye level with the patient.
Distance	Be aware of the distance between you and the patient. Ask for permission before entering your patient's personal space or intimate zone. (This rule may vary among cultures.)
Gestures	Be aware of any body movements or facial expressions you make. Watch your patient's facial expression for indications of how he feels.
Eye Contact	Maintain eye contact with the patient.
Haptics	Use touch to help calm the patient. It can convey compassion and empathy if you are sincere (▶ Figure 4-2).

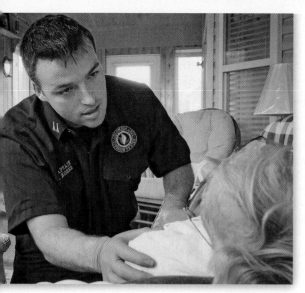

Figure 4-2 A sincere touch can provide comfort to a patient.

- Ask one question at a time, and wait for a response before continuing. Frequently, we are impatient in interviews; rather than listening, we give words to the patient ourselves. Instead of saying "Could you describe the discomfort in your chest?" we say "Is it a sharp pain?" Although the latter yields some information, it may not be the most accurate, and there may be more information available by using the former format.

- Use closed questions (questions calling for a specific response) to clarify responses and obtain specific information. This type of questioning is also important to use if a patient is unable to respond in full sentences.

- Do not ask biased or leading questions. You may miss important information the patient has to offer, and you may inappropriately influence the patient's responses.

- Do not interrupt when the patient is speaking. Remember, what the patient has to say is important.

- Do not talk so much that you fail to actively listen to what the patient has to say.

- Do not provide false assurance to the patient. Be honest, but remain compassionate.

- Do not give inappropriate advice. Your patients view and value your input as a medical professional. Do not offer any form of diagnosis or discourage the patient from seeing a physician and receiving prompt medical treatment.

- Do not ask "why" questions that imply blame. Remain impartial and nonjudgmental.

Besides specific answers to questions, the patient interview can also provide the paramedic with information about other patient considerations. Consider how a proper patient interview might glean information pertaining to the following areas:

- Orientation
- Speech
- Thinking
- Attention
- Concentration
- Comprehension
- Remote, recent, and immediate memory
- Affect
- Autonomic responses
- Facial movements
- Reactive movements
- Grooming movements

Elements as diverse as mental status and physical appearance can be assessed through a proper patient interview. Even subjective findings, such as mood, energy level, and content of thinking, can aid in developing an overall picture of your patient. Consider an interview as not just an opportunity to talk to your patient, but also as a chance to enhance your complete patient assessment.

TRANSCULTURAL CONSIDERATIONS

Culture is composed of the thoughts, communications, actions, and values of a racial, ethnic, social, or religious group. Both the paramedic and the patient bring their cultural experiences into the professional relationship. It is imperative to avoid ethnocentrism (a belief that one's own cultural group is of the most importance) and to respect the patient's culture. According to Bonita Stanton (Kliegman, 2007), the following steps can be used to assist the paramedic in achieving cultural competence:

- Learn to value and understand other cultures, in part through

self-awareness of your own cultural values.

- Learn fundamentals about other cultures, particularly those of the patients with whom you will interact.

- Develop the ability to apply cultural knowledge in patient encounters.

- Seek exposure to cross-cultural interactions.

- Be motivated to achieve all these steps.

The patient's culture affects how information is received, how illness is viewed, and what treatments are preferred. You should be aware of the sick role the patient may fill as part of his cultural beliefs and any types of folk medicines the patient may have used prior to your arrival. As a paramedic, you should understand that the acceptable use of distance and eye contact vary for different cultures, and you should use nonverbal cues to help guide your actions (▶ Figure 4-3).

CHALLENGES IN COMMUNICATION

Challenges in communication can come in different forms. As a paramedic, it is important for you to prepare for, rather than avoid, difficult situations that may cause challenges in communication.

Some specific situations that may cause communication challenges include the following:

> It is important for you to prepare for rather than avoid difficult situations that may cause challenges in communication.

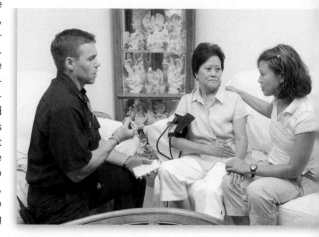

Figure 4-3 A paramedic should try to achieve cultural competence to facilitate communication.

- **Family preference issues.** Respect the family members' desire to help their loved one. Explain the patient's right to make his own decision if the patient is an adult and can provide informed consent. If it is necessary to use a different facility from the one the patient or family wants, explain kindly why using that particular facility is in the patient's best interest.
- **Motivating an unmotivated patient to talk to you.** Try to establish a good rapport. Make sure the patient understands your questions. Use closed questions if the patient has difficulty answering, or does not answer, your open-ended ones. Provide positive feedback.
- **Hostile patients.** Remember, your safety is paramount. Call for additional assistance if necessary. Advise the patient that you are there to help.

Explain the benefits of cooperation. Establish guidelines for appropriate behavior. Conduct the interview as you would for other unmotivated patients.
- **Communicating with children.** Speak in a soft tone and use language that is age appropriate. Speak to children at their eye level. Remember that children may take what you say literally, so be aware of your phrasing of words. Enlist the help of a parent or guardian when interviewing. Allow the child to have a comfort item if it does not impede care. Be honest about painful procedures.
- **Communicating with elderly patients.** Speak directly with your patient in a normal tone. Raise your voice only when a hearing problem exists. Make sure to give your patient time to respond to the questions you ask. Do not be condescending; show respect.

- **Communicating with patients who have disabilities.** If your patient is deaf, see whether he can speak sign language. Use an interpreter if necessary. You can also write notes to obtain information from your patient. When patients have visual impairments, you must explain your actions before they are performed. Patients with cognitive impairments will require you to consider their developmental level in explaining procedures, involving caregivers, and in the nature and complexity of the questions you ask.
- **Communicating with patients who do not speak English.** Language differences may be a barrier encountered by the paramedic when on a call. The use of an interpreter may be necessary. Some services and hospitals use a translation service that is available via telephone.

TRANSITIONING

REVIEW ITEMS

1. The communication technique of _____ redirects the patient's own statements back to him.
   - a. empathy
   - b. clarification
   - c. reflection
   - d. silence

2. Which of the following is an acceptable action when interviewing a patient who does not speak English?
   - a. Raise your voice so the patient can hear you.
   - b. Address only bystanders for information.
   - c. Leave the scene.
   - d. Use an interpreter.

3. Cultural experiences and influences are brought to the patient relationship by _____.
   - a. the patient only
   - b. the paramedic only
   - c. neither the patient nor the paramedic
   - d. both the patient and the paramedic

4. Immediately following the encoding of a message, _____.
   - a. the message should be sent to the receiver
   - b. the sender should provide feedback to the receiver
   - c. the receiver should give feedback to the sender
   - d. the receiver should encode a message to the sender

5. Direct eye contact should be used _____.
   - a. to intimidate your patient
   - b. to show interest and respect for your patient
   - c. regardless of the patient's cultural beliefs

APPLIED KNOWLEDGE

1. List steps a paramedic can take to become more culturally competent.

2. Explain how leading questions can impede effective communication.

3. Explain the process of communication.

4. What communication modifications may be necessary when interviewing a hostile patient?

5. When should an interpreter be used?

6. Why should open-ended questions be used before closed ones when interviewing a patient?

CLINICAL DECISION MAKING

You are called to the residence of a five-year-old male patient for an unknown injury. After determining that the scene is safe, you and your partner approach the residence in uniform with all your equipment. You are met at the door by the patient's mother. You introduce yourself and your partner and indicate that you are there to help.

1. Before entering the residence, what first impressions could you have already made on the mother?

The mother nods and leads you into the kitchen, where you see the child on the floor. There is one man in the room watching you. You ask the mother for her name and her son's name. She says her name is Olga and her son is Giovanni. You note a strong foreign accent when she speaks. As you ask the mother about the reason she called, she appears to have a bewildered look on her face. The woman states that she speaks little English.

2. What could you do to help gain the information you need?

The woman turns to the man and says something in a language with which you are not familiar. The man then identifies himself as a neighbor and offers to help. You thank him. He says the mother called

him after she called the ambulance. He said that her son cut himself on the hand with a kitchen knife. You look at the child, who is holding his hands together, and note a minimal amount of blood on the outside of his left hand.

3. How should you approach and communicate with this patient? What special considerations should you have when addressing a patient his age?

After completing your primary assessment, you advise the mother that her son should be seen by a physician. You anticipate that stitches will be needed, even though you were easily able to control the bleeding and bandage the wound. You found no other significant findings associated with the patient's current condition. You prepare the child for transport and proceed to the hospital; however, the interpreter cannot accompany you.

4. What techniques will you use to communicate with the patient while en route to the receiving facility? Why should you inform the receiving facility about the communication barrier before your arrival?

REFERENCE

Kliegman, Robert. *Nelson Textbook of Pediatrics*. 18th ed. Philadelphia: Saunders Elsevier, 2007.

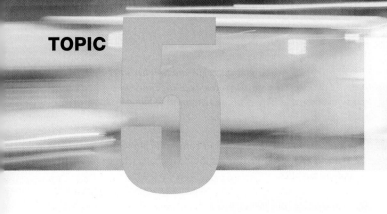

Standard Preparatory

Competency Integrates comprehensive knowledge of EMS systems, safety/well-being of the paramedic, and medical/legal and ethical issues, which are intended to improve the health of EMS personnel, patients, and the community.

RESEARCH: EVIDENCE-BASED DECISION MAKING IN EMS

TRANSITION *highlights*

- *Integration of research into EMS education and practice.*
- *Evidence-based decision making.*
- *The involvement of the paramedic in clinical and EMS systems research.*
- *Scientific theory.*
- *Types of research.*
- *Basics of analyzing and interpreting research.*

INTRODUCTION

Paramedics make choices every day about the care they deliver to their patients. We make choices both in the acute setting and in the long-term debate over protocols and treatment guidelines. Decisions need to be made both in the moment—"Which drug would help my patient the most in this particular situation?"—and in the long term, as well—"Is it worth lobbying our medical director to include this new drug in our protocols?" In each of these cases, research plays a critical role.

The history of EMS is littered with decisions made based on best guesses. For example, consider how the pendulum has swung regarding the importance of pneumatic antishock trousers and resuscitation drugs such as bretylium; what we once thought were the standards of care are now no longer recommended. Consider also the debate surrounding tourniquets. At one point, they were considered a highly dangerous, extreme measure, but now they have been integrated as a far more routine treatment modality. Today EMS has begun to recognize the value of research, especially as it pertains to the decisions that we make. Research enables us to stop guessing.

Not only does quality research demonstrate true efficacy of therapies, but it can also point out the best uses of particular treatments in specific circumstances. Every provider who steps into an ambulance would like to believe that what he is doing is really going to make a difference in the lives of his patients. Research can help us demonstrate this. Moreover, as budgets tighten and managers look for ways to control costs, it is more important than ever to ensure that what we do is both meaningful and cost-effective.

In EMS, however, these are not simple issues. We spend nearly 3 billion dollars each year delivering care, but little of what we do has ever been truly evaluated. This presents some significant problems. How do we know we are being helpful? How do we know that the tools we use are effective? As we mature as a profession, the scientific experimentation to establish facts or measure outcomes, otherwise known as *research*, will offer us an opportunity to factually answer some of these questions and will help us guide our progress to better benefit our patients (▶ Figure 5-1).

This change is not simple. EMS is not an easy field in which to gather research, and serious challenges exist. As a provider, you should understand the value of research not only to your profession, but also to your everyday practice. You can take simple steps to improve your understanding and to help move EMS toward a more evidence-based approach. In this topic, we discuss how EMS research is valuable and how you, as a provider, can improve the role of research in health care.

EMS RESEARCH AND YOU

Knowledge is power. Throughout health care, medicine is moving to a more *evidence-based* approach. This means that outcomes of therapies and interventions are carefully measured to ensure that they have the intended results. When changes are made, decisions are based on clear indications and outcomes that point to meaningful improvements in patient care. As health

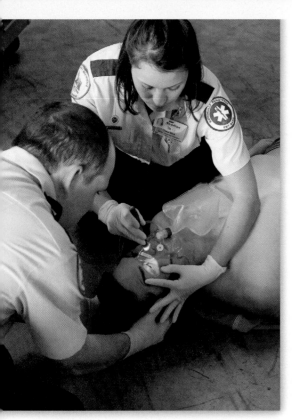

Figure 5-1 Research guides the care we provide.

care matures, more and more progress is based on an evidence-based approach. This means that the interventions we perform and the therapies we deliver must be meaningful and should be measurable. To assess the value of our care, we must turn to research. Quality studies and experimentation will separate important, relevant strategies from frivolous, wasteful endeavors. Consider the following situation:

You work as a paramedic for an ambulance service that has 20 ambulances. Staffing is tight—and the budget is tighter. Tomorrow a new device to treat cardiac arrest will be released, at a cost of $1500 each. The company that created the device claims that it is the most important device the company has ever released and that it will significantly increase cardiac arrest survival rates.

As your company decides whether to buy the device, it must weigh the idea of improving survival rates against the high cost of the device. Of course everyone would like to see patient care improve, but there is a significant cost to implementing this new device. If your company chooses to outfit its entire fleet, it will have to spend $30,000. If the device truly works, it makes a great deal of sense to

purchase it, but if it does not work, the $30,000 could pay for the addition of another paramedic.

How could your service make the correct decision? The answer is quality EMS research. If there exists unbiased scientific experimentation that this device really does double survival rates of cardiac arrest, then this decision would be easy to make. Similarly, if a quality study demonstrates that the device does not improve cardiac arrest survival, then the service could invest its money in more meaningful areas.

If, as a profession, we are committed to an evidence-based approach, we could avoid spending time and money on ineffective therapies and focus our budgets on the elements of care that mean the most. This example is hypothetical, of course, but every day EMS agencies are faced with similar dilemmas. In addition to spending money, consider the dilemmas EMS leaders and providers are faced when developing protocols, adopting new medications and devices, allotting staffing resources, and addressing myriad other questions that desperately need thoughtful answers.

In an age of slick marketing and ever-burgeoning technology, quality research and an evidence-based approach will help us answer questions and expend our resources wisely.

But what about the local level—how does EMS research affect the practice of a single paramedic? Consider your state, regional, or even service-level protocols. Decisions regarding scope of practice, equipment, and medications are made every day. Medical directors, state officials, and services consult relevant research to aid in choosing the paths and procedures that make the most sense.

Consider also the dynamic nature of health care. We know for sure that many of the treatments and therapies you are learning today may prove to be inappropriate on further examination in the future. The history of EMS is chock full of ideas, medications, and other therapies that were considered state of the art until they were thoroughly examined and determined to be incorrect. Understanding how to interpret research will help you, as a provider, stay on the cutting edge of patient care. Decisions are made every day about how we conduct our business.

Understanding research can help you contribute to these discussions.

Even in the moment of patient care, research can be beneficial. Using research to guide immediate decisions used to be the realm only of physicians, but now as paramedics learn to read and effectively interpret research, this door opens to them as well. Consider the recent discussions around the drug vasopressin. This drug may be an option for you in cardiac arrest care as a substitute for epinephrine. In the moment, you might be faced with a decision to use either drug. If you have followed the research, you might know that there is little evidence to support its use in pediatrics, even though it might be available in that circumstance.

The bottom line is that decision makers are consulting EMS research to make choices about your profession. EMS providers at every level are involved in making these decisions, but without a basic understanding of research, providers are routinely excluded from the conversation. Understanding research, even at a very simple level, allows you to speak the language of health care and can deliver a seat at the table for you. The best care possible results from an open dialogue among physicians, administrators, and providers and is best achieved by reviewing quality research.

> To assess the value of our care, we must turn to research.

THE BASICS OF EMS RESEARCH

Someone once said, "Not everything that is researched is true and not everything that is true has been researched." This statement certainly applies in the world of EMS. The dynamic nature of our treatment setting makes research difficult at best. We encounter many obstacles to research that simply are not there in other arms of the health care field. The environment in which we work can be unstable, our encounters are often brief, and our data collection is frequently disjointed and lacks centralization. Furthermore, we face many ethical dilemmas. Obtaining consent from a critical patient is often challenging at best. We do have many opportunities to create valid and important studies on prehospital care—but to do so we must promote best practices of research so our outcomes can truly guide us to high-quality care.

Not all research is created equal. There are good studies and there are bad studies. As we evolve in an evidence-based environment, we should strive to embrace the best practices of conducting and evaluating research. The finer points of medical research are by no means a simple topic, and a thorough examination of how to evaluate research is beyond the scope of this text. However, some broad concepts can be helpful to consider.

Remember that the process of research is the same whether you are an EMS researcher or a scientist in a laboratory. We all rely on the *scientific method*, developed by Galileo almost 400 years ago as a process of experimentation for answering questions and acquiring new knowledge. In this method, general observations are turned into a *hypothesis* (or unproven theory). Predictions are then made, and these predictions, based on the hypothesis, are then tested to either prove or disprove the theory.

For example, you might note that applying a bandage seems to control minor external bleeding. To use the scientific method, you might hypothesize that bandages do indeed control bleeding better than doing nothing at all. You could conduct a randomized control study to test your hypothesis by randomly assigning patients to the "bandage group" or to the "do nothing group." You could then measure the amount of bleeding in each group and compare your results. Although there might be some ethical issues with your study, this experiment would help you prove or disprove the value of bandaging. Furthermore, if your experiment was done properly, your results would hold up if the study was repeated, regardless of who conducted the experiment. That is the value of quality research. Unfortunately, not all research can live up to these quality markers.

In medicine, exacting and comprehensive studies are both difficult and time consuming. In most cases, we make decisions based on a broad variety of different sources. Unfortunately, much of what we do still relies on the "best guess strategy," but as we progress, we rely more and more on research and, in particular, research studies. When making decisions based on evidence (especially patient care decisions), it is clearly best to obtain an opinion based on many studies and

not just a single work. The strength of your conclusion is increased significantly when a variety of studies point to the same conclusion.

The key is to obtain an objective opinion. When more than one study points to the same conclusion, it is more likely to be free from opinion and bias. Many individual studies are clouded by bias, which occurs when research is influenced by prior inclinations, beliefs, or prejudices. Bias influences a study when the outcomes are manipulated to fit an expected outcome instead of being measured objectively against the hypothesis. This can occur when researchers have a financial gain in a particular outcome, but more commonly it occurs simply as a result of poor methods used to conduct the research.

In the true scientific method, outcomes are not bent to conform to previously held notions, but are examined objectively and evaluated based solely on the facts. Valid research embraces this idea and uses methods designed to limit outside influences.

Different methods of research are considered more valid than others. This is typically judged by how well they avoid potential bias and exclude the possibility of error. Consider the following strategies:

Prospective versus retrospective. Retrospective reviews look at events that have occurred in the past. Health care frequently uses retrospective reviews to look back at the outcome of therapies previously performed. In contrast, prospective studies are designed to look forward. Methods are designed to test therapies and outcomes that will occur in the future. Prospective studies are generally easier to control, as rules and regulations can be put in place to control errors and prevent bias. Retrospective studies cannot necessarily be controlled in such a way. Retrospective studies can certainly be considered valid, but a prospective method is generally considered more valid.

Randomization. High-quality studies use randomization. In medicine, this type of study typically compares one therapy against another. Bias is controlled by randomly assigning a therapy to patients, as opposed to having predetermined groups. It also improves objectivity when analyzing

outcomes. In high-quality studies, the researcher and the patients may not even know which therapy they are receiving. This process is called *blinding*. A research study can be either single-blinded (the researcher knows who gets what therapy) or double-blinded (neither the patient nor the researcher knows who gets what therapy). By blinding a study, it is very difficult to influence outcomes in any way, and the results are far more likely to be objective.

Control groups. The use of a control group helps to better evaluate outcomes fairly. In medicine, a control group is commonly a known or currently used therapy. In our previous bandaging study, we compared the bandaging group against a "do nothing" group. In that case, the "do nothing" group would be our control group. Including this group allows us not just to evaluate the outcome of bandaging, but also to compare those outcomes against a different strategy. This comparison adds weight and value to the analysis.

Study group similarity. If a group of patients is being used to test a new treatment, it is important that subjects in that group have a certain degree of similarity. Let us say, for example, that we want to test a new airway device's impact on survival in trauma patients. We have designed and implemented a study to compare the use of the new device against a group of patients who received care without using the device. In our study, paramedics were allowed to choose the patients on whom they wanted to use the new device.

When we look at our results, we find that the device group had a much higher mortality rate. At face, we could assume that this means the device did not work. However, as we analyze the results, we find that the group assigned to the new device was much sicker than the group that did not receive the device. Here, the paramedics just thought it would be better to use the new device on only the worst-off patients. Did more people die because of the device, or did more people die simply because they were hurt worse from the beginning? It is difficult to say—and therein lies the difficulty in comparing two vastly different groups. Consider also the challenges in comparing different age groups, different treatment protocols, or even different genders.

No study can be completely free from bias, but as you have seen, certain methods help to minimize the impact of subjectivity. Because of the dynamic and often sensitive nature of medicine, a large variety of research is used to make conclusions on therapies and treatment. Ideally, systematic reviews guide our most important decisions, but more commonly, a combination of research studies and research methods guides the decisions that are made. Consider the following types of medical research:

Systematic review. In a systematic review, a series of studies pertaining to a single question is evaluated. Their results are reviewed, summarized, and used to draw evidence-based conclusions. It is important to remember that a systematic review is made up of not one, but many different research experiments.

Randomized controlled trials (RCTs). In an RCT, researchers randomly assign eligible subjects into groups to receive or not to receive the intervention being tested. A control group is used to compare the tested theory against a known outcome. In 2000, for example, Marianne Gausche-Hill and her colleagues looked at pediatric intubation in Los Angeles County, California. In their study, children needing airway management were randomized, based on the day of the week, to either an intubation group or a bag-valve-mask (BVM) group. Outcomes of these patients were studied. Objectivity was improved because subjects were randomized and the results were more meaningful, as they could compare outcomes of the intubation group against the control BVM group.

In medicine, drugs are frequently tested in randomized studies using a placebo. To measure the outcome of a drug, patients are frequently randomized to receive either the real drug or a placebo, or "sugar pill," which has no effect. Frequently these studies use a double-blinding process so that even the providers carrying out the study, as well as the patients, do not know which path they are taking. In this type of study, the results of the new medication can be compared against the placebo control group to accurately assess the effect of the therapy.

Cohort/concurrent control/case-control studies In these types of studies, two groups or therapies or patients are compared, but subjects are not necessarily randomized. For example, you might compare the outcomes of one service that uses continuous positive airway pressure (CPAP) against the outcomes of another service that does not. A cohort study might follow patients who have a specific disease and compare them with a group of patients that does not have the disease. In both these studies, you are comparing two groups and have a control group, but the results are not truly randomized. Frequently, case-control studies are retrospective in nature, looking at two groups of events or outcomes that occurred in the past. All these studies can be valid and yield important information, but they also can be prone to bias in that it is difficult to control all aspects of similarity and methods among the different groups.

Case series/case reports. Case studies and case reports review the treatment of a single patient or a series of patients. Frequently they report on unusual circumstances or outcomes. There is no control group, and these reports are always retrospective. They are certainly not as valid as randomized studies, but they often help us formulate larger questions to be investigated.

Meta-analysis A meta-analysis is not truly a study itself, but a compilation of different studies looking at a single topic. A meta-analysis summarizes the work of others and frequently comments on outcomes. In many cases, these are similar to a systematic review, but frequently are of a much smaller scale.

It is important to remember that every study should be reviewed independently. The fact that it is a randomized controlled study does not ensure that its results are valid. That said, methodology does play a role in evaluating a study's importance. The American Heart Association qualifies the validity of research in a linear fashion using a "level of evidence" designation, which assigns varying levels of importance based on the way a study was conducted. This progression is useful in evaluating the importance of data and can be used as a framework for considering the utility of a particular study.

- *Level of Evidence 1.* In this sliding scale, the highest level (most valuable) set of data would result from RCTs or meta-analyses of RCTs.
- *Level of Evidence 2.* Studies using concurrent controls without true randomization. Because they are often retrospective and because the methods are more difficult to control without randomization, these types of studies are often less reliable.
- *Level of Evidence 3.* Studies using retrospective controls. There is little control of these experiments, as the testing is based on events that have already occurred. Because of this, it is difficult to ensure similar circumstances among research subjects. Although the data from retrospective studies may be useful, they can be prone to bias.
- *Level of Evidence 4.* Studies without a control group (e.g., case series). In these studies, only one group is looked at and is not compared to a second group. Here there is no control group against which to examine the results. Important information may be gained, but outcomes are difficult to truly understand without comparing with similar patients who received a different therapy.
- *Level of Evidence 5.* Studies not directly related to the specific patient/population (e.g., a different patient/population, animal models, or mechanical models). These studies are common in EMS and are frequently used to evaluate prehospital treatments. Unfortunately, their data are prone to a wide range of interpretation, as we must make assumptions that what works in different populations or under different circumstances would work in the world of EMS.

Regardless of the type of study you are reading, you should always review research in a way that helps you identify bias or flaws in the

> **Always review research in a way that helps you identify bias or flaws in the methodology.**

methodology. There is certainly a great deal more to learn about the evaluation of medical research, but there are some important questions to consider when reading a study. Consider the following questions:

1. Was the study randomized, and was the randomization blinded?

2. If more than one group was reviewed, were the groups similar at the start of the trial?

3. Were all eligible patients analyzed, and if they were excluded, why were they excluded? Bias often occurs by removing data that lead in a different direction from your hypothesis. Often, the removal of patients from a study can identify potential problems.

4. Were the outcomes really the result of the therapy? Consider the previously discussed example of the new airway device being used in only sicker patients. Occasionally, outcomes can be measured that would have happened randomly. For example, a company could invent a new device that, it claims, would make the sun rise tomorrow at 6:00 AM. Although the company could certainly produce a study that demonstrates the desired outcome, that outcome would have occurred whether the device was used or not. A powerful study is one that can be reproduced with the same results in relatively different circumstances.

5. Is the outcome truly relevant? Many studies show differences among treatment but no real relevance. For example, a study might show that a new medication increases the return of spontaneous circulation in sudden cardiac arrest compared with a placebo control group. Getting a pulse back in more patients is important, but that result is not really relevant if exactly the same number of patients die at the conclusion of care as compared with the control group.

Many good resources on evaluating evidence-based medicine can be found, and there is a great deal more information to learn on evaluating research. Learning more about this topic as a provider will help you to understand the decisions and discussions that are ongoing both in EMS and in health care in general (▶ **Figure 5-2**). Classes, textbooks, and many other tutorials can improve your capability to read and evaluate research. However, there is no better way to learn about research than to become involved in a research study.

> **There is no better way to learn about research than to become involved in a research study.**

YOUR ROLE IN EMS RESEARCH

As previously stated, medicine in general is moving rapidly in a direction guided by evidence-based medicine. In EMS, we face a future in which payment will be based on validated outcomes. Therefore, your role as an advanced life support (ALS) provider in research is especially important.

Aside from reading and discussing research, the ALS provider of the future will be on the front line of conducting research. We now know that the only way to truly prove our worth and prove the importance of our prehospital therapies is to evaluate them through clinical trials. As a provider, there are a variety of ways in which you may be involved in EMS research.

At the simplest level, your good documentation may help improve future studies. As EMS systems begin to collaborate and centralize run report data, this information may help guide any number of potential studies. EMS leaders will consider skills that are used, locations, times of day, and many other reported outcomes as they design the EMS system of the future. The time you take to document your call accurately and thoroughly may be an essential component of evidence-based medicine and may have a significant impact on the decisions that are made regarding how you do business.

You may also take part in a research study. Your service, local hospital, or region may participate and enroll patients in a specifically designed experiment. In this case, it is important to follow all the instructions you are given. Making exceptions or not following the instructions can insert bias or even eliminate your data from being considered. Participating in such a study is an important way to learn more about medical research. Not only might your service benefit from the information learned in the study, but often participation also gives you valuable insight into research methods and procedures.

As you progress as a provider, perhaps you will take part in designing a study. As a paramedic, you are on the forefront of prehospital medicine and can play an important role in shaping the future of our prehospital medicine. Many hospitals and EMS systems conduct research routinely. Your medical director or local state official

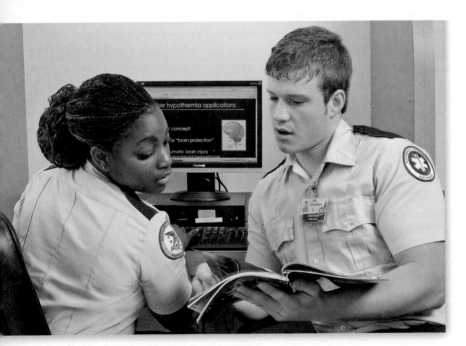

Figure 5-2 Read and evaluate research.

may be able to offer opportunities if you would like to get involved.

The Ethics of Research

As you participate in research, it is essential to include a consideration of ethics as you deal with human participants. In medical research, often the subjects of our studies are real people, and the effects of our studies often can influence their real-world well-being. As passionate as we can be to achieve valid data, we must take care not to coerce subjects into participating.

Quality research is conducted using participants who have granted the reviewers informed consent. Here, the risks and complications of the trial have been clearly outlined prior to enrolling the patient, and it has been made clear that the patient can disenroll from the study at any time.

To ensure ethical behavior, most medical studies are overseen by an institutional review board at the organization that is responsible for patient care (e.g., hospitals or state agencies). This group of reviewers approves research and ensures that the methodology of the study is ethical and responsible. All participants in research must be stewards of ethical conduct and help ensure that the patient's best interest is always kept in mind.

CONCLUSIONS

EMS research is an important part of the future of our profession. Understanding the basic concepts of research offers you a role in shaping that direction. Remember that not all research is created equal. Take the time to learn more about reading and evaluating research literature, and you will improve your own importance to your chosen field. Remember that every EMS provider must play a role in conducting EMS research. Beyond just participating, becoming involved in research development offers a rewarding pathway for enlightened providers.

TRANSITIONING

REVIEW ITEMS

1. Evidence-based medicine means that _____.
   a. you must have evidence of the patient's condition to treat him
   b. your interventions must be measurable and researched
   c. you must present evidence to medical direction to perform interventions
   d. protocols must be pilot-tested and researched before implementation

2. A hypothesis is _____.
   a. the endpoint of a research project
   b. an unproven theory
   c. the procedure used to guide a study
   d. a conclusion

3. A meta-analysis is _____.
   a. a randomized study
   b. a comparison of three or more hypotheses
   c. a compilation of studies looking at a topic

   d. a "blinded" study

4. According to the American Heart Association, a "Level of Evidence 5" means that the study _____.
   a. is not related directly to the patient population
   b. is of the highest value and credibility
   c. did not have a control group
   d. should be used to guide treatment protocols when possible

5. In reference to EMS agencies and providers conducting research, which of the following is true?
   a. EMS providers are not allowed to conduct research.
   b. EMS research is subject to the same rules as in-hospital research.
   c. Research conducted by EMS providers is considered less credible in evaluating prehospital care.
   d. EMS providers may conduct system research but not clinical research.

TOPIC

Standard Anatomy and Physiology

Competency Integrates a complex depth and comprehensive breadth of knowledge of the anatomy and physiology of all human systems.

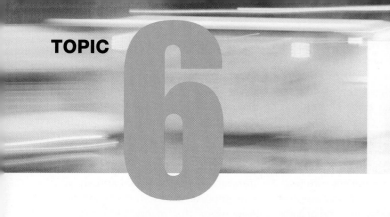

THE CELLULAR ENVIRONMENT AND METABOLISM

TRANSITION *highlights*

- *Understanding how cellular metabolism relates to the daily activities of the paramedic during assessment and management of patients.*

- *Metabolic processes and how they influence the body's structure and function.*

- *Types of cellular respiration and how these activities can either maintain homeostasis or result in death of the patient:*
  - *Aerobic metabolism.*
  - *Anaerobic metabolism.*

- *Clinical illustration of how understanding metabolism and cellular respiration will better prepare the paramedic to understand and interpret medical and traumatic emergencies in the patient.*

INTRODUCTION

To understand anatomy and physiology, you must first understand the cell and how it interacts with its environment. Individual cells are the building blocks of the body; organs and organ systems are created through the combination and interaction of cells. As a result of this composition, the requirements of individual cells represent the requirements of the body in general—and as cellular needs are met, so are the vital necessities of the body. This is a key point of anatomy and physiology, for as a paramedic, you must learn how to recognize exterior signs and symptoms as they relate to dysfunction in the cells.

> **The most basic intention of emergency medical care is to keep the cells alive.**

Although you may be identifying system dysfunction, remember that this also represents a failure to meet the basic needs of individual cells. Signs and symptoms such as altered mental status, cyanosis, and pallor can all point to specific cellular deficiencies. Your treatment strategies should be designed to reverse this process.

The most basic intention of emergency medical care is to keep the cells alive; the most basic treatment strategies are created around this fundamental intention. Establishing and maintaining the airway, ventilation, oxygenation, and circulation are designed to meet and sustain cellular needs. The study of anatomy and physiology is not just theory. It has significant relevance to day-to-day practice as a paramedic. This topic discusses several ways in which anatomy and physiology can be linked to overall patient care.

THE CELL

The human cell is the smallest unit of life. It comprises a series of structures designed to accomplish specific life functions. The outermost layer of the cell is called the *cell membrane*; it is designed to protect and contain the inner contents of the cell while selectively allowing fluid and specific substances, such as ions and nutrients, to cross into and out of the cell. The cell membrane also helps provide structure to the cell and can detect changes in the cellular environment through receptors on its surface.

The internal contents of the cell are called the *cytoplasm*. Cytoplasm is composed of a liquid medium called *cytosol* and functional units called *organelles* (▶ Figure 6-1).

Additional structure of the cell is provided by the cytoskeleton. Microtubules tether organelles in place, and filaments, such as actin and myosin, interconnect the cell membrane with the internal contents of the cell.

The *nucleus* of the cell is the control center where all cellular functions are regulated. The nucleus of a human body cell contains 23 chromosomes, which house DNA, the genetic building

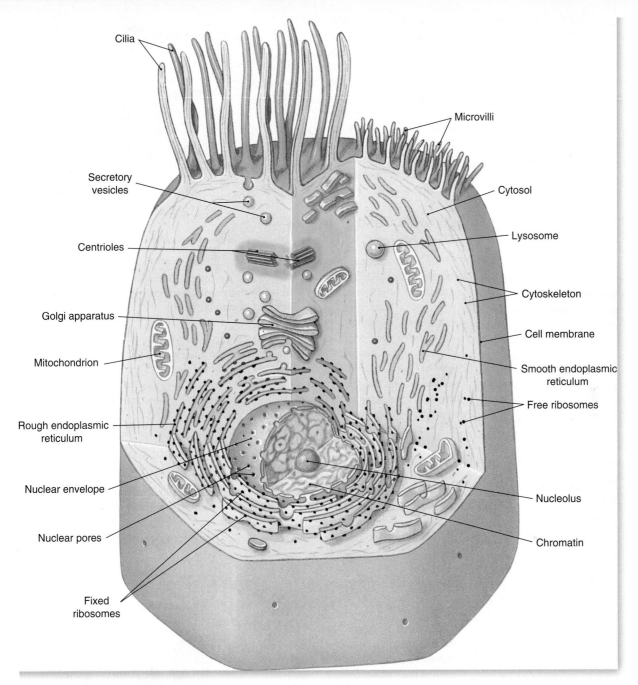

Cilia

Microvilli

Secretory vesicles

Cytosol

Centrioles

Lysosome

Cytoskeleton

Golgi apparatus

Cell membrane

Mitochondrion

Smooth endoplasmic reticulum

Free ribosomes

Rough endoplasmic reticulum

Nuclear envelope

Nucleolus

Nuclear pores

Chromatin

Fixed ribosomes

Figure 6-1 The cell.

blocks of the body. DNA strands contain the code for the synthesis of proteins and therefore are the blueprint for cellular reproduction.

Organelles within each cell provide a specific function. The *endoplasmic reticulum* plays a key role in proteins synthesis. *Ribosomes*, found within the endoplasmic reticulum, use RNA from the cell nucleus to break down proteins for later use. The endoplasmic reticulum also stores cellular materials and assists the cell with intracellular transport.

The *Golgi apparatus* assists the cell with the preparation and secretion of hormones and enzymes and assists with the maintenance of the cell membrane. It helps the cell process to synthesize lipids and proteins for secretion.

Lysosomes assist with digestion of cellular waste products and defend the cell against certain invading bacteria.

The *mitochondria* are responsible for the creation of cellular energy. In general, the body's energy is created by converting the carbohydrates we eat into energy.

Within the cytosol of a cell, glucose molecules are broken down into pyruvic acid molecules. The mitochondria then absorb the pyruvic acid and, with the use of oxygen, convert it into hydrogen and carbon dioxide. Hydrogen is then used to create energy in the form of *adenosine triphosphate* (ATP). It is important to note that when glucose is not available, lipids and protein molecules can be substituted by the cell. This process, called *metabolism*, will be discussed in greater detail in the next section.

The function of each of these individual subunits is critical to the overall life of the cell. Working in concert, these organelles allow the cell to accomplish its individual function and help the body maintain homeostasis.

CELLULAR RESPIRATION AND METABOLISM

Thousands of chemical reactions take place every second in the body's cells; these processes are essential to sustain life. These chemical reactions are collectively referred to as *metabolism*. The sum total of these reactions powers the individual operation of the body cells.

The two types of metabolic processes are catabolism and anabolism. In *catabolism*, molecules are broken down and energy is released. In the previous section, we discussed the breakdown of glucose in the cytosol; this is an example of catabolism. In *anabolism*, larger molecules are formed by synthesizing smaller units. This process releases water and requires some of the energy produced in catabolism. An example of anabolism would be the formation of glycogen from glucose molecules; glycogen is then stored in the liver and other organs for return to the body for later use.

The breakdown reactions (catabolism) must occur at rates that meet the requirements of the reactions that build up or repair cells (anabolism). That is, the reactions that produce energy must be in sufficient supply to support the reactions that consume energy. If a disturbance in this ratio occurs in which the rate of catabolism does not meet the rate of anabolism, cell damage or death will result.

Cellular Respiration

Cellular respiration is the set of the chemical reactions that take place in the cell to convert nutrients into energy in the form of ATP. During cellular respiration, energy is transferred from a glucose molecule and made available for use within the cell. This reaction releases energy and heat. The breakdown of glucose (oxidation) is not only necessary for energy production, but also necessary to maintain body heat. Without an adequate rate of oxidation of glucose molecules in the cells, the body temperature will decrease, eventually leading to hypothermia.

Glucose is a simple sugar converted from the foods we eat. It is the building block of cellular energy and is the primary nutrient of the cell. As stated, the mitochondria convert glucose into ATP, and the cell uses this energy to power the basic functions of life. Without glucose, energy is not created and cell function ceases.

Aerobic Cellular Metabolism

Three distinct but interrelated reactions occur during aerobic cellular metabolism: glycolysis, the citric acid cycle, and the electron transport chain. The term *aerobic* indicates that oxygen is available during the later part of the reaction (▶ Figure 6-2).

Lysis refers to the splitting apart or disintegration of a substance. *Glyco-* is a prefix that refers to glucose. Thus, *glycolysis* is the breakdown of a glucose molecule. Glycolysis is the first process in cellular respiration, which takes a glucose molecule that crosses the cell membrane and breaks it down into two pyruvic acid molecules. During this process, two ATP (energy) molecules are released, along with high-energy electrons. This process is *anaerobic*—it does not require oxygen to be present.

The citric acid cycle, also known as the *Krebs cycle*, occurs in the mitochondria of the cell. The pyruvic acid that was produced during glycolysis enters the mitochondria, in which carbon dioxide, more high-energy electrons, and more ATP are produced. The high-energy electrons are handed off to the electron transport chain, in which electrons are passed along the chain, and energy is transferred to form more ATP.

The final electron carrier is oxygen. With oxygen available, the final byproduct of aerobic cellular metabolism is water (H_2O), carbon dioxide

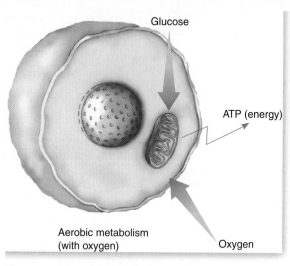

Figure 6-2 Aerobic metabolism. Glucose broken down in the presence of oxygen produces a large amount of energy (ATP).

(CO_2), a large amount of energy (32 to 34 molecules of ATP), and heat. The ATP, water, and heat are necessary for normal cell function; the carbon dioxide is passed to the blood and transported to the lungs, where it is eliminated during exhalation.

Anaerobic Cellular Metabolism

Anaerobic cellular metabolism refers to cellular respiration that occurs without the availability of oxygen (▶ Figure 6-3). Glycolysis does not require oxygen; thus, the

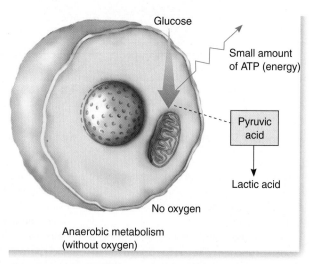

Figure 6-3 Anaerobic metabolism. Glucose broken down without the presence of oxygen produces pyruvic acid, which converts to lactic acid and only a small amount of energy (ATP). A lack of glucose and oxygen will create a disturbance to cellular metabolism and may lead to dysfunction and eventual cell death. Cell dysfunction and death lead to organ dysfunction. When a critical mass of cells dies within an organ, the organ itself then dies.

process still occurs but produces only a very small amount of energy (2 molecules of ATP), high-energy electrons, and two pyruvic acid molecules.

Without oxygen available in the mitochondria for the next reaction to occur, however, hydrogen molecules and the electrons are given back to the pyruvic acid, which then forms lactic acid. Lactic acid builds up within the cell, which inhibits glycolysis and leads to a further reduction in the already minimal production of ATP. The cell lacks the necessary ATP (energy) for normal function, and the environment becomes acidotic. The acid inactivates enzymes necessary to control the metabolic reactions and disrupts the cell membrane. If the integrity of the cell membrane is lost, the cell will die. The lactic acid will also diffuse out of the cell and enter the blood, making it acidotic as well.

Sodium/Potassium Pump

The primary intracellular (inside the cell) ion is potassium (K^+), and the primary extracellular (outside the cell) ion is sodium (Na^+). The cell membrane is less permeable to sodium ions than to potassium ions; thus, the sodium ions have a tendency to stay inside the cell. Sodium has an osmotic effect and draws water. If the sodium were allowed to stay inside the cell, the cell would eventually take on too much water, and the membrane would rupture (lyse), killing the cell.

The *sodium/potassium* (Na^+/K^+) *pump* exchanges three sodium molecules from inside the cell for two potassium molecules located outside the cell. This exchange maintains a normal balance of sodium and potassium and prevents the cell from swelling and rupturing (▶ Figure 6-4).

The Na^+/K^+ pump is an active process and requires energy in order to function. The energy is in the form of ATP. If ATP is not available, the pump does not function properly and allows Na^+ to collect inside the cell. Where sodium goes, water follows it. Therefore, the sodium draws water into the cell, causing it to swell, eventually rupturing the membrane and killing the cell.

CLINICAL APPLICATION OF CELLULAR METABOLISM

For cells to have normal function, an adequate amount of glucose and oxygen must be continuously delivered to them. With adequate delivery, high amounts of cellular energy (ATP), water, heat, and carbon dioxide are produced. The energy is used by the cell to carry out its function, such as muscular contraction or secretion of a hormone. The heat is used to maintain a normal body core temperature. The water is necessary for metabolic processes to occur. The carbon dioxide is transported by the blood and blown off during exhalation.

A lack of glucose and oxygen delivery results in inadequate energy production, a buildup of lactic acid, and a reduction in body heat. The cells may not have enough energy to carry out their normal function, such as forceful muscular contraction or the release of hormones from an endocrine gland. If ATP is not available to fuel the Na^+/K^+ pump, Na^+ stays inside the cell, draws water, causes the cell to swell, and eventually causes the membrane to rupture, leading to cell death.

Cell dysfunction and death lead to organ dysfunction. When a critical mass of cells dies within an organ, the organ itself first fails in its function, and then dies. This results ultimately from inadequate glucose and oxygen getting to cells.

Shock is defined as inadequate tissue perfusion. The inadequate perfusion refers directly to the lack of delivery of adequate amounts of oxygen and glucose to cells. If shock prevails, cells eventually die. A major sign of poor perfusion is

> **Cell dysfunction and death lead to organ dysfunction.**

Sodium/Potassium Pump

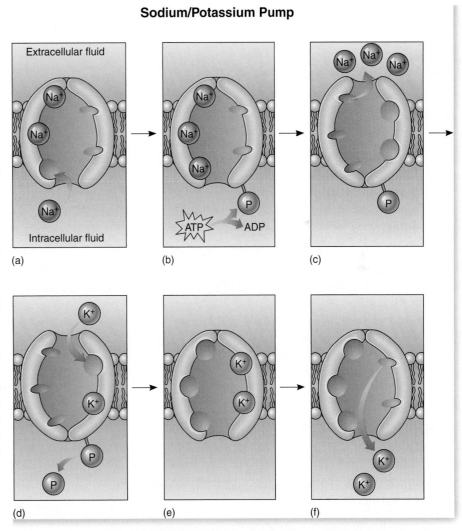

Figure 6-4 The sodium/potassium pump. Energy (ATP) is required to pump sodium (Na^+) molecules out of the cell against the concentration gradient. Potassium (K^+) then moves with the gradient to flow into the cell. Sodium and potassium are exchanged in a continuous cycle, which is necessary for proper cell function. The cycle continues as long as the cells produce energy through aerobic metabolism. When insufficient energy is produced through anaerobic metabolism, the sodium/potassium pump will fail and cells will die.

altered mental status. The lack of oxygen and glucose delivery to the brain cells from poor perfusion—a direct result of the lack of ATP production and the buildup of lactic acid—leads to cerebral cell dysfunction. If the Na^+/K^+ pump fails because of inadequate ATP availability, brain cells begin to rupture and die.

Treatment of Shock

You arrive on the scene of an accident and find two traumatized patients. One is screaming, kicking, and pulling at you when you approach him. He is complaining of excruciating pain to his left humerus, which is fractured and protruding through the skin. His friend is lying quietly, is lethargic, and is not complaining. Which patient would you tend to first?

Most EMS providers select the second patient. It takes a large amount of energy to kick, scream, and complain; thus, the first patient likely has adequate amounts of oxygen and glucose being delivered to his cells. However, his friend has little energy to move or complain. It is likely that his lack of energy is a result of poor ATP energy production from anaerobic metabolism caused by inadequate perfusion of the cells (including the brain) with oxygen and glucose. He is much more likely to be in a shock state than the screaming patient is.

One of the basic principles of shock treatment is to keep the patient warm, even when the ambient temperature is considered hot. Why is hypothermia a problem for the shock patient? It takes energy to maintain normal body temperature and body function. This energy is not available when the patient is in shock. Shock results in the inadequate delivery of oxygen and glucose to cells, which leads to anaerobic metabolism. Aerobic metabolism produces a large amount of heat as a byproduct, whereas anaerobic metabolism produces little heat, resulting in a decrease in the body core temperature. Hypothermia can ensue if the shock state is severe and of a longer duration.

Emergency care of a patient—including airway management, ventilation, oxygenation, bleeding control, administration of glucose and other medication, chest compressions, administration of fluids, and many other treatments—is geared to maintaining an adequate delivery of oxygen and glucose to cells. Lack of either substance may lead to cell, tissue, and organ dysfunction and, ultimately, death.

TRANSITIONING

REVIEW ITEMS

1. If glycolysis were the only component of cellular metabolism occurring, you would expect_____.
   a. excessive production of carbon dioxide
   b. the patient to exhibit little energy
   c. a minimal amount of lactic acid production
   d. the patient to have an increased body core temperature

2. A sudden increase in aerobic cellular metabolism would likely result in _____.
   a. pale, cool skin   b. hypotension
   c. tachypnea   d. bradycardia

3. A lack of the production of ATP would likely lead to _____.
   a. the movement of sodium ions out of the cell
   b. cell dehydration and shrinkage

   c. an increase in cellular activity
   d. cellular swelling and rupture of the membrane

4. The shock patient is at risk of becoming hypothermic because of _____.
   a. dysfunction of the sodium/potassium pump
   b. an increase in lactic acid production
   c. a decrease in glycolysis and aerobic metabolism
   d. an excessive amount of circulating carbon dioxide

5. What must be available in adequate amounts to reverse anaerobic metabolism and restore aerobic metabolism in the cell?
   a. carbon dioxide   b. pyruvic acid
   c. potassium   d. oxygen

APPLIED PATHOPHYSIOLOGY

1. Explain the difference between anabolism and catabolism.

2. Explain the difference between aerobic and anaerobic metabolism to include cellular byproducts.

3. Describe the differences in how the patient with systemic anaerobic metabolism would present, as compared with the patient with aerobic metabolism.

4. List and explain the three distinct and interrelated reactions of aerobic metabolism.

5. Which of the reactions are common to both aerobic and anaerobic metabolism?

6. How much cellular energy production would occur in a patient who had glucose delivery to cells but no oxygen?

7. Explain why glucose is necessary to maintain normal movement of sodium and potassium in and out of the cell.

CLINICAL DECISION MAKING

You arrive on the scene and find a 26-year-old male patient who has been stabbed in the abdomen. A large pool of blood is on the ground near the patient. The patient is not alert and moans in response to a trapezius pinch. His airway is partially occluded with blood and vomit. His respirations are shallow and rapid. His skin is extremely pale, cool, and clammy.

1. After ensuring scene safety, what is your first immediate action on approaching this patient?

2. What are the life threats to this patient?

3. If his airway remains occluded, how would his metabolism be affected?

4. Why is this patient prone to hypothermia?

5. What does the pale, cool, and clammy skin indicate?

6. Why is the patient presenting with an altered mental status?

7. Based on the patient's presentation, what would you expect his cellular ATP production to be?

8. Why is this patient prone to acidosis?

TOPIC

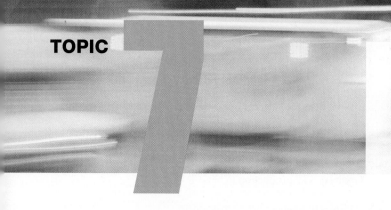

Standard Anatomy and Physiology

Competency Integrates a complex depth and comprehensive breadth of knowledge of the anatomy and physiology of all human systems.

ANATOMY AND PHYSIOLOGY: THE BLOOD

TRANSITION *highlights*

- *Understanding the composition of blood at a cellular level.*
- *Types and function of components:*
  - Plasma.
  - Red blood cells.
  - White blood cells.
  - Platelets.
- *Understanding the complete blood count and the typing of blood.*

INTRODUCTION

The blood is the body's transport mechanism. It carries nutrients, oxygen, and water to the cells to support the vital functions of the body. As a paramedic, you must understand the importance of the blood as it pertains to the physiology of perfusion and the pathophysiology of shock.

Understanding the composition and role of blood is important to understanding the circulatory system in general. When you can anticipate how blood interacts, not only with the other organs of the circulatory system but also with the body as a whole, you can better understand how a loss of blood or another blood-related complication can affect the body's vital capacity. This topic discusses the composition and function of blood and describes its existence within the larger circulatory system.

Blood is composed of formed elements and plasma.

COMPOSITION OF THE BLOOD

Blood is composed of formed elements and plasma. The formed elements, which are cells and proteins, make up approximately 45 percent of blood composition; plasma comprises the remaining 55 percent. The formed elements in the blood include red blood cells, white blood cells, and platelets.

Blood Plasma

Plasma is the yellow-colored liquid medium of blood and comprises the majority of total blood volume. Water makes up 91 percent of plasma; the remainder is made up of small plasma proteins. The primary function of plasma is to suspend and carry the formed elements.

Plasma proteins consist of albumin, antibodies, and clotting factors. Albumin is a large molecule that does not pass easily through a capillary; it plays a major role in maintaining the fluid balance in the blood. Antibodies are produced by the lymphatic system and are responsible for the defense against infectious organisms. Clotting factors include prothrombin and fibrinogen and are key in coagulation of blood from damaged vessels (blood coagulation is described in greater detail later in this topic). Fibrinogen is the most plentiful clotting factor and is the precursor to the fibrin clot.

Red Blood Cells

Red blood cells (*erythrocytes*) make up approximately 48 percent of the blood cell volume in men and 42 percent in women. Red blood cells are created by *hemopoietic tissues* of the bone marrow in a process called *erythropoiesis*. During erythropoiesis, red blood cells are created and mature through different stages. Red blood cells start as *hemocytoblasts*, which are essentially hemopoietic stem cells or basic units of future red blood cells. These stem cells develop and transform into a *normoblast*. The normoblast is the earliest form of a true red blood cell and is developed in the bone marrow. A normoblast develops into a *reticulocyte* and is then released into circulation. At this stage, the cell would be considered an immature red blood cell. These cells typically compose about 1 percent of the red cells in the human body.

The body constantly adjusts the genesis and elimination of red blood cells to provide for adequate oxygen-carrying capacity in the blood. This process is guided by oxygen levels in the body and is designed to ultimately maintain homeostasis. The creation of red blood cells relies on a constant supply of nutrients, including oxygen and iron.

Elimination of red blood cells, also known as *eryptosis*, is accomplished by the spleen, kidneys, and bone marrow. In this process, older red blood cells are destroyed and removed to carefully balance the number of circulating red blood cells to meet the needs of the body.

The cytoplasm of red blood cells contains *hemoglobin*. Hemoglobin is a molecule that contains iron and is primarily responsible for carrying oxygen and delivering it to cells for metabolism. In the presence of oxygen, the iron in this molecule oxidizes and, in a process similar to rusting metal, turns red. This process is responsible for the red coloring of blood.

White Blood Cells

The white blood cells (*leukocytes*) protect the body against infection and eliminate dead and injured cells and other debris. White blood cells are also produced in the hemopoietic tissues of the bone marrow and are generally classified into five different types:

- **Neutrophils.** Neutrophils comprise the largest portion of white blood cells (50 percent to 60 percent). These cells play a very important part in the immune system and are responsible primarily for the destruction and removal of bacterial and fungal invaders of the body. Neutrophils are commonly found in large quantities in pus surrounding an infection.

- **Eosinophils.** Eosinophils are also an important element of the immune system and are also used to deal with invaders to the body. Eosinophils also play a large role in the inflammation associated with hypersensitivity (allergic) reactions.

- **Basophils.** Basophils help the body respond to foreign invaders by releasing histamine. These cells also play a large role in the negative effects of an allergic reaction.

- **Lymphocytes:** Lymphocytes are the key cells of immune response. B cell lymphocytes produce antibodies that help the body recognize invaders. T cell and natural killer cell lymphocytes respond to and destroy foreign invaders.

- **Monocytes.** Monocytes help the immune system in three ways: They

assist antibodies with identifying unwanted invaders, they destroy and remove unwanted materials (similar to that which is done by neutrophils), and they produce cytokines.

Platelets

Platelets, or *thrombocytes*, are not actual cells but, rather, fragments that play a major role in hemostasis (blood clotting and the control of bleeding). When activated, platelets adhere together to form clots and stop bleeding. When specific chemical markers are released into the bloodstream, platelets undergo specific changes. Activation causes platelets to change shape, making accumulation easier. Activation also causes platelets to open specific receptor sites to link with chemicals such as fibrinogen to enhance the clotting cascade. This platelet aggregation essentially plugs a wound to decrease or stop bleeding. Platelets also secrete specific chemical signals to begin the healing process.

Each component of blood plays an important role in ensuring the health of the body as a whole. It is important that you, as a paramedic, understand not only how these functions interact, but also how to ensure that these capabilities are present. Disruption of these functions will typically demonstrate outward signs and symptoms. For example, deoxygenated hemoglobin presents as cyanosis. Depleted platelet counts might present as difficulty controlling bleeding.

Many laboratory tests exist to examine the components of the blood. Although these are not typically performed in the prehospital world, paramedics should be familiar with them and their normal values. Several of these are discussed here.

THE COMPLETE BLOOD COUNT

The complete blood count is a test performed on a sample of blood and is used to determine the presence of key elements of blood composition. Specifically, it examines:

- The total number of white blood cells per unit of blood volume and the types of white blood cells present in the sample

- The actual number of red blood cells per unit of blood volume, the average size of the red blood cells (*mean

corpuscular volume* [MCV]), and the percentage of red blood cells per unit of blood volume (*hematocrit*)

- The variation in the size of red blood cells (*red cell distribution width* [RDW])

- The amount of hemoglobin in the blood, the average amount of hemoglobin inside a red blood cell (*mean corpuscular hemoglobin* [MCH]), and the average concentration of hemoglobin inside the red blood cell (*mean corpuscular hemoglobin concentration* [MCHC])

- The number of platelets in unit of blood volume

Normal values for the complete blood count can be found in **Table 7-1**.

Blood Type and Rh Factor

In addition to testing to determine the composition, blood is also classified by ABO group and Rh factor. The ABO system separates blood into three categories, or types, by the presence or lack of inherited anti-A and anti-B antigens on red blood cells and by specific antibodies that can be found in the blood plasma. This typing is used primarily to assess compatibility in the event of a transfusion. The American Red Cross describes four major blood types:

- **A.** Only the A antigen is present on red blood cells (and B antibody in the plasma)

- **B.** Only the B antigen is present on blood red cells (and A antibody in the plasma)

- **AB.** Has both A and B antigens on red blood cells (but neither A nor B antibody in the plasma)

- **O.** Has neither A nor B antigens on red blood cells (but both A and B antibody are in the plasma)

In addition to looking for specific antigens to classify blood using the ABO system, the Rh, or rhesus, factor is also analyzed. The Rh factor looks for the presence of a specific third antigen and is usually represented as positive (the antigen is present) or negative (the antigen is not present).

HEMOSTASIS

The body goes to great lengths to keep blood within the circulatory system. *Hemostasis* is the process of protecting

TABLE 7-1   Complete Blood Count Normal Values

Test	Normal Value
White blood cells	$4.1–10.9 \times 10^3/\mu L$
(White blood cell differential) Polymorphonuclear cells	35–80%
Immature bands	0–10%
Lymphocytes	20–50%
Monocytes	2–12%
Eosinophils	0–7%
Basophils	0–2%
Red blood cells	$4.3–6.2 \times 10^6/\mu L$ (male) $3.8–5.5 \times 10^6/\mu L$ (female) $3.8–5.5 \times 10^6/\mu L$ (infant/child)
RDW coefficient of variation	11.5–14.5%
Hemoglobin	13.2–16.2 g/dL (male) 12.0–15.2 g/dL (female)
Hematocrit	40–52% (male) 37–46% (female) 31–43% (child)
MCV	82–102 fL (male) 78–101 fL (female)
MCH	27–31 pg/cell
MCHC	31–35 gm/dL
Platelets	$140–450 \times 10^3/\mu L$

the circulatory system from blood loss. Although hemostasis is a complex process, predictable actions occur within a blood vessel when the integrity of the container is challenged.

Under normal circumstances, the endothelial lining of intact blood vessels prevents platelets from grouping together. Chemicals such as nitric oxide and thrombomodulin are regularly secreted to prevent the clotting process from occurring. When the integrity of this inner lining is disrupted—for example, as a result of penetrating trauma—chemical triggers such as von Willebrand factor and tissue thromboplastin are released, and the sequence of hemostasis begins. Hemostasis can be categorized into three distinct phases:

> **Coagulation is designed to be temporary.**

1. **Vasoconstriction.** Thromboxane and systemic hormones, such as epinephrine, are released during the initial phase of hemostasis to cause vasoconstriction. Constriction of the damaged blood vessel (and vessels surrounding the area) shunts blood away from the damage and thereby minimizes loss.

2. **Platelet plugging.** When circulating platelets come into contact with exposed collagen from the inner lining of a damaged blood vessel, they stick and begin to accumulate. This accumulation effectively creates a plug for the hole and can limit blood loss, as the stopper in a drain stops the flow of water. As platelets stick together, they "activate" and secrete their own chemical markers. Chemicals such as thromboxane enhance the attraction among platelets and further assist in gathering other circulating platelets to plug the hole. In cases of unwanted clotting, such as in acute coronary syndrome, aspirin is used to inhibit the effects of thromboxane and prevent platelet aggregation.

3. **Coagulation.** Platelet plugging occurs rapidly and is a relatively quick fix for a ruptured vessel. Coagulation takes longer but produces a more stable, longer lasting fix. Chemical triggers from the damaged area activate self-defense mechanisms to begin a sequence

Coagulation Cascade

The coagulation cascade is a sequence of events: one event triggers the next until the entire sequence is complete. During coagulation, fibrin is introduced to stabilize the platelet plug. The production of fibrin is regulated by chemicals released from the damaged blood vessel and through proteins present in circulating blood. A chemical called *factor X* is activated by the damaged blood vessel and from tissues surrounding the leak. Factor X initiates a series of events that cause coagulation to occur. In the blood, prothrombin is converted to thrombin. Thrombin then converts fibrinogen to fibrin fibers, which are used to envelop the platelet plug with a meshlike net that stabilizes the clot. Calcium also plays a significant role in this coagulation process.

Coagulation is designed to be temporary. Just as secreted chemicals control the creation of clots, specific markers are present early in the production of coagulation that prompt the eventual destruction (lysis) of a clot. The accumulation of fibrin actually inhibits the production of thrombin; therefore, as the level of fibrin increases, the ongoing process of coagulation is limited. Newly healing tissue surrounding formed clots secretes tissue plasminogen activator (tPA). tPA converts circulating plasminogen to plasmin, which, in turn, plays a role in dissolving clots. In pathologic clotting situations, such as acute coronary syndrome, fibrinolytic drugs will be administered and will mirror this clot destruction process.

CONCLUSIONS

The importance of blood to the circulatory system is often overlooked. However, many of the most life-threatening conditions that will face your patients will be tied directly to a problem affecting key components of blood. Subsequent topics in this text will tie pathophysiology to the components of blood, but in general, it is important to consider the role these components play in the vital function of the body as a whole. Consider how disruption will affect larger systems and recognize the outward signs and symptoms of blood dysfunction.

REVIEW ITEMS

1. The liquid medium of blood that comprises roughly 55 percent of its total volume is also known as _____.
   a. plasma
   b. platelets
   c. hemoglobin
   d. fibrin

2. Erythrocytes are also known as _____.
   a. white blood cells
   b. platelets
   c. plasma
   d. red blood cells

3. Erythropoiesis is the process of _____.
   a. creating red blood cells
   b. destroying red blood cells
   c. clotting
   d. dissolving clots

4. Which type of white blood cells is used to fight infection and most commonly found in pus?
   a. eosinophils
   b. basophils
   c. neutrophils
   d. lymphocytes

5. The process used by the circulatory system to prevent the loss of blood is known as _____.
   a. hemostasis
   b. homeostasis
   c. fibrinolysis
   d. eryptosis

APPLIED PATHOPHYSIOLOGY

1. Describe the process of erythropoiesis.

2. Describe the role of lymphocytes.

3. List at least three values assessed during a complete blood count.

4. Describe the common typings of blood as used by the American Red Cross.

5. List the three phases of hemostasis.

6. Describe the process of coagulation.

CLINICAL DECISION MAKING

As you arrive at the scene of a reported gunshot wound, you observe a 22-year-old man staggering and holding a towel against his left shoulder. You note that the towel and his clothes are soaked with blood. There is also a large puddle of blood on the ground. Police on the scene tell you that the wound is spurting blood.

1. After ensuring scene safety, what is your first immediate action on approaching this patient?

2. What are the life threats to this patient?

3. How might this severe blood loss affect cellular metabolism?

The scene is safe, and you begin your assessment. The patient is confused, but answers your questions. You note that the wound is indeed arterial, and blood loss is severe. You also observe that the patient's skin is pale and diaphoretic.

4. What does the pale, cool, and clammy skin indicate?

5. How might this patient's altered mental status be related to blood loss?

You attempt to apply direct pressure to the wound to control bleeding.

6. How would direct pressure assist hemostasis?

7. Given the nature of this type of injury, why might natural hemostasis not be effective?

RESOURCES

The American Red Cross: www.redcrossblood.org/learn-about-blood/blood-types

Hemostasis: www.biosbcc.net/doohan/sample/htm/Hemostasis.htm

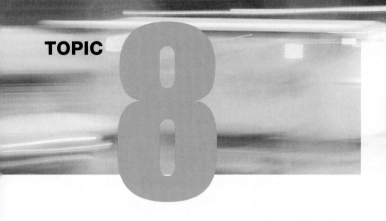

Standard Anatomy and Physiology

Competency Integrates a complex depth and comprehensive breadth of knowledge of the anatomy and physiology of all human systems.

THE NERVOUS SYSTEM

TRANSITION *highlights*

- *The major components of the nervous system.*
- *Differentiation between the central and peripheral nervous system and their roles in maintaining homeostasis.*
- *Clinical application of how the nervous system can affect a patient's physiological presentation.*

INTRODUCTION

The nervous system functions as the "hard wiring" for the body. This system allows the body to receive information from the environment, transport that information to the brain, and process and react to the information gathered. Information from inside the body is also continuously monitored and changed by the nervous system. Thoughts, movements, senses, and reflexes are all results of the actions of the nervous system.

The nervous system, in its entirety, is quite large and has many different components; initially, it is categorized into two large divisions called the *central* and *peripheral nervous systems*. These two components are then further separated into smaller subdivisions. This topic examines the major components, functionality, and building blocks of the nervous system, and then applies that knowledge to the physiology and operation of the senses and reflexes in the body.

NEURONS

The building blocks of every part of the nervous system are small nerve cells, or *neurons*. It can be important to know the anatomy of a neuron in order to understand how its function allows for communication between other neurons and the nervous system

as a whole. This section describes the anatomy of a neuron, how nerves are formed, and the way that they communicate through chemical and electrical signals.

The body of the neuron is called the *soma*. The neuron has a long "leg" called an *axon* and "branches" called *dendrites* that both come off the soma. At the end of the axon are axon terminals with small synaptic bulbs. The dendrites and synaptic bulbs are able to convey information from one neuron to another through the excretion of chemicals or electrical signals. Dendrites take in information and axons transmit information away from the neuron. The *synapse* is a small area between the synaptic bulbs of one neuron and the reception area of another neuron. This gap is created because the two never touch, but are in very close proximity to one another (▶ Figure 8-1).

Myelinated axons are covered in Schwann cells that wrap around them many times. The Schwann cell is made of neurilemma along the outside and the wrapped myelin sheath inside along the axon. Not all axons are myelinated; however, those that have myelin sheaths allow for impulses to move faster down the axon from the neuron body to the synaptic bulbs.

Neuroglia are an important part of the nervous system. Schwann cells, astrocytes, and microglia are a few types of neuroglia. Astrocytes act as the skin of the nervous system. They maintain chemical homeostasis, as well as act as a protective barrier between blood and the nervous system. Microglia engulf microbes and damaged nervous tissue.

Neurons are divided into three types: sensory and motor neurons and interneurons. Sensory neurons bring information from the body back to the central nervous system (CNS). Motor neurons are the opposite of sensory neurons, as they bring messages from the CNS out to the receiving part of the body. Interneurons conduct messages within the CNS. They also work to take in the information from the sensory neurons, process that information, and then send out the appropriate response through motor neurons.

Nerves are grouped axons outside the brain and spinal cord. If each axon were a thread, then a nerve would be a rope

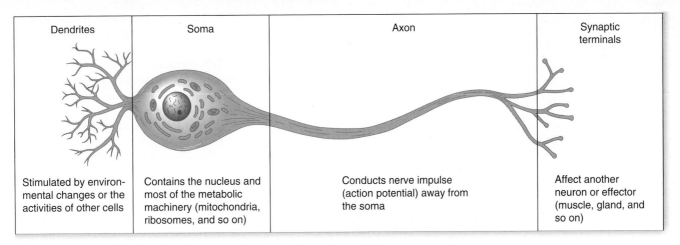

Dendrites	Soma	Axon	Synaptic terminals
Stimulated by environmental changes or the activities of other cells	Contains the nucleus and most of the metabolic machinery (mitochondria, ribosomes, and so on)	Conducts nerve impulse (action potential) away from the soma	Affect another neuron or effector (muscle, gland, and so on)

Figure 8-1 The neuron.

containing hundreds to thousands of threads that are bound together. Sensory nerves contain sensory axons, and motor nerves and mixed nerves contain motor and mixed axons, respectively. The white and gray colors in the brain and spinal cord are due to the composition of the nerves, neurons, axons, and the like. When there is a large amount of myelinated axons, the tract or area is white. Gray color is found in areas with little or no myelin.

Nerves transmit *impulses*, which are changes in charges, to convey information. Charges inside and outside a cell can be changed depending on the concentration of positive and negative ions on each side of the cell membrane. A *polarized* cell is one that has a membrane potential. The typical membrane potential at rest measures –70 mV (Jenkins et al., 2010, p. 370). When the cell depolarizes, it becomes more positive until finally reaching a positive charge, called the *action potential*. Action potential can be compared with a person falling off a diving board. A person can lean a little off a diving board without falling, in the same way that a cell can become slightly positive without having an action potential. The point at which a person leans too far off the diving board to stay on it would be called the *threshold*. Once the threshold point is met, the person falls off the diving board. The threshold in a cell is a relatively positive charge that triggers an action potential. Any charge less than the threshold will not elicit an action potential.

An action potential travels from the trigger zone to the axon terminals along the membrane of the axon. For myelinated axons, the transmission of the action potential down the axon happens by saltatory conduction, a slightly different form of conduction that occurs only in myelinated axons. Here, rather than progressing relatively slowly down the entire axon, the action potential seems to leap from node to node as each area depolarizes to the threshold. This allows for a much faster transmission of the charge than in unmyelinated axons.

The depolarization of the synaptic end bulb results in the release of neurotransmitters into the synapse. The neurotransmitters are released into this open space, where receptors are located on a separate neuron.

As mentioned earlier, the nervous system has two parts: the central and peripheral nervous systems. The CNS consists of the brain and the spinal cord. The spinal cord receives sensory input and provides motor output through spinal nerves. Damage to the spinal cord or spinal nerves creates an interruption in this pathway.

Many factors can cause damage to the nervous system. A deep cut in an extremity, for example, may harm nerves in the peripheral nervous system (PNS). A stroke (sometimes called a cerebrovascular accident) can cause damage to the CNS. Nerve damage can be especially detrimental to the body's natural functions. The PNS can repair itself most of the time, but the CNS can make few repairs. Damaged extremities are more likely to regain function and sensation than damage sustained to the spinal cord.

CENTRAL NERVOUS SYSTEM

The central nervous system (CNS) includes two parts—the brain and the spinal cord—which work in conjunction to maintain homeostasis in the body. Both the brain and spinal cord have complex components that function to transport information that has been gathered, interpret the information, and provide feedback and responses for the body. Injuries to the brain and spinal cord can cause detrimental damage to the body's ability to perform even the most basic of functions, such as breathing and innervation of the heart.

The Brain

The brain is divided into several components: right and left hemispheres, lobes, gray and white matter, and several other divisions and components used to identify the various functions of the brain (▶ Figure 8-2). The divisions of the brain can be based on anatomic landmarks or on the functions of the body controlled by the specific part of the brain.

Surrounding the brain inside the human skull is cerebrospinal fluid (CSF), which is also present in the spinal cord. CSF has several functions: cushioning against force, providing an ideal chemical environment, and circulating nutrients. Areas inside the brain that are CSF-filled spaces, with no dura mater, are called *ventricles*. The brain itself is divided into four lobes: temporal, parietal, occipital, and frontal lobes. The temporal lobe is beneath the temples; the occipital lobe is in the back of the head; the frontal lobe is along the forehead; and the parietal lobes are on the top of the head.

The meninges and blood–brain barrier are two protective structures for the brain. The *meninges* are a covering around the brain and spinal cord.

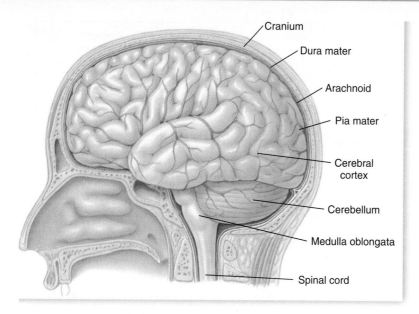

Figure 8-2 Structures of the brain.

The labels on the figure, from top to bottom:
Cranium
Dura mater
Arachnoid
Pia mater
Cerebral cortex
Cerebellum
Medulla oblongata
Spinal cord

Although technically not part of the brain itself, these membranes are important because they are frequently a target for diseases seen in the prehospital setting. The three layers of the cranial meninges are the dura mater, arachnoid mater, and pia mater.

The *blood–brain barrier* is the second protective mechanism for the brain. It allows the passage of some chemicals from blood into the brain while restricting the passage of others. Oxygen and glucose pass through the blood–brain barrier, whereas other harmful substances are prevented from crossing into the brain.

Other parts of the brain include the midbrain, pons, diencephalon, cerebellum, medulla oblongata, basal ganglia, thalamus, and hypothalamus. The *midbrain* extends from the pons to the diencephalon. The *pons* and the midbrain both consist of nuclei, sensory tracts, and motor tracts. The *cerebellum* is a heavily wrinkled part of the brain that sits below the occipital lobe. The cerebellum affects motor functions and a person's gait. The *cerebrum* has sensory and motor areas, and plays a role in emotions. The *medulla oblongata* is part of the brainstem and contributes to cardiac and respiratory functions. The *thalamus* and *hypothalamus* serve several purposes in the well-being of the body. The thalamus relays and processes ascending sensory and descending motor information, whereas the hypothalamus assists in homeostasis of the body by regulating osmotic pressures, glucose levels, hormones, and temperatures. The function of basal ganglia is related to motor function.

PERIPHERAL NERVOUS SYSTEM

The peripheral nervous system (PNS) composes the second set of structures not covered by the CNS. The PNS is divided into two main sections: the somatic and autonomic divisions. The somatic division is generally related to conscious thoughts and movements such as walking. The autonomic division encompasses nonconscious actions—for example, the dilation of blood vessels. Keep in mind that there are exceptions to both divisions in regard to voluntary and involuntary actions.

Somatic Division of the Peripheral Nervous System

The somatic part of the PNS includes the cranial and spinal nerves. The 12 cranial nerves affect most movements of the face. They are used when people speak, chew food, and simply look from left to right. **Table 8-1** gives the name, number, and function of the cranial nerves.

Spinal nerves exit the spine from cervical to coccyx. The nerve pairs are distributed as 8 cervical pairs, 12 thoracic pairs, 5 lumbar pairs, 5 sacral pairs, and 1 coccygeal pair (▶ **Figure 8-3**).

The spinal cord itself has three sensory pathways: the posterior column, spinothalamic, and the spinocerebellar pathways. The posterior column pathway, which forms the white matter on the posterior side of the spinal cord, brings sensory information from the periphery to the cerebral cortex. The spinothalamic pathway brings information from and to the same places, but is the gray matter of the spinal cord. The spinocerebellar pathway is responsible for helping to maintain gait and balance.

Two motor pathways are the pyramidal and extrapyramidal systems. When the motor pathways descend from the cerebrum to the spinal cord, they form the white matter protrusions called *pyramids*, where almost all the axons then cross from the right to left and left to right. This is why an injury on the left side of the brain could cause neurologic problems associated with the right side of the body.

Autonomic Division of the Peripheral Nervous System

Sympathetic and parasympathetic branches compose the autonomic nervous system (ANS). Combined, they allow the body to perform a variety of tasks, both consciously and unconsciously. The "fight-or-flight" response is a well-known saying to describe the sympathetic division, and "rest and digest" describes the parasympathetic. What does that actually mean, though? Throughout the day, emotions and state of being can affect the release of chemicals in the body. These chemicals are designed to cause physiologic changes, as described in the following sections.

SYMPATHETIC BRANCH OF THE AUTONOMIC NERVOUS SYSTEM The sympathetic division of the ANS responds to injury or danger by creating physiologic changes. One of the possible changes includes shunting blood to larger muscle groups and target organs that could be needed to fight or flee. This can be done by dilating the blood vessels to the heart and skeletal muscles, as well as dilating the bronchioles. Heart and respiratory rates also increase. These actions promote the most oxygen entering and being circulated through the body. The adrenal glands release epinephrine and norepinephrine. Dilating the pupils is another response to sympathetic

TABLE 8-1 The Cranial Nerves

Number	Name	Function
I	Olfactory	Sense of smell
II	Optic	Sense of sight
III	Oculomotor	Proprioception, movement of the eyelid, pupil size, and lens shape
IV	Trochlear	Proprioception and eye movement
V	Trigeminal	Sense of touch, pain, and temperature Proprioception and chewing
VI	Abducens	Proprioception and eye movement
VII	Facial	Sense of taste Proprioception, facial movement, tears, and saliva
VIII	Vestibulocochlear	Balance and hearing
IX	Glossopharyngeal	Taste and sensation Proprioception for muscles involved in swallowing food Monitoring blood pressure, blood gases, swallowing, speech, and saliva
X	Vagus	Taste Overseer of the body's blood pressure and respiratory function Sensation and contraction of the abdominal and thoracic organs
XI	Accessory	Proprioception Motor control for swallowing and motor control of the head
XII	Hypoglossal	Proprioception Motor control of the tongue for speech and swallowing

tone. The body decreases its digestion and urination/defecation. The body will also begin to sweat and raise the hairs on the skin. Male reproductive organs respond to the sympathetic division with ejaculation.

PARASYMPATHETIC BRANCH OF THE AUTONOMIC NERVOUS SYSTEM The parasympathetic division plays a major role when people are at rest; it promotes digestion of food and urination/defecation. In a parasympathetic response, the pupils are constricted, and the heart and respiratory rates decrease. The airway and bronchioles are also more constricted, as the body is not preparing for an increase in oxygen demand. In the sex organs, the erection for males is due to the parasympathetic division.

On a clinical note, some medications affect the way the body's sympathetic and parasympathetic divisions work. For example, a beta-blocker medication, such as motoprolol (Lopressor), works to block the beta receptors in the heart. Because sympathetic chemicals released by the body increase the heart rate by affecting the beta receptors in the heart, this medi-

cation may keep blood pressure and heart rate low, even in times of high stress or injury. Always consider how a patient's medications affect the clinical picture. Consider the medication's effects on vital signs, especially those that do not correlate to the patient's pattern of injury or level of anxiety.

SENSES

The purpose of sensations in the body is to be able to relay information about the environment to the nervous system. A person's senses can tell him that fire is hot, which is why he would remove his hand from the flame. This prevents the body from sustaining burn injuries. The body can also respond to chemical changes, such as a decrease in the body's pH level. Compensatory mechanisms for acidosis rely on information from the senses. Without sensation, an individual may not notice that he is in danger.

The basic components of a sense include sensory receptors, sensory neurons, sensory tracts, and sensory areas. Sensory receptors have three types: free nerve endings, encapsulated nerve end-

ings, and separate cells. Free nerve endings are nerve endings with no specialization. Separate cells connect with sensory neurons to convey information. Encapsulated nerve endings, which are surrounded with connective tissue, respond to pressure, touch, and vibration. Sensory neurons conduct impulses from sensory receptors to the CNS. The sensory tract is the path that the neurons take.

The general senses are pain, temperature, touch/pressure/position, and chemical detection. Most of these can be sensed by the largest organ in the body, the skin, which contains pressure, temperature, and pain receptors. Some organs in the body have stretch and chemical receptors. These receptors monitor the chemical composition of the body (chemoreceptors) and monitor pressures in the organs and blood vessels (pressoreceptors).

Sensation is perceived differently throughout the body, because some areas are more sensitive than others. For example, the fingertips are able to distinguish points of two toothpicks that are very close together, whereas the arm may feel one single point.

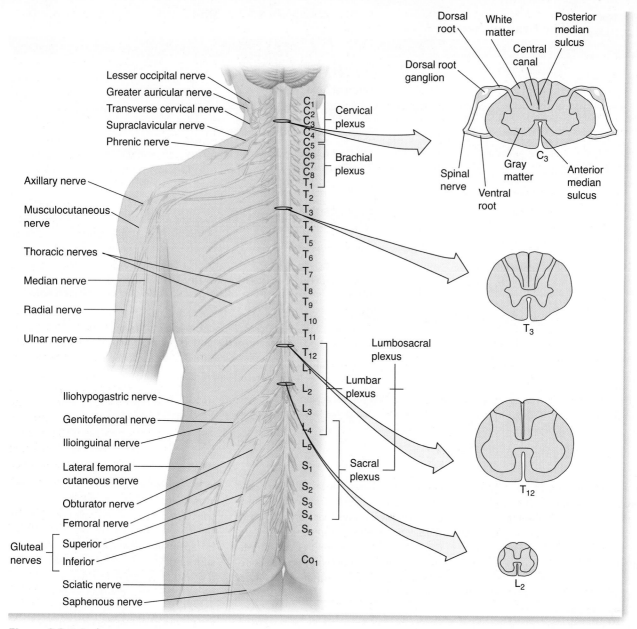

Figure 8-3 Spinal nerves.

Some adaptation can occur with the special senses. For smells, the body is efficient at detecting small amounts of a scent in the air, but quickly becomes adapted to those smells, which then appear less intense. Decreasing sensitivity happens more slowly with taste. The eyes are also able to adapt, which can help in the ability to desensitize the bright sunlight when curtains are first thrown open.

The intensity of pain is often measured by health care providers on scales, such as a number system or pictures of people in pain for children to use. The intensity that the body feels depends on several factors. Intensity will increase with repeated stimulation of a nerve ending that feels pain. Different types of pain can be felt by the body depending on the injuries sustained. The stretching of an organ, for example, will elicit a different pain response from the pain associated with being cut with a knife.

Phantom pain is a phenomenon that occurs when someone feels pain in an extremity that does not exist, or has been amputated. *Referred pain* is pain felt in a different part of the body from the site of injury. Pain is referred because areas in the organ and area of referral contain nerves from the same segment of the spinal cord. Whether it is the pain of a heart attack presenting in the left arm, or pain in the right shoulder to indicate possible gallstones, referred pain is used in medicine every day to diagnose problems in the body.

Close your eyes, and touch your nose. The fact that you know where your hand and nose are, and are able to move your hand to your nose without being able to see either, is due to proprioception. *Proprioception*, or muscle sense, is responsible for telling you what various body parts are doing and where the body is located in space. Without knowing where body parts are oriented in space, people would not be able to perform skills such as walking or guiding a fork full of food to their mouth. Proprioceptors are located in many different parts of the body, including muscle tissue, tendons, and the ears.

Anatomy: Special Senses

THE EYE The eye is made up of several external and internal parts. The eyelids are important protection for the eye. *Conjunctivae* are the mucous membranes that can be seen by pulling down gently on the lower eye lid. An infection of the conjunctiva is called *conjunctivitis* and is common in children. Conjunctivitis can result in red conjunctiva and is therefore often called "pinkeye."

Tears contain salts, water, and lysozyme, an enzyme that fights bacteria. Tears are made in the lacrimal glands, which produce fluid that continues into the lacrimal ducts. From there, the tears are distributed to the eye for natural lubrication. The tears then flow off the eyes and into lacrimal canals. The lacrimal canals move tears into the lacrimal sacs, which then drain into the nasolacrimal duct. Cumulatively, these are known as the *lacrimal apparatus*.

The eyeball itself sits in the orbit of the skull. Several extrinsic muscles move the eye, and intrinsic muscles constrict and dilate the pupils. The *pupil* is the black, center part of the eye. The pupil is surrounded by the *iris*, which is the colored part of the eye. The pupil controls the amount of light entering the eye. The white part of the eye is the *sclera*. The external layer of the eye is the *cornea*, which covers the pupil and iris.

Beneath the cornea is the anterior chamber full of *aqueous humor*, a liquid that provides an ideal chemical environment for the lens and cornea. (Too much aqueous humor creates pressure, which is known as *glaucoma*.) The scleral venous sinus is the part of the anterior chamber that allows the aqueous humor to drain. Behind the anterior chamber is the posterior cavity, which is filled with a gelatinous substance called *vitreous humor*. Vitreous humor helps to maintain the shape of the eye and the correct position of the retina.

Another part of the eye is the *ciliary body*, which includes the ciliary muscles and processes. These connect to the lens with the suspensory ligaments and work to adjust the lens. The *retina* covers the inside of the eye, and the *lens* focuses images on the retina. The image is then transmitted to the brain. (A cataract results from the loss of transparency of the lens of the eye and/or its capsule.) The choroid layer is on top of the retina, and the sclera is the most superficial layer.

At the very back of the retina, where the optic nerve exits, is the optic disk. This is a place where no image can be projected and is thus called the *blind spot*. Another notable part of the eye is the *fovea*, a small indentation in the retina along the posterior part of the eye. The fovea is the area of highest visual acuity and resolution in the eye. Ganglion cells transmit information from the eye. Information is then passed on through ganglion axons at the rear of the eye itself. These axons group together to form the optic nerve.

People see by way of rods and cones that are present on the retina. Rods work in dim light for black and white sight, and cones work in bright light to show colors. All substances that light passes through cause the light to bend in varying degrees. The eye causes the light to refract when entering and leaving the lens, as well as when entering and leaving the cornea. The lens then works with the other angles of bent light to focus the image on the retina.

THE EAR The part of the ear that we see, the *auricle*, is made of cartilage and skin. The auricle directs sounds into the external auditory canal, where they begin their journey into the ear to be heard. The next part of the ear that the sound meets is the *tympanic membrane*, or the eardrum. Three small bones follow the eardrum: the incus, malleus, and stapes. These bones, along with the opening to the auditory tube and two small openings called the oval and round windows, make up the middle ear. The inner ear consists of an intricate set of canals and membranes.

The inner ear has a bony labyrinth that includes semicircular canals, the vestibule, and the cochlea, and is full of perilymph. The inner ear is responsible for hearing and balance. In the bony labyrinth is the membranous labyrinth, which is filled with endolymph. The semicircular canals are above the round window and include medially the saccule and utricle. Medial to the semicircular canals is the cochlea—a spiral organ that contains a coiled sheet of epithelial cells—and about 16,000 hair cells, which are the receptors for hearing.

Physiology: Special Senses

SMELL Smell is a complex process that involves receptors detecting chemicals that are present as odors. Even a very small amount of chemicals can be smelled. Receptors detect the chemicals in the air and send a signal via the nervous system. The signal is transmitted through the olfactory nerves into the brain, where the nerves form the olfactory bulbs.

SIGHT Sight begins with an image—a tree, for example. The image enters the eye and bends when passing through the cornea, and then again when it passes through the lens. The image is portrayed upside down on the retina. When the image is portrayed in front of the retina, a person is nearsighted. When the image focuses behind the retina, the person is farsighted. A part of the lens or cornea having an odd curvature results in astigmatism.

When light reaches the rods it is absorbed by rhodopsin, a photopigment. Cones also have pigments and are responsible for seeing colors. Some people are "color blind." This usually refers to the inability to distinguish red and green from each other. This disease is seen more in males than in females.

When information is transmitted through the optic nerve, it passes through the *optic chiasm*, where some nerves cross from left to right and right to left; after this, the axons become part of the optic tract and move to the brain. Vision is managed in the occipital lobe of the brain; thus, injuries to this lobe can affect people's sight.

HEARING Hearing involves sound waves entering the ear canal to vibrate the eardrum. The vibration causes the small bones of the middle ear to vibrate together, which creates pressure changes in the oval window. The movement of the fluid in the inner ear is transmitted to the vestibule by means of the round window bulging, where the endolymph is then moved in waves. The movement in the endolymph is then transmitted to the basilar membrane, which moves the hair cells of the spiral organ against the tectoral membrane and results in bending of the hair cell microvilli and generation of a nerve impulse.

Some people are born unable to hear, whereas others lose their hearing over time. There are a few different types of hearing loss. *Conductive hearing loss* is due to a problem with the outer or middle ear and is usually treatable (*Hearing Loss—Infants*, 2011). *Nerve deafness* is a process of the middle ear, and involves the transmission of nerve impulses. *Central deafness* involves damage to the auditory nerve and is likely related to a disease process (*Hearing Loss—Infants*, 2011).

While discussing the process for hearing, it is important to mention the equilibrium of the body. Static and dynamic equilibrium are the two types of equilibrium, which is managed by the vestibular apparatus. Movements of cristae and maculae, small hairs located in the spiral organ, are transmitted to the brain, involving the oculomotor, trochlear, abducens, and accessory nerves. Balance is determined by the position of the head and movements of the body.

TASTE Taste is stimulated by chemicals, which can present in five categories: bitter, sour, salty, sweet, and savory. People can distinguish among different tastes because of the taste buds, which pass signals along three cranial nerves—facial, glossopharyngeal, and vagus—and on to the medulla oblongata.

REFLEXES

Reflexes are physiologic responses from the body in response to a stimulus, such as blinking of the eye when something is moving toward the face. Reflexes are divided into different categories, which are determined by the pathway that a stimulus triggers and the resulting reflex follows. Spinal reflexes process information in the spinal cord gray matter. Cranial reflexes integrate stimuli in the gray matter of the brainstem.

Reflexes can also be divided into somatic and autonomic categories. Autonomic reflexes describe the actions and responses of autonomic muscle and glands, whereas somatic reflexes affect skeletal muscles. Somatic reflexes can include the subcategories of stretch and flexor reflexes. When a muscle becomes stretched, a stretch reflex causes that muscle to contract. For example, when a person grabs a hot pan, the reflex is to withdraw the hand. This is protective, preventing the skin from remaining in contact with painful, and likely harmful, stimuli.

CONCLUSIONS

The nervous system is the collector, transporter, and interpreter for the world around us. The nervous system is formed with the building blocks of small neurons, which combine to compose the much larger components of the central and peripheral divisions. The formation of the special senses as structures is important in the way that humans interpret their surroundings and potential life threats. All together, the nervous system is vital for maintaining homeostasis and the ability to move, breathe, think, and understand the environment we live in.

TRANSITIONING

REVIEW ITEMS

1. The small area between the synaptic bulbs of one neuron and the reception area of another neuron is called the_____.
   - a. synapse
   - b. axon
   - c. dendrite
   - d. soma

2. The heavily wrinkled part of the brain that sits below the occipital lobe and affects motor functions and a person's gait is also known as the _____.
   - a. cerebellum
   - b. cerebrum
   - c. medulla oblongata
   - d. thalamus

3. Which of following parts of the brain contributes to cardiac and respiratory functions?
   - a. cerebellum
   - b. cerebrum
   - c. medulla oblongata
   - d. thalamus

4. Which of the following sensory pathways of the spinal cord brings sensory information from the periphery to the cerebral cortex?
   - a. spinocerebellar
   - b. spinothalamic
   - c. posterior
   - d. anterior

5. The part of the ear that can be seen externally is called the _____.
   - a. incus
   - b. auricle
   - c. malleus
   - d. stapes

APPLIED PATHOPHYSIOLOGY

1. When assessing a patient's pupils with a penlight, you note that they did not contract. Which cranial nerve could affect the patient's pupillary response?

2. Which division of the autonomic nervous system will shunt blood to larger muscle groups when a person is preparing to fight or flee from a scary stimulus?

3. What does the myelin sheath of an axon accomplish?

CLINICAL DECISION MAKING

You respond to the home of a 78-year-old female patient. Her family notes that after lunch the patient had difficulty standing up from her chair and now is having difficulty speaking. On arrival, you note that the patient is awake and turns her gaze to you as you address her, but her speech is inaudible. She is breathing and has a radial pulse.

1. What additional elements of the primary assessment would be important to obtain in this particular patient?

2. Based on this limited description of the events, describe your immediate differential diagnosis.

The patient's airway is patent, and her breathing is adequate. A rapid physical examination reveals a right facial droop and a left-sided motor deficit. The patient seems to understand you, but cannot form the words to respond to your questions.

3. Considering the structures of the brain and the components of the nervous system described in this chapter, describe the pathophysiology behind the facial droop.

4. Considering the structures of the brain and the components of the nervous system described in this chapter, describe the pathophysiology behind the motor deficit.

5. Why might the motor deficit be occurring on the opposite side of the facial droop?

Your secondary assessment of this patient includes a more detailed neurologic assessment.

6. Describe the neurologic examination you would conduct, and describe how each step is related to a specific structure or region of the nervous system.

REFERENCES

Jenkins, G., C. Kemnitz, and G. Tortora. *Anatomy and Physiology: From Science to Life.* Hoboken, NJ: John Wiley & Sons, Inc, 2010.

Hearing loss—Infants. (2011). MedlinePlus. Retrieved September 01, 2011, from http://www.nlm.nih.gov/medlineplus/ency/article/007322.htm.

TOPIC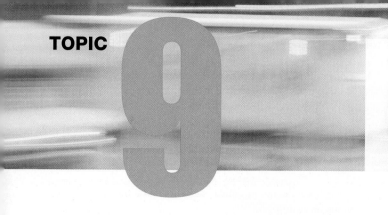

Standard Medical Terminology

Competency Integrates comprehensive anatomical and medical terminology and abbreviations into the written and oral communication with colleagues and other health care professionals.

MEDICAL TERMINOLOGY

TRANSITION *highlights*

- *Review of what comprises a medical term:*
  - Prefix.
  - Suffix.
  - Combining form.
- *Comprehensive list of common medical terms with their definitions.*

INTRODUCTION

At the highest level of prehospital care, precision is essential. The high stakes of paramedic-level intervention require accuracy in assessment, description, and reporting; poor communication has potentially dangerous consequences. Using standardized medical terminology properly can help add precision to all these elements and can improve your communications as a whole.

As a paramedic, your ability to communicate is not just a capability, but also a tool used to accomplish very specific tasks. Just as a mechanic chooses the best tool to tighten a bolt or replace a screw, a paramedic uses specific language to paint an accurate picture and convey a precise message. The terms you choose should be selected carefully to present to your team, your on-line medical direction, or your patient the most accurate description possible. Proper, standardized medical terminology is a key element of any EMS provider's arsenal. Medical terminology is the language of health care; being able to use this language helps us better integrate into the health care team.

> **Medical terminology is the language of health care.**

MEDICAL TERM ORIGINS

Greek and Latin words are commonly used as the basis for modern medical terms. Although these roots often present initial challenges, understanding common components used to form complex terms actually makes interpretation easier. In medicine, many prefixes, suffixes, and combining forms are used to create more complex compound terms. Becoming familiar with the more frequently encountered components will not only help you recognize terminology, but also help you deduce the meaning of words based on their component parts.

In many ways, it is similar to understanding the ingredients in an unfamiliar culinary dish. The name of the dish may be unfamiliar, but knowing the ingredients helps you know exactly what you are eating. Suffixes and prefixes can describe direction or location. Many root words get their meaning from the anatomic structures, organs, and the systems with which they are associated. Recognizing patterns among these terms makes using the terminology easier.

STRUCTURE OF MEDICAL TERMS

Most medical terms have three basic components: prefix, combining form, and suffix. The *combining form* is the subject or foundation of the word that gives the word its essential meaning.

Each combining form consists of two parts: a root and a combining vowel. The *root* is the part of the term that provides the foundation for the rest of the term. *Combining vowels* are joined to the end of a root to connect the root to another root or to a suffix. Combining vowels make the word easier to pronounce. The most common combining vowel is *o*, followed by *i*. A combining vowel is not used if the suffix begins with a vowel.

Some medical terms may contain more than one combining form. For example, the term *cardiovascular* has two combining forms: cardi/o (heart) and vascul/o (vessel).

combining form	+ combining form	+ suffix
cardi/o	+ vascul/o	+ -ar

The *suffix* is the term located at the end of the word. It modifies the root and gives it an additional meaning. In this topic, suffixes appear with a hyphen in front of them, indicating that another term, usually a root, should precede them. For example, the suffix -itis means inflammation. The term *conjunctivitis* can be broken into the combining form conjunctiv/o followed by the suffix -itis. When the suffix is added to the root meaning conjunctiva, the term then refers to inflammation of the conjunctiva.

combining form	+	suffix
conjunctiv/o	+	-itis
(conjunctiva)	+	(inflammation)

A *prefix* is a term that begins the word. It is also used to modify the root. Some terms may not have a prefix, so it is important to memorize which terms are roots and which are prefixes. Throughout this topic, prefixes appear with a hyphen after them, indicating that another term, usually a root word, should follow it. For example, the prefix a- means without. In the word *apnea*, the root *pne(a)* means breathing. By adding the prefix a- to the word, a specific modification has been made, and the meaning is changed to "without breathing."

prefix	+	combining form	+	suffix
a-	+	pne/o	+	-a
(without)	+	(breathing)	+	(condition)

HOW TO READ AND DEFINE MEDICAL TERMS

As other words in English, medical terms are read from left to right. If a term has a prefix, it will be read first and will be followed by the combining form(s) and then the suffix (if one is present). For example, the term *hyperglycemia* contains the prefix hyper-, the combining form glyc/o, and the suffix -emia.

prefix	+	combining form	+	suffix
hyper-	+	glyc/o	+	-emia
(above or excessive)	+	(sugar)	+	(blood condition)

Many medical terms can be defined by determining the meaning of their parts. Unlike the method for reading the term, the definition is derived by determining the meaning of the suffix first, then the prefix, and finally the combining form(s). So in the preceding example of hyperglycemia, the meaning is derived from the suffix -emia (meaning blood condition), then the prefix hyper- (meaning above or excessive), followed by the combining form glyc/o (meaning glucose or sugar). So the meaning of the term *hyperglycemia* would be a blood condition that has an excessive amount of glucose (sugar) in it.

ACCEPTED MEDICAL TERMS AND ABBREVIATIONS

Although breaking down a word into its component parts often can aid in interpretation, the meaning of every accepted medical term is not derived from the sum of its parts alone. Because many terms will be unfamiliar, every paramedic should have access to and use a professional medical dictionary. In many cases, these may be actual books, but modern technology provides many other wonderful resources. Internet sites and smartphone applications all provide viable options to help improve your use of medical terminology.

As you progress throughout your medical career, you will continue to develop your vocabulary and will use many medical terms in your reports and documentation. As is true in learning any language, the more you can use it, the more fluent you will be.

Using Medical Terminology Appropriately

Medical terminology is truly an art form; weaving a precise description based on detailed terms is an important element of paramedic care. However, at times, using complex medical terms may actually cause confusion, as opposed to clarity. You must always consider your audience. A doctor who is familiar with medical terminology greatly benefits from precise terms, but a small child who is unfamiliar with Latin or Greek roots may be confused or frightened by your "medicalese." As a paramedic, you must be conscious of when and how you use complex medical terms and choose the best level of communication to achieve your desired goal. Should you inquire about diaphoresis or should you ask your patient if he is sweaty?

Complex terms can be confusing and sometimes even scary. Terminology can confuse even well-trained providers. If at any time you are unsure of what term to use, remember that you can always fall back on plain language. These choices are not limited to the spoken word; written reports can also fall victim to the confusion of medical terminology. In most cases, using precise terminology is the best course of action, but again, assess your specific situation when considering the best words to use. Abbreviations are frequently used to save time, but be careful, because these too can cause confusion.

Abbreviations

Medical abbreviations are frequently used to consolidate terms and save time. In fact, many services and agencies publish lists of accepted abbreviations suitable for routine use (▶ Figure 9-1; Table 9-1). However, it is important to understand that abbreviations can have more than one meaning and can lead to unclear communication and medical errors. To avoid confusion, you must consider when and where you use abbreviations and use only the abbreviations that are approved for use in your organization. As a point of reference, the Joint Commission has published an official "do not use" list of abbreviations that should *not* be used in your documentation (http://www.jointcommission.org/assets/1/18/Official_Do_Not_Use_List_6_111.PDFt).

COMMON PREFIXES, SUFFIXES, AND COMBINING FORMS

Common prefixes, suffixes, and combining forms are depicted in Tables 9-2, 9-3, and 9-4, respectively. These tables are not all-inclusive, however.

CONCLUSIONS

Like many other tools at the disposal of paramedics, language and accurate communication are important elements of proper patient assessment and care. As a modern EMS provider, these tools must be cultivated and developed in order to provide the best care for your patients.

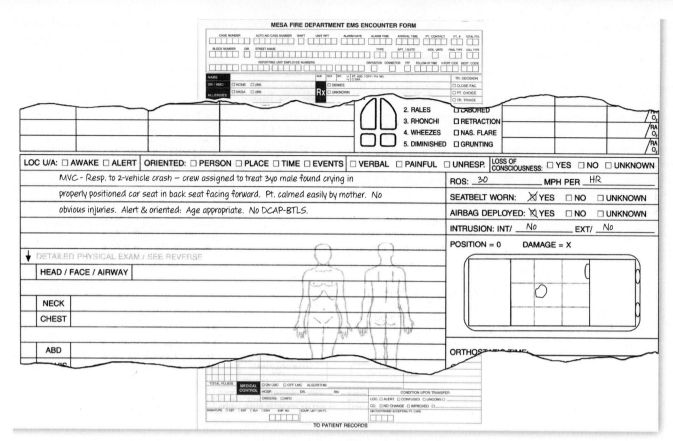

Figure 9-1 Sometimes it will be more convenient to use an accepted medical abbreviation or symbol in your report instead of writing the entire term.

TABLE 9-1	Commonly Used Abbreviations

Abbreviation	Meaning	Abbreviation	Meaning	Abbreviation	Meaning
Δ	change	exam	examination	post	posterior
abd	abdomen/ abdominal	fx	fracture	pt	patient
a-fib	atrial fibrillation	htn	hypertension	reg	regular
		hx	history	rehab	rehabilitation
ant	anterior	incl	including	resp	respiration
approx	approximately	info	information	sx	symptom
bilat	bilateral	irreg	irregular	syst	systolic
ca	cancer	neg	negative	temp	temperature
detox	detoxification (drug)	neur	neurologic	unk	unknown
		norm	normal	w/	with
dr	doctor	ped	pediatric	w/o	without
e.g.	for example	pos	positive	y/o	year old

TABLE 9-2	Common Prefixes in Medical Terms

Prefix	Meaning	Prefix	Meaning	Prefix	Meaning
a-, an-	without	ad-	to; toward, or near	anti-	against
ab-	away from	ante-	before	bi-	two or both

TABLE 9-2 (continued)

Prefix	Meaning
brady-	slow
circum-	around
con-	together or with
contra-	against
de-	from, down, or not
dys-	painful, difficult, or faulty
en-, endo-	within
epi-	upon
eu-	good or normal
hemi-	half

Prefix	Meaning
hyper-	above or excessive
hypo-	below or deficient
infra-	below or deficient
inter-	between
intra-	within
macro-	large
micro-	small
mono-	one
para-	alongside
peri-	around

Prefix	Meaning
poly-	many
post-	after or behind
pre-, pro-	before
quadr/i-	four
sub-	below or deficient
super-, supra-	above or excessive
tachy-	fast
uni-	one

TABLE 9-3 — Common Suffixes in Medical Terms

Suffix	Meaning
-a,	condition of
-ac, -al, -ar, -ary	pertaining to
-acusis	hearing
-algia,	pain
-arche	beginning
-ation	process
-cele	pouching or hernia
-centesis	puncture for aspiration
-dynia	pain
-eal	pertaining to
-ectomy	excision
-emesis	vomiting
-emia	blood condition
-gram	record
-graphy	process of recording
-ia	condition of
-iatrics, -iatry	treatment
-ic	pertaining to
-ism	condition of
-itis	inflammation
-ium	structure or tissue
-lepsy	seizure
-logist	one who specializes in the study of

Suffix	Meaning
-logy	study of
-lysis	breakdown or dissolution
-malacia	softening
-megaly	enlargement
-meter	instrument for measuring
-oma	tumor
-osis	condition or increase
-otomy	cutting or separation
-ous	pertaining to
-plasty	surgical repair or reconstruction
-plegia	paralysis
-pnea	breathing
-rrhage, -rrhagia	to burst forth
-rrhea	discharge
-scope	instrument for examination
-scopy	process of examination
-spasm	involuntary contraction
-stomy	creation of an opening
-tic	pertaining to
-tomy	incision
-tripsy	crushing
-y	condition or process of

TABLE 9-4 **Common Combining Forms in Medical Terms**

Related to the Cardiovascular System

Combining Form	Meaning
angi/o	vessel
aort/o	aorta
arteri/o	artery
ather/o	fatty paste
atri/o	atrium
cardi/o	heart
phleb/o	vein
sphygm/o	pulse
vas/o, vascul/o	vessel
ven/o	vein
ventricul/o	ventricle

Related to the Endocrine and Immune Systems

Combining Form	Meaning
aden/o	gland
adren/o, adrenal/o	adrenal gland
crin/o	to secrete
gluc/o, glyc/o	sugar
hormon/o	hormone
immune/o	safe
ket/o, keton/o	ketone bodies
pancreat/o	pancreas
thalm/o	thalamus
thym/o	thymus gland or mind
thyr/o, thyroid/o	thyroid gland

Related to the Eyes and Ears

Combining Form	Meaning
acous/o, audi/o	hearing
aque/o	water
aur/i	ear
blephar/o	eyelid
cerumen/o	wax
conjunctiv/o	conjunctiva
corne/o	cornea
kerat/o	cornea
myring/o	eardrum
ocul/o	eye
ot/o	ear
retin/o	retina
tympan/o	eardrum

Related to the Gastrointestinal System

Combining Form	Meaning
abdomin/o	abdomen
an/o	anus
appendic/o	appendix
bil/i	bile
bucc/o	cheek
celi/o	abdomen
chol/e	bile
col/o, colon/o	colon
duoden/o	duodenum
enter/o	small intestine
esophag/o	esophagus
gastr/o	stomach
hepat/o, hepatic/o	liver
herni/o	hernia
lapar/o	abdomen
or/o	mouth
peritone/o	peritoneum
phag/o	eat or swallow
proct/o	anus and rectum
rect/o	rectum
splen/o	spleen
stomat/o	mouth

Related to the Integumentary System

Combining Form	Meaning
adip/o	fat
cutane/o	skin
derm/o, dermat/o	skin
hist/o, histi/o	tissue
lip/o	fat
onych/o	nail
seb/o	oil
steat/o	fat
trich/o	hair

Related to the Musculoskeletal System

Combining Form	Meaning
ankyl/o	crooked or stiff
arthr/o, articulo	joint
brachi/o	arm
cephal/o	head
cervic/o	neck
chondr/o	cartilage
cost/o	rib
crani/o	skull
femor/o	femur
kyph/o	humped back
lord/o	bent
lumb/o	lower back
my/o, muscul/o, myos/o	muscle
oste/o	bone
patell/o	patella
pector/o	chest
pelv/i	pelvis
pod/o	foot
radi/o	radius or radiation
stern/o	sternum
steth/o	chest
ten/o, tend/o, tendin/o	tendon
thorac/o	chest
uln/o	ulna
vertebr/o	vertebra

Related to Neurology/Psychology

Combining Form	Meaning
cerebell/o	cerebellum
cerebr/o	cerebrum
encephal/o	entire brain
esthesi/o	sensation
mening/o, meningi/o	meninges
myel/o	bone marrow or spinal cord
neur/o	nerve
phas/o	speech
phob/o	exaggerated fear or sensitivity
phon/o	voice or sound
phren/o	diaphragm or mind
psych/o	mind
schiz/o	split or division

Related to the Reproductive System

Combining Form	Meaning
andr/o	man
balan/o	glans penis

colp/o	vagina
gynec/o	woman
hyster/o	uterus
mamm/o, mast/o	breast
metr/o	uterus
men/o	menstruation
oophor/o	ovary
orch/o, orchid/o	testis (testicle)
ovari/o	ovary
test/o	testis (testicle)
uter/o	uterus
vagin/o	vagina

Related to the Respiratory System

Combining Form	Meaning
aer/o	air or lung
alveol/o	alveolus (air sac)
bronch/o, bronchi/o	bronchus (airway)
bronchiol/o	bronchiole (little airway)
capn/o, carb/o	carbon dioxide
laryng/o	larynx
lob/o	lobe

nas/o	nose
pharyng/o	pharynx
pleur/o	pleura
pne(a)/o	breathing
pneum/o, pneumon/o	air or lung
pulmon/o	lung
rhin/o	nose
sinus/o	hollow
trache/o	trachea

Related to the Urinary System

Combining Form	Meaning
cyst/o	bladder or sac
glomerul/o	glomerulus (small ball)
lith/o	stone
nephr/o	kidney
ren/o	kidney
ur/o, urin/o	urine
ureter/o	ureter
urethr/o	urethra
vesic/o	bladder or sac

Other Common Combining Forms

Combining Form	Meaning
carcin/o	cancer
chrom/o, chromat/o	color
chyl/o	juice
cyan/o	blue
cyt/o	cell
diaphor/o	profuse sweating
dips/o	thirst
erythr/o	red
hem/o, hemat/o	blood
hydr/o	water
leuk/o	white
lingu/o	tongue
lymph/o	lymph
melan/o	black
necr/o	death
ox/o	oxygen
path/o	disease
purpur/o	purple
somat/o	body
thromb/o	clot
tox/o, toxic/o	toxic
xanth/o	yellow

TRANSITIONING

REVIEW ITEMS

1. A patient presents with hypotension. Based on the prefix in the term, you should suspect the patient's blood pressure to be _____.
   - a. above normal
   - b. below normal
   - c. faster than usual
   - d. slower than usual

2. You are called to the residence of a patient in respiratory distress. Dispatch advises the patient has recently had a tracheostomy. Based on this information, you expect to find a(n)_____.
   - a. tube surgically placed in the stomach
   - b. incision into the lungs
   - c. artificial opening in the trachea
   - d. excision of a lobe in the lungs

3. The term referring to the sac surrounding the heart is _____.
   - a. myocardium
   - b. pericardium
   - c. epicardium
   - d. endocardium

4. Which of the following terms refers to difficulty swallowing?
   - a. parenteral
   - b. esophagitis
   - c. dysphagia
   - d. dysphasia

5. A patient is vomiting blood. When documenting this finding, you should use the term _____.
   - a. hematemesis
   - b. rhinorrhea
   - c. hematuria
   - d. diarrhea

APPLIED KNOWLEDGE

1. If a patient has neuralgia, what body system is affected?

2. What does the term *subcutaneous* mean?

3. In what area does a gastroenterologist specialize?

4. If a patient has bradycardia, what does that mean?

5. Where are the suprarenal glands located?

CLINICAL DECISION MAKING

You are called to a nursing home for a 74-year-old male patient complaining of abdominopelvic pain. On arrival, the nurse informs you that the patient had hematemesis, hematuria, and diarrhea that morning. According to the nurse, the patient has a colostomy and has recently had a suprapubic catheter inserted. The nurse states that the patient has a history of gastrointestinal reflux disease, colitis, acute renal failure, hypertension, diabetes, and a previous cerebral vascular attack with residual dysphasia.

1. Based on your knowledge of medical terminology, translate the medical terms and rewrite the preceding passage using common language.

You arrive at a residence of a 68-year-old female patient. As you approach your patient, she tells you she is "not feeling right." You begin to obtain a history and perform your assessment. You discover that she has low blood sugar, high blood pressure, a slow heart rate, difficulty breathing, chest pain, profuse sweating, and a bluish color around her lips. You also find that she had her left lung removed about two years ago. She has had regular checkups by her heart and lung doctor.

2. Based on your understanding of medical terminology, rewrite the passage using professional medical terminology.

Standard Pathophysiology

Competency Integrates comprehensive knowledge of the pathophysiology of major human systems.

INTRODUCTION

The vitally important cell is the basic unit of life and the functional unit of tissues, organs, and organ systems. Disruption of cells leads to dysfunction of the organ system and, ultimately, the organism if the disruption is bad enough. This topic briefly reviews cellular pathophysiology and the changes that occur in the life cycle of the cell (▶ Figure 10-1). Cells exhibit a number of changes, including atrophy, hypertrophy, hyperplasia, dysplasia, metaplasia, and others. This topic discusses each in turn.

CELLULAR ADAPTATION

Atrophy occurs when cells shrink in size. It is often a consequence of disuse, as in the case of skeletal muscle cells during prolonged immobilization in a cast. A lack of use of the cells causes the cells to shrink in volume from a loss of intracellular proteins, a decrease in the number of mitochondria, fewer myofilaments, and a loss of intracellular endoplasmic reticulum. The end result is cells that shrink in size but remain functional, albeit in a less robust manner than normal cells. Atrophy can affect any cell in the body, but is most common in the heart, brain, skeletal muscle, and sex organs.

Hypertrophy occurs when cells increase in size while maintaining the same shape and function. The increased size of the cells leads, in turn, to a net increase in the size of the organ. This increase in size often occurs in relation to a direct challenge facing the cell—for example, myocardial cells in the left ventricle may demonstrate hypertrophy in the face of increased afterload in the setting of heart failure because they must pump (contract) against increased pressures. Hypertrophy is the adaptation that many cells take to meet the increasing demands if they cannot do so by mitotic division. When many cells in the tissue become enlarged, the change may be adaptive (physiologic) or pathologic.

Hyperplasia is an increase in the number of cells because of an increased rate of cell division. Hyperplasia is known to occur in tissues in which damage has been so severe that cell death has occurred, leading to a virtual "vacuum" in which more cells are

needed to meet the functional needs of the tissue and organ system. Hyperplasia may be physiologic or pathologic as well. For example, compensatory hyperplasia occurs in liver transplant patients when the donor is able to regenerate the excised hepatocytes. Hormonal hyperplasia occurs in women during the menstrual cycle and pregnancy, as cells of the uterus and breast increase in number to prepare for implantation of the fertilized ovum. Finally, pathologic hyperplasia can occur when certain hormone-dependent cells of the endometrium grow excessively, leading to excessive menstrual bleeding.

Dysplasia occurs when there are abnormal changes in the size, shape, and organization of mature cells. Dysplasia is also known as atypical hyperplasia. Cells of the cervix and respiratory tract often exhibit these changes. Dysplastic cells are commonly associated with cancerous tissues and may surround them.

Metaplasia is the replacement of mature cells with another type of cells. It is almost always pathologic and may be associated with neoplasia. Examples include chronic changes in the airways of smokers. Evidence suggests that removal of the offending stimulus will result in reversal of the metaplasia.

TRANSITION highlights

- Understanding how ongoing changes within the cell cause functional changes within the human body in the face of illness or injury.

- Differences between adaptive and maladaptive changes in the human body.

- Relation of cellular injury to different pathogens, chemicals, or disease processes that the patient may encounter, leading to interaction with the paramedic.

- Differentiation between chronic injury and acute injury to cells and the different presentations they have in disease states.

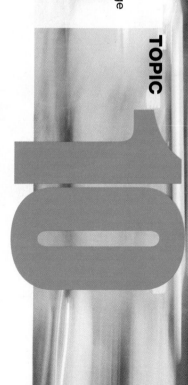

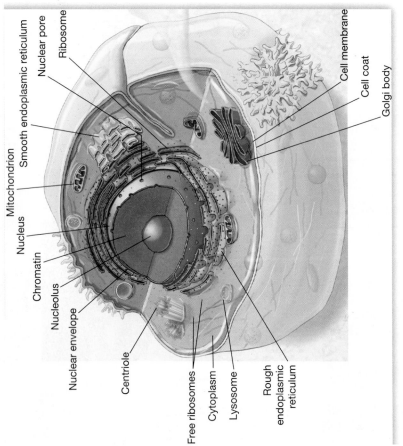

Figure 10-1 The cell—the basic unit of life and the functional unit of tissues.

Apoptosis is not truly a cellular adaptation, but rather represents the end of life for the cell. This is the genetically programmed process of cell death. All cells progress through a cycle of life—some can regenerate through mitosis, some cannot and die. What is important to remember is that this is the normal progression of life for the cell, not a maladaptive pathway.

CELLULAR INJURY

Any variety of internal or external forces can damage cells. Changes in the cell environment (either external or internal) can make it impossible for the cell to survive. Some common mechanisms of cellular injury include ischemia, chemical hypoxia from exposure, or infection. Changes brought about by these factors and many others lead to dramatic changes in the cellular environment and, if internal cellular repair methods are overwhelmed, frequently lead to cell injury and/or death.

Injury to a cell can lead to a number of progressive changes within the cell itself. Such changes can be beneficial for the cell because they enhance survival or can be detrimental, leading to further cellular injury, maladaptive processes, or even cell death. For example, adaptations such as those described in the previous section may allow the cell to survive in the face of increasingly noxious or toxic stimuli. Active cell injury occurs when the stimuli are so intense that the cell itself is damaged, leading to a reaction from various components within the cell. *Reversible cellular injury* occurs when temporary damage occurs to structures within the cell, yet with time, the cell is able to repair this damage and return to baseline or adaptive levels of function. In contrast, *irreversible cellular damage* leads to mitochondrial membrane damage and death of the cell. Another type of cellular damage is *necrosis*, in which cells swell and organelles break down, again with the end result being cell death. Finally, *chronic cell injury* can occur in all types of cells, leading to microalterations within the cell's organelles.

The decision point of whether cell injury is severe enough to cause cellular death relies on a complex interplay between the cell and its host environment. Four common variables that help decide the degree of injury to the cell include the degree to which adenosine triphosphate (ATP) depletion occurs, the presence or absence of oxygen and oxygen-derived free radicals, the presence or absence of intracellular calcium and the loss of a calcium steady state, and defects in cell membrane permeability. These variables, in turn, lead to the three most common forms of cellular injury: hypoxic injury, reactive oxygen species and free-radical-induced injury, and chemical injury.

Hypoxic injury occurs when cells lack oxygen to meet their needs during cellular respiration. Anything that causes a lack of oxygen delivery to tissues—such as ischemia, hypoxemia, anemia, or shock states—can cause hypoxic injury. With even mild hypoxia, cells begin to function differently. Cellular processes are disrupted, membranes become leaky, and the sodium/potassium ATPase pump fails (▶ Figure 10-2). A lack of oxygen leads to a sustained cascade of events that end in cell death. Restoration of oxygen does not always reverse the injury, however.

A specific type of cellular injury called *reperfusion injuries* can occur in diseases such as heart attack and stroke. Although the effects of this specific etiology are not yet fully understood, injury seems to be a specific, secondary consequence of the return of oxygenation.

Free radicals and oxygen-reactive species interact with cells during oxidative stress and cause cellular damage. Free radicals may be produced within the cells themselves or may be part of the extracellular environment. The primary problems caused by free radicals that are understood to date include lipid peroxidation, protein alterations, and alterations of DNA strands. Lipid peroxidation involves destruction of carbon double bonds in lipid membrane layers, causing loss of membrane integrity. Protein alterations and DNA alterations also result from chemical interactions of the free radicals with various parts of these proteins to cause alterations in their structures.

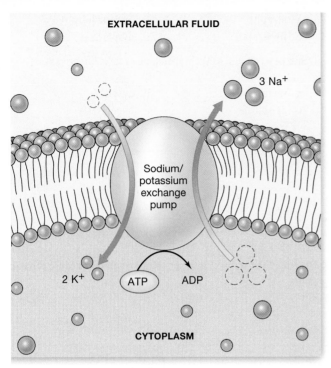

Figure 10-2 Hypoxia disrupts cellular processes, causing cell membranes to become leaky and the sodium/potassium ATPase pump to fail.

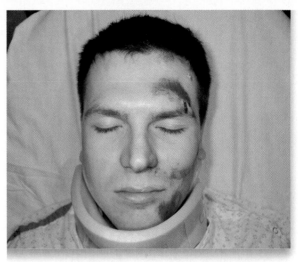

Figure 10-3 Cells can be damaged by physical forces. Blunt trauma can lead to both primary cell injuries (as evidenced by lacerations and bruising) and injuries secondary to inflammation.

Chemical injury occurs to cells when the offending toxin causes biochemical injury to the plasma membrane of the affected cell. The two best-understood mechanisms at this time are free radical and lipid peroxidation injury and injury from direct interaction between the cell membrane or organelles and toxin. Some examples of chemical toxins include carbon tetrachloride, lead, carbon monoxide, ethanol, mercury, and other drugs or chemicals.

Other types of injuries to cells can arise from physical damage, such as from blunt force injuries. Bruises, or contusions, cause local tissue damage as cells at the site of contact are injured first by primary mechanical pressure and then by secondary injury due to pressure from swelling in the area. Edema and local decreases in perfusion from accumulated blood can cause local tissue hypoxia and ischemic injury. Thus, physical injury can also be listed as a cause of cellular demise (▶ Figure 10-3).

Finally, infection, immunologic and inflammatory injury, genetics, physical agents, and nutritional deficiencies may also cause cellular injury. Infectious organisms differ in their abilities to injure a host's tissues by invading and destroying the cells, producing toxins, or causing hypersensitivity states. A highly virulent organism will cause much more disease and distress in the body, and ultimately lead to greater derangements in the cellular environment. Inflammatory and immunologic responses also cause cellular injury from the effects of substances such as histamine, antibodies, lymphokines, complements, and proteases that lead to cellular membrane injury.

Genetic factors can lead to defects in plasma membrane proteins that make cells susceptible to damage or subject other organelles of the cells to damage or disease states. Nutrition can also be a factor in cellular injury from this perspective. If the body does not have the necessary precursor nutrients (proteins, fats, carbohydrates, vitamins, water, etc.), it cannot make healthy, functional cells. Without these functional cells, various disease states occur. Cellular damage can also be caused by injurious physical agents including temperature extremes, illumination, radiation, noise, vibration, changes in atmospheric pressure, mechanical stress, and others.

TRANSITIONING

REVIEW ITEMS

1. Cellular adaption in the form of abnormal changes in the size, shape, and organization of mature cells is known as _____.
   - a. atrophy
   - b. hypertrophy
   - c. hyperplasia
   - d. dysplasia

2. An increase in the size of a cell while it maintains the same shape and function is known as _____.
   - a. atrophy
   - b. hypertrophy
   - c. hyperplasia
   - d. dysplasia

3. A cellular adaption in which the number of cells increases because of an accelerated rate of cell division is known as _____.

    a. atrophy   b. hypertrophy

    c. hyperplasia   d. dysplasia

4. Which of the following describes a cellular condition in which cells shrink in size, often a consequence of disuse?

    a. atrophy   b. hypertrophy

    c. hyperplasia   d. dysplasia

5. Death of a cell due to the normal life cycle is known as _____.

    a. metaplasia   b. dysplasia

    c. apoptosis   d. hyperplasia

APPLIED PATHOPHYSIOLOGY

1. Describe the difference between reversible and irreversible cellular injury.

2. Describe the four common variables that help decide the degree of injury to the cell.

3. Describe the negative consequences (within the cell itself) of a hypoxic cellular injury.

4. Acknowledging that the etiology is not fully understood, describe how reperfusion may actually injure the cell.

5. Describe the two ways in which blunt trauma can cause cellular injury.

CLINICAL DECISION MAKING

A 77-year-old woman complains of three days of weakness, fever, and a cough. On arrival, you note that she is awake and alert, but appears to be slightly short of breath. Her airway is patent and her breathing is labored, with a respiratory rate of 30. She has a strong radial pulse and her skin is warm to touch. While discussing her history, she tells you she has been sick for a month, but worse in the past three days. She notes she was recently diagnosed with cardiac hypertrophy.

1. Given the discussion in this chapter, please describe what is meant by cardiac hypertrophy.

2. How might the hypertrophy be contributing to the patient's current complaint?

3. Given the description of fever and a cough, what other cellular pathophysiology must be considered?

The patient notes that in the past month, she has been severely short of breath and dizzy when climbing her stairs. She tells you, however, that when she is at rest she is fine.

4. How would a hypertyrophied heart affect cardiac output?

5. Why would rest theoretically resolve the dizziness and shortness of breath?

On examination, you note decreased lung sounds on the right side, a persistent, productive cough, and a temperature of 101.5°F. Her SpO_2 is maintained at 89 percent on room air.

6. Given the infectious symptoms, please describe how her lung cells might be injured and the changes that they have undergone as a result of this injury.

7. How might infectious cellular injury be linked to the low pulse oximeter reading?

RESOURCES

McCance, K. L., and S. E. Huether. *Pathophysiology: The Biological Basis for Disease in Adults and Children.* 5th ed. Philadelphia: Elsevier-Mosby, 2006.

Standard: Pathophysiology

Competency: Integrates comprehensive knowledge of the pathophysiology of major human systems.

TOPIC 11

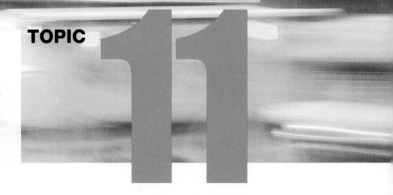

SELF-DEFENSE MECHANISMS AND INFLAMMATION

INTRODUCTION

The human body is constantly bombarded by challenges from within and without. To maintain a healthy organism, the body must defend itself. Innate resistance, sometimes called *native immunity*, includes natural barriers and inflammation. The natural barriers are physical, mechanical, and biochemical lines of defense that work to prevent infection.

The physical and mechanical barriers are self-defense mechanisms consisting of special cells or secretions—for example, mucus and cilia in the respiratory tract, tightly woven epithelial cell layers of the skin, gastric acids of the stomach, or the low temperature of the body's surface. These special adaptations prevent infection by providing an environment too extreme for rapid cell growth and division by pathogens, for example. The end result is a network of interconnected cells that resists intrusion by outside invaders that wish to damage it (▶ Figure 11-1).

The biochemical barriers often work with physical barriers to trap bacteria or other pathogens. Examples of biochemical barriers include sweat, tears, mucus, saliva, and cerumen (ear wax). Specialized cells of the skin and respiratory tree synthesize unique proteins that also help prevent infection and disease, including surfactants, cathelicidins, and defensins. Finally, the normal bacterial flora of the skin and GI tract aid in digestion and produce several chemicals that prevent toxic overgrowths of bacteria or other microorganisms. One needs only to think of a patient with a toxic megacolon from *Clostridium difficile* superinfection after a prolonged course of antibiotic therapy to realize what importance normal flora have in regulating the GI tract.

Equally important to the health of the human body is the phagocytic response of microphages and macrophages. These cellular components ingest and destroy cellular debris and microorganisms rapidly. *Microphages* are the circulating neutrophils and eosinophils in the bloodstream. Neutrophils are specially designed to target bacteria and cellular debris, whereas eosinophils target antibody-rich foreign material. Macrophages work to actively ingest foreign material; they may be fixed to a particular cell or tissue or may roam in the blood and lymphatic system (▶ Figure 11-2).

Natural killer cells are specialized lymphocytes that constantly monitor tissues for invaders by detecting the presence of antigens. When activated by antigens, the natural killer cells create special substances called *perforins*, which destroy the invaders by creating large holes in the cell membrane. The response of natural killer cells is rapid—often more rapid than the response of T or B cells of the immune system—allowing them to slow the spread of infection or eliminate cancer cells.

Interferons are special cytokines (a type of protein produced by the body) that slow viral infections and stimulate the activity of macrophages and natural killer cells. Interferon not only acts locally but also has some hormonal effects that lead to cellular signaling.

The *complement system* is a series of 11 plasma proteins that help improve antibody function. Complement proteins have been shown to accomplish a number of key features in the cell, including attracting phagocytes, stimulating phagocytosis, destroying cell membranes, and promoting inflammation.

THE INFLAMMATORY RESPONSE

The inflammatory response is a complex sequence of interrelated events that is designed to prevent further damage and repair existing damage to cells of the body, when possible

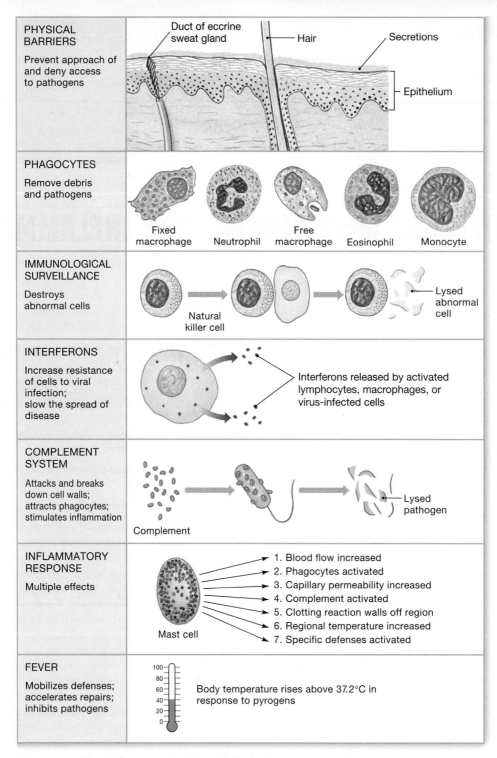

PHYSICAL BARRIERS Prevent approach of and deny access to pathogens	Duct of eccrine sweat gland · Hair · Secretions · Epithelium
PHAGOCYTES Remove debris and pathogens	Fixed macrophage · Neutrophil · Free macrophage · Eosinophil · Monocyte
IMMUNOLOGICAL SURVEILLANCE Destroys abnormal cells	Natural killer cell · Lysed abnormal cell
INTERFERONS Increase resistance of cells to viral infection; slow the spread of disease	Interferons released by activated lymphocytes, macrophages, or virus-infected cells
COMPLEMENT SYSTEM Attacks and breaks down cell walls; attracts phagocytes; stimulates inflammation	Complement · Lysed pathogen
INFLAMMATORY RESPONSE Multiple effects	Mast cell 1. Blood flow increased 2. Phagocytes activated 3. Capillary permeability increased 4. Complement activated 5. Clotting reaction walls off region 6. Regional temperature increased 7. Specific defenses activated
FEVER Mobilizes defenses; accelerates repairs; inhibits pathogens	Body temperature rises above 37.2°C in response to pyrogens

Figure 11-1 The defense mechanisms of the body.

Inflammation is a nonspecific, localized response at sites of cellular injury.

(▶ Figure 11-3). Inflammation is a nonspecific, localized response at sites of cellular injury. It is stimulated by any process that kills cells or damages loose connective tissue. Two phases occur in inflam-mation: the vascular response and the cel-lular response.

Inflammation leads to classic changes in the organism: redness, heat, swelling, and pain. These localized manifestations are the result of cellular changes. When injury occurs, local blood vessels dilate. Increased blood flow to the site of injury brings with it red and white blood cells, plasma proteins, and other chemicals that will be part of the inflammatory response. Capillary permea-bility increases, allowing local edema to form. Mast cells are directly involved in this process, releasing histamine and heparin, which, in turn, provide for the attraction of phagocytic cells, including neutrophils.

In the next stage of the vascular response, fluid leaks from the vessels as

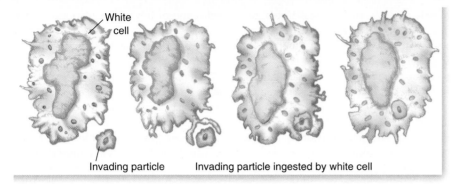

White cell

Invading particle   Invading particle ingested by white cell

Figure 11-2 White blood cells form the basis for the phagocytic response.

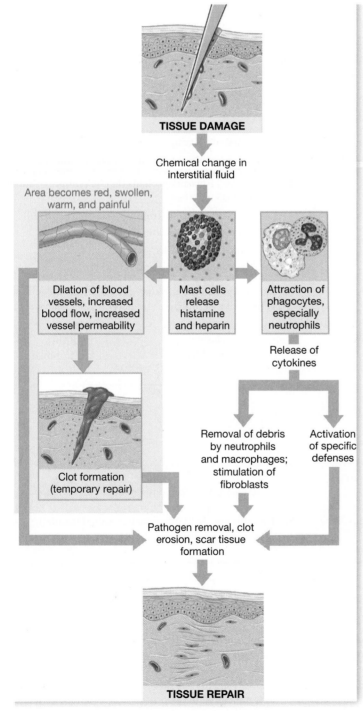

TISSUE DAMAGE

Chemical change in interstitial fluid

Area becomes red, swollen, warm, and painful

Dilation of blood vessels, increased blood flow, increased vessel permeability

Mast cells release histamine and heparin

Attraction of phagocytes, especially neutrophils

Release of cytokines

Clot formation (temporary repair)

Removal of debris by neutrophils and macrophages; stimulation of fibroblasts

Activation of specific defenses

Pathogen removal, clot erosion, scar tissue formation

TISSUE REPAIR

Figure 11-3 The process of inflammation.

biochemical mediators—such as histamine, bradykinin, leukotrienes, substance P, and prostaglandins—stimulate retraction of endothelial cell walls to allow plasma and leukocytes to enter surrounding tissue. This leads to edema at the site. Control of the inflammatory process occurs through the different biochemical mediators that act locally and do not spread to healthy tissue. Toxins are diluted through the influx of plasma and biochemical mediators, as well as the actions of plasma protein systems that contain and destroy bacteria and cellular debris. In addition, macrophages and lymphocytes interact with the adaptive immune response of the body to remove additional pathogens. Finally, the injured area is returned to the prior state of health through drainage by the lymphatic system and epithelial channels, which also help with development of further acquired immunity as T and B lymphocytes are activated when antigens pass through the lymph.

The inflammatory response contains three different plasma protein systems: the complement system, the clotting system, and the kinin system. Each of these systems involves activation of precursor proenzymes that, in turn, activate a cascade of additional biochemical mediators and enzymes. The complement system is a series of special plasma proteins that can destroy pathogens directly or work in concert with the other components of the inflammatory response to defend against bacterial infection.

Although discussion of the complement system is beyond the scope of this topic, the paramedic should remember that acquired immunity from the activation of cellular pathways of the complement system is the result of protein interactions with one of three subpathways: the classical pathway (an antigen–antibody response), the lectin pathway, or an alternative pathway. Cleavage of the proenzymes in these pathways leads to more biologically active substances that can attract or activate these systems and recruit additional biological mediators to the site of inflammation. The end result is an enhanced inflammatory response due to the actions of these chemical messengers.

Manifestations of Inflammation

Local manifestations of inflammation accompany all types of cellular injury. All the typical manifestations of infection are present: heat, redness, swelling, and pain. *Exudate* is a collection of fluid and cellular debris that occur as cells die. Exudate initially is watery but can progress to becoming more thick and clotted. *Pus* is the local collection of purulent exudates from cysts or abscesses.

Systemic manifestations of acute inflammation include fever, leukocytosis, and plasma protein synthesis. Fever is induced by response to specific cytokines such as endogenous pyrogens. *Leukocy-* tosis is a proliferation of leukocytes, primarily neutrophils. Finally, plasma protein synthesis involves release of either pro- or antiinflammatory proteins in the early phases of the immune response that help activate additional biochemical mediators of infection. These biochemical mediators, in turn, activate additional biochemical pathways in a stepwise fashion, leading to additional responses by the body.

Chronic inflammation differs from acute inflammation mainly in the time of activation of the body's response to the stimulus. Chronic infection lasts at least two weeks and may lead to one of four common pathways: persistent acute inflammation, neutrophil degranulation and death, lymphocyte activation, or fibroblast activation. Resolution and repair of the chronic inflammatory state occurs when tissue repair leads to a scar or when lymphocyte and monocyte/macrophage infiltration leads to pus that must be reabsorbed.

TRANSITIONING

REVIEW ITEMS

1. Mucus would be an example of which of the following types of self-defense mechanisms?
   a. mechanical
   b. inflammatory
   c. biochemical
   d. humoral

2. The rapid ingestion and destruction of cellular debris and microorganisms is an example of _____.
   a. a phagocytic response
   b. physical and mechanical barriers
   c. inflammation
   d. leukocytosis

3. Specialized lymphocytes that constantly monitor tissues for invaders by detecting the presence of antigens are known as _____.

   a. macrophages
   b. neutrophils
   c. eosinophils
   d. natural killer cells

4. A series of 11 plasma proteins that help improve antibody function is known as _____.
   a. a biochemical barrier
   b. a phagocytic response
   c. the complement system
   d. the interferon system

5. Special cytokines that slow viral infections and stimulate the activity of macrophages and natural killer cells are known as _____.
   a. interferons
   b. perforins
   c. eosinophils
   d. neutrophils

APPLIED PATHOPHYSIOLOGY

1. Describe how physical and mechanical barriers such as mucus, or even lower external skin temperature, provide protection to the body.

2. Provide an example of a biochemical barrier and discuss how it works with a physical barrier to defend the body.

3. Describe how the phagocytic response defends the body.

4. Describe the vascular component of inflammation.

5. Describe how local inflammation would manifest.

CLINICAL DECISION MAKING

A 22-year-old man has called the ambulance because of leg pain and difficulty walking. On arrival, the patient is awake and alert, but anxious with pain. Your primary assessment notes no deficit with his airway or breathing; although he is slightly tachycardic, his radial pulse is strong, and his skin is warm and dry. The patient complains today of a chronic leg injury. He notes that he stepped on a nail five days ago, *and since then, his foot has become swollen and very painful. He notes that today he cannot walk.*

1. Describe the normal defense mechanisms that the nail defeated as it punctured the skin and introduced foreign matter into the patient's foot.

2. Discuss the likely defense mechanisms that occurred after the nail punctured the foot. How did the body likely respond?

3. What is most likely causing the pain and swelling in the patient's foot?

On examination of the foot, you note significant swelling, redness, and a white, liquid exudate leaking from the wound. The foot is extremely tender to the touch.

4. Describe how the inflammatory response has made the foot red and swollen.

5. Why is the wound leaking the white substance? What is the most likely makeup of this substance?

6. What is the danger of this wound overcoming the body's natural defense mechanisms?

TOPIC

12

Standard Pathophysiology

Competency Integrates comprehensive knowledge of pathophysiology of major human systems.

THE CARDIOVASCULAR SYSTEM

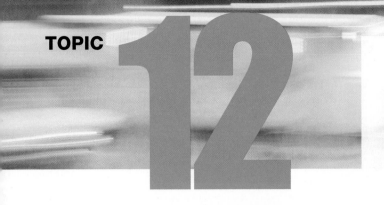

TRANSITION *highlights*

- *Distribution of blood within the vascular compartment and the physiologic determinants that affect movement of fluid into and out of the vascular compartment:*
  - Hydrostatic pressure.
  - Plasma oncotic pressure.

- *Normal cardiac output, and how certain variables can alter it from normal:*
  - Changes in heart rate.
  - Changes in stroke volume.

- *Systemic vascular resistance, and the effects should it become deranged:*
  - Tissue perfusion.
  - Systolic and diastolic blood pressure.
  - Pulse pressure.

- *Microcirculation, and how changes of the aforementioned principles have a positive or negative effect on it.*

- *Blood pressure, and how it becomes deranged from disturbances in the aforementioned principles.*

- *How the autonomic nervous system (sympathetic and parasympathetic) can alter cellular perfusion through manipulation of the aforementioned principles.*

INTRODUCTION

Each component of the cardiovascular system—the heart, the blood, and the blood vessels—plays an essential role in maintaining perfusion in the body. By constantly moving oxygen and nutrients to the cells and returning waste products to the lungs for removal, the delicate balance of homeostasis is maintained.

Although the cardiovascular system has a singular function, maintaining perfusion is a complex task that requires continuous adjustment. For perfusion to be adequate, oxygen must enter the alveoli, cross over the alveolar–capillary membrane, attach to hemoglobin, and be transported via the blood to cells. The blood volume and composition, cardiac function, and vascular resistance all contribute to the movement of oxygenated blood out of the alveolar capillaries and to the cells throughout the body.

The cardiovascular system is extremely relevant to paramedic assessment and care. Integrating cardiovascular anatomy, physiology, and pathophysiology into your assessment will help you recognize and understand the changes that occur in the body when it is faced with challenges. Being familiar with the ways in which the cardiovascular system compensates will help you not only recognize critical situations, but also anticipate further patient deterioration. Understanding pathophysiology and system dysfunction will further provide valuable information as treatment plans are developed. It will not only assist you in understanding outcomes, but also offer valuable data regarding costs, benefits, and potential side effects of therapy.

BLOOD VOLUME

One of the determinants of adequate blood pressure and perfusion is blood volume. An adult has approximately 70 mL of blood for every kilogram (2.2 lb) of body weight. Thus, a patient who weighs 154 lb (70 kg) would have approximately 4,900 mL, or 4.9 liters, of blood volume. Blood volume correlates with body mass; therefore, a larger patient would normally have a greater blood volume. The loss of 1 liter of blood in a 100-lb patient would be much more significant than in a 200-lb patient.

Distribution of Blood

Blood is distributed throughout the cardiovascular system (Table 12-1). The majority of blood is housed within the *venous system*, which is also known as a *reservoir* or *capacitance system*. The venous system is capable of enlarging or reducing its capacity in response to increases or decreases in blood volume. As a patient bleeds, the venous volume is continuously reduced regardless of whether the bleeding is from a vein, an artery, or a capillary.

TABLE 12-1	Distribution of Blood in the Cardiovascular System
Veins	64%
Arteries	13%
Pulmonary vessels	9%
Capillaries	7%
Heart	7%

The venous system is responsible for supplying the right side of the heart with an adequate volume of blood. If the volume entering the right side of the heart is decreased, the amount ejected from the left ventricle, through the arteries, and to the cells is also reduced. Thus, the venous volume plays a major role in maintaining blood pressure and adequate perfusion of the cells. This is discussed in more detail later in this topic. The capillary network is the site of gas exchange occurring with the alveoli or cells.

Hydrostatic Pressure

Hydrostatic pressure is the force inside the vessel or capillary bed generated by the contraction of the heart and blood pressure. Hydrostatic pressure exerts a "push" inside the vessel or capillary—that is, it wants to push fluid out of the vessel or capillary, through the vessel wall, and into the surrounding interstitial space. A high hydrostatic pressure would force more fluid out of the vessel or capillary and promote edema—swelling from excess fluid outside the vessels (▶ Figure 12-1).

For example, if a patient has a left ventricle that is failing and unable to pump blood effectively, the volume and pressure in the left atrium, pulmonary vein, and pulmonary capillaries rise. This occurs because the pulmonary capillaries, pulmonary vein, and left atrium are the pathways by which blood enters the left ventricle.

When the left ventricle fails to empty effectively, blood backs up into the left atrium and pulmonary vessels, which increases the pressure within them. The increased hydrostatic pressure inside the pulmonary capillaries forces fluid out of them. The extruded fluid has a tendency to collect in the spaces between the alveoli and capillaries and around the alveoli, which reduces the ability of oxygen and carbon dioxide to be exchanged across the alveolar/capillary membrane.

This disturbance reduces the blood oxygen content, leading to cellular hypoxia, and also causes the blood to retain carbon dioxide. The fluid will eventually begin to collapse and fill the alveoli, further diminishing gas exchange. This condition is known as *pulmonary edema*.

Plasma Oncotic Pressure

Plasma oncotic pressure, also known as *colloid oncotic pressure* or *oncotic pressure*, is responsible for keeping fluid inside the vessels. A force is generated inside the vessels by large plasma proteins, especially albu-

min, that attract water and other fluids. Opposite to hydrostatic pressure, oncotic pressure exerts a "pull" inside the vessel. A high oncotic pressure would pull fluid from outside the vessel, through the vessel wall, and into the vessel (review Figure 12-1).

A balance between hydrostatic pressure and plasma oncotic pressure must be maintained for equilibrium of fluid balance. The effects of high and low hydrostatic and oncotic pressures are summarized as follows:

- A *high* hydrostatic pressure will push fluid out of a capillary and promote edema.
- A *low* hydrostatic pressure will push less fluid out of the vessel.
- A *high* oncotic pressure will draw excessive amounts of fluid into the vessel or capillary and promote blood volume overload.
- A *low* oncotic pressure will not exert an adequate pull effect to counteract the push of hydrostatic pressure and will therefore promote loss of vascular volume and promote edema (as seen in patients who are malnourished and have low albumin levels).

PUMP FUNCTION OF THE MYOCARDIUM

To have an adequate blood pressure and perfusion, the myocardium must work effectively as a pump. The heart is capable of varying its output to meet a wide range of physiologic demands. It can drastically increase its pump function, up to sixfold. The pump function is typically expressed as the cardiac output. Cardiac output is defined as the amount of blood ejected by the left ventricle in 1 minute. The cardiac output has a major influence on blood pressure and perfusion, as is discussed in the following sections.

Cardiac Output

A normal cardiac output for an adult at rest is 5 to 7 liters/minute. This means that the ventricles will pump nearly the entire blood volume through the vascular system in 1 minute. If a drop of blood left the left ventricle, in 1 minute it should be back at the left ventricle. The cardiac output is determined by the heart rate and the stroke volume. Cardiac output is expressed by the following equation:

Cardiac output
= Heart rate × Stroke volume

Figure 12-1 Hydrostatic pressure pushes water out of the capillary. Plasma oncotic pressure pulls water into the capillary.

Labels in figure: Arteriole, Venule, Hydrostatic pressure pushes water out., Plasma oncotic pressure pulls water in., H_2O, H_2O, Capillary

Heart Rate

The *heart rate* is defined as the number of times the heart contracts in 1 minute. The heart has the property of *automaticity*, meaning it can generate its own impulse. This is achieved through the conduction system, with the *sinoatrial (SA) node* being the primary pacemaker. The heart rate can also be influenced to increase or decrease its rate of firing by several factors outside the heart, primarily hormones and the autonomic nervous system, composed of the sympathetic and parasympathetic systems. The influence of the autonomic nervous system on the heart rate is summarized as follows:

- An *increase* in stimulation by the sympathetic nervous system *increases* the heart rate.
- A *decrease* in stimulation by the sympathetic nervous system *decreases* the heart rate.
- An *increase* in stimulation by the parasympathetic nervous system *decreases* the heart rate.
- A *decrease* in stimulation by the parasympathetic nervous system *increases* the heart rate.

The sympathetic and parasympathetic nervous systems exert control over the heart rate through the cardiovascular control center located in the brainstem. The cardiovascular control center is composed of the cardioexcitatory center and the cardioinhibitory center. The cardioexcitatory center increases the heart rate by increasing sympathetic stimulation and decreasing parasympathetic stimulation. The cardioinhibitory center decreases the heart rate by decreasing sympathetic stimulation and increasing parasympathetic stimulation.

Direct neural stimulation provides an immediate response in the heart rate and force of ventricular contraction. In addition, stimulation of the sympathetic nervous system may cause the release of epinephrine and norepinephrine from the adrenal gland located on top of the kidney. The release of these hormones may take a few minutes; however, the response will be sustained as long as the hormones are continuously released and circulating. The beta$_1$ properties in the epinephrine will cause an increase in the heart rate and force of contraction.

Stroke Volume

Stroke volume is defined as the volume of blood ejected by the left ventricle with each contraction. Stroke volume is determined by preload, myocardial contractility, and afterload.

PRELOAD   *Preload* is the pressure generated in the left ventricle at the end of diastole (the resting phase of the cardiac cycle). Preload pressure is created by the blood volume in the left ventricle at the end of diastole. The available venous volume, which determines the volume of blood in the ventricle, consequently plays a major role in determining preload. An increase in preload generally increases stroke volume, which in turn increases the cardiac output. Preload determines the force necessary to eject the blood out of the ventricle.

MYOCARDIAL CONTRACTILITY   As blood fills the left ventricle, the muscle fibers stretch to house the blood. The stretch of the muscle fiber at the end of diastole determines the force available to eject the blood from the ventricle. This is known as the *Frank-Starling law of the heart*. As the blood volume increases in the left ventricle, the increased stretch in the muscle fibers generates a commensurate increase in contraction force. In short, the volume of blood in the ventricle automatically generates a contraction forceful enough to eject it. The effectiveness of fiber stretch is limited, however. In the case of a severely dilated ventricle where the fibers are overstretched, the Frank-Starling law no longer applies, and the heart begins to fail.

To have an adequate stroke volume, the left ventricle must be able to generate enough force to effectively eject its blood volume. An increase in myocardial contractility will increase the stroke volume and improve cardiac output. Conversely, a decrease in myocardial contractility will lead to a decrease in stroke volume and a resulting decrease in cardiac output.

For example, a patient with congestive heart failure will have a decrease in contractile force of the left ventricle that is likely to result in diminished cardiac output. A patient who has suffered a heart attack will have a deadened portion of cardiac muscle that will no longer contribute to the contractile force. If the area of necrosis is large, the contractile force will be significantly reduced, with a proportional decrease in stroke volume and cardiac output.

AFTERLOAD   *Afterload* is the resistance in the aorta that must be overcome by contraction of the left ventricle to eject the blood. The force generated by the left ventricle must overcome the pressure in the aorta to move the blood forward. A high afterload places an increased workload on the left ventricle. A chronically elevated diastolic blood pressure will create a high afterload, generating an increased myocardial workload that could lead to left ventricular failure over time.

In general, a decrease in either the heart rate or stroke volume will decrease the cardiac output:

- A *decrease* in heart rate causes a *decrease* in cardiac output.
- A *decrease* in stroke volume causes a *decrease* in cardiac output.

The effects of heart rate, blood volume, myocardial contractility, autonomic nervous system stimulation, hormone release, and diastolic blood pressure on cardiac output are as follows:

- A *decrease* in heart rate will *decrease* cardiac output.
- An *increase* in heart rate, if not excessive, will *increase* cardiac output.
- A *decrease* in blood volume will *decrease* preload, stroke volume, and cardiac output.
- An *increase* in blood volume will *increase* preload, stroke volume, and cardiac output.
- A *decrease* in myocardial contractility will *decrease* stroke volume and cardiac output.
- An *increase* in myocardial contractility will *increase* stroke volume and cardiac output.
- Neural stimulation from the sympathetic nervous system will *increase* heart rate, myocardial contractility, and cardiac output.

Direct neural stimulation provides an immediate response in the heart rate and force of ventricular contraction.

A decrease in myocardial contractility will lead to a decrease in stroke volume and a resulting decrease in cardiac output.

- Neural stimulation from the parasympathetic nervous system will *decrease* heart rate, myocardial contractility, and cardiac output.
- Beta$_1$ stimulation from epinephrine will *increase* heart rate, myocardial contractility, and cardiac output.
- Beta$_1$ blockade (e.g., a patient on a beta blocker) will block beta$_1$ stimulation and *decrease* heart rate, myocardial contractility, and cardiac output.
- An extremely high diastolic blood pressure will *increase* the pressure in the aorta, requiring a more forceful contraction to overcome the aortic pressure and a higher myocardial workload, and it may weaken the heart and decrease the cardiac output over time.
- A *decrease* in the diastolic blood pressure will *decrease* the pressure in the aorta, require a less forceful contraction to overcome the aortic pressure, and reduce the myocardial workload, which may improve the cardiac output in a weakened heart.

A faster heart rate may increase cardiac output; however, if the rate is extremely fast, the cardiac output may actually decrease. With excessively fast heart rates, usually greater than 160 beats per minute (bpm) in the adult patient, the time between beats is so short that there is not enough time for the ventricles to fill. This reduces the preload, which in turn reduces the cardiac output.

SYSTEMIC VASCULAR RESISTANCE

Systemic vascular resistance is the resistance that is offered to blood flow through a vessel. As a vessel constricts (decreases its diameter), resistance inside the vessel increases, which typically increases pressure inside the vessel. Conversely, as a vessel dilates (increases its diameter), resistance inside the vessel decreases, which typically decreases pressure inside the vessel.

Vessel size influences blood pressure. *Vasoconstriction* decreases vessel diameter, increases resistance, and increases blood pressure. *Vasodilation* increases vessel diameter, decreases resistance, and decreases blood pressure.

Pressure within the vessels is greatest during cardiac contraction (systole) and least during cardiac relaxation (diastole). The basic measure of systemic vascular resistance is the diastolic blood pressure because it is assessed during the relaxation phase, indicating the resting pressure within the vessels. Systolic blood pressure, created by the wave of blood ejected from the left ventricle during contraction, increases the pressure within the vessels beyond their resting pressure.

An abnormally high diastolic blood pressure is not a desirable condition. The diastolic blood pressure is the pressure inside the arteries and the aortic root immediately prior to contraction of the left ventricle. The higher the diastolic blood pressure, the greater the resistance to blood being ejected from the left ventricle. That means the left ventricle has to work harder to pump the blood out against a higher diastolic pressure. If the diastolic blood pressure is chronically elevated, it will eventually cause the heart to fail. It is all related to resistance of flow and harder workloads.

For example, a person is given two weights to lift simultaneously. The weight in the right hand weighs only 1 lb, whereas the weight in the left hand weighs 10 lb. Which extremity and muscle would become fatigued and fail first if the person were asked to continuously lift the weights? Obviously the left arm lifting the 10-lb weight would fatigue and fail first, because the muscle is working against a greater resistance.

Relate this example to the heart of a patient with a chronically elevated diastolic blood pressure. The high resistance to blood flow causes the left ventricle to work harder to pump the blood out. If the left ventricle has to contract chronically against the high resistance, it eventually weakens and fails. This condition is known as *left ventricular failure* or *congestive heart failure*.

The autonomic nervous system influences the systemic vascular resistance. Direct neural stimulation from the sympathetic nervous system causes the vessels to constrict, increasing vessel resistance and pressure. Parasympathetic nervous system stimulation causes the vessels to dilate, reducing resistance and pressure. In addition, the epinephrine and norepinephrine that are released by the adrenal gland in response to sympathetic stimulation have alpha properties. Alpha$_1$ receptor stimulation causes the vessels to constrict, increasing the vessels' resistance and pressure.

If the volume of blood inside a vessel decreases, one way to maintain the pressure is to decrease vessel size and increase resistance. When blood is being lost and overall volume is decreasing, vessels will usually compensate for this loss by continuing to constrict to raise resistance and pressure. Blood pressure may thus be maintained at a normal level, making it appear as if no volume has been lost. That is why it is so important not only to evaluate the vital signs in a patient with blood loss, but also to look for signs of poor perfusion. A drop in pressure is a late finding as blood is lost.

Think back to preceding topics and the discussion of cellular metabolism. As vessels decrease in size to maintain blood pressure, they do so at the expense of cellular perfusion. As the vessels constrict, less blood flows through them and less oxygen is delivered to the cells. As oxygen delivery decreases, the cells change from aerobic to anaerobic metabolism.

The loss in energy is often noted in the patient's general appearance at the scene. The patient with poor perfusion is typically quiet and reserved and may actually appear sleepy. The patient who is screaming and yelling and constantly moving about must have a great deal of energy to do so. An adequate delivery of oxygen and glucose to the cells is necessary to produce this amount of energy. Be careful not to mistake this high level of patient energy with the agitation and aggression experienced by patients whose brain cells are hypoxic.

The effects of the autonomic nervous system on systemic vascular resistance are summarized as follows:

- Sympathetic stimulation causes vasoconstriction, which *decreases* vessel diameter and *increases* systemic vascular resistance.
- Parasympathetic stimulation causes vasodilation, which *increases* vessel diameter and *decreases* systemic vascular resistance.
- The alpha$_1$ properties in epinephrine and norepinephrine, released in response to sympathetic stimulation, cause vasoconstriction, which *decreases* vessel diameter and *increases* systemic vascular resistance.

> It is important not only to evaluate the vital signs in a patient with blood loss, but also to look for signs of poor perfusion.

Systemic Vascular Resistance Effect on Pulse Pressure

Systolic blood pressure is a relative indicator of cardiac output, whereas diastolic blood pressure measures the systemic vascular resistance. If the systolic blood pressure is decreasing, it is an indication of diminishing cardiac output. The following describes the effect of systemic vascular resistance on diastolic blood pressure:

- An *increase* in the systemic vascular resistance will *increase* the diastolic blood pressure.
- A *decrease* in the systemic vascular resistance will *decrease* the diastolic blood pressure.

The *pulse pressure* is the difference between the systolic and the diastolic blood pressure readings. If the patient has a blood pressure of 132/74 mmHg, for example, the pulse pressure would be derived by subtracting the diastolic from the systolic. In this case, the pulse pressure would be 58 mmHg (132 − 74 = 58). A *narrow pulse pressure* is defined as being less than 25 percent of the systolic blood pressure reading. In this case, a narrow pulse pressure would be less than 33 mmHg (132 × 25% = 33 mmHg).

In the patient with blood or fluid loss, a narrow pulse pressure is a significant sign. As a patient loses blood, the following occurs:

- Blood loss *decreases* venous volume, which *decreases* preload, which *decreases* stroke volume, which *decreases* cardiac output.

The systolic blood pressure begins to decrease from the drop in cardiac output. One way the body attempts to compensate for the decrease in blood pressure is by increasing the systemic vascular resistance, which elevates diastolic blood pressure.

You will see the following in the blood pressure reading:

↓

Systolic blood pressure

Diastolic blood pressure

↑

| Narrow pulse pressure |

Although blood pressure may appear to be within normal limits, the narrow pulse pressure may warn you of a dropping cardiac output from blood or fluid loss and a rising systemic vascular resistance as an attempt to compensate for the decreasing pressure.

For example, a patient with suspected bleeding in the abdomen presents with a blood pressure of 108/88 mmHg. Based on normal blood pressure ranges, this blood pressure falls well within a normal range and may not alarm you. However, if you look at the pulse pressure, it is only 20 mmHg (108 − 88 = 20 mmHg).

A normal pulse pressure would be greater than 25 percent of the systolic blood pressure. In this case, a normal pulse pressure would be 27 mmHg or greater (108 × 25% = 27 mmHg). Thus, this patient has a narrow pulse pressure, which may be an indication of a dropping cardiac output from a decrease in venous volume and preload and an increasing systemic vascular resistance to compensate for the decrease in pressure.

By just looking at the patient's blood pressure, you could easily say it is normal. When considering the pulse pressure, as well as other signs of perfusion—such as skin color, temperature, condition, and mental status—you might reclassify it as abnormal.

MICROCIRCULATION

Microcirculation is the flow of blood through the smallest blood vessels: arterioles, capillaries, and venules (▶ Figure 12-2). As mentioned previously, the veins and venules primarily serve a capacitance function by pooling blood as needed and supplying it to the heart as necessary to maintain cardiac output. Arteries branch into arterioles, which are at the terminal ends of the arteries. The arterioles, which are made up of almost all smooth muscle, control the movement of blood into the capillaries.

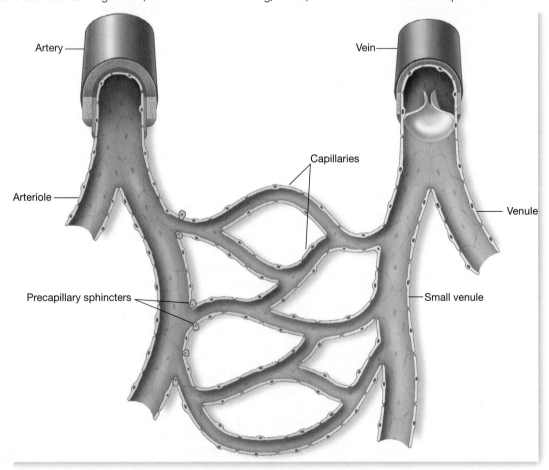

Figure 12-2 Microcirculation is the flow of blood through the smallest blood vessels: arterioles, capillaries, and venules. Precapillary sphincters control the flow of blood through the capillaries.

- Vasoconstriction *decreases* the flow of blood into the capillaries, and vasodilation *increases* the capillary blood flow.

The true capillaries are the sites of exchange between the blood and the cells of nutrients, oxygen, carbon dioxide, glucose, waste products, and metabolic substances. *Metarterioles* are often described as thoroughfares or channels that connect the arterioles and venules. True capillaries branch from the metarterioles. Precapillary sphincters control the movement of blood through the true capillaries. If the precapillary sphincter is relaxed, blood moves through the capillary. If the precapillary sphincter is contracted, the blood is shunted away from the true capillary. The precapillary sphincters help to maintain arterial pressure and control the movement of blood through the capillary beds.

Three regulatory influences control blood flow through the capillaries: local factors, neural factors, and hormonal factors. Local factors are found in the immediate environment around or within the capillary structure—for example, temperature, hypoxia, acidosis, and histamine. A cold temperature would cause the peripheral arterioles to constrict and precapillary sphincters to close, shunting blood away from the capillaries in an attempt to reduce the blood exposure to the cold environment. The opposite would be true in a warm environment, in which the arterioles would dilate and the precapillary sphincters would open to shunt the blood to the periphery, where it can cool.

Neural factors are associated with the influence of the sympathetic and parasympathetic nervous systems on the arterioles and precapillary sphincters. Sympathetic nervous stimulation would cause the arterioles to constrict and precapillary sphincters to close. Parasympathetic nervous stimulation would cause the arterioles to dilate and the precapillary sphincters to open.

Hormonal factors are associated with control of the movement of blood through the capillaries. For example, the alpha$_1$ stimulation from epinephrine causes the arterioles to constrict and the precapillary sphincters to close.

In a resting state, the local factors predominantly control blood flow through the capillaries. When adaptation is necessary, the neural factors will change the capillary blood flow. Hormones are usually responsible for a sustained effect on the arterioles and capillaries.

BLOOD PRESSURE

As previously noted, the systolic blood pressure is a measure of cardiac output. The diastolic blood pressure is a measure of systemic vascular resistance. The body's compensation mechanisms are geared toward maintaining pressure inside the vessel and perfusion of the cells.

Blood pressure (BP) is derived by multiplying two major factors: cardiac output (CO) and systemic vascular resistance (SVR).

$$BP = CO \times SVR$$

Both the cardiac output and systemic vascular resistance have a direct effect on blood pressure, which is summarized as follows:

- An *increase* in cardiac output will *increase* blood pressure.
- A *decrease* in cardiac output will *decrease* blood pressure.
- An *increase* in the heart rate will *increase* the cardiac output, which will *increase* blood pressure.
- A *decrease* in the heart rate will *decrease* the cardiac output, which will *decrease* blood pressure.
- An *increase* in the stroke volume will *increase* the cardiac output, which will *increase* blood pressure.
- A *decrease* in the stroke volume will *decrease* the cardiac output, which will *decrease* blood pressure.
- An *increase* in systemic vascular resistance will *increase* blood pressure.
- A *decrease* in systemic vascular resistance will *decrease* blood pressure.

Perfusion of cells is linked to blood pressure. To maintain adequate perfusion, the blood must be pushed with enough force to constantly deliver oxygen and glucose to the cells and remove carbon dioxide and other waste products. The general effect of blood pressure on perfusion is as follows:

- An *increase* in blood pressure will *increase* cellular perfusion.
- A *decrease* in blood pressure will *decrease* cellular perfusion.

Regulation of Blood Pressure by Baroreceptors and Chemoreceptors

Blood pressure is monitored and regulated by both baroreceptors and chemoreceptors.

BARORECEPTORS *Baroreceptors*, located in the aortic arch and carotid sinuses, are stretch-sensitive receptors that detect changes in blood pressure. As the pressure inside the vessels changes, it decreases or increases the stretch of the fibers of the baroreceptors. The baroreceptors, having thus detected the change in blood pressure, send impulses to the cardioregulatory and vasomotor centers in the brainstem to make compensatory alterations in blood pressure. The cardioregulatory center consists of the cardioexcitatory (cardioacceleratory) center and the cardioinhibitory center, which control heart rate and force of cardiac contraction. The vasomotor center controls the vessel size and resistance through vasoconstriction and vasodilation.

An increase in blood pressure prompts the baroreceptors to signal the brainstem to alter heart function and vessel size to decrease blood pressure. The cardioinhibitory center responds by sending parasympathetic nervous system impulses that cause the heart to decrease heart rate and myocardial contractility. A decrease in myocardial contractility decreases stroke volume. A decrease in stroke volume and heart rate decreases cardiac output. A decrease in cardiac output decreases blood pressure. The vasomotor center responds by parasympathetic impulses to dilate the blood vessels. Vasodilation increases the vessel diameter and decreases the systemic vascular resistance, which decreases blood pressure.

A decrease in blood pressure prompts the baroreceptors to signal the brainstem to alter heart function and vessel size to increase blood pressure. The cardioexcitatory and vasomotor centers send out sympathetic nervous system impulses to increase the heart rate and myocardial contractility and to constrict the vessels. The increase in heart rate increases the cardiac output. The increase in myocardial contractility increases the stroke volume, which increases the cardiac output. An increase in cardiac output increases blood pressure. Vasoconstriction decreases blood vessel diameter and increases the systemic

> **Vasodilation increases the vessel diameter and decreases the systemic vascular resistance, which decreases blood pressure.**

vascular resistance, which increases blood pressure.

CHEMORECEPTORS As discussed previously, the chemoreceptors monitor the content of oxygen, carbon dioxide, and hydrogen ions, as well as the pH of blood. The greatest stimulation to change blood pressure occurs when the oxygen content in arterial blood decreases. An increase in the carbon dioxide level and a decrease in the pH (more acid) have a much lesser effect on increasing blood pressure. When the oxygen content in the arterial blood falls, the carbon dioxide level increases or pH decreases (more acid in the blood), and the brainstem triggers the sympathetic nervous system through the cardioexcitatory center and vasomotor centers to increase blood pressure by increasing the heart rate, myocardial contractility, and vasoconstriction.

The increase in blood pressure is intended to improve the delivery of oxygen to the brain cells and to remove more carbon dioxide. These changes account for the signs you may observe as a paramedic. An early sign of hypoxia is pale, cool, clammy skin and an increase in heart rate. The pale, cool skin is from vasoconstriction, and the increase in heart rate is from sympathetic stimulation of the SA node.

A decrease in blood pressure and oxygen content in the blood will also trigger the release of a cascade of hormones from different endocrine organs. This is discussed in greater detail in Topic 24: Shock.

Maintaining aerobic metabolism is essential for the cells, the organs, and the patient to survive. In summary, to maintain aerobic metabolism of cells, the following must be adequate:

- Oxygen content in ambient air
- Patency of the airway
- Minute ventilation
  - Ventilatory rate
  - Tidal volume
- Alveolar ventilation
  - Ventilatory rate
  - Tidal volume
- Perfusion in the pulmonary capillaries
  - Venous volume
  - Right ventricular pump function
- Gas exchange between the capillaries and the alveoli
- Content of blood
  - Red blood cells
  - Hemoglobin
  - Plasma
- Cardiac output
  - Heart rate
  - Preload
  - Stroke volume
  - Myocardial contractility
  - Afterload
- Systemic vascular resistance
  - Sympathetic nervous system stimulation
  - Parasympathetic nervous system stimulation
  - Gas exchange between the capillaries and the cells

TRANSITIONING

REVIEW ITEMS

1. A dramatic increase in the pressure and blood volume in the pulmonary capillaries would likely lead to _____.
   a. bronchospasm
   b. pulmonary edema
   c. a decrease in heart rate
   d. hypotension

2. Which of the following clinical signs would you expect the patient to exhibit in response to a decrease in the plasma oncotic pressure?
   a. hypertension
   b. bradycardia
   c. peripheral edema
   d. jugular venous distention

3. Preload is primarily determined by _____.
   a. venous blood volume
   b. pressure in the aortic root
   c. cellular uptake of glucose
   d. alveolar ventilation

4. Your patient has just received albuterol by nebulizer for bronchospasm. As a side effect of the medication, you would likely see an increase in the heart rate owing to _____.
   a. parasympathetic stimulation
   b. reduction in the oxygen content in the blood
   c. beta$_2$ stimulation of the sinoatrial node
   d. trace amounts of beta$_1$ in the nebulized drug

5. Which of the following signs would directly indicate an increase in systemic vascular resistance?
   a. a decrease in heart rate
   b. a decrease in systolic blood pressure
   c. a widened pulse pressure
   d. pale, cool skin

APPLIED PATHOPHYSIOLOGY

1. Define hydrostatic pressure and plasma oncotic pressure.

2. List, define, and describe the factors that determine the cardiac output, systemic vascular resistance, and blood pressure.

3. Describe the influence of the sympathetic nervous system and parasympathetic nervous system on the cardiac output and blood pressure.

4. Define microcirculation, and describe how it affects blood pressure and perfusion.

5. Identify the location and describe the role of the baroreceptors.

6. Discuss how the chemoreceptors influence changes in blood pressure.

CLINICAL DECISION MAKING

You arrive on the scene and find a 46-year-old man who fell while bicycling for exercise. He has an open midshaft femur fracture. Blood is spurting from the wound. The patient responds slowly when you call out his name. His respiratory rate is 24/minute. His radial pulse is very weak. His skin is extremely pale, cool, and clammy. His blood pressure is 94/76 mmHg, and heart rate is 131 beats per minute.

1. Following scene safety, what is your first immediate action after approaching this patient?

2. What are the life threats to this patient?

3. Why is the patient's mental status deteriorating, and why is he responding so poorly?

4. How is the spurting blood affecting the perfusion of the cells?

5. What is causing a decrease in the systolic blood pressure?

6. Is the pulse pressure narrow? If so, describe why.

7. Why is the skin pale, cool, and clammy?

8. Why is the heart rate 131 bpm?

9. Are the cells of this patient likely undergoing aerobic or anaerobic metabolism? Why?

10. Why does the patient have such a lack of energy?

LIFE SPAN DEVELOPMENT

TRANSITION *highlights*

- Brief overview of how understanding life span development can help the paramedic when dealing with differing age brackets.

- Identification of the revised age brackets when discussing life span development.

- Explanation of the common characteristics of each developmental age bracket:
  - Physiologic development.
  - Psychological maturation.
  - Normal vital signs.
  - Assessment tips.

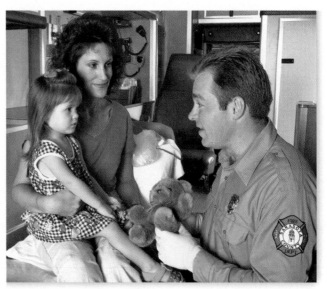

Figure 13-1 Modify your approach to fit the patient's stage of development.

INTRODUCTION

From the time we are born to the time we die, human beings experience ongoing and often significant changes through the process of aging (Table 13-1). Both physical and psychosocial changes present a wide array of anatomic and developmental difference. Life span changes are an important consideration in medicine. As a paramedic, you should be familiar with important milestones of both growth and development and use these expectations as points of reference in your assessment.

Understanding life span changes provides your patient interaction with valuable baselines and helps you adapt your expectations to the current level of your patient's capabilities. Although these changes can often vary from person to person, having a rough idea of what you can expect from your patient is always helpful in determining the patient's current health status (▶ Figure 13-1).

NEONATES AND INFANTS

Some of the most rapid growth and development occur during the neonate and infant period in a child's life. As the child ages, changes will continue to occur in every system of his body.

TABLE 13-1	Stages of Development
Stage of Development	**Age Range**
Neonate	Birth to 1 month
Infant	1 month to 1 year
Toddler	1 to 3 years
Preschooler	3 to 6 years
School age	6 to 12 years
Adolescence	12 to 19 years
Early adulthood	20 to 40 years
Middle adulthood	41 to 60 years
Late adulthood	61 years and older

At birth, the neonate usually weighs around 3 kg, 25 percent of which is the head. The infant cranium has fontanels, which allow room for rapid growth of the brain during this time. Some of the birth weight is lost during the first week of life, but with proper breast or formula feedings it is quickly regained. After this initial period, the weight will continue to increase as the infant is able to consume soft, then solid, foods after the primary teeth emerge.

The neonate is primarily a nose breather. An infant's airways are shorter and narrower than those of adults, making the infant more susceptible to airway obstruction. The immune system is immature, and the passive immunity acquired from the mother will be retained for only about the first six months. Immunizations normally are administered after birth and continue to be provided throughout childhood.

The infant's nervous system allows for normal movement and sensation, but at this age the infant is not capable of localizing pain. Reflexes such as blinking, rooting, sucking, and grasping are present at birth and allow for the infant's survival.

Infants also experience psychosocial changes during this period. Their primary relationships involve those who fulfill their needs. By the end of this stage, the infant will be able to recognize the faces of parents and family. The infant will usually cry when separated from caregivers. An infant will also cry in response to pain, a basic need, or anger. Some of the developmental milestones for an infant appear in Table 13-2.

TABLE 13-2	Developmental Milestones for Infants		
Age	Gross Motor Skills	Visual–Motor, Problem Solving Skills	Language, Social, Adaptive Skills
1 month	Raises head slightly from prone position Makes "crawling" movements	*Birth:* fixes visually *1 month:* grasps tightly, follows to midline	Looks at faces Alerts to sounds
2 months	Holds head in midline Lifts chest	No longer clenches fist tightly Follows objects past midline	Smiles socially (after being talked to or touched) Recognizes parent
3 months	Holds head up steadily Supports on forearms in prone position	Holds hands open at rest Follows in circular fashion	Makes cooing (long vowel) sounds Reaches for familiar people or objects Anticipates feeding
4 months	Rolls front to back Supports on wrists and shifts weight	Reaches with both arms together Brings hands to midline	Laughs, orients to voice Enjoys looking at surroundings
5 months	Rolls back to front Sits while supported	Transfers objects from hand to hand	Makes sound combinations ("ah-boo") Orients to sounds laterally
6 months	Sits unsupported Puts feet in mouth when supine	Unilateral reach Uses "raking" grasp	Babbles Recognizes strangers
7 months	Creeps, "scoots"	*7–8 months:* inspects objects *7–9 months:* feeds self with fingers	Orients to sounds indirectly
8 months	Sits up Crawls		Says "Dada" indiscriminately
9 months	Pivots when sitting Pulls to stand "Cruises"	Uses "pincer" grasp Holds bottle Pokes with forefinger Makes gestures Waves bye-bye Throws objects	Says "Mama" indiscriminately Understands "no" Starts to explore environment Plays gesture games ("clap hands, clap hands")
10 months			Says "Dada" and "Mama" discriminately Orients to sounds directly
11 months			Says one word other than "Dada" and "Mama" Follows one-step command with gesture
12 months	Walks alone	Uses mature pincer grasp Releases grasp voluntarily Makes pencil marks on paper	Uses two words other than "Dada" and "Mama" Runs several unintelligible words together Comes when called Imitates actions Cooperates with dressing
13 months			Uses three words
14 months			Follows one-step command without gesture

Note: Milestones vary and are designed to provide a general guideline.

Tips for Assessment of Neonates and Infants

- The infant's fontanels (when sunken) may provide an indirect estimate of hydration.
- Look at both the chest and abdomen when assessing an infant's respirations.
- Look for symmetrical movement of the extremities during your assessment.
- Keep the infant warm and dry.
- Suspect an underlying cause if the infant continues to cry excessively after needs have been met.
- Keep the parent calm. The infant is an expert in body language.
- Distractions such as toys and penlights are useful tools to help provide emotional control of the infant during the assessment.
- Smile to help reassure the infant.

TODDLERS AND PRESCHOOLERS

Toddlers continue to grow physically throughout this period. The musculoskeletal system increases in density, and the child's weight will taper by the end of this period. The brain is the fastest-growing part of the child's body and will

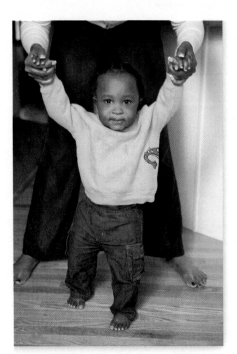

Figure 13-2 A young toddler begins to exhibit improved motor skills and problem-solving abilities.

TABLE 13-3	Developmental Milestones of Toddlers	
Physical Skills	**Social Skills**	**Cognitive Thinking**
• Walks alone	• Imitates others' actions	• Finds objects even when hidden behind or under other objects
• Pulls objects while walking	• Aware of self as distinct from others	• Sorts objects by shape, color
• Stands on tiptoe	• Enjoys company of other children	• Plays "pretend"
• Learns to run		
• Begins to kick a ball		

TABLE 13-4	Developmental Milestones of Preschoolers	
Physical Skills	**Social Skills**	**Cognitive Thinking**
• Runs easily	• Imitates adults and other children	• Makes simple mechanical toys work
• Climbs well	• Shows affection for friends	• Sorts objects by shape, color
• Walks up and down stairs	• Understands the concept of taking turns	• Puts together 3- and 4-piece puzzles
• Bends over without falling	• Learns to share	• Understands elementary number concepts
• Kicks balls	• Grasps idea of "mine" and "yours"	
• Pedals a tricycle		

reach 90 percent of its adult weight by the end of this period. Toddlers acquire some fine motor skills during this period. These children acquire active immunity, as they are exposed to various pathogens. It is during this period that toddlers will be potty trained.

Children in this age group are able to communicate with language. They can form sentences and tend to take each word literally. They develop friendships and participate in playtime. Playing allows a child to engage in new activities, solve problems, and develop social skills (▶ Figure 13-2).

Toddlers will often experience separation anxiety about their parents. These children frequently have misconceptions about illnesses and injuries, and many believe their behavior may have caused the problems. Some developmental milestones for toddlers and preschoolers appear in Tables 13-3 and 13-4.

Tips for Assessment of Toddlers and Preschoolers

- Speak softly and use language the child can understand.
- Allow the child to touch the equipment before you use it.
- Allow the parent to stay with the child if possible.
- Praise and reassure the child. This will help build a positive rapport.
- Allow the child to have some control over his experience, such as picking which ear you examine first.
- Use a toy or favorite object to help calm the child.

SCHOOL-AGE CHILDREN

Children in school continue to grow and change. Many experience some discomfort as their bones increase in size and density.

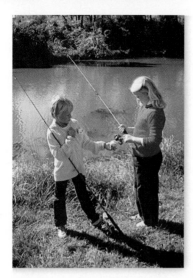

Figure 13-3 School-age children participate in a wide variety of activities and use their experiences to develop skills to solve problems.

They lose their primary teeth and begin to replace them with permanent ones. Their brain function continues to increase.

Children in this age group are able to communicate in various forms. They can read and write. During this period, they develop their own self-concept and begin to compare themselves with their peers. Many participate in a wide variety of extracurricular activities and use their experiences to develop skills to solve problems (▶ Figure 13-3). They understand concepts of pain, death, and illness but usually are afraid when such events occur.

Tips for Assessment of School-Age Children

- A child may have misconceptions about how much you can do. Answer and address the child's concerns and fears honestly.
- Communicate with the child at his level.
- Explain procedures to the child before doing them.
- Gain information from both the child and parent. Make sure you include the child in your conversation.
- Continue to provide choices for the child as long as it does not impede emergency care.

ADOLESCENTS

Adolescents continue to grow—usually in spurts—during this period. Usually this growth ends at age 16 for girls and 18 for boys. It is during this stage that the adolescent will go through puberty and experience significant sexual development. The female adolescent will begin menstruation, her breasts will enlarge, she will grow pubic and axillary hair, her hips will widen, and her waist will get smaller. The male adolescent will grow facial, pubic, and axillary hair, his voice will deepen, his shoulders will broaden, his muscles will increase in size, and his penis and testicles will grow. Both genders will experience hormonal changes during this time.

Adolescents desire to be treated as adults, and they value their privacy. They are capable of making many types of decisions, but they still require parental consent for treatment. Many adolescents participate in risky behaviors during this period and view themselves as invulnerable. Conflicts in family relationships, especially with parents, are common during this time. Adolescents' sense of identity and self-esteem are influenced drastically by their body image and peer relationships (▶ Figure 13-4).

Tips for Assessment of Adolescents

- Begin by interviewing the parent and adolescent together, then gain consent from the parent to finish the interview and assessment in private with the adolescent.
- Conduct the interview and assessment as you would for an adult.
- Remain unbiased and nonjudgmental.

EARLY ADULTHOOD

During early adulthood, peak physical condition is obtained; then the physical condition begins to slow down. Fat is stored, weight is gained, and muscle tone is decreased in the adult body. The habits and routines established during this period affect the quality of health and life.

It is during early adulthood that many individuals complete school,

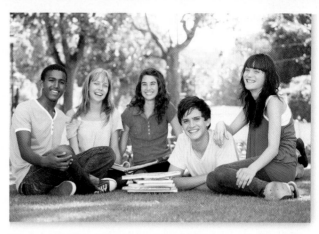

Figure 13-4 Adolescents' sense of identity and self-esteem are influenced by their body image and peer relationships.
(© Monkey Business Images/Shutterstock)

begin careers, and leave their parents' homes. Many adults will choose to marry and start families of their own. These adults typically have the highest levels of job stress but are usually more capable of coping with the stress than they were when they were younger.

MIDDLE ADULTHOOD

During middle adulthood, the body experiences varying amounts of degradation but is usually capable of functioning at high levels. Chronic illnesses, vision and hearing changes, and cardiovascular concerns are common during this time. Women experience menopause during this period, and many will lose height because of osteoporosis.

Most adults during this period accomplish their personal goals. Some delay seeking help for their own health issues so they can help their parents or children. They are aware of time, and tend to create goals for the remainder of their lives. It is during this period that their children usually leave home and they become grandparents.

LATE ADULTHOOD

During late adulthood, the rate of occurrence of disease and illness increases, and body systems continue to deteriorate. The workload and size of the heart increase, and the functional blood volume decreases. The lung capacity and diffusion of gases in the alveoli are diminished. The loss of neurons in the brain can result in problems with memory and movement. Sensory functions also decrease, and many individuals will require aids to help compensate for the loss. The gastrointestinal system functions less effectively; problems with absorption, constipation, and hydration are common in this age group. Adults during this period have decreased metabolism and renal functions. Many older adults will have underlying chronic conditions that may exist outside of the current emergency.

Older adults face challenges that they may have not experienced before (▶ Figure 13-5). They reflect on their lives and consider their death or those of their loved ones. Some older adults have difficulty finding self-worth. Many are forced into retirement and have to make difficult housing and living decisions. Finances may influence the ability of some of these adults to receive certain health care benefits and remain compliant with their medications.

> The paramedic should know the common ranges of vital signs for every age group.

Tips for Assessment of Adults in Middle or Late Adulthood

- Speak in a normal tone unless you are certain that the patient has a hearing problem.

- Allow extra time for the patient to formulate a response to your questions.
- Do not assume that every elderly patient has cognitive or physical problems.
- Show respect for the patient and listen attentively to the patient's needs.

NORMAL VITAL SIGNS

It is very important to assess vital signs on every patient multiple times to identify trends and obtain a more accurate physiologic assessment of the patient. The paramedic should know the common ranges of vital signs for every age group. By knowing the usual values for each group, it is possible to identify when they are not within the norm and incorporate that knowledge into your emergency care.

Table 13-5 shows the normal vital sign ranges during each stage of development.

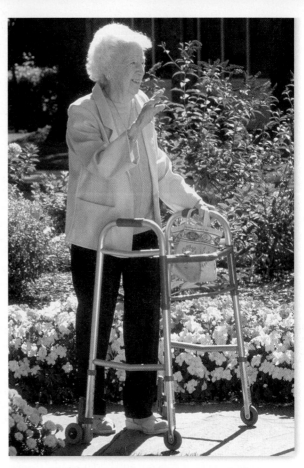

Figure 13-5 Many older adults face new challenges, but the ability to learn and adjust continues throughout life.

TABLE 13-5 Normal Vital Signs

Stage of Development	Pulse (beats per minute)	Respirations (breaths per minute)	Blood Pressure (average mmHg)	Temperature (degrees Fahrenheit)
Infancy: at birth	100–180	30–60	60–90 systolic	98–100
Infancy: at 1 year	100–160	30–60	87–105 systolic	98–100
Toddlers	80–110	24–40	95–105 systolic	98.6–99.6
Preschoolers	70–110	22–34	95–110 systolic	98.6–99.6
School age	65–110	18–30	97–112 systolic	98.6
Adolescence	60–90	12–26	112–128 systolic	98.6
Early adulthood	60–100	12–20	120/80	98.6
Middle adulthood	60–100	12–20	120/80	98.6
Late adulthood	Depends on patient's physical and health status	Depends on patient's physical and health status	Depends on patient's physical and health status	98.6

Modified from Bryan E. Bledsoe, Robert S. Porter, and Richard A. Cherry, *Paramedic Care Principles & Practice*, 3rd ed. Upper Saddle River, NJ: Pearson/Prentice Hall, 2009.

TRANSITIONING

REVIEW ITEMS

1. You are assessing a toddler. You expect his pulse rate to be between _____ times a minute.
   - a. 80 and 110
   - b. 60 and 100
   - c. 100 and 160
   - d. 65 and 110

2. By what age should an infant be able to sit unsupported?
   - a. 2 months
   - b. 4 months
   - c. 6 months
   - d. 8 months

3. During which stage does significant sexual development occur?
   - a. school age
   - b. adolescence
   - c. early adulthood
   - d. middle adulthood

4. Which of the following occurs during late adulthood?
   - a. The blood volume increases.
   - b. The blood volume decreases.
   - c. The size of the heart decreases.
   - d. The lung capacity increases.

5. A neonate's head weighs about ____ percent of the entire body weight.
   - a. 10
   - b. 40
   - c. 15
   - d. 25

APPLIED KNOWLEDGE

1. List the stages of development and their corresponding ages.

2. Explain the significance of knowing the milestones for each age group.

3. What physical changes occur to adolescents during puberty?

4. Why is it important to use age-appropriate language during your assessment?

CLINICAL DECISION MAKING

You arrive at a residence for a child who fell. You are met by an adolescent, who states she was babysitting her 2-year-old niece. She says she put the child down for a nap in her crib about an hour earlier. She says she was talking to her boyfriend on the telephone when she heard a loud thump. When she ran into the room, she saw the child on the floor crying.

1. What types of responses to your questions should you expect from the adolescent?

2. Is the mechanism of injury described by the teen a reasonable one based on the child's age?

The teen states she picked up the child and tried to comfort her, but it didn't work. She says she just kept calling for Mama and holding her arm. She called the parents, who were out of town, and then called the ambulance.

3. How should you approach the child?

4. What techniques can you use to establish a good rapport with the toddler?

You talk to the parents on speakerphone as you approach the child. You perform your primary and secondary assessments.

5. What vital signs do you expect your patient to have?

6. What do you know about the bones of a toddler?

7. How do you expect the patient to respond to you?

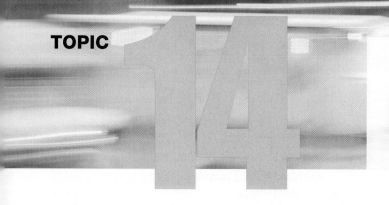

Standard Public Health

Competency Applies fundamental knowledge of principles of public health and epidemiology, including public health emergencies, health promotion, and illness and injury prevention.

PUBLIC HEALTH AND EMS

TRANSITION *highlights*

- *Introduction to public health and its determining components, and what they mean to the paramedic.*

- *Differences between public health and individual patient care.*

- *Important milestones public health has achieved, identifying many of those that have directly affected EMS.*

- *Interface between EMS and public health principals.*

INTRODUCTION

Public health is a complex, diverse field composed of people from different backgrounds. Because of its complexity, public health is hard to define. According to the world-renowned public health leader C. E. A. Winslow, who wrote in 1920, public health is

> The science and art of preventing disease, prolonging life, and promoting health and efficiency through organized community effort for the sanitation of the environment, the control of communicable infections, the education of the individual in personal hygiene, the organization of medical and nursing services for the early diagnosis and preventive treatment of disease, and for the development of the social machinery to insure everyone a standard of living adequate for the maintenance of health, so organizing these benefits as to enable every citizen to realize his birthright of health and longevity. (Winslow, 1920)

Winslow's definition was also referenced in the seminal report "The Future of Public Health" (Institute of Medicine, 1988), which outlined the mission and functions of public health. The mission of public health, accord-

The core functions of public health include assessment, policy development, and assurance.

ing to the Institute of Medicine (IOM), is "fulfilling society's interests in assuring [*sic*] conditions in which people can be healthy." Then, in 1994, the U.S. Public Health Service (USPHS) released the document "Public Health in America" with the intent to provide a consensus on definition, vision, and function for public health professionals as well as the public.

According to the USPHS document, the mission of public health is to "promote physical and mental health and prevent disease, injury, and disability" by preventing epidemics and the spread of disease, protecting against environmental hazards, preventing injuries, promoting and encouraging healthy behaviors, responding to disasters and assisting communities in recovery, and ensuring the quality and accessibility of health services (USPHS, 2008).

These definitions reflect the core concepts of public health, with an emphasis on prevention. To perform the missions given by the IOM and the USPHS, governmental agencies and private organizations must lead organized efforts to do so. However, government agencies are charged with a major role in ensuring that the mission, core functions, and essential services of public health are achieved.

The core functions of public health addressed at all levels of government include assessment, policy development, and assurance, which are carried out through public health's multiple arms: epidemiology, biostatistics, health policy and management/ health administration, behavioral or social science/health education, and environmental health.

Assessment, including epidemiology and biostatistics first and foremost, is the systematic collection, assembling, analyzing, and availability of information on the health of the community. *Policy development* entails the development of policies and plans that support individual and community health efforts, enforcement of laws and regulations, and research for new solutions; it involves all arms of government and public health. *Assurance*, generally led by the health policy and management/ health administration arm, ensures the provision of health services through the involvement of policy makers and the public in the decision-making process (Institute of Medicine, 1988). These core functions are executed through the 10 essential public health services shown in Table 14-1.

TABLE 14-1 — Core Functions of Public Health and Essential Public Health Services

Core Functions	Essential Public Health Services
Assessment	Monitor health status to identify community health problems
	Diagnose and investigate health problems and health hazards in the community
	Inform, educate, and empower people about health issues
Policy Development	Mobilize community partnerships to identify and solve health problems
	Develop policies and plans that support individual and community health efforts
Assurance	Enforce laws and regulations that protect health and ensure safety
	Link people to needed personal health services and ensure the provision of health care when otherwise unavailable
	Ensure a competent public health and personal health care workforce
	Evaluate effectiveness, accessibility, and quality of personal and population-based health services
Assessment Policy Development Assurance	Research for new insights and innovative solutions to health problems

Source: Centers for Disease Control and Prevention, National Public Health Performance Standards Program, www.cdc.gov/od/ocphp/nphpsp/index.htm.

PUBLIC HEALTH VERSUS INDIVIDUAL PATIENT CARE

Public health is a unique field in that it partners with many health professions to ensure a healthy population. As a result, public health is often confused with many other professions that may have similar goals and missions. One of the most frequent partnerships occurs between public health and the medical profession.

Although public health and the medical profession work closely to ensure healthy individuals, and both are grounded in science (Afifi and Breslow, 1994), the two entities view health differently (see Table 14-2).

Public health centers on the prevention of disease, injury, or disability *before* diagnosis of a condition in an entire population. Public health views disability or health conditions as a consequence of numerous factors, including behavioral, biological, social, economic, cultural, environmental, and psychological (Institute of Medicine, 2003).

In contrast, the medical profession deals with the acute care of ill individuals *after* the onset of symptoms and/or disease. The medical profession views disease or disability as a result of an issue within the body or mind of the individual (Byock, 1999). In recent years, however, the medical profession has begun to discourage these views and instead has sought to incorporate aspects of disease prevention into the medical practice. In addition, public health continually uses the expertise of the medical profession in dealing with disease epidemics, including cancer, obesity, influenza, and others.

ACHIEVEMENTS OF PUBLIC HEALTH

Many major improvements in health have been accomplished through public health measures. An excellent way to understand the influence that public health has had on the lives of many is to review the greatest achievements of public health. According to the *Morbidity and Mortality Weekly Report* (Centers for Disease Control and Prevention, 1999), the following are the greatest public health achievements:

- Vaccination, resulting in the eradication or elimination of smallpox and poliomyelitis, and control of measles, rubella, tetanus, diphtheria, chickenpox, and human papillomavirus (HPV), among others
- Motor vehicle safety, resulting in a decrease in fatalities owing to laws regulating seat belt use, child safety seats, and drinking
- Safer workplaces, decreasing worker injury fatalities as a result of improved safety equipment, machinery, and devices, ventilation, and other regulatory efforts
- Control of infectious diseases, through improved water and sanitation practices and advanced scientific and technological advances
- Decline in deaths from coronary heart disease and stroke, from health education and promotion efforts targeting risk factor reduction, increased numbers and better trained emergency medical providers
- Safer and healthier foods, the consequence of hand washing, sanitation, decreased microbial contamination, refrigeration, pasteurization, and pesticides
- Healthier mothers and babies, owing to improved prenatal care, nutrition practices, hygiene, and vaccinations
- Family planning, providing options allowing men and women to better control family size and pregnancies through contraception and fertility measures
- Fluoridation of drinking water, preventing tooth loss and decay
- Recognition of tobacco use as a health hazard, resulting in increased health

TABLE 14-2 — Public Health versus Medicine

Public Health	Medicine
Population health	Individual health
Emphasis on prevention of disease in a population through health promotion and health education	Emphasis on diagnosis and treatment of a patient following onset of symptoms
Health conditions, diseases, and disabilities are caused by multiple factors, both internal and external	Health conditions, diseases, and disabilities are caused by problems within the body or mind
Health professionals from various backgrounds working in many settings in the community	Physicians with various specialties working primarily in health care settings

education and promotion efforts and laws to prevent smoking

Further explanation of public health achievements is shown by the trends in leading causes of mortality in the 21st century in the United States. The leading causes of death in 1900 are a stark contrast to the leading causes of death today. In 1900, the top three causes of death were pneumonia and influenza, tuberculosis, and diarrheal diseases, and the average life expectancy at birth was 47.3 years of age (Arias, 2007; National Center for Health Statistics, n.d.). In 2006, however, heart disease, cancer, and stroke were the top three causes of death, and the average life expectancy at birth had increased by 30 years to 77.7 years of age, with 20 of those years attributed to public health measures (Heron et al., 2009).

> **Public health functions as an intersectoral system in which all entities work together to deliver essential public health services within communities.**

PUBLIC HEALTH LAWS, REGULATIONS, AND GUIDELINES

Although health is viewed as a right of all individuals, it was not a part of the U.S. Constitution. Health was viewed as a primary responsibility of the states. Thus, most public health activities are implemented by state and local governments, although all levels—national, state, and local—are responsible for ensuring a healthy population. Therefore, state and local governments have developed mechanisms to prevent disease, promote health, and protect the health status of their residents by ensuring organized community efforts through enforcement of public health laws, regulations, and guidelines (Institute of Medicine, 2003; Kocher, 2009; Mensah et al. 2004a, 2004b).

These mechanisms include disease surveillance to monitor disease, injuries, and disability; health screenings and testing; health education and promotion; access to and quality of health care services; vaccinations; and ensuring safe and sanitary conditions (Institute of Medicine, 2003).

EMS INTERFACE WITH PUBLIC HEALTH

Preventing, promoting, and protecting the health of a population is no small undertaking; it requires the collective responsibility of all public, private, and voluntary organizations, in addition to individuals and informal associations. As such, public health functions as an intersectoral system in which all organizations and entities contribute and work together to deliver essential public health services within communities (Centers for Disease Control and Prevention, 2005).

In 1996, the *EMS Agenda for the Future* envisioned EMS being fully integrated with health care providers, public health, and public safety in treatment and surveillance activities (National Registry of Emergency Medical Technicians, 1996). In 2002, the National Public Health Performance Standards Program (Centers for Disease Control and Prevention, 2007) unveiled a diagram demonstrating the interrelationships in the public health system. ▶ Figure 14-1 shows the role of the EMS along with other organizations

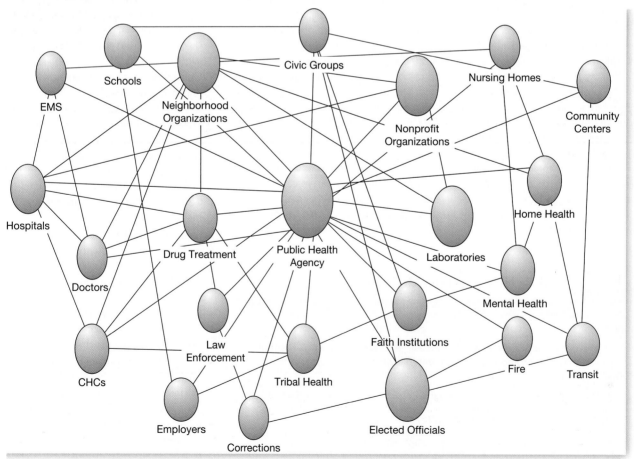

Figure 14-1 EMS has a role among other members of the interrelated public health system.

and entities in the local public health system.

Public health and EMS are partners in ensuring the health of the public. EMS assists public health through multiple functions, both in treatment of the public and in monitoring health and the conditions in which people live. The role of EMS is essential in all levels of prevention. In *primary prevention*—prevention of disease and disability within the community—EMS helps with health promotion and public health education efforts to prevent driving under the influence; inform about risk factors for chronic disease; prevent falls; educate about fire injury prevention; promote seat belt, car seat, and helmet use campaigns; and provide correct, relevant, and timely information to communities (▶ Figure 14-2).

During prevention of disease progression, or *secondary prevention*, the role of EMS includes screening to identify those at risk and to minimize disease complications; reporting any potential public health concerns; maintaining safe home environments for children; ensuring public access to automated external defibrillators (AEDs) to help those at high risk for heart attacks; and, of particular and growing importance in recent years, emergency management planning. For example, EMS has been identified by states and local public health agencies to assist with surveillance, mitigation, and response activities in pandemic influenza planning (Centers for Disease Control and Prevention, 2009).

In addition, in disease management and rehabilitation, or *tertiary prevention*, EMS provides treatment and acute care to the community.

THE PUBLIC HEALTH PARAMEDIC

The role of today's paramedic is expanding rapidly; the future seems to include many advances into the world of public health. As leaders of prehospital medicine, paramedics have already experienced the forefront in the areas discussed previously, but as our profession evolves, more opportunities to partner with other professionals move us closer to the *EMS Agenda for the Future*'s vision of complete integration into the world of public health. Not only will paramedics continue with the successful ongoing strategies such as data collection, public education, and disease reporting, but the ability of paramedics to reach a wider population base may also make our particular skill set even more valuable.

Many rural communities have realized that paramedics can be used for more than just responding to an emergency. In areas where those emergencies are few and far between, an opportunity exists to use the existing scope of paramedic practice to help enhance primary care and preventive capabilities. In these communities, paramedics participate in valuable public health activities such as vaccination administration, preventive evaluation, and routine follow-up care.

As simple as these tasks may seem, without community paramedics these services would not be provided. As policy makers evaluate budgets and allocate resources carefully, community paramedics, as an arm of the public health community, may be an increasingly reasonable option to consider.

CONCLUSIONS

The mission of ensuring the health of the population can be undertaken only through collaborative resources and the efforts of multiple agencies, or the public health system, in which EMS personnel play a vital function. EMS supports public health not only through providing individual treatment and acute patient care, but also through surveillance activities and by assisting in the prevention of diseases and disability and reducing the need for further medical care. Continued integration of public health efforts is necessary for responding appropriately to the threats of chronic and infectious disease.

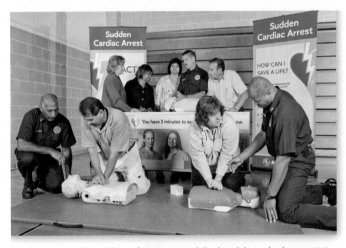

Figure 14-2 The roles of EMS in public health include participation in public education programs and health screenings.

TRANSITIONING

REVIEW ITEMS

1. A primary role of EMS that relates directly to the mission of public health is _____.
   a. preventing epidemics through vaccination programs
   b. preventing consumer injuries through education programs
   c. adhering to strict medical direction
   d. implementing quality improvement programs

2. Providing run sheet data on the incidence of gunshot wounds in a particular geographic area would most likely be used directly by which of the following public health arms?
   a. policy development
   b. epidemiology
   c. health administration
   d. behavioral health education

3. The difference between public health and the medical profession is that public health focuses on _____.
   a. prevention of a disease, injury, or disability before diagnosis of a condition in an entire population
   b. treatment of a disease or injury after the onset of signs and symptoms or the diagnosis of the condition
   c. prevention of illness or injury, focusing on individuals in a particular group
   d. the disease or disability as a result of an issue within the body or mind of the individual

4. To which of the following greatest public health achievements has EMS contributed significantly?

   a. elimination of smallpox through vaccination
   b. control of infection through sanitation
   c. decline in coronary heart disease and stroke deaths
   d. healthier mothers and babies through prenatal care

5. Most public health activities are governed by _____.
   a. the U.S. Constitution
   b. the executive branch of the government
   c. federal agencies
   d. state and local laws

REFERENCES

Afifi, A. A., and L. Breslow. "The Maturing Paradigm of Public Health." *Annual Review of Public Health* 15 (1994): 223–235.

Arias, E. "United States Life Tables, 2004." Centers for Disease Control: *National Vital Statistics Reports* 56 (2007). www.cdc.gov/nchs/data/nvsr/nvsr56/nvsr56_09.pdf.

Byock, I. R. "Conceptual Models and the Outcomes of Caring." *Journal of Pain and Symptom Management* 17 (1999): 83–92.

Centers for Disease Control and Prevention. "Ten Great Public Health Achievements—United States, 1900–1999." *MMWR* 48 (1999): 241–243.

Centers for Disease Control and Prevention (2005). *Building Our Nation's Health System: National Public Health Performance Standards Program.* www.cdc.gov/od/ocphp/nphpsp/PDF/FactSheet.pdf.

Centers for Disease Control and Prevention (2007). *National Public Health Performance Standards Program: User Guide.* www.cdc.gov/od/ocphp/nphpsp/PDF/UserGuide.pdf.

Centers for Disease Control and Prevention (2009). *Interim Guidance for Emergency Medical Services (EMS) Systems and 9-1-1 Public Safety Answering Points (PSAPs) for Management of Patients with Confirmed or Suspected Swine-Origin Influenza A (H1N1) Infection.* www.cdc.gov/h1n1flu/guidance_ems.htm.

Heron, M., D. L., Hoyert, S. L., Murphy, et al. (2009). *National Vital Statistics Reports. Deaths: Final Data for 2006.* National Center for Health Statistics. www.cdc.gov/nchs/data/nvsr/nvsr57/nvsr57_14.pdf.

Institute of Medicine. *Future of Public Health.* Washington, DC: National Academy Press, 1988.

Institute of Medicine. *Future of Public Health in the 21st Century.* Washington, DC: National Academy Press, 2003.

Kocher, P. (2009). *Key Concepts of U.S. Law in Public Health Practice.* PowerPoint presentation. www2.cdc.gov/phlp/NCCDPHP_Workshop/materials.asp.

Mensah, G.A., R. A. Goodman, S. Zaza, et al. "Law as a Tool for Preventing Chronic Diseases: Expanding the Spectrum of Effective Public Health Strategies, part 1." *Preventing Chronic Disease* (2004a). www.cdc.gov/pcd/issues/2004/jan/03_0033.htm.

Mensah, G.A., R. A. Goodman, S. Zaza, et al. "Law as a Tool for Preventing Chronic Diseases: Expanding the Spectrum of Effective Public Health Strategies, part 2." *Preventing Chronic Disease* (2004b). www.cdc.gov/pcd/issues/2004/apr/04_0009.htm.

National Center for Health Statistics (n.d.). *Leading Causes of Death, 1900–1908.* www.cdc.gov/nchs/data/dvs/lead1900_98.pdf.

National Registry of Emergency Medical Technicians (1996). *EMS Agenda for the Future.* www.nremt.org/nremt/about/emsAgendaFuture.asp.

U.S. Public Health Service (2008). *Public Health in America.* www.health.gov/phfunctions/public.htm.

Winslow, C. E. A. "The Untilled Fields of Public Health." *Science* 51 (1920): 23.

Standard Pharmacology

Competency Integrates comprehensive knowledge of pharmacology to formulate a treatment plan intended to mitigate emergencies and improve the overall health of the patient.

TOPIC

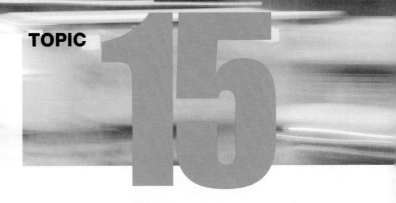

MEDICATION ADMINISTRATION

INTRODUCTION

As prehospital care advances in the 21st century, so has the use of pharmacology in the prehospital environment. Today's paramedics have access to a wide array of medications that can have profound treatment effects. As prehospital pharmacology evolves, however, the professional responsibility associated with handling and administering medication increases.

Paramedics today are shouldered with great responsibility. Modern providers have been afforded trust not only to competently administer medications that have powerful benefits for the patient, but also to be aware of the potent side effects and dangerous consequences associated with medication errors. Paramedics must accept that trust into the core of their professionalism and endeavor to maintain their knowledge base and skill set. Patient safety must be the center of concern. Medications, once given, are difficult to undo. Therefore, safe use of pharmacology must be a tactic addressed in a preemptive manner—that is, safety must be considered before administering the medication, not afterward.

The strategies associated with safe medication administration must also include continuing education to remain proficient with a rapidly changing list of medications. Prehospital pharmacology is a dynamic field of study that is updated constantly as science evolves. Paramedics cannot rest on what they learned in their original licensure education, as medications are removed and added to the formulary regularly. The medications used by paramedics even five years ago are vastly different when compared to the medications available to today's prehospital providers. Professionalism demands that as prehospital pharmacology advances, paramedics maintain, improve, and enhance their capabilities to utilize these medications.

It is important to note that the professional responsibility of safe medication administration is not just a system responsibility, but also a personal obligation. Although there are standardized medications outlined in the education standards, formularies and protocols for medication use vary from state to state and often from region to region. You, as a paramedic, must be

TRANSITION *highlights*

- *Patient safety strategies associated with medication administration.*
- *Responsibilities of paramedic-level pharmacology.*
- *Prevention of medication administration errors.*
- *Review of nontraditional medication routes.*

thoroughly familiar with the rules and regulations regarding prehospital pharmacology in your area.

PATIENT SAFETY

As paramedic, you will have great responsibility with medication administration. As Topic 2 discussed, studies in the hospital setting have shown that medication errors are surprisingly common. This likely carries over to EMS.

A medication error may be an error in dose, route, rate of administration, or administering a medication to an allergic patient. A medication may also be administered to a patient whose condition does not match what the drug is intended for.

The following points will help you reduce medication errors in your practice:

- Be familiar with all medications you carry and the relevant information for each (indications, contraindications, dose, route, etc.). Carry a reference or have reference information available in the ambulance. Know your protocols.
- Many medication containers look similar. Be sure you have obtained the medication you intend to administer and double-check before administering it (▶ **Figure 15-1**).
- When speaking with medical direction, verify all medication orders back to the physician and wait for confirmation. Write

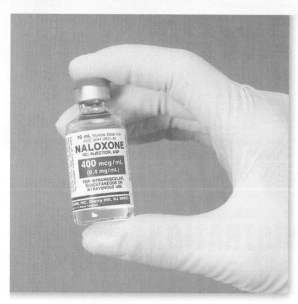

Figure 15-1 **Check the medication.**

down the medication, dose, route, and time of the order.

- Verify the amount and concentration of all medications before you administer them. Some medications, such as epinephrine and dopamine, can be present in different concentrations.
- Calm down and concentrate. Stress robs you of IQ points, and many of the situations in which medication administration will be necessary are stressful. Take steps to concentrate before administering medications. Double-check drug math, review resources, and do whatever is necessary to maintain accuracy.
- Work as a team. Monitor all actions going on around the patient. Your partner or crew should do the same. Good teamwork can help prevent errors. Many paramedics verify the medication, dose, and route again with a partner before administration.
- Do not practice while fatigued. Fatigue is a significant contributing factor in many medical errors.

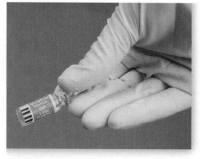

Figure 15-2 **Double-check the concentration and expiration date.**

- Errors should be prevented. If an error does occur, however, be sure to report it immediately to the emergency department and to a supervisor within your organization. You should also follow your department's guidelines for documenting errors.

The Five Rights of Medication Administration

Most likely you learned the five rights of medication administration in your original paramedic class, but when it comes to patient safety, they are certainly worth reviewing. Even though they may seem to be repetitive, taking these steps before administration of a medication significantly decreases the likelihood of error.

1. **Right medication.** Is this medication the correct one to administer for this patient? Should this specific drug be used to treat this specific situation? Is it the correct concentration?

2. **Right dose.** Is this the correct amount to administer? Can you check a reference, such as a protocol book, or read back an order (▶ Figure 15-2)?

3. **Right time.** Is it appropriate to administer this medication now? How quickly/slowly should the medication be administered?

4. **Right route.** What is the most appropriate way to administer this medication?

5. **Right patient.** Is it appropriate to administer this medication to this patient? Are the indications present? Are there any contraindications?

Many paramedics are taught more than five "rights." Other considerations include "right evaluation, documentation, reassessment" and the "right to refuse." Assuredly, there is no such thing as overthinking patient safety.

MAINTAINING COMPETENCY

Pharmacology is an ever-evolving science. Medications used to fight illness and injury are constantly reviewed, updated, and eliminated. As a paramedic, you must take steps to ensure that your knowledge base meets and exceeds the current standards of care. In most cases, medication administration in EMS is guided by protocol; as such, you must first and foremost be familiar with the regulations guiding your practice. Remember that protocols are updated often, and it is your responsibility as a paramedic to make sure your information is current.

Although most paramedics must adhere to local rules and regulations, other standards may be important. For example, the American Heart Association Guidelines for Cardiopulmonary Resuscitation and Emergency Cardiovascular Care are a common source that many states use to form local and regional protocols. These guidelines are updated every four years and are a good source to review the applicable science associated with cardiovascular medications.

In Topic 5, we discussed the value of research. In the science of pharmacology, research is a key source of information. Peer-reviewed journals are constantly evaluating new medications and the efficacy of long-standing therapies. Although these new trends may not allow you to alter your protocol-based treatments, keeping up with research may help you anticipate (and participate) in upcoming change.

Advances in Medication Administration

Not all changes in pharmacology are associated with medications themselves. In recent years, paramedics have adopted a number of changes associated with the delivery of medications; as an EMS professional, you should be familiar with these as well.

INTRAOSSEOUS ADMINISTRATION Even 10 years ago, the intraosseous (IO) route was thought to be limited to pediatric emergencies only. It was once thought that the bones of an adult were too tough to penetrate and that circulation was limited in the intermedullary space. Research and experience have proven these facts to be resoundingly false, and the IO route for medication administration has proven to be a valuable method of administering medications in an emergency. Modern technology, such as powered devices (▶ Figure 15-3), have allowed paramedics quick access to the

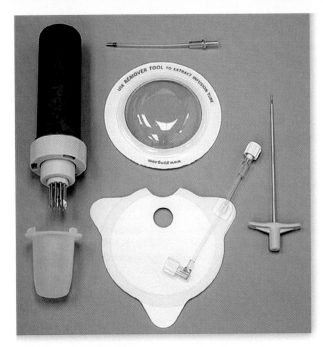

Figure 15-3 The EZ-IO (Vida-Care Corporation).

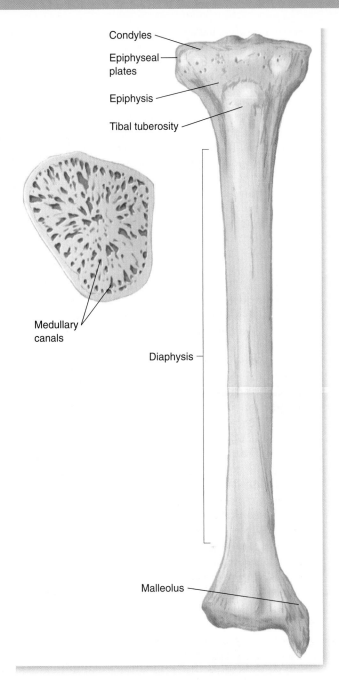

Condyles
Epiphyseal plates
Epiphysis
Tibal tuberosity
Medullary canals
Diaphysis
Malleolus

Figure 15-4 The intermedullary space of the tibia.

marrow space within the bone; research has proven that medication administration via this route is safe and effective.

In most cases, any prehospital medication can be administered through the IO route; effective onset times have been shown to be similar to those for the intravenous route. Although fluids may require pressure to be delivered and often will require more time to administer volume, central circulation can be reached rapidly by accessing this route. Furthermore, accessing intermedullary space (▶ Figure 15-4) may be far easier than accessing the intravascular space in times of circulatory collapse. The marrow space is noncollapsible and will remain a viable option for access even though an IV is unavailable.

The IO route is often more challenging to push volumes of fluid quickly and most frequently will require pressure to enhance the infusion. Consider diluting very viscous fluids such as 50% dextrose before administering it (always follow local protocols).

Accessing the IO space is very much dependent on the tool you are using; you should always follow the manufacturer's recommendations when you use a specific device. There are, however, some common elements that will help you make IO access more successful.

- Avoid the temptation to use a skill just because you can. Instead, use IO when indications point to the best benefit. IO

is not designed to replace IV therapy skills. Although it can be used safely as an emergent alternative, you should first look for possible IV access unless there is a specific contraindication (e.g., major burns, circulatory collapse). Again, always follow local protocol.

- Have a high regard for aseptic/sterile procedure. Although IO is commonly used in an emergency situation, you should always approach this skill in a way that is as sterile as possible.

- With whatever device you are using to access the marrow space, be prepared to stop penetration once you break through the cortex of the bone. In many cases, especially in pediatric patients, it will be easy to penetrate through both sides of the bone. Care should be taken to recognize proper placement and avoid overpenetration.

- Confirm placement by aspirating bone marrow. Remember that in most cases, this marrow will look like blood. Remember also that a failure

to aspirate bone marrow does not always indicate a misplaced IO needle. Attempt to flush before removing the needle.

- Flush with normal saline before administering medications. Typically at least 5 mL of normal saline is recommended to clear the catheter before medications are administered. It has been demonstrated that this is very important to keeping the IO clear and viable in the short-term setting.

- Use pressure when infusing volume. Just as the IO is a noncollapsible site, it is also a nonexpandable site. You will need to overcome the intrinsic pressure within the bone in order to administer fluid. Use a pressure bag or manual pressure when delivering infusions.

Complications can be associated with an IO infusion. If you have completely penetrated the bone, fluid can leak into the local tissues. This is identified with the same methods you would use to identify an infiltrating IV. Look for local swelling and fluid accumulation. It is also possible to fracture the bone in the process of accessing the IO space. In most cases, this will be evident on insertion, but may also lead to infiltrating fluid into local tissues.

INTRANASAL ADMINISTRATION The intranasal route has gained popularity with certain drugs in recent years. Specifically, it can be advantageous because of its relatively fast absorption rate and the safety of avoiding the use of needles. The intranasal route accesses the very vascular mucous membranes of the nasal passages and can introduce medications quite rapidly. Because of the relatively rich circulatory supply to the nasal tissue, medication absorption often can be faster with intranasal administration than with the intramuscular and subcutaneous routes. Absorption can be affected, however, by preexisting nasal conditions, trauma, and recent use of vasoconstrictors, such as cocaine.

The intranasal route is often preferred because it does not use needles. Unlike subcutaneous or intramuscular adminis-tration, intranasal delivery uses a small syringe that is inserted into each nostril without the necessity of sharps. This can be particularly important when administering medications under suboptimal conditions, such as to a patient who is having a seizure.

Intranasal access is most effective when medications are introduced as a mist rather than as a pure liquid. To do this, most intranasal protocols use an atomizer device attached to a small syringe. This device produces the misting effect and helps distribute the medication more effectively. The effectiveness of intranasal administration is also enhanced by dividing the medication between two nostrils. This effectively increases the amount or surface area with which the medication interacts. Most protocols call for such a technique.

Common prehospital medications that can be delivered via the intranasal route include midazolam, naloxone, fentanyl, and ketamine. Glucagon may also be an option. Most intranasal protocols will also use a higher dose of medication compared with that used in the intravenous route. The intranasal route typically requires a higher dose to maintain bioavailability of the drug as it absorbs in the nasal passages. This dosing can vary from drug to drug, so always be sure to follow local protocol.

To deliver an intranasal medication:

1. Place the patient in a supine or recumbent position.

2. Draw up the medication into a small syringe (1 mL, 3 mL) (most protocols will call for half the medication dose to be administered to each nostril).

3. Remove any needle and place the atomizer device onto the syringe (if an atomizer is not available, simply use the syringe, but ensure a rapid push delivery during administration).

4. Insert the syringe/atomizer in one nostril and rapidly compress the plunger to expel the medication. Deliver half the dose.

5. Insert the syringe into the other nostril and deliver the second half of the dose.

6. If medication is running out of the patient's nose, compress the nostrils to contain the runoff.

7. Document the medication administration and evaluate your patient.

CONCLUSIONS

In the time it takes to publish this text, there will be at least one advance in pharmacology, if not many, that could potentially affect EMS. Given the potential consequences of an error in medication administration, this fact should weigh heavily on you. Medication administration is an important responsibility of all paramedics and must be taken seriously. Be current in your knowledge base, be safe in your administration, and continue to educate yourself on the dynamic world of prehospital pharmacology.

TRANSITIONING

REVIEW ITEMS

1. You are treating a 6-year-old boy in cardiac arrest. In the stress of the moment, you are finding it difficult to calculate the correct dose of epinephrine. You should _____.
   a. just estimate based on the size of the patient
   b. use a reference, such as a length-based resuscitation tape
   c. divide the adult dose in half and administer that
   d. not administer the medication

2. Medical direction gives you an order to administer a dopamine drip. Which of the following would be the most effective strategy to avoid a medication error?

   a. Write down the dose and specific instructions.
   b. Repeat the order back to the doctor.
   c. Speak the order out loud.
   d. Repeat the order to your partner.

3. While preparing to administer a dopamine drip, you notice that your drug box contains two different concentrations and you are unsure of which one to use. You should _____.
   a. use the higher concentration
   b. use the lower concentration
   c. not administer the medication
   d. contact medical direction for clarification

4. During a cardiac arrest, you accidently administer one dose of 1:1000 epinephrine instead of the 1:10,000 epinephrine outlined in your protocol. You should _____.

    a. continue with the correct dose and report the error to a supervisor immediately

    b. ignore the error, as the patient will likely die anyway

    c. continue with the correct dose and report the error only if the patient dies

    d. stop resuscitation immediately and contact medical direction

5. The intranasal route is considered safer than the intramuscular route because _____.

    a. its effects are slower

    b. it uses a lower dose of medication

    c. it does not use a needle

    d. it uses a smaller needle

APPLIED KNOWLEDGE

1. Describe three methods you could employ to help avoid medication errors.

2. List the five rights of medication administration.

3. Describe why it is important to flush an IO before medication administration.

4. Describe why it is important to administer half the dose of a medication to each nostril during intranasal administration.

CLINICAL DECISION MAKING

A 3-year-old boy is found having a tonic–clonic seizure. Bystanders note that the child has been seizing now for roughly 8 minutes. Your protocols indicate that you should stop any seizure lasting longer than 5 minutes.

1. If you could not recall the dose of anticonvulsant, what resources would you have to identify the correct answer?

2. Would the intranasal route be preferred under the circumstances—and, if so, why?

As your partner attempts to draw the medication up for administration, he seems confused.

3. What steps would you take to ensure patient safety?

4. How might the five rights of medication administration be used in this scenario?

TOPIC
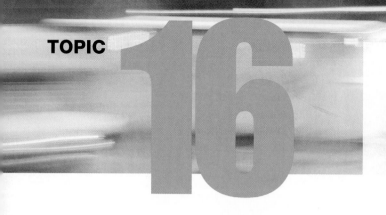

Standard Pharmacology

Competency Integrates comprehensive knowledge of pharmacology to formulate a treatment plan
intended to mitigate emergencies and improve the
overall health of the patient.

PARAMEDIC MEDICATIONS

TRANSITION *highlights*

- *Review of the paramedic formulary.*
- *New approach with traditional prehospital medications.*
- *Overview of the debate swirling around specific prehospital medications.*

INTRODUCTION

For years the list of prehospital medications administered by paramedics has remained relatively stable. Although resuscitation medications seemed to move in and out of favor, the core group of drugs essentially remained the same. In recent years, however, the standard set of paramedic medications has undergone a new scrutiny based on newly available research, and for the first time, thinking on these medications has begun to shift. Fundamental truths we once blindly accepted with regard to medications such as oxygen are now cast in a different light. Widely used medications such as morphine and furosemide are now being replaced or pushed aside.

Regardless of the national debate, you must always adhere to your local protocols. However, it is also important to familiarize yourself with the new research and recognize how prehospital pharmacology is evolving in the modern world. Although your formulary may be fixed within a protocol, the application and indications of a particular medication may have evolved through the emergence of new and better research.

This topic reviews key discussions pertaining to current prehospital medications. It is intended not to supersede local regulations or protocols, but to introduce paramedics to new information regarding medications and to describe the various debates pertaining to emergency pharmacology that are occurring on the national stage.

OXYGEN RECONSIDERED

For 50 years, supplemental oxygen has been the staple of the EMS formulary. Providers were routinely trained that there is no such thing as too much oxygen and that high-flow delivery systems can be applied in every prehospital situation. Recently though, new research has pointed out that these universal truths may not be so universal after all (▶ Figure 16-1).

The fact still remains that hypoxic patients require oxygen. No research has ever proposed withholding oxygen from a patient with low saturation. Certainly if a patient is in need of oxygen, he should be given it. That said, new information seems to point out that there is such a thing as *too much* oxygen and that unmitigated administration may actually be harmful.

Too much oxygen, also referred to as *hyperoxia*, may be harmful. Although this is still somewhat theoretical, some experts propose that hyperoxia leads to systemic vasoconstriction and a release of free radicals (charged oxygen atoms) in the body. Free radicals may be responsible for cellular destruction, particularly

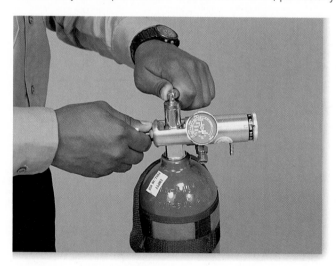

Figure 16-1 Use of supplemental oxygen is being reconsidered.

in already ischemic tissues, and vasoconstriction can exacerbate certain ischemic conditions, such as acute coronary syndrome and stroke.

These theories have some grounding in research. In 2010, the American Heart Association (AHA) scientific review conducted during the update to its guidelines for cardiopulmonary resuscitation and emergency cardiovascular care examined a series of small studies looking at the effects of oxygen on cardiac patients. The AHA concluded that the evidence showed "no benefit and potential harm" from administering continued high-flow oxygen to patients with saturations above 94 percent. As a result, the 2010 guidelines suggest that "there is insufficient evidence to support [oxygen's] routine use in uncomplicated [acute coronary syndrome]. If the patient is dyspneic, hypoxemic, or has obvious signs of heart failure, providers should titrate therapy, based on monitoring of oxyhemoglobin saturation, to ≥94%." The 2010 guidelines also suggest this titrated approach to oxygen therapy in the treatment of stroke and in neonatal resuscitation.

Research has also reached into other areas of EMS care. A study conducted in Australia and published in 2010 in the *British Medical Journal* describes oxygen delivery to chronic obstructive pulmonary disease (COPD) patients. In this research, oxygen administration was randomized into either 8 to 10 liters per minute (lpm) of oxygen or titrated oxygen to keep saturations between 88 percent and 92 percent. In the titrated group, mortality was significantly lower than in the high-flow group.

Although all this research needs to be developed further, it does emphasize the logical premise that oxygen is a drug and, as with any drug, thought must be given to its administration. Again, no one is asserting that paramedics should withhold oxygen from hypoxic patients, but perhaps we should not continue unfettered administration once saturations have normalized. As always, follow your local protocol.

ACUTE PULMONARY EDEMA MEDICATIONS

In recent years, the treatment of acute pulmonary edema (APE) has also come under more rigorous scrutiny. Whereas once there was a routine cocktail of nitroglycerine, morphine sulfate, and furosemide, there is now a far more measured approach.

Morphine Sulfate

It was once believed that morphine sulfate should be administered to APE patients because of its vasodilatory properties. It was thought that morphine possessed properties similar to those of nitroglycerine, and preload would be reduced by its administration. As it turns out, this idea really is not true. In fact, the vasodilatory effects have been more recently referred to as anecdotal. Moreover, although morphine may provide an anxiolytic effect (i.e., it calms patients down), it can also depress the respiratory drive and lead to higher intubation rates and increased mortality. Growing concern also exists over the potentially cardiac toxic properties of morphine.

In theory, the administration of morphine may actually decrease cardiac output. Anxiolysis may still benefit patients suffering from APE, but there are better medications to use for that purpose than morphine. Low-dose benzodiazepines, such as midazolam or diazepam, can provide the calming effect without the negative side effects of morphine.

Furosemide

Furosemide (Lasix) was traditionally administered to APE patients with the idea that diuresis would benefit their hypervolemic state. In many cases, paramedics gave high doses, often doubling the patient's daily dose in one bolus administration. Although diuresis can benefit some heart failure patients, it turns out that many acute pulmonary patients (in some studies, as many as 50 percent to 60 percent) are not, in fact, hypervolemic at all, but normovolemic; therefore, the removal of fluid secondary to diuresis leads to *hypovolemia* that must be corrected. Furthermore, furosemide is an unforgiving medication.

The diagnosis of APE is a challenging one, and statistically speaking, there is a high probability of error. The administration of furosemide for conditions such as exacerbated COPD and pneumonia has been shown to increase mortality, and as these are conditions frequently misdiagnosed as APE, furosemide can be dangerous. Furosemide

can still be useful in treating APE, but its use seems to be limited to patients who are known to be hypervolemic. Many experts view this as a difficult, if not impossible, distinction to be made in the prehospital realm and therefore question the ongoing utility of furosemide as a paramedic medication.

CARDIAC ARREST MEDICATIONS

The care of cardiac arrest is most commonly guided by the American Heart Association Guidelines for Cardiopulmonary Resuscitation. Every four years, that agency conducts a lengthy scientific review. Although the conclusions reached by the AHA are not necessarily definitive, in most cases they are grounded in some form of evidence. The following medications have been recently reviewed by the AHA and have remained a cause of much debate and research with respect to appropriate care of cardiac arrest:

- **Atropine.** The 2010 AHA Guidelines for Cardiopulmonary Resuscitation removed atropine sulfate from the asystole and pulseless electrical activity (PEA) treatment algorithm. According to the guidelines, "available evidence suggests that the routine use of atropine during PEA or asystole is unlikely to have a therapeutic benefit. For this reason atropine has been removed from the cardiac arrest algorithm."

- **Vasopressin.** Vasopressin is a non-adrenergic peripheral vasoconstrictor that can be used in a vasopressor role to treat cardiac arrest. It is often used to take the place of either the first or second dose of epinephrine in adult cardiac arrest. Numerous controlled trials have been conducted to assess the efficacy of this drug, but none thus far has shown it to be significantly better or different than standard epinephrine in the treatment of cardiac arrest. As such, the 2010 AHA Guidelines for Cardiopulmonary Resuscitation suggest that vasopressin can be used interchangeably with epinephrine in either the first or second dose.

- **Sodium bicarbonate.** Sodium bicarbonate has been a controversial drug for many years, often with many followers advocating or deriding its use. Although the evidence is still incomplete, there seems to be growing research pointing against its use in cardiac arrest. In fact, the scientific review conducted by the AHA concluded that "the majority of studies showed no benefit or found a relationship with poor outcome."

OTHER CONTROVERSIAL MEDICATIONS

Other prehospital medications are controversial in select circles. Examples include the following:

- **Thiamine.** Once a perennial component of the "coma cocktail," thiamine is now being described by some experts as an ineffective waste of resources. Its use was originally designed to reverse the effects of thiamine deficiency commonly seen in chronic alcohol abusers and to enhance the body's ability to metabolize dextrose in the event of hypoglycemia. However, the incidence of thiamine deficiency (especially Wernicke encephalopathy) seems to be rather rare; furthermore, to effectively correct this syndrome, thiamine would need to be administered over days. The relatively minor impact of prehospital administration appears not to have a major impact on patient outcomes.

- **Procainamide.** Procainamide is an antidysrhythmic used for the treatment of wide complex tachycardias. It has gone in and out of favor multiple times in the past 20 years. It seems, however, to be back in favor. In the AHA science review, at least "one randomized comparison found procainamide to be superior to lidocaine (1.5 mg/kg) for termination of hemodynamically stable monomorphic VT." It is important, however, to remember that procainamide should be avoided in patients with prolonged QT and congestive heart failure.

CONCLUSIONS

Paramedics should anticipate that these debates will continue. Pharmacology has been, and will continue to be, an evolving science. Although sometimes frustrating, these changes in the end are intended to provide the best care to our patients. Part of the professional obligation that must be accepted when wearing a paramedic's patch is the ongoing education necessary to remain current with prehospital medications.

TRANSITIONING

REVIEW ITEMS

1. True or false: You should avoid high-flow oxygen in patients with low oxygen saturation.
   - a. True
   - b. False

2. According to current research, which of the following patients would not require oxygen?
   - a. a chest pain patient with an oxygen saturation of 94 percent
   - b. a hypovolemic shock patient with pale skin and altered mental status
   - c. a hypotensive cardiogenic shock patient
   - d. a patient with exacerbated COPD and an oxygen saturation of 87 percent

3. A 67-year-old man presents in acute pulmonary edema. According to current research, which of the following medications would be appropriate to administer?
   - a. nitroglycerine
   - b. morphine
   - c. furosemide
   - d. dextrose

4. Which of the following is an actual effect of furosemide in acute pulmonary edema?
   - a. vasodilation
   - b. vasoconstriction
   - c. diuresis
   - d. anxiolysis

5. According to the AHA Guidelines, which of the following medications would be appropriate to administer to a patient in asystole?
   - a. atropine
   - b. vasopressin
   - c. procainamide
   - d. sodium bicarbonate

APPLIED PATHOPHYSIOLOGY

1. Describe why it is inappropriate to administer morphine sulfate to a patient in acute pulmonary edema.

2. Describe why it is inappropriate to administer furosemide to a normovolemic patient in acute pulmonary edema.

3. Describe why you would consider titrating oxygen to 94 percent when treating an ACS patient.

4. Describe the role of vasopressin in cardiac arrest.

CLINICAL DECISION MAKING

A 65-year-old man complains of chest pain. You find him pale, diaphoretic, and clutching his chest. He describes the pain as sharp and steady and denies any other symptoms. His vital signs are pulse 100, respirations 24, blood pressure 148/90 mmHg, and O_2 saturation 94 percent on room air.

1. Describe how you would use supplemental oxygen with this patient.

After you move the patient on a stair chair, he now begins to complain of difficulty breathing. He becomes agitated, and you note a new onset of crackles when you auscultate lung sounds.

2. Describe the medications you would use to treat this patient.

3. Would you use furosemide? Why or why not?

RESOURCES

Austin, M., K. Wills, L. Blizzard, et al. "Effect of High Flow Oxygen on Mortality in Chronic Obstructive Pulmonary Disease Patients in Prehospital Setting: Randomised Controlled Trial." *British Medical Journal* 341 (2010): c5462.

Bledsoe, B. *Prehospital Pharmacology: A Common-Sense Approach.* Retrieved July 22, 2011, from www.bryanbledsoe.com.

Cabello, J., A. Burls, J. Emparanza, et al. "Oxygen Therapy for Acute Myocardial Infarction." *Cochrane Database of Systemic Review* 6 (2010).

Delooz, H. H., and P. J. Lewi. "Are Inter-center Differences in EMS-Management and Sodium-Bicarbonate Administration Important for the Outcome of CPR? The Cerebral Resuscitation Study Group." *Resuscitation* 17 (1989): S161–S172; discussion S199–S206.

Gorgels, A. P., A. van den Dool, A. Hofs, et al. "Comparison of Procainamide and Lidocaine in Terminating Sustained Monomorphic Ventricular Tachycardia." *American Journal of Cardiology* 78 (1996): 43–46.

Gueugniaud, P. Y., J. S. David, E. Chanzy, et al. "Vasopressin and Epinephrine vs. Epinephrine Alone in Cardiopulmonary Resuscitation." *New England Journal of Medicine* 359 (2008): 21–30.

Hoffman, J. R., and S. Reynolds. "Comparison of Nitroglycerin, Morphine and Furosemide in Treatment of Presumed Prehospital Pulmonary Edema." *Chest* 92 (1987): 586–593.

Meine, T. J., M. T. Roe, A. Y. Chen, et al. "Association of Intravenous Morphine Use and Outcomes in Acute Coronary Syndromes: Results from the CRUSADE Quality Improvement Initiative." *American Heart Journal* 149 (2005): 1043–1049.

Mukoyama, T., K. Kinoshita, K. Nagao, and K. Tanjoh. "Reduced Effectiveness of Vasopressin in Repeated Doses for Patients Undergoing Prolonged Cardiopulmonary Resuscitation." *Resuscitation* 80 (2009): 755–761.

O'Connor, R., W. Brady, S. Brooks, et al. "Part 10: Acute Coronary Syndromes: 2010 American Heart Association Guidelines for Cardiopulmonary Resuscitation and Emergency Cardiovascular Care." *Circulation* 122 (2010).

Peacock, W. F., J. E. Hollander, D. B. Diercks, et al. "Morphine and Outcomes in Acute Decompensated Heart Failure: An ADHERE Analysis." *Emergency Medicine Journal* 25 (2008): 205–209.

Tang, W. H. "Pharmacologic Therapy for Acute Heart Failure." *Cardiology Clinics* 25 (2007): 539–551.

Wenzel, V., A. C. Krismer, H. R. Arntz, et al. "A Comparison of Vasopressin and Epinephrine for Out-of-Hospital Cardiopulmonary Resuscitation." *New England Journal of Medicine* 350 (2004): 105–113.

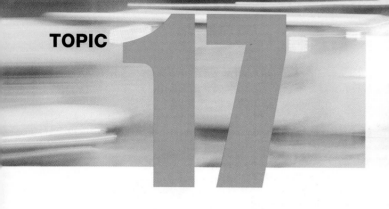

Standard Airway Management, Respiration, and Artificial Ventilation

Competency Integrates complex knowledge of anatomy, physiology, and pathophysiology into the assessment to develop and implement a treatment plan with the goal of ensuring a patent airway, adequate mechanical ventilation, and respiration for patients of all ages.

AIRWAY ASSESSMENT AND DECISION MAKING

TRANSITION *highlights*

- *Delineating between respiratory distress and respiratory failure.*

- *Signs and symptoms that illustrate ventilatory adequacy or inadequacy.*

- *How to determine when or when not to ventilate, based on signs and symptoms.*

- *Approaching the treatment of respiratory failure.*

- *Review of the paramedic airway treatment options.*

- *Integration of treatment options to the most appropriate airway circumstance:*
  – *Matching dysfunction to the correct treatment pathway.*

- *Core treatment interventions for a patient suffering from a disturbance to the airway.*

INTRODUCTION

One of the most significant findings an EMS provider can recognize is respiratory failure. Every level of EMS provider is taught to use the primary assessment to rapidly identify airway deficiencies and correct problems when they are found. This is no less true now that you are a paramedic. However, your thinking must become slightly more sophisticated when it comes to airway management.

Assessment and recognition of airway dysfunction is still most important, but now you must learn to link the findings of your assessment to a decision-making process. Because of the wide array of interventions you can deploy, you must use the information you gather to choose the most appropriate treatment option. As opposed to the purely algorithmic approach of the EMT, your approach must be goal oriented. For example, if your patient has

an obstructed airway, you will not have time to escalate through all your potential airway treatment devices. Rather, you must progress rapidly from basic obstructed airway procedures to specifically advanced procedures, such as surgical airway placement. That is not to say that an algorithmic approach is not valuable. On many occasions, you will use an escalating process; however, as a paramedic, you should guide your airway management based on the outcomes you wish to achieve. Each step should be taken based on assessment findings and evaluated for its desired effect. This is indeed a thinking person's game.

This topic discusses the process by which you will use airway assessment to guide your treatment. It discusses the most important goals of airway management and the assessment findings associated with those outcomes, and focuses primarily on critical thinking. Although treatment is certainly linked to this topic, specific treatment modalities will be discussed in the two topics that follow this one; for more information concerning many of the treatment options discussed here, continue reading.

PATHOPHYSIOLOGY

Respiratory dysfunctions are typically the result of either an obstruction of air movement, such as something in the way, or changes in the respiratory structures that affect the movement of oxygen and carbon dioxide. Occasionally, both these issues play a role. Respiratory dysfunctions can be further classified as either upper or lower airway problems. Upper airway issues affect the airway structures above the glottic opening (▶ Figure 17-1), and lower airway disorders affect the structures found from the trachea to the alveoli.

Upper Airway Dysfunction

The classic upper airway problem is the obstructed airway. When we think of this, we often picture a child choking on a small toy. However, far more commonly, upper airway obstruction is the result of poor airway muscle tone resulting from altered mental status. When the brain is not functioning properly, the muscles and nerves that protect the airway fail. This failure frequently results in an inability to keep an airway open. For example, when

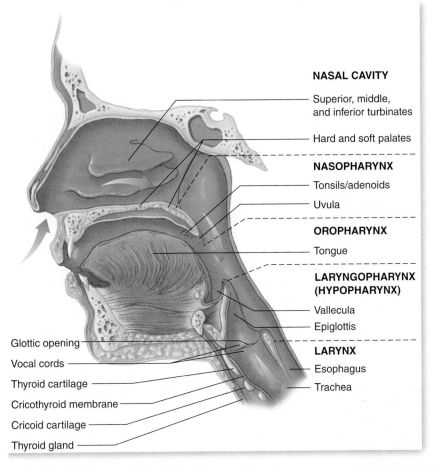

NASAL CAVITY

Superior, middle, and inferior turbinates

Hard and soft palates

NASOPHARYNX

Tonsils/adenoids

Uvula

OROPHARYNX

Tongue

LARYNGOPHARYNX (HYPOPHARYNX)

Vallecula

Epiglottis

LARYNX

Esophagus

Trachea

Glottic opening

Vocal cords

Thyroid cartilage

Cricothyroid membrane

Cricoid cartilage

Thyroid gland

Figure 17-1 Anatomy of the upper airway.

lying supine, a patient with an altered mental status may relax the muscles of the upper airway too much and allow the epiglottis to fall back and cover the glottic opening (▶ Figure 17-2).

The upper airway can also be affected by structural changes. Airflow can be impeded by swelling in and around the larynx. Conditions such as burns, infection, anaphylaxis, and even direct trauma can cause laryngeal edema and inflammation and result in a rapid decrease in the size of the glottic opening, significantly obstructing airflow.

Lower Airway Dysfunction

The most common cause of lower airway dysfunction is bronchoconstriction. A number of diseases and disorders, such as asthma and anaphylaxis, can cause the bronchiole passages to spasm and constrict. Even small changes in the diameter of these tubes can cause tremendous resistance to airflow that can seriously decrease the movement of air.

In addition to bronchoconstriction, other disorders can structurally change how gas is exchanged in the alveoli. Problems such as congestive heart failure, near drowning, and even altitude sickness can cause

the fluid portion of the blood to cross the alveolar membrane and interfere with the diffusion of oxygen and carbon dioxide. This pulmonary edema thickens the alveolar membrane, collapses some alveoli, and even (in late stages) can fill the alveoli themselves. Infections such as pneumonia can cause similar dysfunction. In these cases, the alveoli can be obstructed by pus and other byproducts of infection, causing a similar gas exchange issue.

AIRWAY ASSESSMENT

When assessing a patient with respiratory distress, the most important goal may not be to determine the exact nature of the disorder. The need to recognize respiratory failure and support ventilation may be far more important.

The primary assessment is a critical component of the assessment in any patient. It is even more important in a patient with respiratory distress. It begins by ensuring the patency and security of the airway: Is it open? Is air moving at all? Breathing and the ability to speak are key findings, for if a person can speak then at least at some level air is moving through the airway. Consider also the quality of the patient's speech. Is the voice hoarse or raspy? This can indicate a threatened airway due to inflammation. Stridor (inspiratory or expiratory) can be an ominous sign as well.

If the airway is not open, you must take steps to open it. Beyond the immediate moment, you must also consider the future: Will it stay open? Is the ongoing security of this airway threatened, and if so, what steps are necessary to reverse that course?

Consider the pathophysiology. What is causing the potential obstruction to airflow? In many cases, you can expect the condition to get worse. Consider burns or trauma to the neck. In these cases, swelling threatens the airway over time. Partial foreign body airway obstructions can rapidly progress to complete obstructions. Consider other findings that might point to a threatened airway. Decreasing mental status is a very important threat to the airway. Consider also voice changes over time and the emergence of new findings, such as stridor. Every patient needs a clear path for air to move. If this path is obstructed or threatened, steps must be taken to secure it.

When assessing breathing, you also must consider multiple elements. First,

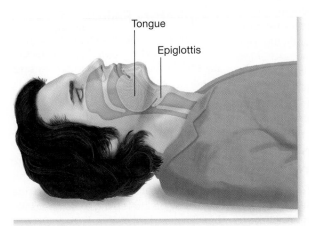

Tongue

Epiglottis

Figure 17-2 Loss of control of the upper airway may occur, for example, when the muscles of the upper airway relax too much and the epiglottis is allowed to fall back and cover the glottic opening.

you must ensure that the patient actually is breathing; but second, you must further ensure that the patient's breathing is adequate to meet the needs of his body. "Look, listen, and feel" will quickly provide an answer to the first question, but for the second question you must engage in some critical thinking.

Remember that the goals of breathing are twofold. The body must oxygenate, but it must also ventilate by removing carbon dioxide. Any breathing assessment must keep these goals in mind. Look for signs of hypoxia, including altered mental status, cyanosis, and poor oxygen saturation. Look for signs of poor ventilation, including altered mental status, poor air movement, and increasing end-tidal carbon dioxide.

> **When assessing breathing, always keep minute ventilation and alveolar ventilation in mind.**

Always keep minute ventilation and alveolar ventilation in mind when assessing breathing. You must ask yourself continually how much air is actually reaching the alveoli each minute. Remember that minute volume is composed of both rate *and* volume. Breathing within an acceptable rate is important, but again, you must consider how much volume is being moved down to the alveoli in each breath. In addition, keep in mind the concept of dead space.

In the primary assessment, you need to look at the adequacy of breathing (▶ **Figure 17-3**). How fast or slow is the patient breathing? Quickly listen to both sides of the patient's chest. This is the time not for a thorough examination of lung sounds but, rather, for a quick assurance that air is moving in and out on both sides. It takes only seconds to determine whether volume is inadequate. Sounds of dysfunction are also rapidly identified with even a quick listen. For example, are there wheezes that might identify bronchoconstriction? Consider also the patient's ability to speak. If he must take a breath after every word, his minute volume has been seriously challenged.

Finally, as an advanced provider, you may be tempted to move on to advanced modalities such as medications and intravenous lines. Resist this temptation until the primary assessment is complete and all immediate life threats have been addressed.

Respiratory Distress

When a person experiences a challenge to respiratory system function, the body responds in a predictable manner: It compensates. As in shock, the brain takes specific steps to help overcome the deficit caused by the offending issue. When the brain senses increasing carbon dioxide and low oxygen, the respiratory center in the medulla increases the respiratory rate. Additional muscles in the neck, chest, and abdomen (accessory muscles) are engaged to assist with breathing (▶ **Figure 17-4**). The sympathetic nervous system tells the heart to beat faster and stronger.

These compensatory mechanisms can be easily identified in your assessment of breathing. What is the respiratory rate? How hard is the patient working to breathe? Look at the patient's chest: Is the patient using accessory muscles? All these findings indicate the body's effort to compensate. As with compensated shock, these measures can often sustain normal body function temporarily and hold off the challenge.

When respiratory compensation works, we deem the patient to be in respiratory *distress*—that is, he is challenged, but the compensatory efforts are sustaining normal function despite the problem. A patient in respiratory distress will exhibit signs of the challenge, such as tripod positioning, accessory muscle use, and increased respiration rate, yet he should also be showing signs that these measures are allowing normal function. The patient's brain should be oxygenated, and therefore he should have a normal mental status. He should not be showing signs of profound hypoxia, such as cyanosis. The key to differentiating respiratory distress from respiratory failure is identifying that normal function.

Respiratory Failure

Unfortunately, the body's compensation is limited. Some respiratory challenges exceed the body's ability to compensate. Other times, compensation simply fails over time. Keep in mind that when we ask muscles to do more work, more oxygen is required. If hypoxia is already a challenge, the muscles of compensation can help for only a short time. Respiratory *failure* occurs when compensation fails. At this point, the challenge continues and the body may be attempting to compensate, but function has been affected. Oxygen may not be getting distributed, carbon dioxide is being retained, and the muscles of respiration tire. As a paramedic, you must be ever vigilant to recognize

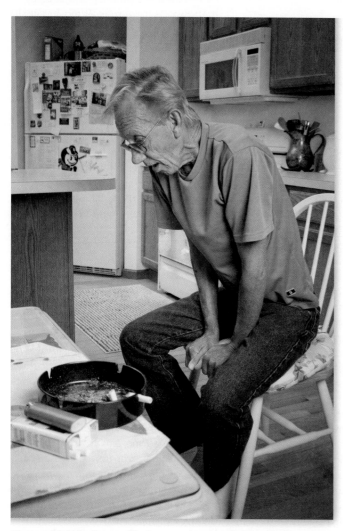

Figure 17-3 Patient suffering respiratory distress, indicated by his tripod position.

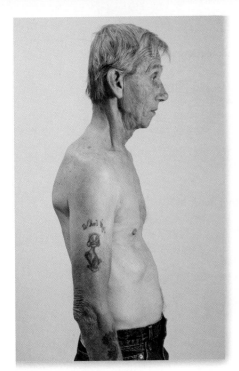

Figure 17-4 Barrel chest in an emphysema patient.

respiratory failure because it demonstrates that what the patient is doing on his own is not enough.

A patient in respiratory failure exhibits signs and symptoms similar to those of a patient in respiratory distress. He will have a challenge, he will be compensating, but he will not be meeting his needs. Look for signs that compensation has failed. Altered mental status is a key indicator. Anxiety, combativeness, somnolence, and even unconsciousness all point to hypoxia and hypercapnia. Look for additional signs of hypoxia, such as cyanosis and low oxygen saturation. These findings are especially worrisome if they occur despite supplemental oxygen. Look for other signs of failure, including signs of respiratory fatigue. Respiratory muscles need oxygen and eventually fail as they become hypoxic. Look for slowing rates, irregular patterns, and gasping as indicators of respiratory failure (▶ **Figure 17-5**).

Remember that a patient in respiratory failure may indeed be breathing. Consider the following example:

You are assessing a 14-year-old asthma patient. He has been having an attack for roughly an hour now. You assess his airway and find that he has a patent airway, but he has difficulty speaking. He is breathing at a rate of 54 breaths per minute. You find him in tripod position; when you look at his chest you note

retractions and other accessory muscle use. When you listen to his chest you can barely hear any air movement at all. His fingernails are blue. When you attempt to engage him with questions, you note that he has a very sleepy affect.

This young man is in respiratory failure. He is compensating for his asthma, as evidenced by his respiratory rate, his use of accessory muscles, and his position, but those compensatory mechanisms are not working, as demonstrated by his altered mental status and cyanosis. This patient needs immediate help.

It is important to also remember that identifying respiratory distress does not require diagnosing a specific respiratory dysfunction. You may identify failure (and take action) long before you have time to accurately complete a differential diagnosis. Luckily, the treatment for respiratory failure is, for the most part, the same regardless of what disorder is causing it.

USING ASSESSMENT TO GUIDE TREATMENT

Quality airway assessment not only allows for recognition of a problem, but also feeds information to a critical decision-making process. Modern paramedics can deploy a host of devices and interventions to address even the most complex airway issues, but to determine the best treatment modality, the paramedic must weigh costs and benefits and consider the usefulness of a treatment in the context of the assessment findings. Airway management must be grounded in critical thinking. Using the right tool in the right circumstance depends on linking evaluation to critical thinking.

Paramedics should always consider pathophysiology. The first steps in any decision-making process are assessment based. What is going wrong? Use external signs and symptoms to recognize system-level pathophysiology. Although this might seem complicated, it can be fairly simple. For example, you encounter an unconscious patient with snoring respirations. Your primary assessment identifies the snoring. Your knowledge of pathophysiology helps you determine that snoring is caused by relaxed muscles of the airway causing turbulent air movement in the upper airway. You can then feed this information into a few milliseconds of decision making and determine that airway positioning, or perhaps an airway adjunct, would be the best treatment modality for this patient. Sometimes the process

is slightly more complicated, but the assess–think critically– decide model is vital to accomplishing the most appropriate treatment for your patient.

> **Respiratory *failure* occurs when compensation fails.**

Goals of Airway Management

In the primary assessment, you assess the basic, most vital functions of the respiratory system. You assess the ability to move air (airway), and you assess the ability to exchange oxygen and carbon dioxide (breathing). You further assess whether these functions are being achieved (respiratory distress vs. respiratory failure). The goals of airway management should be linked to these key functions.

Given this idea, three key goals should be kept in mind: secure/protect the airway, oxygenate the patient, and ventilate the patient. Although these three key goals have many subcategories, these outcomes should provide the basis for any treatment strategy. In a simplified overview, this means that if the airway is unsecured, secure it. If the patient is not oxygenating, oxygenate him. If the patient is not ventilating, you must ventilate for him. Of course, this process is far more complicated, but it helps greatly to keep these key concepts in mind as you proceed.

OUTCOME-BASED MANAGEMENT

For many years, airway management has been taught in a linear fashion—that is, to always start at step one before going to step two. We now recognize that this may not be the best approach and that in many situations, step two may be more appropriate than step one. This is called *outcome-based management* and depends on critical thinking. In the process of making a treatment plan, you should not only link assessment findings to a desired outcome, but also keep pathophysiology in mind. For example, if your goal is to definitively secure the airway of a burn patient, a laryngeal mask airway (LMA) would not be aggressive enough. In this case, swelling could occur below the area the LMA has secured and could still threaten the long-term patency of the airway. Here, endotracheal intubation (ETI) would be more appropriate.

Adequate breathing:
Speaks full sentences;
alert and calm

Nonrebreather mask or nasal cannula

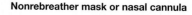
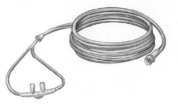

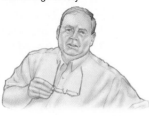

Increasing respiratory distress:
Visibly short of breath;
Speaking 3–4 word sentences;
Increasing anxiety

Nonrebreather mask

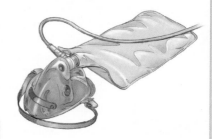

Key decision-making point:

Recognize inadequate breathing
before respiratory arrest
develops.

Assist ventilations
before they stop altogether!

Severe respiratory distress:
Speaking only 1–2 word sentences;
Very diaphoretic (sweaty);
Severe anxiety

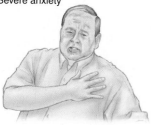

Assisted ventilations
Pocket face mask (PFM),
bag-valve mask (BVM), or
flow-restricted, oxygen-powered
ventilation device (FROPVD)

Assist the patient's own
ventilations, adjusting the
rate for rapid or slow
breathing

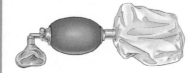

Continues to deteriorate:
Sleepy with head-bobbing;
Becomes unarousable

Respiratory arrest:
No breathing

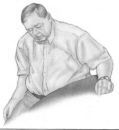

Artificial ventilation
Pocket face mask (PFM),
bag-valve mask (BVM), or
flow-restricted, oxygen-powered
ventilation device (FROPV)

Assisted ventilations at
12/minute for an adult or
20/minute for a child or infant

Figure 17-5 The continuum of breathing ranges from normal, adequate breathing to no breathing at all. It is essential to recognize the need for assisted ventilations even before severe respiratory distress develops.

In many treatment situations, a progressive approach is appropriate. You may start out with basic interventions only to recognize a need for further, more advanced treatment. However, critical thinking—not always an escalating algorithm—should guide your treatment. Instead of working through every tool in the airway management toolbox, paramedics must match the particular dysfunction to the best tool suitable to fix it.

What is the most effective method of airway management? The method that keeps air moving in your patient. Airway management needs to be a dynamic process that varies depending on assessment findings. No one method should be applied universally. Outcome-based management moves away from a hard-and-fast, inflexible algorithm and allows you to skip inappropriate treatment options in favor of the most appropriate tool for the job.

Opening/Securing the Airway

Securing the airway is a complex decision-making pathway with both short-term and long-term considerations. In many ways, this is one of the most challenging decisions a paramedic will face. Topic 19 discusses the invasive airway management decision-making process in detail, but in the meantime, here are some important points to consider:

- **Frequently, basic airway interventions are most appropriate to open and even secure an airway.** Maneuvers such as head positioning (head tilt–chin lift and jaw thrust), suction, and basic airway adjuncts often afford rapid and complete correction of airway compromise with minimal risk of complications. Although you may have many reasons to escalate, these basic interventions should not be forgotten.
- **Short-term versus long-term management must be considered.** Although you must always consider the clinical course of the patient, frequently prehospital airway concerns can be considered short term and as a result, short-term interventions may be appropriate. For example, cardiac arrest still remains the most common reason for securing an airway; although these airways are profoundly unsecure, short-term interventions are most appropriate (at least initially).

All airway maneuvers must be reviewed in a cost–benefit analysis. In cardiac arrest patients, intubation might provide the most secure airway, but the necessary interruption in chest compressions while the tube is placed makes its initial costs higher than its initial benefit. In this case, a blind insertion airway device, such as a King airway or an LMA, would be more appropriate, as its placement does not interrupt compressions. Although these blind insertion devices are typically intended for short-term airway security, in many ways cardiac arrest requires short-term management.

On the other hand, paramedics are frequently faced with long-term airway management situations. Burn patients' long-term needs have been discussed previously. Consider also the needs of a respiratory failure patient. If a patient has become so fatigued because of increased respiratory effort that he cannot continue breathing on his own, relatively long-term ventilation will be necessary. In this case, it might be more appropriate to move to intubation early, as that is the likely clinical course.

- **Consider the nature of the disorder.** When choosing a treatment pathway, you must consider the pathophysiology against which you are trying to defend. What are you faced with immediately? As stated earlier, a severe foreign body airway obstruction requires very rapid, very specific airway interventions. If foreign body airway maneuvers are unsuccessful, you must move to the next most aggressive option at your disposal. For many paramedics, this next step will be a surgical airway, even though many other airway tools are skipped over. Consider also the ongoing nature of the problem. Will the issue get worse (such as with a burn), and what is the expectation of potential interventions? A patient with epiglottitis might benefit from intubation, but accessing the hypopharynx might also accelerate the obstruction of the airway.

- **Consider the cost–benefit equation.** All interventions have potential costs. You must weigh those costs against the desired gain. Does the benefit outweigh the risk?

Oxygenating and Ventilating Your Patient

Ensuring oxygenation and ventilation are essential goals of any airway management intervention. Commonly these goals are linked to securing the airway and often can be accomplished with just that intervention. In other cases, however, more aggressive treatments may be necessary. Once the airway is open, you must next address the breathing aspect of your primary assessment (Figure 17-5).

If the patient is in respiratory failure, you must rapidly move to positive pressure ventilation. What the patient is doing on his own is not meeting his body's metabolic needs. In this case, a minimum of bag-mask ventilation will be essential. When moving to positive pressure ventilation, you will need to determine the importance of securing the airway as well. Sometimes this will be important, but in other situations basic bag-mask ventilation may suffice. For example, in a study in southern California, Marianne Gausche-Hill and her colleagues found that in a short-term setting, bag-mask ventilation was as successful as intubation in pediatric patients with respiratory arrest. Remember that the key here may be to ensure oxygenation and ventilation; this may or may not require more aggressive airway management.

With few exceptions, respiratory failure requires assisting the patient with a bag-valve mask (▶ Figure 17-6). You must take over when the patient's own respiratory

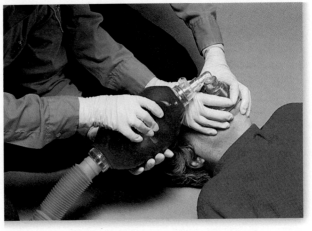

Figure 17-6 Two rescuers deliver bag-valve-mask ventilation.

system has failed. The two goals for this assisted ventilation are improving oxygenation and improving ventilation. Once again, consider minute volume. In a patient breathing exceptionally fast, your goal is not to slow down the rate, but to increase a diminished tidal volume. With every third, fourth, or even fifth breath, you will deliver a positive pressure breath with a tidal volume greater than the patient is able to achieve on his own. In many cases, positive pressure ventilation can reverse the effects of poor oxygenation and ventilation, but in some situations, you may also have to address the root cause of the disorder. Additional pharmacologic treatments may be necessary. Positive pressure ventilation is discussed in further detail in Topic 18.

The treatment goals when dealing with a patient in respiratory distress are to support the compensatory efforts of the patient and work on reversing the challenge. Remember, a patient in respiratory distress is compensating for a respiratory challenge and—at least so far—this compensation is successful. Supplemental oxygen to normalize saturation is important (▶ Figure 17-7). Remember, however, the discussion in Topic 16, "Paramedic Medications," that described the potentially negative effects of hyperoxia. Always remember that oxygen is a drug and, as such, judgment is required in its administration. Use oxygen to achieve a desired effect and titrate when that effective goal is reached. Supplemental oxygen can be delivered in many ways. Nonrebreathers and nasal cannulas are most common, but also consider the role of Venturi systems as well as continuous positive airway pressure (CPAP). Remember also that oxygen is delivered in high quantity when connected to a bag-mask device.

After you ensure that the status is respiratory *distress* and not *failure*, you should use your assessment to better determine the nature of the dysfunction and treat the root cause. As a paramedic, your approach now will be to focus on a treatment plan that helps reverse the pathology of the oxygenation and ventilation imbalance. For example, bronchodilators might be used to reverse bronchospasm and nitrates might be used to treat acute pulmonary edema. This definitive treatment will most likely be key to resolving any disturbances in the long-term sense. Respiratory treatment will be discussed in greater detail in later topics, but it is extremely important that these definitive treatments be considered in any airway management plan.

Unfortunately, oxygenation and ventilation issues are never simple and need to be considered in the context of larger, more complicated issues. Occasionally, oxygenation and ventilation problems are the result of poor airway security. For example, a head-injured patient with decreased mental status has poor airway muscle control and occluded airflow. Here, the oxygenation and ventilation problem can be resolved by simply opening and securing the airway.

More commonly, oxygenation and ventilation problems result from more complex pathophysiology. For example, a patient with acute pulmonary edema cannot oxygenate or ventilate because of changes in the alveolar capillary membrane and fluid in the alveoli. Because he is profoundly hypoxic and has mental status changes, he also cannot maintain his airway. Here, treatment must begin with securing the airway, but it must also include positive pressure ventilation to account for respiratory failure, as well as definitive medical treatment to reverse the acute pulmonary edema. Even simply securing the airway may be complicated. Perhaps this patient has poor mental status but intact protective reflexes in his airway. Although he likely needs ETI for both airway security and long-term positive pressure ventilation, this procedure will be extremely difficult unless paralytics are available for rapid sequence intubation. The level of airway management here needs to be determined based not just on patient needs, but also on crew capabilities.

CONCLUSIONS

Airway management is a challenging process in the prehospital world, but you have the tools to make it possible and safe. Unfortunately, there is no page from a textbook that can apply to all the different scenarios that can confront you. Rely on assessment and critical thinking and always weigh the costs and benefits as you develop your plan.

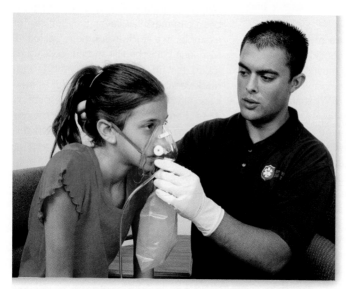

Figure 17-7 Provide oxygen via a nonrebreather mask to the patient who is breathing adequately but with difficulty (respiratory distress).

TRANSITIONING • • • • • • • •

REVIEW ITEMS

1. Which of the following problems would be designated as an upper airway disorder?
   a. laryngeal edema caused by anaphylaxis
   b. bronchoconstriction caused by asthma
   c. destruction of the alveoli caused by emphysema
   d. pulmonary edema caused by congestive heart failure

2. You are assessing a patient who has a hoarse voice and poor air movement after being struck in the throat by a baseball. Given the primary assessment, which of the following would be your most important next step?

    a. Apply a cold pack to the neck for pain management.

    b. Prepare for intubation and a possibly surgical airway.

    c. Ask the patient to sip cool water.

    d. Continue on to your secondary assessment.

3. Which of the following signs would help you differentiate respiratory distress from respiratory failure?

    a. altered mental status

    b. increased respiratory rate

    c. accessory muscle use

    d. increased heart rate

4. You are treating a patient in respiratory failure. Which of the following treatments should you complete first?

    a. Complete a thorough secondary assessment.

    b. Deliver supplemental oxygen with a nasal cannula.

    c. Begin chest compressions.

    d. Deliver positive pressure ventilations with a bag-valve mask.

5. You are treating a patient in acute pulmonary edema. After ensuring that he is *not* in respiratory failure and applying supplemental oxygen, what should you do next?

    a. Administer nitrates and CPAP.

    b. Prepare for intubation.

    c. Administer positive pressure ventilations with a bag mask device.

    d. Prepare for a surgical airway.

APPLIED PATHOPHYSIOLOGY

1. List three ways in which the body compensates for a respiratory challenge.

2. Explain how these compensatory methods may be recognized in an assessment.

3. Discuss why compensation might fail in a patient with hypoxic respiratory distress.

4. Describe the approach to airway management for a person in respiratory distress (not respiratory failure).

CLINICAL DECISION MAKING

You are assessing a 65-year-old female patient with chronic obstructive pulmonary disease (COPD). Her family says that she has had shortness of breath for three days, but "she is much worse today." You find the patient sitting upright, looking scared, and unable to speak.

1. What indications does your general impression give you that this woman's condition may be critical?

Your patient has a patent airway and is breathing 48 times per minute. She has lung sounds bilaterally but is moving little air, with a prominent wheeze. Her radial pulse is 128, her skin is wet, and she is confused (this is not her normal state).

2. Is this patient in respiratory distress or respiratory failure? Please discuss why you feel this way.

3. Based on your primary assessment, are any immediate interventions necessary? If so, what are they?

4. Explain the pathophysiologic cause for the following:

    a. Confusion

    b. Wheezing

    c. Increased heart rate

The family reports to you that the patient also has a history of acute pulmonary edema secondary to congestive heart failure (CHF).

5. Based on your primary survey, is it important to determine if this patient is currently in APE or exacerbated COPD? Why or why not?

6. If you determined that this patient was in APE, how would it change your immediate interventions?

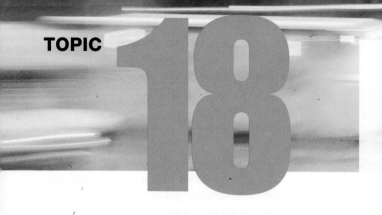

Standard Airway Management, Respiration, and Artificial Ventilation

Competency Integrates complex knowledge of anatomy, physiology, and pathophysiology into the assessment to develop and implement a treatment plan with the goal of assuring a patent airway, adequate mechanical ventilation, and respiration for patients of all ages.

NONINVASIVE AIRWAY INTERVENTION

TRANSITION *highlights*

- *Core treatment interventions for a patient suffering from a disturbance to the airway.*

- *Oxygen therapy revisited.*

- *Positive pressure ventilation revisited.*

- *Use of continuous positive airway pressure (CPAP) during prehospital management of a patient with respiratory distress.*

INTRODUCTION

Today's paramedics possess a wide array of tools for airway management. From simple airway adjuncts to surgical airways, interventions span the spectrum from noninvasive to invasive. As Topic 17, "Airway Assessment and Decision Making," discussed, paramedics must use assessment and critical thinking to decide which tool is right for a specific patient.

Far too often, paramedics catch themselves in a web of technology. In a desire to use the skills they have now earned or to experience a particular procedure, paramedics too often replace fundamental basic skills with the technology of advanced interventions. Although sometimes this is appropriate, advanced invasive skills often bring with them the highest risk of complication for the patient. Judgment should rule the day. Just because you *can* perform a skill does not mean that you *should*. In many cases, the least invasive skill may be the most appropriate intervention of all and may suffice even though more advanced procedures are available.

This topic picks up where Topic 17 left off. Here, we discuss moving from decision making to treatment. Noninvasive therapies are discussed and placed in the context of airway management decision making.

> In many cases, basic noninvasive maneuvers are the most appropriate interventions.

DON'T FORGET THE BASICS

As a paramedic, you have earned the right to perform many advanced airway skills. Endotracheal intubation, needle decompression, and surgical airways may all be within your scope of practice. Especially in the early stages of your career, it makes sense that you to want to use these skills. However, appropriate airway management means using the techniques and interventions that best serve your patient, not the ones that best serve your ego. In many cases, basic noninvasive maneuvers are the most appropriate interventions. As a paramedic, you must weigh the costs and benefits to determine the best treatment plan for your patient.

Consider the following situations:

- **Cardiac arrest.** Cardiac arrest accounts for a large majority of airway management skills and heretofore was the single largest indication for endotracheal intubation. However, new research is demonstrating that this invasive skill may not be the most appropriate way to manage a cardiac arrest patient's airway. We now know that the most important element of cardiac arrest care is the performance of uninterrupted, quality chest compressions. We further know that endotracheal intubation, no matter how skillfully performed, interrupts those chest compressions. As such, the procedure may actually have a negative impact on resuscitation efforts. This does not mean that intubation is absolutely contraindicated, but it does likely mean that it would be more reasonable under the circumstances to use a tool that accomplishes nearly the same goal without interrupting compressions.

- **Traumatic brain injuries.** There is at least limited evidence that multiple intubation attempts in patients with traumatic brain injuries can lead to hypoxia, and this hypoxia can lead to worsened outcomes. Again, this does not mean that intubation should not be used in this patient category, but it does point out a larger cost in the cost–benefit analysis.

- **Pediatric patients.** It has been demonstrated that in a short-term setting, bag-mask ventilation has similar outcomes to endotracheal intubation in pediatric respiratory arrest patients. Considering the infrequency of skill opportunities and the relatively high risk of intubation, perhaps we should prioritize bag-mask ventilation when managing the airways of our youngest patients.

Advanced procedures such as endotracheal intubation certainly play an important role in the right circumstances, but that time and place should be carefully examined in the airway management decision-making process. In some cases, they are most appropriate. In some cases, they will need to be used when basic maneuvers fail. In other situations, however, basic noninvasive interventions may be the most appropriate option.

Remember also that basic interventions often must precede advanced techniques. Preoxygenation should come before any advanced airway. Suction is a vastly underutilized skill. Frequently, advanced skills can be avoided simply by performing quality basic interventions. Continuous positive airway pressure (CPAP), for example, can prevent the need for future endotracheal intubation. As a paramedic, you must consider all your tools when making airway management decisions and not forget the ones you learned in EMT class.

The Most Difficult Intervention of All: Doing Nothing

Although most commonly airway management steps should be taken, in a small subset of patients it may be more important to not attempt airway management than to be aggressive. This can be incredibly challenging to the paramedic, but recognizing these situations is important when making airway management decisions. In the cost–benefit analysis, you must judge the benefit of your procedure against the potential negative side effects. In some cases, these negative outcomes can outweigh the benefit. Consider the following example:

A 36-year-old male presents with a four-day history of fever and now complains of difficulty breathing. He has difficulty speaking, and you note that his airway is dependent on him sitting upright in a sniffing position. As long as he maintains this position, he can keep his airway open, but even a move to a semi-Fowler position causes occlusion. The fever and complaint suggest an upper airway infection; indeed, this patient's airway is significantly threatened. Ideally, intubation would be used to secure the airway; however, serious risks are associated with that procedure in this patient. With a positionally patent airway, it might be better to transport this patient and allow airway management to be performed under optimal circumstances. We know by his external signs that intubation is likely to be difficult and may lead to complete occlusion. Is the benefit worth the risk?

Cost–benefit analysis must weigh many factors, not just the condition of the patient. As a paramedic, you must also consider crew capabilities (the ability to perform a surgical airway would certainly be a consideration in the patient discussed here), equipment, and transport time before undertaking any advanced skill. Again, just because you *can* do not mean you *should*.

SUPPLEMENTAL OXYGEN REVISITED

Hypoxia kills. As an EMS provider, one of your most important roles is to prevent this life-threatening condition. Supplemental oxygen can be a valuable tool in this role. However, you must also remember that oxygen is a drug, and it must be used correctly to avoid complications associated with its administration.

In your initial training, you may have learned that there is no such thing as too much oxygen. Recent research has demonstrated that this may not necessarily be true—although hypoxic patients certainly need oxygen, continued high-flow oxygen beyond normal oxygen saturations may cause a condition called *hyperoxia*. Hyperoxia is theorized to cause harm through two potential problems. It may cause a systemic vasoconstriction that limits essential blood flow. It also releases free radicals into the bloodstream that many consider to be cardiac toxic. At least in theory, cardiac output can be affected.

Recent research has supported the theory of negative effects of hyperoxia. In a study conducted in Australia, oxygen delivery was randomized in chronic obstructive pulmonary disease (COPD) patients. Cohorts of these patients were given either 8 to 10 liters per minute (lpm) of oxygen or titrated oxygen to keep saturations between 88 percent and 92 percent. In the titrated group, mortality was significantly lower than in the high-flow group.

You should always follow local protocol, but many experts currently recommend that oxygen be titrated to normal saturation levels (typically 94 percent to 95 percent). The American Heart Association (AHA), in its 2010 Guidelines for Cardiopulmonary Resuscitation and Emergency Cardiovascular Care, concluded that the evidence showed "no benefit and potential harm" from administering continued high-flow oxygen to patients with saturations above 94 percent. The guidelines suggest that "there is insufficient evidence to support [oxygen's] routine use in uncomplicated ACS. If the patient is dyspneic, hypoxemic, or has obvious signs of heart failure, providers should titrate therapy, based on monitoring of oxyhemoglobin saturation, to ≥94%." The AHA also makes similar recommendations for stroke patients and in the setting of neonatal resuscitation.

Of course, titrating oxygen requires accurate saturation evaluation capabilities (which are not always available in low perfusion states). When it is possible, though, it makes sense to evaluate your patient and adjust treatments based on improvement and current needs. That means it may be possible to maximize oxygen saturation with a variety of different delivery devices. The best choice might be a nonrebreather mask, but it also might be a nasal cannula or a Venturi mask. The key is to use good judgment (and follow local protocol).

POSITIVE PRESSURE VENTILATION REVISITED

Positive pressure ventilation is an incredibly important skill used to correct respiratory failure, and paramedics must be aggressive with its application. However, new information points out that positive pressure ventilation does come at a cost, and paramedics must evaluate its potentially negative side effects when working through the airway management decision process. Positive pressure ventilation is still the only real way to move air into a nonbreathing patient; however, consideration of its negative aspects should reinforce the importance of proper technique.

The body normally uses negative pressure to bring air into the chest. The diaphragm contracts, the intercostal muscles flex, and negative pressure is created in the chest cavity to pull air in through the glottic opening. With mechanical ventilation, an opposite mechanism is used to move air into the lungs: Positive pressure is applied externally to force air in.

Positive pressure ventilation sometimes disrupts normal body functions. For example, the heart uses the negative pressure of breathing to assist with filling. When positive pressure is applied, the heart can no longer rely on the negative pressure, and often filling is decreased. This can drop cardiac output. The esophagus is also not designed for positive pressure air entry. Because it is an expandable tube, positive pressure ventilation often drives air into the stomach. This gastric insufflation can lead to pressure on the diaphragm and decreased lung capacity.

> **Positive pressure ventilation is essential for a patient who is not breathing or is in respiratory failure.**

Despite these difficulties, positive pressure ventilation is essential for a patient who is not breathing or is in respiratory failure. Keeping the following side effects in mind will help you improve your positive pressure ventilation technique.

- **Minimize the effect of positive pressure.** Ventilate with only enough volume to raise the chest wall. Doing this helps minimize the effects of positive pressure on the heart and can increase cardiac filling.

- **Keep gastric insufflation in mind.** Always use an airway adjunct (when possible). Airway adjuncts help create better channels for air and help

avoid forcing air into the esophagus. Although you may also consider using cricoid pressure (the Sellick maneuver) to compress the esophagus during ventilation (▶ Figure 18-1), recent evidence has cast some doubt as to the value of this procedure, and the AHA has significantly limited its recommendations for cricoid pressure in its 2010 guidelines.

- **Hyperventilation kills.** Ventilate at appropriate rates (12–20/minute for children and 10–12/minute for adults). This helps prevent gastric insufflation as well as preventing the unnecessary removal of too much carbon dioxide, which can lead to cerebral vasoconstriction and reduced blood flow to the brain.

The cost–benefit analysis of positive pressure ventilation is an important one. Your ability to identify respiratory failure effectively is essential. Even more essential, however, is your decision to act on that problem. Far too often, respiratory failure is identified but allowed to worsen because of indecision. Always remember that your assessment is more than just a gathering of information; it is a very important element of making critical decisions.

Bag-Mask Device and Cardiac Arrest

Is there a need for intubation in cardiac arrest? The answer is a resounding "maybe." As stated previously, we know that intubation interrupts compressions and, as a result, may negatively affect the resuscitation effort. But it may also be necessary to effectively manage the airway. For some patients, bag-mask ventilation may not be an effective means to move air. Head position, obesity, and trauma may all present situations in which bag-mask ventilation may be insufficient. The better alternative would most commonly be a blind insertion airway device, such as a King airway or a laryngeal mask airway, but in some cases bag-mask ventilation will suffice.

Bag-mask ventilation in a short-term setting can provide

adequate oxygenation and ventilation to your patient. Potential risks include gastric insufflation and an unsecure airway, but in some settings the benefit might outweigh the risk. Consider the previously discussed pediatric patient. In this case, bag-mask use has proven to be an effective alternative, and in cardiac arrest states there is little need to move immediately to intubation.

In general, the airway management decision-making process must assess the efficacy of current interventions. It must assess the success or failure of initial steps. If bag-mask ventilation is successful, the paramedic must then judge the benefits and costs of moving to a more aggressive step.

CONTINUOUS POSITIVE AIRWAY PRESSURE

CPAP is a technology that uses positive pressure in a different manner from a bag-mask system. The positive pressure created by a CPAP system does not force air in but creates a constant, slight flow of air against which the patient will breathe. This "wall of resistance" will often make the work of breathing easier, keep alveoli open, and make breathing more effective (▶ Figure 18-2).

A variety of different CPAP systems are available. In general, CPAP systems create a higher flow of air by mixing oxygen with room air (although some systems use just room air). For years, sleep apnea patients have used positive pressure to keep open the soft tissues of the hypopharynx and prevent snoring. In EMS, that pressure is used to "pneumatically splint" open lower airways and the alveoli.

Uses of CPAP

CPAP is most commonly used to treat acute pulmonary edema (APE). By pressurizing the inside of the alveoli, the fluid of pulmonary edema is prevented from crossing the alveolar membrane. It also helps prevent the collapse of alveoli under the weight of the edema. By potentially reducing the negative pressure in the chest, CPAP can also decrease preload and therefore reduce the heart's workload. As we will discuss soon, this preload reduction can be both helpful and dangerous. CPAP should be used in concert with other APE therapies. Its combination with nitrates provides an effective "one-two punch" against pulmonary edema. CPAP has been proven to rapidly improve APE in

Figure 18-1 Applying cricoid pressure (Sellick maneuver) with positive pressure ventilation.

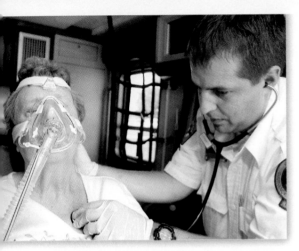

Figure 18-2 Continuous positive airway pressure (CPAP) is used for the awake and spontaneously breathing patient who needs ventilatory support. (© *Ken Kerr*)

some patients and, in many cases, to prevent the need for intubation.

CPAP is also used to treat other forms of respiratory distress. Keeping small airways open via the pneumatic splint tends to increase oxygenation and decrease the sensation of difficulty breathing. Keeping the alveoli from collapsing also leads to increased surface area for gas exchange. These effects can help a variety of respiratory disorders, including bronchospasm and pneumonia. Many CPAP systems allow for the inclusion of bronchodilators while administering CPAP, but bronchodilator treatments should not be traded for CPAP in patients with bronchospasm. Bronchodilators here are the most important therapy and should be the first choice if a choice must be made. Indications for CPAP vary from system to system, so always follow local protocol.

Applying CPAP

CPAP is *not* artificial ventilation. If the patient cannot maintain an airway or breathe on his own, he is *not* a candidate for CPAP. Many patients will need more aggressive treatments. Always use a thorough patient assessment to make the correct treatment choice.

Just as with a bag mask, the positive pressure of CPAP can also drop cardiac output by counteracting the negative filling pressure of the heart. Therefore, you should never apply CPAP to a hypotensive patient. Follow local guidelines for minimum systolic blood pressure values.

CPAP can also be psychologically difficult for a patient. A mask is strapped to the face of a patient who is already having difficulty breathing. Often a patient will not tolerate this treatment. CPAP should never be forced. Consider allowing the patient to hold the mask on his face before strapping it on. Often, when the patient feels the effects, he will be more likely to allow the strap.

CPAP can be rapidly beneficial, but not every patient will get better after its application. Reassessment is critical. Many times CPAP will be applied to patients who are close to respiratory failure. These patients sometimes progress to respiratory failure and will need more aggressive treatment. Remember also that hypotension can be a side effect.

CONCLUSIONS

Noninvasive airway procedures are an important element of airway management. Paramedics should always consider these procedures as an essential element of any airway management plan. Although these topics are covered routinely in lower-level licensure programs, it is important for paramedics to stay current with new philosophies, adapted treatment strategies, and more modern indications.

TRANSITIONING

REVIEW ITEMS

1. A 65-year-old male patient is found in respiratory failure. He is nearly unconscious, cyanotic, and clearly fatigued. His vital signs are pulse 130, respirations 4, blood pressure 160/100 mmHg. To treat this patient, you should first _____.
   a. perform endotracheal intubation
   b. administer positive pressure ventilations with a bag mask
   c. administer supplemental O₂ with a nonrebreather mask
   d. administer a bronchodilator treatment via nebulizer

2. Cardiopulmonary resuscitation (CPR) is being performed on a 2-year-old female patient. Bag-mask ventilations are causing chest rise with clear lung sounds. As a paramedic you should _____.
   a. perform endotracheal intubation
   b. perform a surgical airway
   c. cease ventilations and perform compression-only CPR
   d. continue with bag-mask ventilations

3. Which of the following would be considered a negative side effect associated with hyperoxia?

   a. decreased blood pressure   b. bradycardia
   c. systemic vasoconstriction   d. hypoglycemia

4. First responders are treating a 59-year-old man who complains of chest pain. They are managing his airway with a nasal cannula. His saturation is maintained at 94 percent. You should _____.
   a. deliver positive pressure ventilations with a bag-mask
   b. continue supplemental oxygen with a nasal cannula
   c. replace the nasal cannula with a nonrebreather mask
   d. remove the nasal cannula

5. Which of the following vital signs would rule out the use of CPAP?
   a. respiratory rate of 4/min
   b. respiratory rate of 40/min
   c. blood pressure of 198/100 mmHg
   d. heart rate of 140

APPLIED PATHOPHYSIOLOGY

1. Describe the theory of hyperoxia. How might hyperoxia negatively affect the body?

2. Describe how positive pressure ventilation is different from the way a person normally breathes.

3. List three negative side effects of positive pressure ventilation.

4. Describe a scenario in which bag-mask ventilation might be preferable to endotracheal intubation.

5. Describe how CPAP improves oxygenation and ventilation.

CLINICAL DECISION MAKING

A 65-year-old man has called EMS after waking from sleep with severe shortness of breath. He is very sweaty, and you note he is obviously struggling to breathe. He is awake, but is only able to speak in short sentences because of his dyspnea. He tells you, "I feel like I'm going to die." His wife tells you that "he was fine at bedtime last night." You begin your assessment as your partner applies oxygen.

1. Is this patient in respiratory failure? What additional information will you require to make this decision?

Your patient has a patent airway and is breathing 50 times per minute. You note crackles over all fields when you listen to his lung sounds and recognize accessory muscle use in his neck and chest. The patient is agitated, but alert. His vital signs are pulse 136, respirations 50, blood pressure 200/116 mmHg. His pulse oximetry is 86 percent.

2. Based on your primary assessment, are any immediate interventions necessary? If so, what are they?

3. Is positive pressure ventilation warranted in this patient? If so, how would you administer it?

4. What, if any, is the role of supplemental oxygen in this patient? If warranted, how would you administer it?

The patient's wife states that the patient had a heart attack one year ago and has a history of hypertension and high cholesterol. She notes that the patient was feeling weak yesterday but was otherwise fine at bedtime.

5. Based on your findings, what, if any, medications would you administer?

Standard Airway Management, Respiration, and Artificial Ventilation

Competency Integrates complex knowledge of anatomy, physiology, and pathophysiology into the assessment to develop and implement a treatment plan with the goal of ensuring a patent airway, adequate mechanical ventilation, and respiration for patients of all ages.

TOPIC

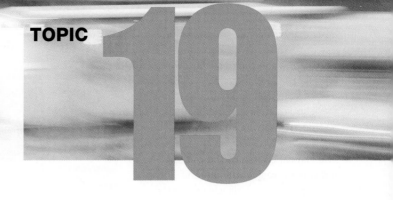

INVASIVE AIRWAY MANAGEMENT

INTRODUCTION

The paramedic scope of practice represents the pinnacle of prehospital airway management. When basic skills fail, the paramedic is called on to intervene with more advanced—and typically more invasive—procedures. Skills such as endotracheal intubation (ETI) and surgical airways represent definitive management and are used to secure the most difficult and threatened airways.

Just as with any other airway management skill, the decision to move to invasive procedures should be made after careful consideration of the costs and benefits of the intervention. In making an airway management decision, paramedics should consider invasive techniques in the context of a larger toolbox and choose the intervention that makes the most sense given the circumstances of the problem.

Although the advanced skill set represents a wider capability, it brings with it a larger responsibility and greater risk to the patient. This responsibility, particularly with respect to ETI, has been a point of controversy in recent years. ETI success rates and complications, as well as the negative outcomes of other advanced procedures, have led to a reexamination of ETI's importance and perhaps a new prioritization of invasive airway techniques. A new reverence for invasive skills has emerged; paramedics not only should be familiar with the ongoing debate, but should also incorporate these valid concerns into their airway management decision-making process.

PROGRESSING TO INVASIVE AIRWAY MANAGEMENT

As Topics 17 and 18 discussed, the airway management decision must take a number of factors into account. First, assessment should identify the problem at hand. The primary assessment is used to identify airway and breathing issues and typically will be the point at which airway interventions take place. Next, use pathophysiology to determine the most appropriate method to resolve the issue. Finally, consider other circumstances to create the best treatment plan for the patient.

TRANSITION *highlights*

- *Decision making and the invasive airway.*
- *Review of blind insertion airway devices.*
- *The endotracheal intubation dilemma.*
- *Preserving endotracheal intubation in the paramedic scope of practice.*

This consideration must include costs and benefits of the procedure, risks, crew capabilities, equipment on hand, and a variety of other situational data. Although this seems complex, experienced paramedics make this decision daily and typically it is made in a matter of seconds.

The decision to undertake an invasive procedure should be made with the most forethought, for typically these procedures carry with them the highest level of risk. This does not mean they are a last resort, but that they be reserved for situations in which their benefit clearly outweighs their risk. Consider the following indications for invasive airways:

- **More basic maneuvers have failed.** This situation could include patients who cannot be ventilated using a bag-mask device or a situation in which less invasive procedures did not accomplish the desired result.

- **Invasive airways are indicated by the pathophysiology of the situation.** In some situations, invasive procedures are indicated. For example, burn patients with the risk of glottic edema obstructing their airway need immediate ETI. Less invasive procedures will not resolve the pathophysiology of the edema.

- **Invasive airways represent the better choice given an analysis of the circumstances.** In some circumstances, basic maneuvers could work, but invasive procedures simply represent the better choice. A patient with severe bleeding around the airway could theoretically be managed with a bag mask and continuous suctioning, but securing the airway with ETI would be the better alternative.

- **The clinical course of the patient indicates invasive maneuvers.** Some situations dictate a clinical course for the patient that involves advanced procedures. A patient in respiratory failure will need to be placed on a ventilator to resolve respiratory muscle fatigue. This is not a short-term airway, but one that will require relatively long-term management. In this case, ETI would be the more appropriate choice, as it represents the better long-term option.

> **No airway should be approached in a predetermined manner.**

In the end, no airway should be approached in a predetermined manner. Each circumstance must be evaluated individually and a plan tailor-made to suit its own particulars.

Cost–Benefit Analysis (in General)

All invasive airway interventions should take place only after a careful cost–benefit analysis. Invasive procedures may represent the highest level of airway management, but in most cases they also represent the highest level of risk. **Table 19-1** lists some of the general benefits and risks of advanced airway maneuvers.

> **Preserving intubation should be a priority for all paramedics.**

Definitive airway management can be critically important. In many cases, the benefits of invasive procedures will outweigh the risks. Providers must recognize those circumstances but at the same time resist temptation to apply invasive procedures to situations for which basic maneuvers would be equally effective.

THE ENDOTRACHEAL INTUBATION DILEMA

When performed correctly, ETI represents the highest level of prehospital airway management. No airway is more secure than an endotracheal (ET) tube. When the tube is properly placed, the trachea is definitively isolated and air is prevented from getting into the stomach. ETI truly represents a definitive airway. Why, then, is this procedure so controversial? Shouldn't definitive airway management be the goal for every patient with an unsecure airway?

To answer these questions successfully, we must also look at the downside of ETI. As a procedure, it carries many risks, not the least of which is patient death. Unrecognized esophageal intubation actually prevents air from reaching the lungs and rapidly results in hypoxia and death unless it is resolved quickly. Although it is difficult to determine how often this happens, numerous studies have reported poor success rates. Although each study has its specific limitations, prehospital success rates of 60 percent to 90 percent seem to be more the norm than the exception. When you consider the potentially disastrous consequences, any success rate less than 100 percent is too low. Other complications of ETI include hypoxia induced during tube placement, increased intracranial pressure, and trauma to the tissues of the airway. All these are important, but pale in comparison to the risk misplaced tubes represent.

Low success rates are a function of a variety of factors. Poor initial training, infrequent use of the procedure, and nonexistent continuing education opportunities all contribute to the prevalence of negative outcomes. Furthermore, it is increasingly difficult to improve these circumstances. Operating rooms (ORs), where paramedics obtain their original training, are more frequently using blind insertion devices instead of ETI for short-term anesthesia. This limits the opportunities paramedic students have for training. Liability questions and competition from other professions have also limited the OR experience for many paramedic students. Intubation is a technical skill and just as with any other technique, lack of use decreases skill. In many cases, especially in rural states, paramedic use of ETI is limited to only a few times (if any) each year. Finally, ongoing education requirements are often loosely defined. Ongoing training opportunities face the same challenges as initial education.

When one considers the educational challenges in context with the difficult situations in which paramedics are charged with performing the skill, it is no wonder that success rates are as low as they are. As a result, the paramedic scope of practice faces some very real challenges.

As a profession, we cannot continue to perform a high-risk skill at the success rates that have been reported. Success rates must improve or the skill will be assuredly removed from our arsenal of airway management. Unfortunately, the desperate situations for which intubation is necessary are not going away. The burn patients, the respiratory failure patients, and the trauma patients will still need intubation, so we must do our best to make the necessary changes.

Preserving intubation should be a priority for all paramedics, and proactive steps must be taken.

Preserving Intubation in the Paramedic Scope of Practice

Intubation can be preserved by undertaking three major philosophical shifts. First, we need to recognize and admit that we have a problem. Second, we need to better select the situations in which intubation is used. Third, we must concentrate on improving ET confirmation. Of course we must consider other steps, such as selecting who intubates and providing higher quality initial education, but the main three are within the grasp of every

TABLE 19-1	Benefits and Risks of Advanced Airway Procedures
Benefits	**Risks**
Definitive airway management	Inappropriate placement
Secure airway	Hypoxia from the procedure
Minimal gastric insufflation	Time of procedure
Minimal aspiration	Training and skill maintenance
Long term	Equipment requirements
Nonpositional	Crew requirements

provider and should be a priority for those who wish to keep the skill.

1. **Recognize the problem.** Many paramedics are fond of making excuses. "It wasn't my fault," "The tube must have become displaced when we moved the patient," and "That study is flawed" are common excuses made for what seems to be an indisputable issue. If we wish to move forward, we must recognize that, at a minimum, we have a major concern for the safety of our patients and, at a maximum, we have a major problem. Either way, we will begin to face real solutions only after admitting that there is an issue.

2. **Select appropriate patients.** Not every patient who has an airway issue needs intubation. Because the procedure has a high risk, it should be reserved for patients who will gain the greatest benefit. Although this may not change overall success rates, it will allow paramedics to focus attention where that attention is needed and limit the risk to the highest reward.

3. **Improving confirmation is an essential step to preserving intubation.** Esophageal intubation will never be fully resolved, but with appropriate confirmation, paramedics can recognize 100 percent of the times that it occurs. Paramedics should focus on technical means of confirmation and remove the human factor from the equation.

These steps are important to paramedics at every level. Although some of the key elements are system-level changes, each provider shares a responsibility.

Intubation Indications Revisited

Because ETI is a high-risk skill, it should be reserved for situations in which its benefit is most meaningful. Patients should be selected by the highest need and greatest benefit, not just because the skill is available. Unfortunately for many paramedics, this was not the approach they were taught. For many years, licensure programs taught new paramedics that intubation was the standard of care for specific disorders and that in these cases, the skill should be performed regardless of the circumstances.

Take, for example, cardiac arrest care. For years, the paramedic standard of care

was intubation. Paramedics intubated cardiac arrest victims often before even starting cardiopulmonary resuscitation (CPR). Now, new information has changed this approach greatly. As cardiac arrest outcomes are studied, it is recognized now that intubation may actually be detrimental to the initial resuscitation attempt. Intubation attempts interrupt chest compressions and cause unnecessary drops in both cerebral and coronary perfusion pressures. In a more modern approach, intubation should be replaced when possible by blind insertion airway devices (BIADs) that need not interrupt compressions as they are inserted. This does not mean that intubation is entirely contraindicated in cardiac arrest patients—it may be necessary if other airway control measures fail—but it does mean that it should be limited to unusual circumstances or to later stages of the resuscitation.

This revisionist approach is not limited to cardiac arrest; in numerous other situations, ETI is no longer a foregone conclusion. Rather than concentrate on when intubation is not indicated, however, let us consider a few situations in which intubation still remains an essential skill. Consider the following indications:

- **Airway edema.** Intubation is very important in protecting the airway of patients at risk for increased edema or laryngeal inflammation. Burn patients, neck trauma patients, and even some anaphylactic patients are candidates for high-priority intubation. Periglottic devices such as King airways and laryngeal mask airways (LMAs) simply do not protect against this edema.

- **Respiratory failure.** Although this indication is less certain than the previous one, a patient with exhausted muscles of respiration generally will require intubation. Resolution of this pathology will typically require protracted time on a ventilator, and intubation remains the best long-term airway management tool.

- **Acute pulmonary edema refractory to CPAP.** If CPAP cannot reverse the effects of pulmonary edema, then the positive pressures of intubation are generally considered the next best option. Again, this is by no means a certainty, but most periglottic devices are unable to sustain the level of airway pressure that ETI can.

- **Severely threatened airways.** This is a broad category, but generally includes patients whose airways are threatened by pharyngeal bleeding or other uncontrolled secretions. Periglottic devices may help, but generally do not offer the same level of protection.

There are, of course, other indications. As always, use assessment and critical thinking to make airway management decisions. Invasive techniques such as ETI should be considered one of many tools capable of completing the task at hand. You should also always follow local protocols.

Intubation Confirmation

Confirmation is critical. If every ETI were confirmed to 100 percent certainty, then esophageal intubation would disappear. Prehospital ETI is performed in some of the least optimal circumstances in medicine, but nonetheless it is essential. Because of the frequently austere circumstances, it is reasonable to conclude that errors occur. This is why confirmation is so important. Positive confirmation recognizes and corrects all the errors that happen. Using technological confirmation further takes away human stress, vanity, and incompetence.

The gold standard for ET tube confirmation is waveform capnography, in which exhaled carbon dioxide is measured and graphically represented. Tubes are confirmed by both the presence and waveform of end-tidal carbon dioxide ($ETCO_2$). This is significant because capnography offers both an objective and a real-time evaluation of the ET tube. Other confirmation methods are limited by time and circumstances, but capnography offers almost definitive findings. Capnography can have limitations, however. Patients in cardiac arrest or in very low perfusion states produce minimal exhaled carbon dioxide. This can present a false negative on the capnography. Capnography is also an expensive technology.

> **The gold standard for endotracheal tube confirmation is waveform capnography.**

A less-expensive variation of $ETCO_2$ monitoring is qualitative $ETCO_2$ measurement, otherwise known as CO_2 detectors. These devices use paper that changes color in the presence of CO_2. They are attached to the end of ET tubes to detect CO_2 during ventilation. These devices are generally limited to short-term use and are not nearly as sensitive as capnography. Nonetheless, they have been proven to detect 100 percent of misplaced tubes. Despite issues with false negatives, CO_2 detectors represent an important alternative when capnography is not available.

Other confirmation devices exist, but none is as specific as capnography or even CO_2 detectors. However, they can be used in concert with these devices and can certainly be utilized if CO_2 detection is not available. Esophageal detector devices, auscultation of lung sounds, and visualization of condensation in the tube during exhalation each can be an important addition to the confirmation arsenal.

There is no one perfect method of ETI confirmation. As such, you should always incorporate multiple methods to achieve definitive confirmation. Capnography should be paired with lung sounds, and CO_2 detectors should be combined with tube condensation to maximize safety.

BLIND INSERTION AIRWAY DEVICES

Blind insertion airway devices (BIADs) are a general category of airway adjuncts so named because they do not require specialized equipment, such as a laryngoscope, to insert. They are designed to offer a simple alternative to ETI and provide a level of protection from aspiration by (at least in theory) isolating the glottic opening. A variety of types of BIADs exists; they all manage the airway in slightly different ways. In general, they require limited training and do not interrupt chest compressions when used during cardiac arrest care.

Although they are designed to be an alternative to ETI, BIADs are not always an appropriate or superior alternative to ETI. BIADs are not definitive airway protection. Although they add some level of defense against secretions and vomiting, they do not fully isolate the trachea in the manner that ETI does. When definitive airway management is necessary (airway burns, laryngeal edema, etc.), these devices should not be substituted for ETI. As with intubation, these devices require specific training. Furthermore, the insertion of a BIAD can elicit a gag reflex and stimulate the vagus nerve, causing bradycardia.

In general, BIADs can be divided into two categories: esophageal obturation and supraglottic devices.

- **Esophageal obturation.** With devices that use esophageal obturation, the glottic opening is isolated by blocking the esophagus and by blocking the backflow of air in the hypopharynx. The most common devices that use esophageal obturation are the dual-lumen CombiTube® and the King LT® airway. Both these devices can be inserted with the patient's head in a neutral position. They are inserted blindly to a depth based on the patient's size. In each device, a distal balloon is inflated to obstruct the opening to the esophagus and a second balloon is inflated to obstruct the hypopharynx. With both these balloons inflated, the glottic opening becomes the only pathway for positive pressure air. As the glottis is now isolated, it is at least theoretically protected from secretions, blood, and other foreign substances.

  Most esophageal obturation type devices are size dependent. In fact, the dual-lumen airway cannot be used in pediatric patients and the King LT airway also has a minimum size. Airways that enter the esophagus should not be used in patients with known esophageal disease or esophageal bleeding. They should also not be used in patients who have ingested a caustic substance. Esophageal obturation devices can dislodge after patient movement. The placement of esophageal obturation devices is confirmed by the ability (or inability) to obtain chest rise while ventilating through the device. If the device is placed properly, normal ventilations should result in movement of the chest. If they are placed improperly, no chest rise will be visible. As always, follow local protocol and manufacturers recommendations for proper placement and use of particular devices.

- **Supraglottic devices.** The laryngeal mask airway is the most common supraglottic airway; although there are a series of variations, this device serves as the flagship for this category. A supraglottic airway is a BIAD that achieves airway management by creating an internal seal around the glottic

opening. They move air in a manner similar to an external mask used in positive pressure ventilation. With an external mask, a seal is created to isolate the mouth and nose and force positive pressure air into the airway. In a supraglottic airway, the seal is created internally around the glottic opening. Positive pressure air is therefore forced into the trachea. Creating this internal seal also adds a level of protection to the glottic opening. As long as the seal is maintained, the glottic opening is reasonably protected from secretions and foreign matter.

Most supraglottic airways are size dependent and must be matched to an appropriately sized patient. Supraglottic airways somewhat limited by the fact that they are not intended for high airway pressures and can dislodge when pressures exceed 30 mmHg. Movement of the patient can also frequently dislodge this type of airway. Positive confirmation is also achieved by visualizing chest rise and the ability to ventilate the patient. $ETCO_2$ monitoring can also be used for definitive confirmation.

BIADs can be an excellent alternative to intubation. Although they do not secure the airway as well as intubation, in many situations BIADS may be the preferred method of airway management. We have already discussed the advantages of using a BIAD in cardiac arrest care, but consider also situations in which intubation may be difficult or suboptimal. For example, instead of attempting a difficult, out-of-position intubation on a person trapped in a car, why not insert a BIAD and intubate later when conditions are more favorable? As with any device, BIADs are simply another tool to consider as the airway management decision is made.

CONCLUSIONS

Although a paramedic can use many tools during airway management, the most important tool to use is the brain. Gone are the days of cookbook airway management in which one intervention is applied universally. Proper airway management requires a careful combination of critical thinking and patient assessment. Airway procedures should be used based on what is best for the patient and what outcome is most important.

TRANSITIONING

REVIEW ITEMS

1. Which of the following rationales would be an appropriate reason to escalate to endotracheal intubation in airway management?
   a. The airway is unsecure; thus, a tube is necessary.
   b. We have been using a BIAD for a long time, and now a tube must be placed.
   c. Basic maneuvers have failed to establish a patent airway.
   d. Intubation is always used in cardiac arrest patients.

2. Which of the following is the most significant risk of endotracheal intubation?
   a. unrecognized esophageal intubation
   b. rising intracranial pressure
   c. trauma to the airway
   d. cervical spine movement

3. Which of the following would best describe why intubation should not be used initially in cardiac arrest care?

   a. Intubation causes bradycardia.
   b. Intubation interrupts chest compressions.
   c. Intubation can drop blood pressure.
   d. Intubation can cause a rise in intracranial pressure.

4. Which of the following patients would be the best candidate for endotracheal intubation?
   a. an 81-year-old woman in cardiac arrest
   b. a 22-year-old suffering from airway burns
   c. a 59-year-old man with decreasing mental status
   d. a 42-year-old man trapped in a vehicle with poor air movement in his chest

5. Which of the following would be described as an esophageal obturation type of BIAD?
   a. an endotracheal tube
   b. a laryngeal mask airway
   c. a Cobra PL airway
   d. a King airway

APPLIED PATHOPHYSIOLOGY

1. Describe three general risks of invasive airway maneuvers.

2. Describe three general benefits of invasive airway maneuvers.

3. Describe two steps you can take to help preserve ETI in the paramedic scope of practice.

4. Describe a situation in which a blind insertion airway device would be more appropriate than ETI.

CLINICAL DECISION MAKING

You are assessing a 65-year-old female patient with chronic obstructive pulmonary disease (COPD). Her family says that she has had shortness of breath for three days, but "she is much worse today." You find the patient sitting upright, looking scared, and unable to speak.

1. What indications does your general impression give you that this woman's condition may be critical?

Your patient has a patent airway and is breathing 48 times per minute. She has lung sounds bilaterally but is moving little air, with a prominent wheeze. Her radial pulse is 128, her skin is wet, and she is confused (this is not her normal state).

2. Is this patient in respiratory distress or respiratory failure? Please discuss why you feel this way.

3. Based on your primary assessment, are any immediate interventions necessary? If so, what are they?

4. Explain the pathophysiologic cause for the following:
   a. Confusion
   b. Wheezing
   c. Increased heart rate

The family reports to you that the patient also has a history of acute pulmonary edema secondary to congestive heart failure (CHF).

5. Based on your primary survey, is it important to determine if this patient is currently in APE or exacerbated COPD? Why or why not?

6. If you determined that this patient was in APE, how would it change your immediate interventions?

TOPIC

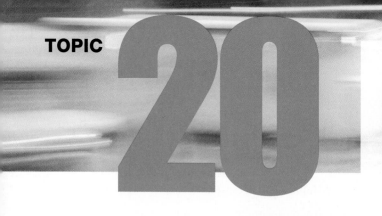

Standard Patient Assessment

Competency Applies scene information and patient assessment findings (scene size-up, primary and secondary assessment, patient history, reassessment) to guide emergency management.

CRITICAL THINKING

TRANSITION highlights

- *Definition of critical thinking and how it relates to the paramedic.*
- *Difference between clinician and technician as it pertains to the role of critical thinking in the prehospital environment.*
- *Importance of determining patient life threats.*
- *Developing a differential diagnosis based on assessment phases and assessment findings:*
  - *Scene size-up.*
  - *Primary assessment.*
  - *Secondary assessment.*
  - *Reassessment.*
  - *Monitoring devices.*
- *Constructing care plans based on the paramedic's assessment findings and differential diagnoses.*

INTRODUCTION

The ability to think critically is desired by EMS providers at every level—and may largely be a measure of clinical success. However, the concept is not easily defined, quantified, or taught.

Your initial EMT class presented a patient assessment process to you that looked like a neat diagram. You likely thought that was the way assessment would go. Experience has taught you that those guides were just that—guides—and that many variables are considered in assessment. In your advanced-level classes, pathophysiology was introduced to your assessment and your questions began to take on a deeper purpose. You were no longer just the "eyes and ears of the hospital" but rather were now gathering information for making patient care decisions. You now began to understand why you were asking the questions.

With new skills and medications, you also realized that new and different clinical decisions must be made for each patient.

When it comes to assessment, different paramedics could assess the same cardiac patient, and there would be just as many ways to ask the history questions and do a physical assessment. The only steadfast rule is to address life threats first.

As an introduction, consider the following example of how you may use critical thinking in everyday life. It is not limited to medicine.

While starting your car, it did not want to start up. When the car finally started, it ran rough. It bucked and sputtered. Then the "check engine" light came on. You are about to go on a long drive, so you had to make a decision or two.

The car was relatively new and well maintained. There were no odors, no unusual sounds, and no stains on the floor indicating leaking fluids. The gas gauge was between one-quarter full and empty. The weather had been rainy for weeks.

You questioned whether you should take the car on the trip or bring it to the shop. You decided that driving it would not cause damage. Bringing it to the shop would cost hundreds in diagnostics, which you did not want if they were unnecessary.

You decide to drive your car to a gas station, put in some dry gas, and fill the tank. After doing that, you drive it around town for a few minutes to see if the car runs better. It does. The "check engine" light turns off, and you go to the meeting uneventfully.

This real-life example demonstrates the components of a critical thinking process: identifying a problem (chief complaint), gathering facts (history and physical exam), identifying possibilities and narrowing these possibilities to probabilities (differential diagnosis), developing a plan, evaluating risks versus benefits, and implementing the plan.

This topic focuses on the thinking process—that is, how to get to the treatment choices, rather than on the treatment itself.

CRITICAL THINKING DEFINED

Chapman et al., in *Rosen's Emergency Medicine* (Elsevier, 2001), describe the critical thinking process as having three parts: medical inquiry (history, physical exam, and diagnostic testing), clinical

TECHNICIAN VERSUS CLINICIAN

EMS is summoned by a 73-year-old woman who is having difficulty breathing. The crew arrives to see the woman sitting in the tripod position, with her feet dangling over the side of her bed. She states that she suddenly developed difficulty breathing.

While obtaining a pertinent history and administering oxygen, the patient's medications of Duovent and Nasonex are discovered. The patient responds that her doctor recently gave her the medications for allergies. She said that she went to the doctor for wheezing about 10 days ago. Her only history is that of hypertension, for which she has not refilled her prescription in some time.

She does, in fact, have some scattered wheezes, and her blood pressure is on the high side.

From this point on, the technician and clinician take different approaches.

The technician hears wheezes, notes that there is a treatment for recently diagnosed wheezes, and either administers the inhaler or provides albuterol by small-volume nebulizer.

The clinician uses a differential diagnostic process to identify causes for the patient's condition. Through this process, and the accompanying respiratory and cardiac workup, it is determined that the patient has had a recent weight gain, complained about abdominal fullness, had difficulty breathing when walking up stairs at home, and began sleeping in her chair because of orthopnea. She quit smoking many years ago and denies occupational or other exposure to respiratory toxins.

This information, combined with the history of hypertension—a risk factor for heart failure—led the clinician to correctly determine that the patient was experiencing acute pulmonary edema secondary to heart failure and to begin appropriate therapy. The earlier diagnosis of allergies was made based on the early presence of wheezing—which is also an early sign of congestive heart failure (CHF). Knowledge of pathophysiology is a crucial foundation to an effective differential diagnostic process.

Note that the technician-versus-clinician discussion is not an attack on any specific level of provider. In fact, technicians and clinicians are both found within each level of provider.

A paramedic who is a thinking clinician is able to identify patients who are stable or unstable and require prompt transport. The paramedic/clinician also makes decisions such as when to call for support or air-medical evacuation, when to perform a rapid extrication, and when to immobilize the patient before removing him from the vehicle.

In most cases, clinicians are not created in class—they are developed on the street through experience, continuing education, and clinical mentoring.

Regardless of your level of training, strive to be a clinician.

---

decision making (a cognitive process that evaluates information to diagnose or manage a patient's condition), and clinical reasoning, which involves both medical inquiry and clinical decision making.

In fact, proper decisions are made only after evaluating necessary, accurate information. The relationship between decision making and reasoning is a continuous process—a feedback loop, rather than a straight line from assessment to care. New information is evaluated as it is obtained and applied to the body of knowledge about the patient's condition and filtered through practicality, risks, and benefits.

The concept of critical thinking is more than a process; it is a mind-set. As part of this discussion, it is a good time to revisit the difference between a technician and a clinician. In context to this topic, the ability to apply clinical reasoning to a patient problem belongs exclusively to the clinician.

A technician is not expected to use high levels of reasoning skills. Technicians are strictly protocol driven and respond in a specific way when a certain group of signs and symptoms appears.

Clinicians, however, gather pertinent information from many sources, evaluate that information carefully, and develop a treatment plan from protocols or a series of protocols that will benefit the patient (see "Technician Versus Clinician").

THE PARAMEDIC AS CLINICIAN

There is a difference between a clinician and a technician in EMS. Part of the difference involves the amount of training and experience possessed by a provider. The second, and perhaps the most important, is the mind-set of the clinician.

The clinician is not satisfied by observing superficial information or apparent patterns. Clinicians look at each patient as a challenge or puzzle and seek out pertinent assessment information, even about patients who appear to have an obvious presenting problem.

Consider a challenging patient presentation and a decision you may have to make as a paramedic. You are called to a patient with respiratory distress. The patient has a history of CHF and chronic obstructive pulmonary disease (COPD). You have the ability to administer medications that would be appropriate for both these conditions, but how will you know which condition to treat? Assessment and thinking will get you there.

Look at this from another perspective—yours, as a patient. Who would you want for your primary care provider? Would you want someone who came in, did a few perfunctory tests, and made an assumption and a treatment decision based on this scant information? Or would you prefer the person who listened to you, considered a variety of possibilities (differential diagnosis, discussed later), looked to find the most likely cause of your condition, and tested and treated you accordingly? Like most people, you would choose the latter, the clinician.

TREAT LIFE THREATS FIRST

The primary assessment is vitally important. EMT class does not prepare students for the critical patients who will be seen and the immediate interventions necessary for their survival. Advanced training now adds other modalities, such as advanced airways, that can distract from these vital initial steps of ABC. In fact, opening the airway, checking for breathing, and looking for and controlling bleeding are a small portion of this initial process.

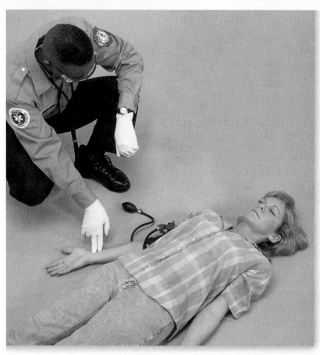

Figure 20-1 The primary assessment must be completed before any diagnostic steps are taken.

> **The differential diagnostic process is fueled by solid initial training, quality continuing education, field experience, and clinical mentoring.**

The primary assessment (▶ **Figure 20-1**) is a foundation for the entire call and cannot be completed without touching the patient. Something as simple as noticing cool, moist skin and a rapid pulse early in the call alerts you to shock long before taking vital signs.

During the primary assessment, you should also be able to identify breathing problems (this requires exposing the patient, a stethoscope, and, in some cases, palpation or percussion), including pneumothorax, open chest injury, and inadequate breathing; identify shock (by a quick note of skin condition, pulse rate, and quality); and decide whether the patient is a load-and-go priority.

Patient care is part of this early process, including oxygen, ventilation, bleeding control, and care for shock if necessary.

THE DIFFERENTIAL DIAGNOSTIC PROCESS

Even though we are not given the full spectrum of diagnostic modalities that in-

hospital clinicians have, we do have an ever-expanding toolbox and a significant arsenal of treatments to employ based on our assessment findings. Sometimes called a *presumptive* or *field diagnosis*, differential diagnosis is an important responsibility because the clinician makes treatment decisions based on it.

The differential diagnostic approach is a hallmark of advanced-level providers. The modalities you are allowed to perform are based on sound assessment and decisions leading to a valid differential diagnostic process. This process is fueled by solid initial training, quality continuing education, field experience, and clinical mentoring at any level of EMS certification or licensure.

Consider the following case: You are called to a patient who complains of chest pain (▶ **Figure 20-2**). The 55-year-old man has a history of angina and hypertension. He describes the pain as slightly to the left of center of his chest, tearing in nature, and radiating to his throat. It is different from any angina he has had in the past. He

took one nitroglycerin tablet without relief. You complete his vital signs and find that his pulse is 104, blood pressure 180/104 mmHg, respirations 20 and slightly labored. His skin is warm and slightly moist.

Following protocol, you would likely have the ability to administer a second and a third nitroglycerin tablet.

But is this truly cardiac pain?

The clinician listens to the patient and gets a thorough description of the pain. Although it appears to be cardiac because of the radiation to the throat, it is atypical for the patient and thus worthy of additional assessment.

To be most effective, the provider—at any level—uses a differential diagnostic approach. In this approach, the provider develops a list of possible causes of the chest pain. This might include myocardial infarction, pneumonia, pneumothorax, pulmonary embolus, proximal aortic dissection, and trauma (rib fracture, muscle pull).

Methods of evaluating and narrowing possibilities down to probabilities exist at all levels of EMS practice for those who think like clinicians. Even if treatment options for each condition are not available, the information obtained from the examination will allow you to promptly alert the hospital about potentially serious conditions.

The goal of the differential diagnostic process is to narrow a wide range of possibilities down to probabilities. Consider the following to either rule out or include any of the following in this patient's differential diagnosis:

Differential Diagnosis	Include in or Exclude from Presumptive Diagnosis by:
Cardiac event (ischemia, infarct)	Detailed history Absence of finding other conditions during assessment process
Pneumonia	Fever, chills, malaise Cough, may be productive Gradual onset
Pneumothorax	Sudden onset (spontaneous pneumothorax) Lung sounds Pain may be pleuritic
Proximal aortic dissection	Pain characteristic (location, description) Difference in radial pulse strength, quality Blood pressure differences between arms
Pulmonary embolus	Recent immobilization Pain or discomfort in legs (deep vein thrombosis)
Trauma	History of injury (fall, lifting) Description of pain Pain on palpation or movement

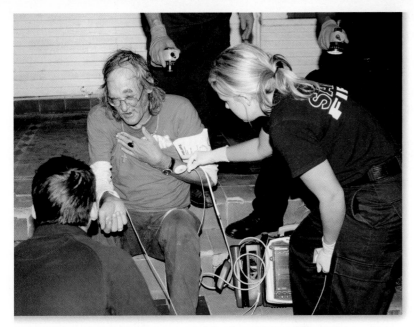

Figure 20-2 Chest pain is one complaint for which a differential diagnostic approach is important.

After development of the list of differentials, the actual exams and history items do not add significant initial time and are clinically very relevant.

The patient denies trauma. The area is nontender to palpation. He denies immobilization, fever, cough, or other illness. Lung sounds are present, clear, and equal bilaterally. The exam reveals a radial pulse deficit, with a blood pressure in the left arm now at 180/100 mmHg, whereas the pressure in the right arm is 130/80 mmHg.

Your presumptive diagnosis now shifts to an ascending aortic aneurysm. Suddenly, aspirin and a second nitroglycerin tablet are not looking as appealing as they did a few minutes ago.

This process is not without pitfalls, of course. The clinician must also know the pitfalls and balance risk versus benefits appropriately (the clinical reasoning process). For example, it has been reported that 10 percent to 15 percent of patients who have myocardial infarction have pain that is reported as pleuritic or affected by movement. It would be unwise to rule out any condition or to advise against treatment and transport based on any single finding. The clinician should also realize that ascending aneurysms occur in an extremely small percentage of the population. One should not expect to see that a lot—but it is crucial to be able to identify it when it is present.

ASSESSMENT: AN ONGOING PROCESS

An experienced provider realizes that rarely will the first planned assessments be enough. The finding from the first assessments will bring up additional questions— or even take the provider in an entirely different direction (▶ Figure 20-3).

New paramedics like it when a question is answered. Experienced paramedics like it when a question brings about two more questions.

In fact, the assessment process is dynamic and directly linked to the differential diagnostic process described previously. Although it is not the scope of this topic to discuss every possible history and assessment technique, the following are some high-yield favorites:

- **In the SAMPLE history, look for key information**—especially in "events." It is last in the old SAMPLE sequence but among the first in importance. Especially valuable in cases involving altered mental status, the events can be an important piece of the puzzle in building a clinical case for seizure versus simple fainting versus more serious pathologies. Specifically, probe for prodromal signs and symptoms such as dizziness, weakness, palpitations, changes in skin color, temperature, and condition before the episode, and whether the patient was able to lower himself to the ground or dropped like a rock. Often, patients will be able to describe a feeling of their vision closing in, described as a blackout or "whiting out."

- **Listen to lung sounds properly and in a setting where it is possible to hear them.** Although we wish to make diagnostic decisions based on these sounds, the assessment performed is often inadequate. Many providers listen to lung sounds over one or two locations (often only anteriorly), and that is all. Lung sounds must be listened to for a full cycle and in multiple locations. The patient should breathe

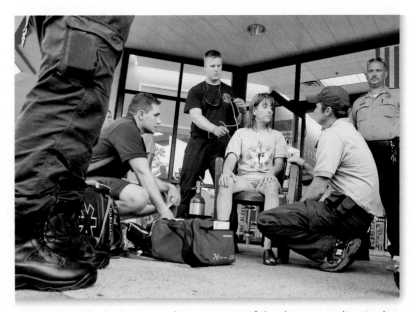

Figure 20-3 The history provides a majority of the diagnostic clues in the medical emergency.

in and out deeply with the mouth open. With wheezes and other lung sounds, it is incomplete to note merely that they are present; it should also be noted where in the respiratory cycle these sounds are heard. Because of the structure of the lungs, if you have not auscultated posteriorly, you have not heard the lower lobes.

- **Use orthostatic vital signs— safely.** Orthostatic vital signs are somewhat misunderstood and are often misapplied. The general concept is to take the vital signs of a supine patient. Ideally, the patient should have been supine for about 10 minutes prior to the exam. Have the patient stand, and take the vital signs immediately. Take them again 2 minutes later. Pulse elevation of 10 to 20 beats per minute or blood pressure decrease of 10 to 20 mmHg may indicate blood or other significant volume loss. Be sure to support the patient. If the patient feels dizzy or faint, stop the test and consider it positive. Rates indicating hypovolemia may vary in the elderly and in those taking medications that slow the pulse, such as beta blockers.

- **Consider risk factors.** This is a standard practice for in-hospital clinicians but is used less in the field. Smoking, diabetes, obesity, hypercholesterolemia, and hypertension are all significant risk factors for myocardial infarction and stroke. Even though these are not the definite smoking gun we would like for diagnosis, when weighted properly they may make the difference in some precautionary treatment and transport decisions.

EMBRACE CONTRADICTIONS AND CHALLENGES

If every patient came with a diagnosis, EMS would be boring. Patients often throw us curves—and only the clinicians among us are there to catch them. Remain open to the fact that patients may have coexisting conditions. Pneumonia and urinary tract infections are common causes of sepsis. Medications mask the reactions to illness and injury. Geriatric patients present differently in many disease states. Occasionally the patient's complaint is not even the most serious problem you uncover.

It is up to the clinician to determine what findings are important, and in what proportion.

DEVELOP CAREFUL, STRATEGIC, DYNAMIC CARE PLANS

To many providers, especially those new to their level of certification, care is about performing modalities. Experienced providers, however, know that care is a carefully balanced event. It is balanced between need and risk, standing order and online consult, and present need at the scene versus consideration of hospital care down the line. In some cases, oxygen and calming are prudent, powerful treatments.

Care plans fit into the continuum of clinical reasoning in that constant monitoring for therapeutic benefit or adverse reaction is necessary—and that the patient's response to a particular modality may be diagnostic.

Each patient contact is a clinical mystery waiting to be solved and an educational experience that builds the foundation of a true clinician.

TRANSITIONING

REVIEW ITEMS

1. The concept of differential diagnosis is best described as narrowing _____.
   a. probabilities to probabilities
   b. possibilities to probabilities
   c. chief complaint to differentials
   d. differentials to diagnostics

2. Which of the following is *not* part of the clinical thinking process?
   a. clinical reasoning
   b. medical inquiry
   c. clinical decision making
   d. ethical inquiry

3. The difference between a technician mind-set and a clinician mind-set is best described as follows:
   a. The clinician identifies a narrow pattern of signs and symptoms and provides scripted treatment protocols, whereas the technician synthesizes information from various sources and applies treatments from protocol or protocols as necessary.
   b. The technician identifies a narrow pattern of signs and symptoms and provides scripted treatment protocols, whereas the clinician synthesizes information from various sources and applies treatments from protocol or protocols as necessary.
   c. Technicians rarely use online medical direction, largely depending on protocols and assessment findings to determine care plans. Clinicians are driven mostly by online medical direction.
   d. Clinicians are most closely related to the Advanced Practice Paramedic concept and have skills and knowledge similar to those of physician extenders.

4. Differential diagnosis possibilities for respiratory distress would likely include all of the following *except* _____.
   a. myocardial infarction
   b. pulmonary embolus
   c. cerebrovascular accident
   d. COPD exacerbation

5. Orthostatic hypotension is defined as a(n) _____ of _____ beats per minute in pulse.
   a. increase, 5–10
   b. decrease, 5–10
   c. increase, 10–20
   d. decrease, 10–20

6. To auscultate the lung bases you must listen _____.
   a. anteriorly
   b. laterally
   c. medially
   d. posteriorly

7. How are risk factors used as part of differential diagnosis?
   a. To confirm that a condition is present
   b. As backup to differential diagnosis
   c. As a factor to weigh into the differential diagnosis
   d. Risk factors are not a significant factor in differential diagnosis.

8. Which of the following should be performed as part of a primary assessment/life threat determination?
   a. obtaining a blood pressure
   b. palpating the femur
   c. obtaining a history of current events
   d. administering oxygen

9. Determining the exact details around a syncopal episode would be done during which part of the SAMPLE history?
   a. signs and symptoms
   b. allergies
   c. pertinent past history
   d. events

10. Differential diagnosis for chest pain might include all of the following *except* _____.
    a. hypertension
    b. aortic aneurysm
    c. pulmonary embolus
    d. pneumonia

APPLIED PATHOPHYSIOLOGY

You are called to a patient with an altered mental status. You begin a differential diagnostic process and come up with the possible causes listed in the following table. For each cause, list the pathophysiologic processes that could cause altered mental status. Hypoglycemia is included as an example in the first row.

Potential Cause of Altered Mental Status	Pathophysiology
Hypoglycemia	The brain cannot tolerate a lack of glucose as a fuel even for a short time. Hypoglycemia causes brain cell dysfunction.
Stroke	
Sepsis	
Seizure	
Head injury	
Hypoxia	

CLINICAL DECISION MAKING

Your ambulance is called to a motor vehicle collision in which a car has been T-boned while turning left. You are presented with three occupants between the two cars. Two are reporting injury. After performing a scene size-up and requesting an additional ambulance and personnel, your triage leads you to an approximately 20-year-old woman who is lying on the ground. She was the restrained passenger who took the impact directly into her door.

You note between 12 and 15 inches of intrusion into her passenger space. Your primary assessment reveals a rapid pulse and respirations.

Your crew administers oxygen and gets vital signs, while you perform a rapid secondary exam. You note no signs of injury during your exam (the patient denies pain, she has adequate respirations without chest pain or tenderness, her abdomen is soft and nontender, and no bone or spine injury is noted). The patient is upset about the crash but is rational and not anxious.

Vital signs are reported as pulse 124 and regular, respirations 28, blood pressure 118/68 mmHg, pupils equal and reactive, skin cool and dry.

1. What role does mechanism of injury play in your decision making in reference to the patient's initial priority and status determination?

2. How does your knowledge of anatomy help you to predict injury patterns and organ involvement?

3. What do the vital signs tell you about the patient's status? Do you believe the patient is in shock? Why or why not?

4. If you had a local hospital 10 minutes away and a trauma center 30 minutes away, to which would you choose to transport this patient? What factors affect your decision?

Standard Patient Assessment

Competency Integrates scene and patient assessment findings with knowledge of epidemiology and pathophysiology to form a field impression. This includes developing a list of differential diagnoses through clinical reasoning to modify the assessment and formulate a treatment plan.

TOPIC

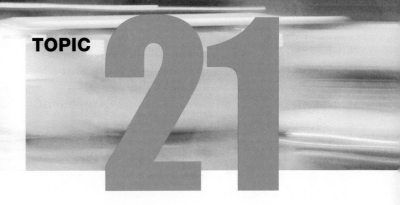

PATIENT ASSESSMENT

INTRODUCTION

If you can learn only one thing in EMS, you should learn to think critically. Critical thinking allows decisions to be made based on the clinical picture presented to you and helps you to prioritize interventions in the best interest of the patient. For the EMS provider, patient assessment is the basis of critical thinking. A quality patient assessment identifies necessary decisions and feeds information into the ongoing cost–benefit analysis. It is, in fact, the most important tool a prehospital provider can use. Just as a chef must learn to use a knife and a barber must learn to use scissors, a paramedic must become an expert in patient assessment skills to truly master prehospital medicine. A skilled provider learns to recognize information from a multitude of sources. They learn that although physical findings and technological readings are important, vital information can also be found by looking at the scene and by talking to the patient. A skilled clinician takes clues from all aspects of the situation at hand. Furthermore, experienced providers learn that patient assessment is an ongoing process and not a one-time event. Injured and ill patients are dynamic, and nature and ever-changing conditions pose ongoing threats. Finally, the most excellent providers learn to adapt their patient assessment skills as new technologies and strategies emerge. They adopt new devices and continually hone their craft to offer the patient only the best prehospital medicine.

This topic is designed to review the key elements of patient assessment. It is not intended to be a comprehensive set of instructions. In particular, the topic focuses on terminology and steps designed to be universal to all types of patients. Although it discusses some of the differences in assessment procedures for trauma and medical patients, this review is designed to be broad based in nature and not specific to a single etiology.

TERMINOLOGY CHANGES

As EMS education evolves, the process of patient assessment is constantly examined. Although the basic principles have remained the same, terminology is updated frequently to reflect the most current educational strategies. This topic will introduce you to the patient assessment process as outlined in the National

TRANSITION highlights

- *Update of assessment terminology to meet National EMS Education Standards nomenclature.*
- *Increased importance of scene assessment.*
- *Review of the primary assessment process.*
- *Importance of a body system approach.*
- *Important questions to ask the patient when assessing a certain body system given the patient's complaint(s).*
- *Importance of performing a reassessment.*
- *Comparison of the secondary assessments for medical and trauma patients.*
- *The importance of trending vital signs.*
- *Reinforcement of the critical thinking and differential diagnosis.*

EMS Education Standards. It is important to note that the terminology used in these standards may differ from the way you were taught in your initial training.

If you took your initial EMT-B class after 1994, you learned a scripted approach to assessment. You likely learned a scene size-up, initial assessment, and rapid trauma exam or focused assessment, followed by a detailed, then an ongoing, assessment. Your advanced classes and subsequent practice likely refined this model.

The National EMS Education Standards do not provide this scripted approach. The standards do include a scene size-up, which is very similar to the existing size-up, and a primary assessment, which is similar to the existing initial assessment. Missing from the standards is the detailed information on executing the subsequent hands-on assessments. The standards do include a

TABLE 21-1	Comparison of the Assessment Flow in Prior Curricula and National EMS Education Standards (Trauma Assessment)

Prior Curricula	National EMS Education Standards
Scene size-up	Scene size-up
Initial assessment	Primary assessment
Rapid trauma exam	Secondary assessment
Focused exam	Secondary assessment
Detailed assessment	Secondary assessment
Ongoing assessment	Reassessment

reassessment, which is similar to the existing ongoing assessment.

For the medical patient, the Education Standards describe a body systems approach. For example, if a patient has chest pain or discomfort, you will assess the cardiac and respiratory systems. A patient with an altered mental status will require the examination of several systems to determine the potential cause and choose the correct interventions.

As an experienced provider, you may notice new EMTs, Advanced EMTs, and paramedics using this updated terminology. It is always helpful to review these new approaches, but remember that the essence of patient assessment has stayed the same. The vital elements you learned and use every day are still essential to quality patient care. Table 21-1 compares the prior EMS curricula terms with the new National EMS Education Standards terminology.

SCENE SIZE-UP

Scene size-up is not new to patient assessment, but its importance cannot be overstated. A quality scene size-up first and foremost ensures the safety of the EMS providers and then provides important clues to the situation at hand. As an advanced provider, you may now be increasingly required to consider scene management priorities as well.

Safety

Scene size-up must always include a safety review. This is true for both medical and trauma patients. Before approaching the scene, a paramedic must consider dispatch information and then rapidly assess the scene for any potential threats. Scene size-up must include an assessment of threats to the crew, to the patient, and to bystanders. All providers must be responsible for identifying threats and taking appropriate protective action. A full discussion on safety is beyond the scope of this topic, but nonetheless, its importance must be emphasized.

Scene Management

As a paramedic, other providers will look to you to lead the call in many cases. As such, scene management may be an important priority to consider immediately. In an incident command model, you may be tasked with providing other incoming units with a size-up. You must immediately identify the number and types of patients and consider the need for additional or specialized resources. It may be important to examine access to and egress from the scene, and organize the response accordingly. Finally, you may need to consider the necessary level of personal protection before approaching the patient.

Scene Management for the Trauma Patient

A significant change associated with scene size-up of the trauma patient is the consideration of mechanism of injury. In the past, mechanism of injury was used as a significant predictor of injury and was a formative part of the early decisions EMS providers made. Now, although mechanism of injury is still part of the puzzle, it is considered of less prognostic value. Mechanism of injury was once a singular factor in determining whether a patient should receive a rapid examination and be expedited from the scene. Under new trauma triage guidelines issued by the Centers for Disease Control and Prevention (CDC), mechanism of injury is actually the third consideration in trauma triage. Examples of the guidelines are as follows (the complete CDC trauma triage decision scheme can be found in ▶ Figure 21-1):

1. **Physiologic criteria.** Does the patient have physiologic signs of instability, including a diminished Glasgow Coma Scale (GCS) score (<14), a decreased systolic blood pressure (<90 mmHg), or respirations <10 or >29 per minute? If so, the patient should be transported to a trauma center.

2. **Anatomic criteria.** Does the patient have anatomic signs of serious injury? These include penetrating injuries to the head and torso, flail chest, multiple long bone fractures, and other significant injuries. These injuries indicate the need for transport to a trauma center.

3. **Mechanism of injury.** Has the patient experienced a fall (adult >20 feet, child >10 feet or two to three times the child's height), ejection from a vehicle, or a death in the same passenger compartment or significant intrusion of damage into the passenger compartment? In many cases, you will have already decided to transport to a trauma center, but if not, these mechanisms will indicate that transport to a trauma center is warranted.

4. **Special patient or scene considerations.** These include the age of the patient, pregnancy, some additional specific injuries, and the judgment of the EMS provider.

Although the significance of mechanism of injury has been reduced, it has not been eliminated. The decision scheme simply places it in a more practical place—and more in line with the way we work in the field. Mechanism of injury still has a primary role in initially determining whether cervical spine stabilization should be maintained.

If your assessment reveals an unstable patient (altered mental status or hypotension), the patient is clearly injured. The same holds true for specific injuries found during assessment. When a patient has a significant mechanism of injury, he may or may not be injured. Research has yet to show a definitive correlation between mechanism of injury and actual injury.

Scene Size-Up and the Medical Patient

As with every patient, you will use a scene assessment to identify clues that may help identify treatment priorities for your patient. With trauma patients, we focus attention on mechanism of injury. With

FIELD TRIAGE DECISION SCHEME: THE NATIONAL TRAUMA TRIAGE PROTOCOL

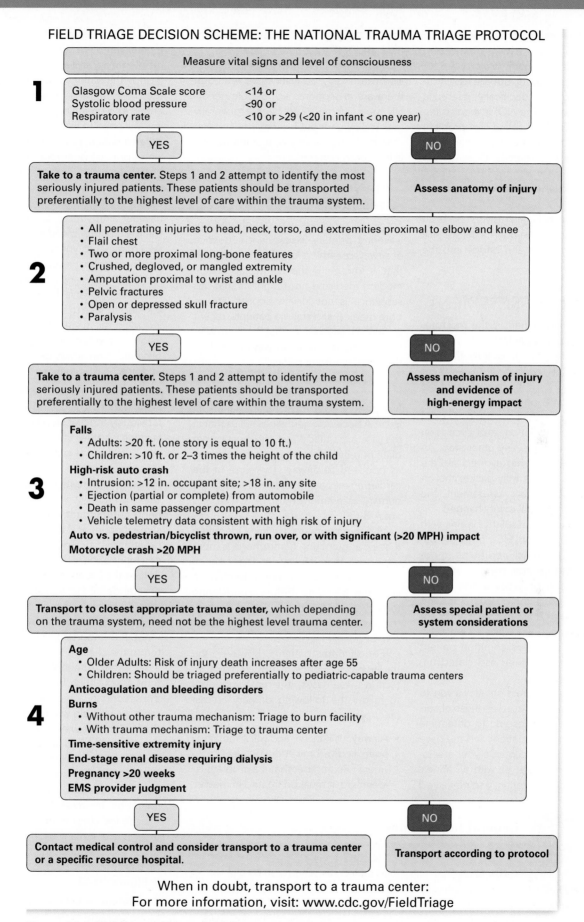

1 Measure vital signs and level of consciousness

Glasgow Coma Scale score   <14 or
Systolic blood pressure   <90 or
Respiratory rate   <10 or >29 (<20 in infant < one year)

YES → Take to a trauma center. Steps 1 and 2 attempt to identify the most seriously injured patients. These patients should be transported preferentially to the highest level of care within the trauma system.

NO → Assess anatomy of injury

2
• All penetrating injuries to head, neck, torso, and extremities proximal to elbow and knee
• Flail chest
• Two or more proximal long-bone features
• Crushed, degloved, or mangled extremity
• Amputation proximal to wrist and ankle
• Pelvic fractures
• Open or depressed skull fracture
• Paralysis

YES → Take to a trauma center. Steps 1 and 2 attempt to identify the most seriously injured patients. These patients should be transported preferentially to the highest level of care within the trauma system.

NO → Assess mechanism of injury and evidence of high-energy impact

3
Falls
• Adults: >20 ft. (one story is equal to 10 ft.)
• Children: >10 ft. or 2–3 times the height of the child
High-risk auto crash
• Intrusion: >12 in. occupant site; >18 in. any site
• Ejection (partial or complete) from automobile
• Death in same passenger compartment
• Vehicle telemetry data consistent with high risk of injury
Auto vs. pedestrian/bicyclist thrown, run over, or with significant (>20 MPH) impact
Motorcycle crash >20 MPH

YES → Transport to closest appropriate trauma center, which depending on the trauma system, need not be the highest level trauma center.

NO → Assess special patient or system considerations

4
Age
• Older Adults: Risk of injury death increases after age 55
• Children: Should be triaged preferentially to pediatric-capable trauma centers
Anticoagulation and bleeding disorders
Burns
• Without other trauma mechanism: Triage to burn facility
• With trauma mechanism: Triage to trauma center
Time-sensitive extremity injury
End-stage renal disease requiring dialysis
Pregnancy >20 weeks
EMS provider judgment

YES → Contact medical control and consider transport to a trauma center or a specific resource hospital.

NO → Transport according to protocol

When in doubt, transport to a trauma center:
For more information, visit: www.cdc.gov/FieldTriage

Figure 21-1 CDC Trauma Triage Guidelines.
Source: Morbidity and Mortality Weekly Report, Vol. 58, No RR-1 (2009).

medical patients, we focus primarily on the nature of illness (NOI). (Considering the NOI is likely a common practice for experienced providers, but the new Education Standards specifically reference this terminology.) The NOI is the first impression of the kind of medical problem your patient has. This can be determined from a variety of sources. Dispatch will begin this process with the information it relays to you. You may also get information from family members or bystanders as you approach. Finally, as you approach the patient and arrive at his side, you will get this information and bridge into the primary assessment.

PRIMARY ASSESSMENT

The primary assessment is the most important element (aside from safety) in any patient assessment. It is truly the one component of the patient assessment that remains consistent, regardless of the etiology or type of patient. For all patients, we must ensure the basic needs of oxygenation, ventilation, and circulation before moving on to any other step. Although terminology has evolved and the acuity of the patient may dictate the urgency of the primary assessment, the basic components have not changed.

The primary assessment begins with a general impression. How does the patient look? This initial step helps to determine whether the patient appears responsive and provides a first glance at patient positioning (e.g., holding c-spine, clenched fist to chest) and general appearance (e.g., pale, anxious). Table 21-2 describes common patient presentations and their associated underlying conditions.

The general impression allows you to gather information based on these observations alone. It helps you to determine the criticality of the patient and the pace with which you will continue your assessment. In some cases, as with an apneic patient or with a potentially spine-injured

patient, the general impression may identify immediate treatment needs.

Remember that the general impression can largely be instinctual. Although there are exceptions, sick people generally look sick and well people generally look well. If your gut instinct is telling you that the person is very ill, that impression is frequently correct.

Sequence of the Primary Assessment

For years, providers were taught the unwavering primary assessment sequence of airway–breathing–circulation. Although that is frequently the correct approach, modern medicine has taught us that this sequence is not always appropriate. In both medical and trauma patients, recent evidence has shown us that there are specific situations in which airway may not be the most important priority.

In apneic and pulseless patients, we have now learned that airway is not the first priority. The most recent American Heart Association guidelines tell us that in the case of cardiac arrest, the most immediate priority is compressions (circulation), as opposed to airway. Therefore in the cardiac arrest patient, the sequence of the primary assessment must be C-A-B and not A-B-C.

In trauma patients, we have identified that exsanguinating hemorrhage is more important than airway. In the case of massive bleeding, you must take steps to stop the bleeding before considering the airway. Again, this is a case in which the sequence would be C-A-B and not A-B-C.

For all other patients, however, the traditional sequence of ABC remains intact. In these cases, it is most important to follow the following primary assessment procedure:

- **Airway.** Is it open, and will it remain open if I divert my attention elsewhere? Remember that if a problem is identified, it must be treated immedi-

ately. Remember also that decreasing mental status is a key threat to airway maintenance, and assessment must include the patient's ability to maintain the airway. If the patient is alert, oriented, and breathing, it is likely that you will need to take no action here. When a patient has an altered mental status or noisy (sonorous or gurgling) breathing, you must open the airway and suction as necessary. This is especially important in trauma patients who have facial trauma or direct laryngeal trauma that may bleed into the airway. As a paramedic, your assessment must also include what level of airway protection is necessary. If the airway is threatened, what is the most appropriate step to take to secure it? This may include basic maneuvers, but may also involve advanced airways, such as blind insertion airway devices or even endotracheal intubation.

- **Breathing.** Is the patient breathing? Is the patient's breathing adequate? Obviously the first step here is to determine whether the patient is breathing, but of equal importance is the assessment of adequacy. Many patients will be breathing but breathing with respiratory failure. The latter patients need urgent intervention in the same manner as if they were not breathing at all. Topic 17, "Airway Assessment and Decision Making," describes the breathing assessment in greater detail, but you should know that this evaluation is an essential component of the primary assessment. It is important also to briefly listen to the chest in the primary assessment. Although you will perform a more thorough auscultation in the secondary assessment, a quick listen now will help you to rapidly assess tidal volume as well as identify any absent or diminished lung sounds. This is especially important in the case of trauma patients, as tension pneumothorax is a deadly but correctable condition. It may also be important to expose the chest to identify accessory muscle use and any injuries or deformities. Of course, the situation will dictate the importance of this step (▶ Figure 21-2).

- **Circulation.** Is the patient circulating blood? A rapid pulse check can quickly answer this question. Consider first assessing a radial pulse, as its presence

TABLE 21-2	General Impressions
If you see . . .	**It may mean . . .**
Patient clutching closed fist to chest: Levine's sign	Chest pain or discomfort usually high on the 1–10 scale and potentially severe
Tripod position	Significant respiratory distress
Anxious or restless patient	Hypoxia
Poor skin color (pale) and condition (moist)	Shock, hypoglycemia

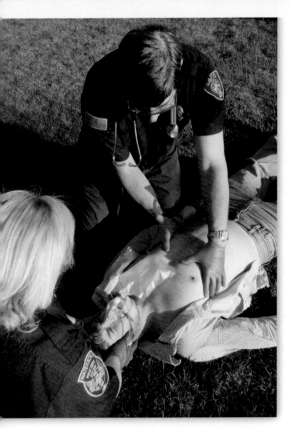

Figure 21-2 Assess the chest during the primary assessment.

gives you some information on blood pressure. Although older attempts to associate a radial pulse with a specific blood pressure have proven to be inaccurate, it is still true that a lack of a radial pulse is generally associated with a poor blood pressure. Pulse checks can also help rapidly identify life-threatening tachycardias and bradycardias that must be dealt with immediately. Look for gross bleeding; remember that this also includes a quick sweep of bulky clothing to identify hidden hemorrhage. Assess the skin; pale skin can be a clue that points to shock. Remember that supporting circulation is essential if deficits are found. This may include cardiopulmonary resuscitation (CPR), bleeding control, and volume replacement when appropriate.

- **Disability.** Disability generally implies a brief neurologic assessment. In most cases, this is completed simply by talking to the patient. What is the patient's mental status? Is the patient able to move his extremities? A more thorough examination will be necessary, particularly in cases of spinal injuries or brain injuries, but at this point you are looking for the immediate life threat.

- **Expose.** In multisystem trauma patients, you must visualize the entire patient in a search for life-threatening injuries. In other patients, you will expose based on situational necessity. For example, you should examine the abdomen of a patient complaining of abdominal pain. Use good judgment to determine the need to remove the patient's clothing.

- **Priority determination.** What are the patient's status and his transport priority? Is the patient stable, potentially unstable, or unstable? At this point, you will decide on your patient's general status and make decisions based on that status. If your patient is unstable, he will be rapidly assessed and transported from the scene, with spinal considerations, to an appropriate destination. Stable patients will be assessed, fully immobilized, and transported routinely to the hospital. The wide range of potentially unstable patients will be treated more expediently than stable patients, who will receive more care on scene than unstable patients.

- **Baseline vital signs/other key assessments.** After assessing the previous elements, it is important to obtain a baseline set of vital signs. This information will not only provide a sense of immediate patient status, but also establish a baseline for later trending. In some systems, this baseline assessment may also include other evaluations such as 12-lead electrocardiogram (ECG) and even blood glucose analysis (particularly in the case of an altered mental status).

SECONDARY ASSESSMENT

The secondary assessment comprises the further evaluation of the patient after the primary assessment has been completed. It is important to note that a secondary assessment may never be completed if more immediate treatment concerns are identified in the primary assessment. For example, if a patient has an

exsanguinating hemorrhage you may never complete a more detailed physical examination, as all your resources may be dedicated to controlling bleeding. That said, the secondary assessment is an important element of any patient assessment and provides a great deal of information to the paramedic's critical-thinking process.

The secondary assessment can be divided into different sections and may be different among different types of patients.

History Taking

Obtaining a patient history is a dynamic process and may be obtained through a variety of sources. Patient history provides us with a wealth of knowledge and is arguably the most important element aside from the findings of the primary assessment. A proper history can not only identify the current problem, but also provide insight into previous problems and provide linkage for how those previous problems relate to the issue at hand. Patient history is an absolute priority in a medical patient (as much of the patient assessment will rely on these findings) (▶ Figure 21-3), but it should not be dismissed in the trauma patient. Although in

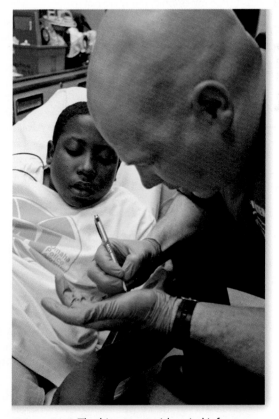

Figure 21-3 The history provides vital information for the medical patient.

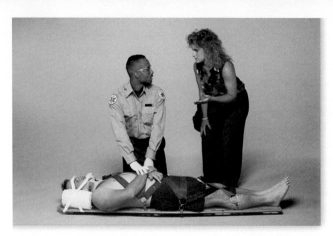
Figure 21-4 Patient history is an important element of trauma assessment.

trauma, physical findings are often more important, patient history can provide valuable information and point out compounding factors that can influence care (▶ Figure 21-4).

It is beyond the scope of this topic to reteach the entire process of taking a patient history. However, the following section reviews some simple steps used to make history taking more effective and insightful. When obtaining a patient history, consider the following:

- **Events.** Because it is at the end of the SAMPLE mnemonic, many do not use this important concept to its fullest. Patients do not always know which things they should tell you. For example, with patients who suddenly passed out, it is important to know whether they were active or sitting. Patients may report that they were standing when they actually just went from a sitting to a standing position suddenly. The patient's activities and observations about the onset are also significant. Patients may recall specific feelings before an event (e.g., "whiting out" or an aura before a seizure). Remember, this is also an important element for trauma patients. Although the mechanism of injury may demonstrate the events, often other factors may have played a role. Although the patient fell down the stairs, for example, was he dizzy with chest pain before the fall? Always carefully explore the events with any patient.

- **Onset.** There is a significant difference in medical diagnosis between gradual and sudden onset. Using respiratory distress as an example, patients who have respiratory distress

with a slow onset, pleuritic pain, and fever likely have a condition such as pneumonia. Patients who have a history of chronic obstructive pulmonary disease (COPD) often have a respiratory infection for a day or several days, which triggers an acute exacerbation. Patients who have a sudden onset are more likely to have an acute condition such as an asthma attack, aortic dissection, or a myocardial infarction (MI). The classic presentation of a patient experiencing a worsening of congestive heart failure is a patient who calls because he suddenly cannot breathe. A careful history usually reveals weight gain, increasing orthopnea, dyspnea on exertion, and edema for days or even weeks before the call to EMS. (It is worth noting, though, that a rapid change in blood pressure can rapidly precipitate congestive heart failure or "flash pulmonary edema.")

- **Medications.** It is not enough to ask about medications or copy down the names from containers you find. Medications themselves often play a role in the patient's condition, for a number of reasons. Patients often self-adjust their medication doses because of side effects or financial concerns. A recent change in medication, especially with antihypertensives and cardiac medications, can cause syncope or other medical problems. Remember to ask about over-the-counter medications. Medications can also affect trauma patients and play a role in traumatic injuries. A patient on beta blockers, for instance, may be in shock, but tachycardic. Certain other medications may make patients more susceptible to heat or cold.

- **Risk factors.** In addition to the traditional information related to SAMPLE, consider other relevant information, such as risk factors related to the current condition. For example, a person with a recent history of a deep vein thrombosis is at high risk for a pulmonary embolism. A

patient with a history of hypertension is at risk for stroke. Risk factors may also include personal habits such as smoking or drug use and even family history.

Physical Examination

The Education Standards organize physical examination around a "body systems" approach. This is true in both trauma and medical patients. Remember that your approach to physical examination may differ depending on the etiology of the illness or injury, but it still should be a comprehensive assessment.

PHYSICAL EXAMINATION OF THE TRAUMA PATIENT In trauma patients you may choose to focus on an isolated injury or rapidly move head to toe in the case of a severely injured person. Table 21-3 describes the different approaches to physical examination of a trauma patient based on patient stability.

It is important to complete a comprehensive physical assessment in trauma patients, as often the obvious injury is not the most life-threatening problem. A body systems approach not only allows to work from head to toe, but also considers the major systems of the body. ▶ Figure 21-5 describes a comprehensive physical assessment of a trauma patient.

PHYSICAL EXAMINATION OF THE MEDICAL PATIENT In medical patients, attention is focused on the system that is likely the root cause of the patient's problem, but other body systems should also be considered to ensure a thorough assessment and to identify additional findings pertinent to the problem at hand.

Table 21-4 describes how a patient's chief complaint can help focus a physical examination toward a specific body system.

In many ways, assessment of a medical patient will combine both history and physical findings. Understanding the pathophysiology of a specific disease process will help guide assessment. Paramedics must understand enough about the specific complaint and possible causes to choose the correct body system exam or exams to perform. In medicine, this is called a *differential diagnostic approach* (discussed in Topic 20, "Critical Thinking"). The clinician thinks of all the

TABLE 21-3 · Secondary Assessments of Unstable and Stable Patients

Secondary Assessment—Unstable Patient	Secondary Assessment—Stable Patient
Purpose: To perform a rapid exam that will help identify major injuries and end with the patient being placed on a spine board.	*Purpose:* To perform a head-to-toe assessment on a stable patient to determine a full picture of the patient's injuries.
Further examination can be done en route if time permits.	*-or-* To assess a single injured area on a patient if the mechanism of injury and chief complaint indicate the injury is isolated.
Maintain c-spine stabilization throughout.	Maintain c-spine stabilization if indicated.
Rapidly examine the following: • Head • Neck • Chest • Abdomen • Pelvis • Extremities • Posterior	Examine in detail (when indicated): • Head • Face • Neck • Shoulders/clavicles • Chest • Abdomen • Pelvis • Lower extremities • Upper extremities • Posterior

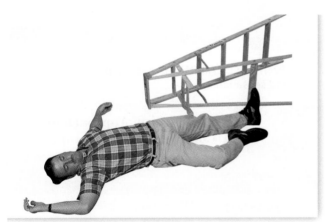

PHYSICAL EXAMINATION OF THE TRAUMA PATIENT

a. Take Standard Precautions.
b. Reassess mechanism of injury (MOI). If it is not significant (e.g., patient has a cut finger), focus the physical exam only on the injured part. If the MOI is significant:
 • Continue manual stabilization of the head and neck.
 • Reconsider transport decision.
 • Reassess mental status.
 • Perform a trauma assessment.
c. Rapidly assess each part of the body for the following problems (say "Dee-cap B-T-L-S" as a memory prompt): Deformities, Burns, Contusions, Tenderness, Abrasions, Lacerations, Punctures/Penetrations, Swelling

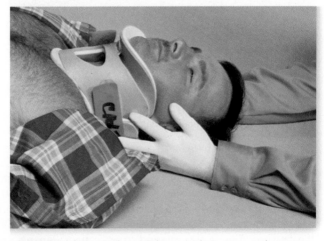

NECK: DCAP-BTLS plus jugular vein distention and crepitation (then apply cervical collar).

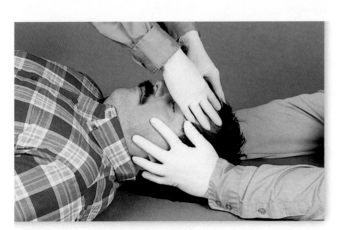

HEAD: DCAP-BTLS plus crepitation.

Figure 21-5 Secondary assessment is a head-to-toe examination.

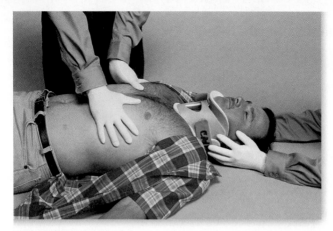

CHEST: DCAP-BTLS plus crepitation, paradoxical motion, and breath sounds (absent, present, equal).

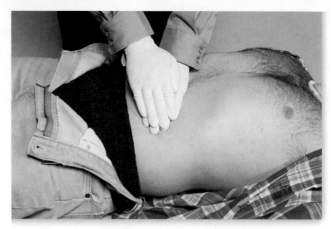

ABDOMEN: DCAP-BTLS plus firm, soft, distended.

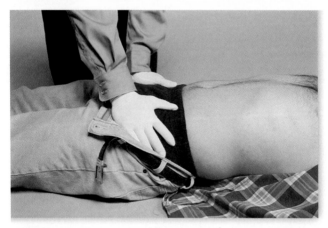

PELVIS: DCAP-BTLS with gentle compression for tenderness or motion.

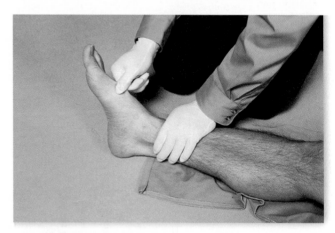

EXTREMITIES: DCAP-BTLS plus distal pulse, motor function, and sensation.

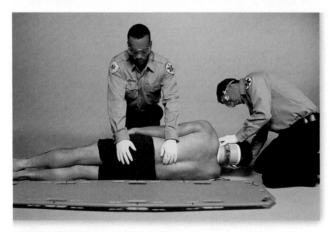

POSTERIOR: DCAP-BTLS. (To examine posterior, roll patient using spinal precautions.)

Figure 21-5 (*Continued*)

TABLE 21-4	Body System Approach to Common Medical Complaints
Complaint/ Presenting Problem	**Body Systems to Examine**
Difficulty breathing	Respiratory Cardiac
Chest pain or discomfort	Cardiac Respiratory
Altered mental status	Endocrine Neurologic Scene evaluation
General malaise	Will require more focused history to determine systems
Syncopal episode	Cardiac Respiratory Endocrine Neurologic
Abdominal pain or discomfort Seizure	Gastrointestinal Neurologic If patient does not come out of the seizure or has an ongoing altered mental status, add endocrine and cardiac

possible causes for a patient complaint (within reason), performs examinations to either rule in or tentatively rule out causes, and makes a treatment decision based on the findings. This is also referred to as going from *possible* to *probable* causes.

In a medical patient, the way you perform a secondary exam will depend on a number of factors, the most important of which is the patient's overall status. Patients who have an altered mental status, problems with the ABCs,

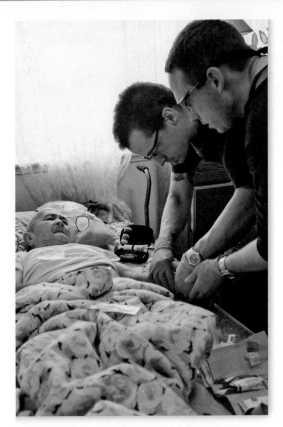

Figure 21-6 The on-scene secondary assessment is expedited when the patient is unstable.

any condition that could lead to instability (e.g., cardiac or respiratory difficulties), or any condition that requires prompt transport to appropriate facilities (e.g., patients with MI or stroke) will be expedited from the scene after a primary assessment and a quick history and physical exam (▶ Figure 21-6). The remainder of the history and physical examination will be provided en route.

In stable patients—and those without critical complaints—you will take more time on the scene to do a complete history and examination.

Vital Signs

Vital signs—or, more important, *trends* in vital signs (see Table 21-5)—are crucial in determining the severity and progression of your patient's condition. The traditional vital signs include the following:

- Pulse
- Respirations
- Skin color, temperature, and condition
- Blood pressure
- Pupils

Although we frequently think the importance of vital signs in trauma patients, obtaining and trending vital signs are of equal importance in medical patients. Consider the following points when assessing the vital signs of medical patients:

- **Watch vital signs for shock.** Although it is easy to think of shock and trauma going together, medical patients can also experience shock. GI bleed, late sepsis, anaphylaxis, and MI are potential causes of medical shock.
- **Pay attention to the respiratory rate.** It is easy to gravitate more toward pulse, blood pressure, and skin color. Respirations are a key vital sign and one of the earliest changes in shock—but respirations will also be an indication of acid–base balance. Patients with diabetic ketoacidosis and those who have overdosed on aspirin (acetylsalicylic acid) will have rapid, deep respirations in an attempt to rid the body of acids.
- **Check pupils.** Pupils may be the only indicator of a narcotic overdose (although not every narcotic causes pinpoint pupils) and may also help alert you to intracranial bleeds that occur spontaneously (as opposed to those from trauma).
- **Trends are best.** Always take and evaluate multiple sets of vital signs.

Pulse oximetry is in such common use that it is frequently considered a sixth vital sign. Use caution when obtaining pulse oximetry readings on patients who are hypoperfusing, however, as the readings are frequently inaccurate. The hemoglobin in the blood may be 100 percent saturated, but this is of minimal value diagnostically when the patient is severely hypovolemic.

Pulse oximetry will likely have a greater role in patient assessment and care, as more protocols specify oxygen delivery amounts and devices based on oximetry readings. Unstable trauma patients and any patient suspected of being hypovolemic will still receive high-concentration oxygen via nonrebreather mask when breathing adequately, and positive pressure ventilation with oxygen when necessary for inadequate or absent breathing.

Vital signs are monitored frequently, depending on the patient's status. Generally, the patient's vitals are rechecked approximately every 15 minutes (and at least twice) when the patient is stable and every 5 minutes when the patient is unstable—transport time and priorities permitting.

Noninvasive blood pressure (NIBP) devices (▶ Figure 21-7) are being used more frequently in the field and are specifically mentioned in the Education Standards. NIBP devices are convenient in that they automatically measure the patient's blood pressure at preselected intervals.

You should always take one manual blood pressure during the call—preferably at the beginning—to compare with the NIBP reading. Because the NIBP is a mechanical device, it may occasionally display an incorrect or erroneous reading.

TABLE 21-5	Vital Sign Trends in Traumatic Conditions					
	Pulse	Respirations	Blood Pressure	Pulse Pressure	Skin
Shock	Increase	Increase	Decrease (late)	Narrows	Becomes cool and clammy
Increasing intracranial pressure (late)	Decrease	Irregular	Increase	Widens	Varies
Anxious, uninjured patient calming down	Decrease	Decrease	May decrease or remain the same	No significant change	Becomes warm and dry

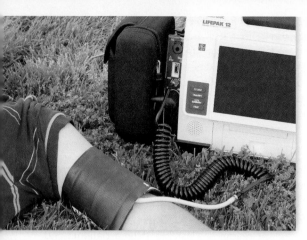

Figure 21-7 Noninvasive blood pressure (NIBP) monitor.

Obtaining an occasional manual blood pressure will help reduce the impact of the erroneous readings, especially in hypotensive patients.

REASSESSMENT

Patient assessment is not a one-time event. Injured and ill patients change over time, and reassessment is necessary to recognize changes that occur in your patient. Reassess your patient frequently. This will help to observe trends in the patient's condition and help you recognize decompensation and worsening problems. In the absence of higher priorities (e.g., suction or ventilating your patient), your reassessment will cover the following components when applicable and time permits:

- Reevaluate components of the primary assessment.
- Reevaluate the chief complaint and/or injuries.
- Recheck vital signs.
- Verify that all interventions are still effective.
- Reassess the effect of interventions performed.

Reassessment should be performed approximately every 15 minutes for stable patients and every 5 minutes for unstable patients when time and priorities permit (▶ **Figure 21-8**).

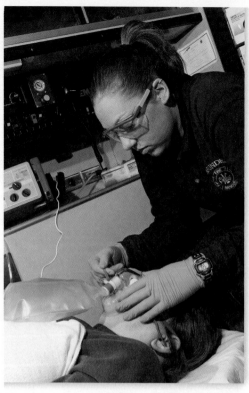

Figure 21-8 Reassessment is done en route to the hospital and performed every 5 minutes for the unstable patient and every 15 minutes for the stable patient.

TRANSITIONING • • • • • • • • • •

REVIEW ITEMS

1. Your patient's blood pressure has increased, his pulse has decreased, and his pulse pressure has widened. He likely has _____.
   a. sepsis
   b. spinal shock
   c. hypovolemic shock
   d. increasing intracranial pressure

2. Pulse oximetry may not be relevant in trauma cases because _____.
   a. hemoglobin no longer carries oxygen when the patient is in shock
   b. the hemoglobin is saturated but the patient has reduced volume
   c. the hemoglobin will be saturated with carbon dioxide instead of oxygen
   d. a special probe is necessary to detect carboxyhemoglobin in trauma cases

3. Observing skin color, temperature, and condition in the primary assessment _____.
   a. helps identify shock early
   b. is primarily a sign of myocardial infarction
   c. is of little value in a medical patient
   d. is primarily used for identifying patients with heat emergencies

4. Your trauma patient is unstable. En route to the hospital, he began bleeding into his airway. You were unable to reassess the patient after 5 minutes because you were performing suction almost constantly. You are concerned because your run report will not contain a second set of vital signs. What should you do?
   a. Note the reason for the single set of vitals in your narrative.

b. Because you saw that the pulse oximeter reflected a pulse, you should use that number and use the other vital signs from the initial set you took.

c. Make up a set of vitals that match the patient's declining condition.

d. Do nothing. It was not your fault.

5. What is the primary difference in secondary assessment between a stable and an unstable patient?

a. location the exam is performed

b. speed of the exam

c. thoroughness of the exam

d. level of responsiveness of the patient

APPLIED KNOWLEDGE

For each of the following body systems, choose one complaint or patient presentation that would cause you to examine it.

Looking at things from a different angle helps learning and application.

Body System	Patient Presentation or Complaint
Respiratory	
Cardiac	
Endocrine	
Neurologic	

CLINICAL DECISION MAKING

You are called to a patient who was stabbed by his wife. You drive to the patient's neighborhood while the EMS dispatcher is trying to determine whether police have arrived on scene yet. As you round a corner, you observe what appears to be the patient out on the sidewalk. He is clutching his chest, his hand bloody.

1. What are the risks of approaching the scene?

2. What do you do to remain safe?

The police arrive on scene quickly and secure it. There is no sign around of the wife. Because the patient is standing at the street, you bring him into your ambulance. He looks anxious and pale. His breathing is labored. He is still clutching at his chest with a bloody hand.

3. Assuming the wound to his chest is the only injury, what would you expect to find in the primary assessment?

4. What care would you perform in the primary assessment?

After your assessment and care in the primary assessment, you perform a secondary assessment, which reveals no further injuries. During transport to the hospital, you perform an initial set of vital signs and then reassess the patient on a regular basis.

5. If the patient were to have a worsening of his chest injury, how would you expect his vital signs to trend?

6. How would you balance any advanced life support care versus assessment and transport? What are your priorities?

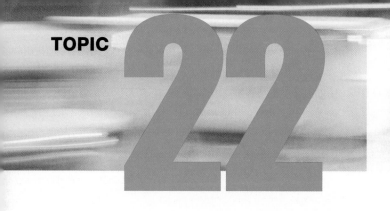

Standard Patient Assessment

Competency Integrates scene and patient assessment findings with knowledge of epidemiology and pathophysiology to form a field impression. This includes developing a list of differential diagnoses through clinical reasoning to modify the assessment and formulate a treatment plan.

PATIENT MONITORING DEVICES

TRANSITION *highlights*

- *Indications, contraindications, and rationales for using common patient monitoring devices in the prehospital environment.*
- *Information provided by patient monitoring devices.*
- *Interpretation of data to help improve or revise a plan of care.*
- *Acquisition of single-lead ECG strips, as well as 12-, 15-, and 18-lead electrocardiograms (ECGs).*
- *Correct use of pulse oximeters, CO-oximeters, continuous waveform capnography, and specialty point-of-care testing units.*

INTRODUCTION

In our fast-paced, technological world, the variety of electronic devices at our disposal increases on an almost daily basis. Medical care a century ago was dominated by the listening skills of the physician. Patient assessment included an accurate history and a hands-on physical assessment, but the cornerstones of diagnostic therapy included a stethoscope, a thermometer, a watch, and a mercury sphygmomanometer. Much has changed in medicine in the past century—and these changes continue today.

Modern paramedic assessment uses a wealth of diagnostic aids (Table 22-1). Patient monitoring devices will never replace a thorough history or hands-on assessment, but the diagnostic data that patient monitoring devices can supply to EMS providers serves to increase the accuracy and reliability of a "field diagnosis." Tools that were once reserved for the hospital are now rapidly becoming part of the front lines of field EMS evaluation and treatment. *Point-of-care testing* is the buzzword for testing performed at the patient's bedside, outside the traditional clinical laboratory.

CARDIAC MONITORS

Since the early days of EMS, cardiac monitoring and defibrillation have been mainstays of advanced life support care. The wonders of modern electronics have allowed smaller and more portable devices over time. Gone are the days of the simple single-color oscilloscope. Today's paramedic can expect to encounter a wide variety of sophisticated monitors that can include everything from simple, single-lead electrocardiogram (ECG) monitoring to multiple ECG leads with invasive pressure monitoring. Common conditions requiring continuous cardiac monitoring in the field are summarized in Table 22-2. A full examination of cardiac monitoring is beyond the scope of this text; however, every paramedic should be competent in the basic skills. Here are some

TABLE 22-1	EMS Monitoring Devices and Strategies		
Cardiac	**Respiratory**	**Other Monitors**	**Point-of-Care Tests**
Single- or multiple-lead ECG monitors	Pulse oximetry	Thermometers (digital and hypothermic)	Cardiac enzyme testing
Diagnostic ECG monitoring (12-, 15-, or 18-lead ECGs)	Pulse CO-oximetry	Blood glucose monitors	Portable laboratory units
	Capnography or capnometry	Lactate monitors	

TABLE 22-2	Conditions that May Require Continuous ECG Monitoring

Chest pain or pressure

Palpitations or suspected dysrhythmias

History of cardiac disease or disorder

Hypertension

Altered mental status

Respiratory difficulty

Chest trauma

Multisystem trauma

Fluid and electrolyte disturbances

Dialysis patients

Syncope/presyncope

key principles of cardiac monitoring to keep in mind:

- Continuous cardiac monitoring is designed to evaluate the patient for changes in cardiac rhythm over time.
  - *Remember:* Cardiac monitors collect data about the electrical activity of the heart, not its mechanical ability. Always treat the patient, not the monitor.
- Modern cardiac monitors may display ECG rhythms in either diagnostic or monitor quality.
  - All monitors contain filters to limit artifacts.
  - Is your monitor calibrated correctly? Most autocalibrate today, but to be accurate, both the paper speed and amplitude must be set appropriately:
    - Standard paper speed for a diagnostic tracing is 25 mm/sec.
    - Standard calibration is 1 mV = 10 small vertical boxes.
  - Diagnostic quality filters show the best representation of the actual ECG rhythm and act as a continuous diagnostic lead strip off a 12-lead ECG.
  - Know the fidelity of your default monitor display; do not overinterpret specific parts of the rhythm (e.g., ST segment changes).
- Select your monitor leads to give you the best information for the given patient situation.
  - Lead II often shows P waves the best and is frequently considered the best for detecting atrial activity.

- Lead V₅ often shows ST segment elevation in the ventricles the best and is often considered the best lead for monitoring ventricular dysrhythmias.
- Lead positioning is important.
  - Consistent ECG interpretation requires standardized placement of electrodes on the body. Exact and appropriate geographic placement is essential.
  - Attach ECG electrodes to lead wires first for ease and patient comfort during application.
  - Apply electrodes over muscle areas, being careful to spread the conductive gel evenly and push down with a slight degree of pressure to ensure good contact.
    Variations in lead position (e.g., chest leads moved secondary to pacing pads in place) should be noted on the tracing (▶ Figure 22-1).
- Skin preparation is often overlooked but is essential for good-quality rhythm strips and tracings.

  - Clean, dry, oil-free skin allows for the best electrode adhesion.
  - Electrodes must be fresh, with intact conductive gel.
  - Do not hesitate to gently rough up the skin by briskly rubbing with a 2 × 2 gauze and/or an alcohol prep.
  - Muscle artifact can be minimized by coaching patients to relax progressively from head to feet. Another helpful tip is to have the patient contract all skeletal muscles tightly for 30 to 60 seconds and then go as limp as possible. During the time the muscles are repolarizing, acquire your ECG.

Telemetry Transmission and the ECG

Although telemetry transmission is not a new concept, the importance of communicating ECG find-

ings in the care of acute coronary syndrome is driving a revival of sorts. Transmission technology varies from system to system. It can include wired or wireless systems and may incorporate cellular and digital communication systems. Unfortunately, many paramedics view telemetry requirements as a distrust of paramedic ECG interpretation skills; however, they should rather view telemetry as an opportunity to add a second and even a third level of interpretation to improve diagnostic accuracy. Many studies have demonstrated that paramedics can interpret ECG tracings accurately; however, more examination always improves diagnostic capability.

Interpretation in conjunction with on-line medical control may further enhance the paramedic's capability when faced with particularly complex rhythms or disease states, especially when treatment options are at high risk (e.g., atrial fibrillation with suspected Wolff-Parkinson-White syndrome).

> Cardiac monitors collect data about the electrical activity of the heart, not its mechanical ability.

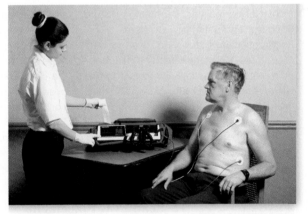

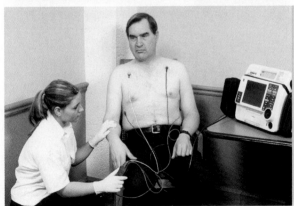

Figure 22-1 12-lead ECG placement.

Documentation of ECG Findings

Documentation is another important element of cardiac monitoring. Most ECG monitors print on thermal-type paper, which fades with time. Inquire whether your agency makes provisions for electronic storage of ECG strips, either by direct upload into the run report or in some other way. When in doubt, it is wise to photocopy strips, as photocopies do not fade in the heat or when exposed to light. Accurate documentation requires two patient identifiers on the strip—the patient's full name and date of birth, at a minimum—for safety.

Diagnostic ECG Acquisition: 12-, 15-, and 18-Lead Monitors

Diagnostic ECG acquisition is the placement of multiple ECG leads in prescribed patterns to collect a standardized tracing. A 12-lead ECG, then, has certain rules for interpretation that allow the paramedic to interpret and diagnose a variety of conditions in the field, including myocardial ischemia, acute ST segment elevation myocardial infarction (STEMI), profound electrolyte disturbances, atrial and ventricular abnormalities, conduction disturbances, and similar problems. The additional data that cannot be obtained over single- or multiple-lead nondiagnostic monitoring are vitally important to the paramedic in many situations, but they can often be potentially lifesaving when STEMI is identified.

Remembering the maxim that in an acute myocardial infarction (MI), "time is muscle" is crucial to the paramedic in the field. Acquisition of a diagnostic-quality 12-lead ECG has been proven in numerous studies to shorten both "door-to-drug" and "door-to-balloon" times in urban, rural, and suburban EMS systems. In many systems, acquisition of an initial diagnostic 12-lead ECG by EMS allows a tiered triage of acute coronary syndrome (ACS) patients to appropriate cardiac interventional centers. Frequently this triage system provides for bypassing an emergency department completely in order to directly deliver the patient to the catheterization lab. EMS and advanced cardiac care hinges on acquisition of 12-lead ECGs in the field to start the treatment process; today's paramedics must be thoroughly comfortable acquiring and interpreting diagnostic-quality 12-lead ECGs.

DIAGNOSTIC LEAD ECG POSITIONING Of great importance in the use of 12-lead ECGs is rigid adherence to standard lead positioning. For example, deviations of one or more intercostal spaces can cause axis changes on the ECG, leading to ECG changes that the paramedic may wrongly interpret as actual pathology when in fact they may be caused by lead misplacement. A standard 12-lead ECG is acquired from 10 electrodes on the body: six unipolar chest (precordial) leads that are placed on the anterior chest to view the myocardium; a ground lead (which may be placed anywhere as a reference point); and three bipolar limb leads that are placed on the distal limbs in the standard reference positions. These standardized reference positions are outlined in Table 22-3.

It is imperative that the paramedic remember that failure to acquire an accurate tracing because of lead misplacement can cause serious problems for the health care team, potentially including inappropriate therapies such as fibrinolytics when prehospital use of these agents is approved under local/state protocols.

For some patients suspected of experiencing certain types of cardiac emergencies, additional diagnostic information can be obtained through the acquisition of 15- and 18- lead ECGs, also known as right-sided and posterior ECGs, respectively. Table 22-4 contains the standard positions for obtaining right-sided and posterior leads.

RESPIRATORY MONITORING IN EMS

Even though most information about a patient's respiratory status is gained through observation, inspection, palpation, and auscultation of breath sounds, respiratory monitoring devices are an important adjunct to collecting data about cellular use of oxygen, oxygen transport, and ventilation status. Two main categories of respiratory monitoring devices are of interest to the paramedic: pulse oximeters and CO-oximeters, which measure saturation of hemoglobin, and capnography/capnometry devices, which reflect ventilatory status.

Pulse Oximetry

Oxygenation monitoring takes place primarily through the use of a noninvasive monitor called a *pulse oximeter*. Pulse oximetry uses infrared light to detect the percentage of hemoglobin molecules that are fully saturated with a substance at each of four binding sites on the hemoglobin molecule. Pulse oximeters have several limitations: they cannot tell what is bound

TABLE 22-3	12-Lead ECG Placement
Lead	**Anatomic Placement**
V_1	4th intercostal space just lateral to the sternum, right side
V_2	4th intercostal space just lateral to the sternum, left side
V_3	Midpoint between V_2 and V_4
V_4	5th intercostal space midclavicular line, left side
V_5	5th intercostal space anterior axillary line, left side
V_6	5th intercostal space midaxillary line, left side

TABLE 22-4	18-Lead ECG Placement
Lead	**Anatomic Placement**
V_4R	5th intercostal space mid-clavicular line, right side (use V_3 lead)
V_5R	5th intercostal space anterior axillary line, right side (use V_2 lead)
V_6R	5th intercostal space mid-axillary line, right side (use V_1 lead)
V_7	5th intercostal space posterior axillary line, left side (use V_4 lead)
V_8	5th intercostal space mid-scapula line, left side (use V_5 lead)
V_9	5th intercostal space paraspinal line (midway between V_8 and the spine), left side (use V_6 lead)

to them (oxygen vs. carbon monoxide or another substance); they do not tell total oxygen-carrying capacity, because hemoglobin values are not routinely measured; and they are influenced by a variety of conditions, such as ambient light, nail polish, exposure to certain chemicals, dysfunctional hemoglobin states (sickle cell anemia or methemoglobinemia), low perfusion states, and others. Use of the pulse oximeter in EMS provides a baseline assessment and can help track changes in the patient's respiratory status over time if trends are used. Like all the technology described in this topic, the paramedic must be a "thinking cook" when evaluating machine values in the face of the patient's clinical presentation.

Pulse oximetry should be considered for any patient with airway or respiratory issues, all cardiac patients, shock patients, and those with altered mental status. As a tool for the paramedic clinician, it allows an estimation of the oxygen reservoir from which the cells of the body have to draw for cellular respiration. The paramedic must remember, however, that as any measurement, it has its limitations, as discussed earlier (▶ Figure 22-2).

Capnography

The opposite side of the respiratory monitoring coin is capnography or capnometry, also known as *end-tidal CO₂ monitoring*. This type of monitoring is relatively new to EMS, having come to the forefront in the past few years. Originally developed in the operating room for monitoring ventilatory status and airway placement, its use in EMS has come a long way from simple monitoring of

endotracheal tube position. Today's paramedics are expected to consider end-tidal CO_2 monitoring as a front-line tool in the arsenal for monitoring the patient with moderate to severe respiratory distress. This noninvasive technology allows the paramedic to obtain several important factors in the respiratory patient: true respiratory rates, because each exhaled breath is measured by the machine; estimates of total alveolar CO_2; estimates of tidal volume and depth of breathing in a breath-to-breath fashion; estimates of total end-tidal CO_2 as measured at end expiration by either a noninvasive collection device or an airway sensor in the patient with an advanced airway in place; and, finally, waveform analysis during capnography of inspiration and expiration, which may provide the paramedic with clues to possible causes of respiratory distress, including bronchospasm, rebreathing, inadvertent extubation, and others.

Pulse CO-Oximetry

The final respiratory monitoring technology that the paramedic needs to be aware of is the pulse CO-oximeter. These units are specialized devices that analyze hemoglobin using infrared light in a much broader way then the standard pulse oximeter. Specifically, these units are able to differentiate between fully oxygenated hemoglobin molecules, partially oxygenated hemoglobin molecules, methemoglobin, and carboxyhemoglobin. Useful in the evaluation of any patient with a known or suspected toxic inhalation injury (e.g., closed space fires, suicide attempts, suspected carbon monoxide poisonings), these units provide a rapid screening tool for several conditions that mimic adequately saturated hemoglobin.

OTHER MONITORS

Other monitors that EMS providers encounter include devices such as thermometers, glucometers, and serum lactate monitors. The advent of low-cost, accurate digital thermometers

has allowed EMS providers to obtain readings of a patient's temperature in the field. Conditions such as heat exhaustion, hypothermia, and flu-like symptoms are obvious cases for which obtaining a temperature is appropriate, but other situations, such as suspected sepsis and certain toxic exposures, also use temperature as a fundamental part of the field workup.

Perhaps the most widely used clinical point-of-care test in EMS today is the glucometer. These electronic units use a blood sample and specially calibrated reagent stick to read a patient's blood glucose. In widespread use by patients and providers alike, glucometers provide a rapid screening method to estimate a patient's serum glucose. For patients, home insulin dosing may be managed with these monitors. For EMS providers, glucose may be administered to the symptomatic hypoglycemic patient, hypoglycemia as an antecedent of altered mental status may be ruled out, and additional therapies may be undertaken per local protocol for the hyperglycemic patient.

A third group of point-of-care testing devices that the EMS provider may encounter are portable serum lactate monitors. These devices, similar to glucometers, detect elevated levels of lactate in whole blood. As a byproduct of anaerobic metabolism, lactate or lactic acid signals that the body is not metabolizing glucose effectively. This often can signal anaerobic metabolism and the development of shock states. Currently, a number of EMS systems nationwide are instituting medical shock protocols that help identify conditions such as sepsis and sepsis shock through elevated serum lactate levels.

Other point-of-care tests that the EMS provider may encounter include serum or whole blood chemical assays for specific lab tests, such as tests for cardiac markers, including myoglobin, troponin, and creatine kinase. These simple tests allow providers to place a small amount of blood on a specially coated test platform, wait a prescribed time period, then read the results. The majority of these kits function similarly to a home pregnancy test kit,

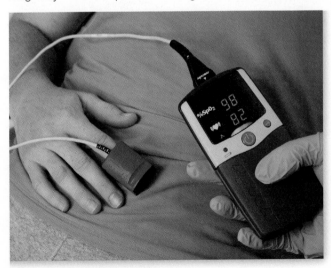

Figure 22-2 **Pulse oximeter.**

with built-in diagnostic/calibration strips. In the future, EMS providers may perform many different tests to aid in the diagnostic process as these technologies become more widespread.

At the more advanced end of point-of-care testing are portable laboratory units. Developed originally for settings such as physicians' offices and the military, these units have started to enter EMS to a limited extent. These units use special cartridges similar to those described previously to perform certain banks of tests, each with its own controls. Some of the tests of interest to EMS providers include cardiac enzyme testing, complete blood counts, blood chemistry panels, lipid panels, coagulation panels, and arterial or venous blood gases. Though not widely deployed in EMS as yet, they offer the utility to certain specialty transport applications of providing almost real-time information about critical care patients that can allow the EMS team to adjust therapies en route.

TRANSITIONING

REVIEW ITEMS

1. Point-of-care testing refers to testing that is _____.
   a. completed at a laboratory
   b. completed as the patient is transferred to the emergency department
   c. completed at the patient's bedside
   d. completed following initial hospital care

2. Which of the following is an accurate description of the role of a cardiac monitor?
   a. It is used to measure the strength of contraction of the heart.
   b. It is used to evaluate electrical activity in the heart.
   c. It is used to measure a patient's pulse rate.
   d. It is used to rapidly identify cardiac arrest.

3. Properly placing cardiac monitor leads is essential to ensure _____.

   a. the ability to assess mechanical function in the heart
   b. the ability to properly defibrillate the patient
   c. an accurate ability to assess blood pressure in the patient
   d. accurate and consistent interpretation of electrical activity

4. Which of the following devices uses infrared light to detect the percentage of hemoglobin molecules that are fully saturated at each of four binding sites on the molecule?
   a. pulse oximeter   b. capnograph
   c. spirometer   d. cardiac monitor

5. Which of the following is measured by capnography?
   a. alveolar CO_2 b. arterial CO
   c. venous O_2 d. serum lactates

APPLIED PATHOPHYSIOLOGY

1. Describe the key elements of skin preparation prior to utilizing a cardiac monitor.

2. Explain the difference between standard pulse oximetry and CO-oximetry.

3. Describe why a serum lactate monitor might be used.

CLINICAL DECISION MAKING

An 83-year-old female nursing home patient is found by staff to be "not acting right." Staff members note her mental status to be altered and say that she "feels hot." On arrival, you find the patient in bed. She is confused, and you note a rapid respiratory rate.

1. Describe the key elements of the primary assessment that would be necessary in this patient.

2. Describe how a pulse oximeter might be useful in the assessment of this patient.

The patient has a patent airway, and she is breathing at a rate of 38 breaths per minute. You have difficulty finding her radial pulse, but *note a rapid carotid pulse at 120 beats per minute. You also note that the patient's skin looks very mottled.*

3. Would assessing the patient's temperature be important, and if so, why?

4. What is the role of a cardiac monitor in this patient?

5. What information would a lactate monitor provide in this type of patient, and why might that information be useful?

Standard Shock and Resuscitation

Competency Applies fundamental knowledge to provide basic and selected advanced emergency care and transportation based on assessment findings for a patient in shock, respiratory failure or arrest, cardiac failure or arrest, and postresuscitation management.

TOPIC

23

CARDIAC ARREST AND RESUSCITATION

INTRODUCTION

Today, the wealth of information on the treatment of cardiac arrest far exceeds that in any other period in the history of prehospital medicine. Research is booming, and new strategies and tactics are evolving rapidly. It is certainly an exciting area of paramedic care, but with this evolution comes distinct responsibilities for providers to stay current and learn how new trends can affect the care they deliver.

Although the data set is still immature, evidence-based trends are driving the modern care of the out-of-hospital cardiac arrest patient. Debates about specific therapies may be ongoing, but immutable truths have begun to emerge. The first and foremost of these truths is that successful resuscitation is centered around quality, uninterrupted chest compressions and that for all the paramedic drugs and interventions, this basic skill is most meaningful.

The second evidence-based truth is that early defibrillation is essential. Research has demonstrated that these two links in the American Heart Association (AHA) chain of survival are most important when considering outcomes. Coupling early defibrillation with ongoing chest compressions maximizes the chance of successful resuscitation.

Many other therapies have evolved around these two truths. A changing paradigm of on-scene care is evolving. Furthermore, we are now realizing just how important postarrest care is as well.

As a paramedic, you must integrate these dynamic changes and recognize that treatment modalities will likely change as research continues on. Although you will most likely be driven by local protocol, it is essential that you understand the best strategies for caring for cardiac arrest.

EPIDEMIOLOGY

Cardiovascular disease is the most prevalent chronic condition in the United States, as well as the leading contributor to death. It has been said that cardiovascular disease is actually a "young person's" disease process that results in "old age" complications. In other words, the way a younger person treats his body

TRANSITION *highlights*

- *Frequency of annual cardiac arrest rates and similar trends over the past several years.*

- *Pathophysiologic changes that occur in cardiac arrest; how quickly cells may become injured and die.*

- *Electrical changes to the heart that accompany cardiac arrest.*

- *Relationship between cardiac arrest and the metabolic changes that lead to cellular damage and death.*

- *Assessment findings indicative of cardiac arrest, and findings suggestive of a patient who may go into cardiac arrest.*

- *Importance of prehospital interventions and why they are successful in reversing cardiac arrest.*

- *The best way to integrate care interventions for a successful reversal of cardiac arrest:*
  - Difference in management of witnessed and unwitnessed cardiac arrests.
  - Provision of high-quality CPR.
  - Automated external defibrillator operation.
  - Proper airway and ventilation.
  - Importance of not interrupting compressions.

in the present time will have a direct impact on disease presence and progression by the time he reaches late adulthood. In fact, with many cardiovascular disease processes, the first clinical indication of its presence may well be the patient's first heart attack, stroke, or even sudden cardiac arrest (SCA).

The statistics representing cardiovascular disease are as alarming as the disease process itself. It has been estimated that more than 62 million Americans have some form of cardiovascular disease (this number does not include those yet to be diagnosed). As the result of cardiovascular disease, 1.5 million people will suffer a heart attack each year, which will result in cardiac arrest and the death of 500,000 of them.

Studies from 2009 indicate that up to 350,000 patients each year suffer cardiac arrest within one hour following the onset of the signs and symptoms, which means that the majority of cardiac arrests will occur in the prehospital environment—in fact, about 60 percent of all cardiac arrests are treated by EMS. In a more sobering light, about once every minute someone will collapse from SCA.

> **About once every minute someone will collapse from sudden cardiac arrest.**

SCA is not always caused by cardiovascular disease. Statistics described previously have shown that cardiovascular disease is the leading cause of arrest; however, approximately 30 percent to 35 percent of cardiac arrests occur because of other etiologies. These include traumatic injuries (head and chest), nontraumatic hemorrhage (gastrointestinal [GI] bleeds, aortic rupture, intracranial bleeds), drug overdoses (accidental or purposeful), and pulmonary embolism.

> **During cardiac arrest, the normal electrical impulses are usually absent or disrupted, or the mechanical response to the electrical impulse does not occur.**

Regardless of etiology, all cardiac arrest patients require the same assessment and treatment goals: rapid identification and assessment, airway maintenance, support of absent breathing, artificial circulatory support, provision of electrical therapy as warranted, and attempts at reversing or remediating the offending cause of the arrest situation.

PATHOPHYSIOLOGY

To better understand the signs and symptoms of cardiac arrest, the paramedic must first understand the basic pathophysiologic underpinnings related to the condition. *Cardiac arrest* (also known as *cardiopulmonary arrest* or *circulatory arrest*) is the cessation of normal circulation of the blood; if this is unexpected (as it often is), it can be termed a *sudden cardiac arrest*.

With cardiac arrest, ventricular contraction is absent or ineffective, resulting immediately in the cessation of blood flow and systemic circulatory failure—in fact, it is the final common pathway to human death. Although it is often difficult to determine the cause of cardiopulmonary arrest at the time of presentation, a working differential diagnosis of the causes can be formulated based on the patient's history, physical examination, and automated external defibrillator (AED) rhythm analysis.

With stoppage of the heart, blood flow ceases and no oxygenated blood is being delivered to the capillary beds of the body. Lack of blood flow initially causes pulselessness and unresponsiveness in the patient, but the lack of oxygen supply to the body's cells results in irreversible tissue damage and death.

All organs have different susceptibilities to ischemic injury from cardiac arrest, with the brain being the most vulnerable. Literature suggests that brain damage occurs after 4 to 6 minutes of normothermic cardiac arrest, and the damage is irreversible. The heart is the second most susceptible organ to ischemic injury. The renal, GI, musculoskeletal, and integumentary systems are much more resistant to ischemia than the heart and brain; these organs rarely sustain irreversible damage in patients who are successfully resuscitated. As such, for the best chance of survival and neurologic recovery, immediate and decisive treatment is imperative.

Cardiac arrest can also be caused by multiple etiologies, either medical or traumatic. As discussed, the primary risk factor for an acute coronary syndrome is coronary artery disease. Although cardiac arrest is commonly caused by an acute coronary syndrome, it can also be caused by myriad other conditions. For example, a traumatized patient may be in arrest following severe head trauma or significant blood loss.

A person who accidentally or intentionally overdoses on his medication may be in arrest owing to the effects of the medication or asphyxia. Even stroke or seizure patients may go into cardiac arrest secondary to permanent brain damage from inadequate oxygenation of cerebral tissue.

It is also important to note the common changes that occur to the electrical conduction system of the heart when a person experiences cardiac arrest, as specific treatment modalities may be necessary based on the heart rhythm. During cardiac arrest, the normal electrical impulses are usually absent or disrupted, or the mechanical response to the electrical impulse does not occur. In most situations of cardiac arrest caused by cardiovascular disease, instead of smooth, coordinated contractions the heart often shows a different type of electrical activity, most commonly the uncoordinated twitching known as *ventricular fibrillation*, which cannot produce any ventricular contraction.

Conversely, in some situations in which the cause of arrest was hemorrhagic or trauma related, the heart might show organized electrical activity without evidence of actual mechanical contraction or blood flow because of the loss of volume or direct damage to the heart muscle itself. The final common pathway in these and other arrest scenarios is that after cardiac arrest has existed for several minutes, the heart will eventually cease all electrical activity and the patient will "flatline" (an electrocardiogram [ECG] rhythm known as *asystole*). Asystole is the least viable rhythm, which most often leads to an unsuccessful resuscitation attempt.

Tissue metabolic concerns also must be taken into account when managing any patient in cardiac arrest. Research has indicated that, during cardiac arrest, the metabolic demands of the cells are no longer being met secondary to the lack of perfusion. Despite this, the cells still attempt to maintain functioning as long as possible with the residual oxygen and metabolic substrates remaining in the adjacent bloodstream. Eventually, the normal cellular activity and ongoing creation of energy (adenosine triphosphate [ATP]) becomes so deranged from a lack of perfusion that the cells cease aerobic metabolism in favor of anaerobic metabolism in an attempt to maintain ATP production.

The consequence of this metabolic shift is the creation of overwhelming acidosis that actually hastens ongoing cellular damage and death. This has a clinical consideration regarding the management of cardiac arrest (the provision of cardiopulmonary resuscitation, artificial ventilation, and defibrillation), based on the estimated downtime of the patient and whether or not bystander cardiopulmonary resuscitation (CPR) was started prior to EMS arrival. These considerations will be discussed more thoroughly in the "Emergency Medical Care" section of this topic.

The discussion thus far has centered on cardiac arrest in the adult patient. However, cardiac arrest can also occur in the pediatric patient—the most common etiologies are acute airway/breathing compromise or body system trauma. In children, the presenting cardiovascular change is typically caused by airway/breathing compromise with resulting bradycardia, which, left untreated, will eventually deteriorate into asystole. However, in about 15 percent to 20 percent of pediatric cardiac arrests, the patient may present with ventricular tachycardia or fibrillation, which is managed with the AED. Thus, the need for rapid defibrillation should be considered in children who meet AED utilization criteria with SCA not preceded by respiratory symptoms.

ASSESSMENT FINDINGS

Dispatch may provide information that will lead you to suspect cardiac arrest. Reports that a patient has no pulse or that emergency medical responders are performing CPR clearly indicate cardiac arrest. But also be alert to the possibility of cardiac arrest in calls to patients with other complaints, including chest pain or discomfort, difficulty in breathing, seizures, unresponsiveness, or serious motor vehicle crashes or other significant trauma.

Often the patient in cardiac arrest is not hard to identify. During the primary assessment, the paramedic will note the patient in cardiac arrest to be unresponsive, pulseless and apneic, and frequently cyanotic. The determination of pulselessness is commonly determined in a large core body artery, at either the carotid or femoral locations. Determining pulselessness can be difficult; therefore, a pulse check should be limited to 10 seconds or less. According to the 2010 American Heart Association Guidelines for Cardiopulmonary Resuscitation and Emergency Cardiovascular Care, unresponsiveness and absence of breathing or absence of normal breathing should be the key assessment indicators of cardiac arrest.

Health care providers perform pulse checks simultaneously with assessment for unresponsiveness and apnea or agonal respirations.

Usually following cessation of blood flow, the patient will lose consciousness within 15 seconds; this may be followed by brief seizure activity. A near-immediate loss of bowel/bladder control may also occur with the onset of arrest. Agonal or gasping respirations may last up to 60 seconds. Pupils also typically dilate within 60 seconds of arrest.

Dependent lividity and rigor mortis, which are also associated with cardiac arrest patients, will not develop for hours after cardiac arrest occurs. If those signs are present, they are indicative of a prolonged downtime; in these cases, the patient should not be resuscitated. The following are the most important clinical indications of cardiac arrest:

- Unresponsiveness (usually occurs about 10 to 15 seconds after the heart stops)
- Absence of breathing or normal breathing (breathing may last up to 60 seconds following arrest)
- No detectable pulse (central)

Historical information gathered from on-scene family or bystanders may provide key information regarding etiology and potential outcome. If the cardiopulmonary arrest is witnessed, there exists a potential for bystander/health care provider CPR, which increases the likelihood of a successful resuscitation. If the cardiac arrest occurs prior to arrival of the EMS, then information obtained from family, bystanders, or other emergency personnel may provide key information that will assist in resuscitation of the patient. Important historical information includes the following questions:

- Was the arrest witnessed?
- How quickly was CPR started?
- Was an AED used?
- How much time passed since the arrest was first recognized (remembering that such estimates are often inaccurate)?
- What was the patient doing at the time of arrest and during the several hours just prior to the arrest?
- What are the patient's past medical history and current medications?

Not all patients with chest pain will experience cardiac arrest, nor will all unre-

sponsive or traumatized patients. What is important to note is that these patients can rapidly deteriorate to cardiac arrest. In these situations, in which the patient is suspected to be in critical condition, it may be best to bring the monitor/defibrillator from the ambulance to the patient on initial approach.

EMERGENCY MEDICAL CARE

Although medical direction and protocol will ultimately determine what interventional steps are recommended or taken, the paramedic should follow the current guidelines for cardiopulmonary resuscitation as written by the AHA. Remember also the importance of the "chain of survival," which underscores the importance of a systematic approach toward cardiac arrest management.

The 2010 American Heart Association Guidelines for Cardiopulmonary Resuscitation and Emergency Cardiovascular Care emphasize the need to begin chest compressions in the cardiac arrest patient immediately and minimize any interruptions once the chest compressions are begun. Quality chest compressions provide around 25 percent of normal circulation and help cells stay alive as the heart arrhythmia is corrected. Appropriately performed chest compressions sustain adequate cerebral perfusion pressure (which perfuses brain tissue) and adequate coronary perfusion pressure (which perfuses heart muscle). Not only are these essential to sustain life, but they have also proven to be at least theoretical predictors of successful resuscitation.

Because of the importance of chest compressions, the standard ABC sequence of initial assessment is altered to CAB in suspected cardiac arrest patients. In cardiac arrest, chest compressions (C) are initiated immediately; after 30 compressions, the airway is opened (A), and the first two ventilations (B) are delivered. This sequence reduces the delay to first compressions and restores coronary and cerebral perfusion pressure as soon as possible. The following are key treatment considerations during the management of a patient in cardiac arrest:

1. Witnessed versus unwitnessed cardiac arrest. If the EMS personnel did not witness the cardiac arrest, immediately initiate CPR beginning with

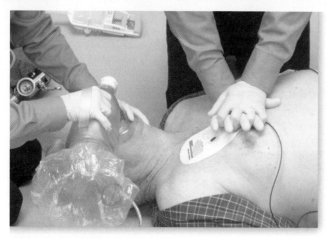

Figure 23-1 Direct ventilation with high-concentration oxygen.

chest compressions. Attach the monitor/defibrillator but continue compressions until you are ready to analyze the rhythm. Cease compressions to analyze and defibrillate if necessary, and then return immediately to chest compressions following the defibrillation (or following the analyzation if a nonshockable rhythm is identified). CPR is then continued in 2-minute cycles (5 cycles of 30 compressions and 2 ventilations). At the conclusion of the 2-minute cycle, the rhythm will be analyzed again and a pulse check performed if an organized rhythm is identified.

If the paramedic witnessed the cardiac arrest, the goal is to defibrillate within 3 minutes from the onset of cardiac arrest (or as soon as possible). As in an unwitnessed arrest, chest compressions should be initiated while the monitor defibrillator is prepared, but they should not delay immediate defibrillation when indicated.

2. Open the airway, insert an oropharyngeal airway, and ventilate the patient with a bag-valve mask and 100 percent oxygen (▶ Figure 23-1). Ventilate the patient carefully, being sure not to exceed the recommended ventilation rate of one ventilation after every 30 compressions (8 to 10/minute). Research has indicated that overventilation (ventilations that are either too fast or deliver too large a tidal volume) is detrimental to cardiac output in arrested patients. Remember, in the cardiac arrest patient, chest compressions precede opening the airway and ventilation (CAB). Adequate resources are often available in the prehospital setting to perform airway management simultaneously with chest compressions. The key is to not interrupt or compromise the effectiveness of chest compressions at any time.

In nonarrest states, blood is returned to the heart via muscular contraction of the muscles that "milk" the veins in conjunction with the one-way valves in the veins' lumina. Blood also returns to the heart via gravity from the head and upper torso and because of the negative intrathoracic pressure created during spontaneous breathing (known as the *cardiothoracic pump*). In a cardiac arrest, obviously the patient will be motionless, which eliminates blood return facilitated by muscular contraction. Furthermore, the arrested patient is typically in a supine position; therefore, gravity cannot facilitate blood return to the heart. Finally, if the patient is apneic and positive pressure ventilation (PPV) is being provided, there is minimal generation of negative intrathoracic pressure during the recoil of chest compressions to facilitate blood flow to the lungs.

Although the first two influences (supine position and lack of motion) cannot realistically be mediated by the paramedic, the third influence (provision of PPV) and its effect on the cardiothoracic pump can be at least minimized by providing ventilations at a rate of 8 to 10 per minute, with a tidal volume just sufficient to achieve visible chest rise. Only after an advanced airway is in place should ventilations be delivered asynchronously to chest compressions at a rate of 8 to 10 ventilations per minute. In support of this, it has been shown through recent research that, historically, the patient in cardiac arrest has been overventilated by care providers, which in turn diminishes cardiac output states during compressions by altering cardiac preload. Ultimately, it was shown that overventilation is negatively correlated with cardiac arrest survival rates.

As a paramedic, you may also have to make a decision about the most appropriate method to manage the airway. Although the airway in cardiac arrest patients is by default unsecure, definitive airway management in the form of endotracheal intubation (ETI) may not be the most appropriate intervention. Even though the net result of ETI is a secure airway, the process of placing the tube likely interrupts chest compressions for an unacceptable length of time. Because chest compressions are so vital to a successful outcome, the paramedic must weigh the benefit of a secured airway against the cost of interrupted compressions. Remember also that blind insertion airway devices such as the King airway and the laryngeal mask airway do not interrupt compressions and may provide a viable alternative to ETI in the cardiac arrest setting.

3. Assess the pulse and provide cardiac compressions. As noted previously, assess a core pulse location for determining whether cardiac compressions are warranted. Traditionally, the carotid pulse is used for this determination, but some research has shown that lay providers and health care providers alike may have trouble determining whether the pulse is present or absent in a hemodynamically unstable or critical patient. Therefore, quickly (maximum 10-second count) assess the pulse (▶ Figure 23-2). This is done correctly by being sure to assess the pulse on the same side as the paramedic, assessing with the fingertips of the first and second digit (do not use the thumb), and never assessing for carotid

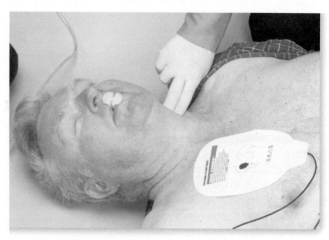

Figure 23-2 Checking the patient's carotid pulse (maximum 10 seconds).

pulses simultaneously on each side of the neck. If the patient is unresponsive, with no breathing or agonal breathing, and a central pulse cannot be quickly located, immediately begin chest compressions. Do not waste precious compression time trying to ensure that the patient is pulseless. Chest compressions delivered to patients who are not pulseless rarely lead to significant injury.

The second concern with assessing the pulse and providing compressions is the fashion in which the paramedic delivers external compressions. Since 2005, the AHA has been advocating "push hard, push fast" to underscore the importance of high-quality compressions in increasing survival rates of arrested patients. It has been well documented in previous research that even perfectly performed compressions can achieve only a small portion of normal cardiac output. It has been more recently documented in the literature that shallow compressions, slow compressions, or frequent interruptions of compressions result in reduced cardiac output, which ultimately translates into poor survival rates. Research has shown that compressions that are delivered at a rapid rate (100/min) and depress the sternum to a depth of at least 2 inches with complete recoil of the chest wall will optimize the effectiveness of compression.

The paramedic must also realize that any interruption of compressions, even for brief periods, causes the cardiac output and coronary perfusion to drop to

nothing. On resumption of compressions it can take up to 45 seconds of constant compressions to return cardiac output to what it was prior to ceasing compressions. As such, always minimize the number of times you have to stop compressions and minimize the length of time compressions have to be stopped (this is also why the compression/ventilation ratio is now 30:2 and why the initial focus in cardiac arrest is on chest compressions).

Advocating and performing the "push hard, push fast" approach to compressions at a 30:2 ratio is correlated with increased cardiac output and is correlated with higher survival rates in arrested patients.

4. Examine other cardiac arrest considerations. Additional CPR adjuncts and interventions may become more commonplace during prehospital management of arrested patients. One device is a mechanical CPR adjunct that will alleviate one person from performing CPR. Because it is mechanical in nature, it may provide more consistent compressions; however, no adjunct to date has been proven to be superior to standard manual CPR (▶ **Figure 23-3**).

5. Consider postarrest care. Cardiac arrest is but a symptom of a larger problem; although it requires immediate resuscitative efforts, paramedics should never lose sight that there is some underlying cause that made the arrest occur. Once resuscitation is successful,

paramedics should rapidly shift their focus toward identifying and treating this cause. The most likely concern (and most likely cause of cardiac arrest) is acute coronary syndrome. Paramedics should consider a 12-lead ECG following return of a perfusing rhythm and also consider transport to an appropriate facility capable of restoring coronary blood flow or treating other underlying causes. Another intervention is the use of therapeutic hypothermia during the postarrest resuscitation phase. It has been learned through controlled clinical trials that by carefully lowering the body core temperature, metabolic demands decrease, edema diminishes, and increased survival rates have been realized. This intervention is implemented into some EMS protocols and, as a paramedic, you may initiate this therapy. Always follow local protocols.

OTHER ADVANCED CARDIAC LIFE SUPPORT CHANGES

The 2010 AHA Guidelines for Cardiopulmonary Resuscitation and Emergency Cardiovascular Care contain several other changes that are significant to paramedic-level care. The highlights include the following:

- **Removal of atropine from the asystole and pulseless electrical activity treatment algorithm.** The 2010 Guidelines state, "Available evidence

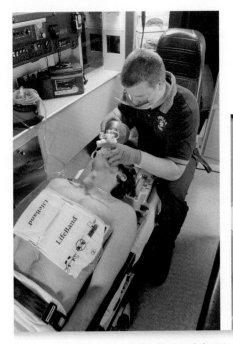
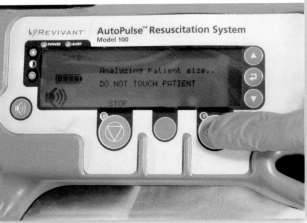

Figure 23-3 The AutoPulse™ Model 100: (A) applied to a patient; (B) close-up view.

suggests that the routine use of atropine during PEA or asystole is unlikely to have a therapeutic benefit. For this reason atropine has been removed from the cardiac arrest algorithm."

- **Waveform capnography in cardiac arrest.** Recent research has shown that using waveform capnography in cardiac arrest care may be valuable. During cardiac arrest, CO_2 is not returned to the lungs; therefore, $PETCO_2$ (exhaled CO_2) will be relatively nonexistent. When chest compressions are initiated, blood flow to the lungs is at least partially restored and $PETCO_2$ should become detectable. $PETCO_2$ therefore correlates well with cardiac output during chest compressions; trending can be used to assess the adequacy of CPR and, according to the 2010 Guidelines, "optimize compression depth and rate and detect fatigue in the provider performing compressions." Abrupt sustained increase in $PETCO_2$ during CPR can also indicate the return of spontaneous circulation.
- **Vasopressin.** Topic 15, "Medication Administration," discussed the role of vasopressin in cardiac arrest. However, in summary, it can be said that vasopressin is a nonadrenergic peripheral vasoconstrictor that also causes coronary and renal vasoconstriction. It is used in cardiac arrest care to provide effects similar to epinephrine (although through a slightly different mechanism). The 2010 Guidelines note:

Because the effects of vasopressin have not been shown to differ from those of epinephrine in cardiac arrest, 1 dose of vasopressin 40 units IV/IO may replace either the first or second dose of epinephrine in the treatment of cardiac arrest. Although there is little evidence to suggest vasopressin performs better than epinephrine, some systems may implement this drug into their prehospital formularies.

Although specific chronological interventions for the management of a cardiac arrest patient in the prehospital environment were not discussed in their entirety, the previous discussion was intended to address the current research and physiology regarding cardiac arrest management and how to maximize the effects of the interventions to improve resuscitation rates. Treatment for the patient in cardiac arrest must be delivered in a timely manner, without error. Failure to do so will invariably lead to lower success rates in patient resuscitation.

When caring for a patient in cardiac arrest, always do your best in each of the interventions you are providing. Remember to "push hard, push fast" with compressions so that the brain and heart can still receive blood flow during arrest management. Ensure adequate ventilations, and provide oxygen during the arrest as well. Minimize the amount of time that CPR is interrupted.

The AED should be used specifically as addressed earlier in this topic so that patients in ventricular fibrillation or pulseless ventricular tachycardia will have the greatest opportunity for survival. Patients in nonventricular fibrillation cardiac arrest should also receive this high level of care so that they, too, may have the greatest chance for survival.

The person with impending cardiac arrest, in cardiac arrest, or just coming out of cardiac arrest is probably one of the most challenging and dynamic patients the paramedic will ever encounter. The situation requires a thorough understanding of the body, application of multiple skills simultaneously, and coordination of multiple EMS providers—all done in the shortest time possible so the patient can be transported to the hospital for definitive care.

TRANSITIONING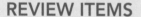

REVIEW ITEMS

1. Of the following clinical findings, which is most reliable for determining whether the patient is in cardiac arrest or not?
   a. unresponsiveness
   b. brief seizure activity
   c. agonal breathing pattern
   d. absence of a core pulse

2. What is the most significant contributor to cardiac arrest in the prehospital environment?
   a. trauma
   b. cardiovascular disease
   c. gastrointestinal hemorrhage
   d. occlusion of a cerebral artery

3. A patient is found in cardiac arrest; no bystanders or family were present. All that is known is that it took EMS 8 minutes to arrive. Given this, the first intervention should be to _____.
   a. start CPR
   b. attach the defibrillator
   c. contact medical direction
   d. initiate ventilations at 12 per minute

4. Which of the following would best describe why a blind insertion airway device (BIAD) might be preferred to endotracheal intubation in the treatment of a cardiac arrest patient?
   a. A BIAD secures the airway more definitively.
   b. Insertion of a BIAD does not interrupt chest compressions.
   c. Endotracheal intubation improves blood return to the heart.
   d. Hyperventilation is more likely when an endotracheal tube is in place.

5. Overventilation of the patient in cardiac arrest can have what detrimental effect?
   a. inability to properly compress the sternum
   b. failures of the AED to read the cardiac rhythm correctly
   c. decrease in cardiac output achieved through compressions
   d. hyperventilation causing hyperoxemia, which damages the central nervous system

APPLIED PATHOPHYSIOLOGY

While nearing the end of your 12-hour night shift, you are paged for a possible cardiac arrest in a 67-year-old man. On arrival at the scene nine minutes later, the family member who found the patient states that he was "fine last night." Currently nothing is being done for the patient, who is in fact pulseless and apneic. The patient is still warm to the touch, there is cyanosis to the fingertips and hands, and no rigor or dependent lividity is present.

1. Should the paramedic initiate CPR or apply the defibrillator first, assuming that both could be done simultaneously?

2. Explain your rationale in support of your answer to the preceding question. What clinical condition or change in the circumstances would have to be present for you to change your answer?

3. Describe the anticipated physiologic benefit(s) for each of the interventions that may be administered to a patient suffering from a cardiac arrest:

   a. PPV delivered at a rate of 10–12/min

   b. Providing compressions at a rate >100/min

   c. Use of defibrillation after CPR has been initiated in an unwitnessed cardiac arrest

4. What three clinical findings are most reliable for determining that an adult patient is in cardiac arrest?

5. What are four or five specific questions regarding the patient's history that the paramedic should try to ascertain as rapidly as possible when confronted with a patient in cardiac arrest?

6. What is the most common underlying etiology to pediatric cardiac arrest, and what is typically the presenting cardiac rhythm in these patients?

CLINICAL DECISION MAKING

You are transporting to the hospital a 59-year-old obese patient with a history of hypertension and diabetes secondary to chest pain. Thus far, you have placed the patient in a position of comfort, administered oxygen via nonrebreather mask, and assisted in the administration of two doses of nitroglycerin. While reassessing the patient's vital signs, he moans loudly and then suddenly loses consciousness. You then witness him experiencing a mild full-body seizure that lasts about 10 seconds. You can visually see the patient is now apneic, and his skin is rapidly becoming ashen in color.

1. Based on the information provided, what assessment parameter should the paramedic determine first, before initiating any other patient care interventions?

2. What cardiac rhythm disturbance does this patient most likely have?

After confirming that the patient is unresponsive to external stimuli and is apneic and pulseless, as you reach for the defibrillator, the ambulance stops and paramedic from a backup unit from the same EMS company climbs into the back of the ambulance with you, and you are again en route to the hospital with lights and sirens.

3. What are your immediate interventions? Support your answer with an understanding of the metabolic changes seen in cardiac arrest.

After another 5 minutes of transport time toward the hospital, you now have an airway in place, compressions are ongoing, and the patient is receiving positive pressure ventilation via bag-valve mask attached to high-flow oxygen. You notice that your partner is ventilating the patient at a rate of about 18 per minute.

4. Is this an appropriate rate for an adult patient in cardiac arrest? If not, what is the appropriate rate?

5. What detrimental effects, if any, may occur secondary to the overventilation of a patient in cardiac arrest?

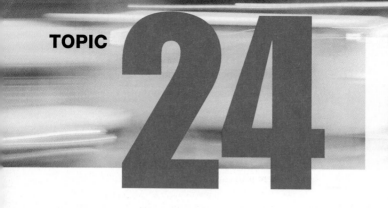

Standard Shock and Resuscitation

Competency Integrates a comprehensive knowledge of the causes and pathophysiology into the management of shock, respiratory failure, or arrest with an emphasis on early intervention to prevent arrest.

SHOCK

TRANSITION *highlights*

- *Review of the speculative rates for hypoperfusion and shock, including mortality rates.*

- *Aerobic and anaerobic metabolism and its relation to hypoperfusion.*

- *The final common pathway of a hypoperfusive state leading to cellular death.*

- *Pathologic basis of the cellular stages of shock:*
  - *Initial stage.*
  - *Compensatory stage.*
  - *Progressive stage.*
  - *Refractive stage.*

- *Etiologies of shock and comparison with the aforementioned general pathophysiology.*

- *Comparison of common assessment parameters as they present according to the etiology of shock.*

- *Treatment strategies for managing a patient with hypoperfusion and shock, regardless of the etiology of the disturbance.*

> **Hypoperfusion can be characterized as a global diminution of perfusion to the body's cells.**

INTRODUCTION

In 1743, while describing a state of poor tissue perfusion from battlefield injuries, a young French surgeon used the phrase "shock and agitation" in his written description of the clinical syndrome that a soldier experienced after being struck by a bullet, and the term *shock* was born. The term was quickly adopted by the Germans and the French and was initially used exclusively in connection with describing wounds and inju-

ries. As time passed, however, the word became associated with other medical conditions, such as insulin shock, electrical shock, spinal shock, burn shock, psychiatric use, and, in the effects of war, as shell shock.

Despite the medical community's attempt to remove this term because of its now varied meanings, it is still used widely today to describe myriad conditions causing patient instability.

In the traditional sense of the word, *shock* describes what occurs at the cellular level when the supplies of oxygenated blood and metabolic nutrients are insufficient to meet the body's needs, while removal of cellular waste products from this metabolic activity is simultaneously inadequate. Essentially, when cells become injured and die from shock, widespread tissue death results. With significant tissue death, the associated organ begins to dysfunction. Organ dysfunction will subsequently result in body system disturbances, and if the disturbance is grave enough, the death of the patient will ensue from this cellular "shock."

Although the term *shock* will probably never leave the lexicon of medical terms, more recently *hypoperfusion* has been introduced to better reflect what is actually happening at the cellular and tissue level and is gaining more widespread acceptance in the medical community.

EPIDEMIOLOGY

As discussed, hypoperfusion can be characterized as a global diminution of perfusion to the body's cells. Because adequate perfusion necessitates three components (adequate heart function, adequate blood supply, and adequate vascular tone) to exist properly, hypoperfusion can occur from the failure of one or more of these components—which would initially be caused by some emergency. For example, a myocardial infarction (MI) could weaken the heart muscle to a point at which it can no longer maintain an adequate cardiac output level, which in turn can cause hypoperfusion to cells, which enter into a shock state and die.

As such, it is difficult to get a precise reflection of the incidence or prevalence rates for hypoperfusion in general because of the varied etiologies and interpretations of the syndrome. It has been speculated that in the United States more than 1 million cases of hypoperfusion (from various etiologies) are seen annually in emergency departments. Mortality rates from hypoperfusion in general have been reported to consistently exceed 20 percent, with some specific etiologies of shock causing up to 90 percent mortality.

PATHOPHYSIOLOGY

Hypoperfusion from any etiology (cardiac, volume, or vascular) is a multifaceted clinical and physiologic syndrome that can disrupt normal homeostatic mechanisms along many dimensions. Despite the uniqueness of each etiology of hypoperfusion, all of them share one final pathway: the deterioration in cellular oxygenation and buildup of cellular waste in the terminal tissue beds. Although this syndrome does have clinical markers, hypoperfusion is truly a cellular disturbance that results in a cascade of events that progress from cellular and tissue death, to organ breakdown, to system failure, and ultimately to global dysfunction and patient death.

Early medical literature characterized shock as "a momentary pause in the act of death." Because the cell and microcirculation are the first to suffer the insult from hypoperfusion and inadequate oxygenation, it is best to have a functional knowledge of how the cell and microcirculation normally operate before introducing the pathophysiologic changes from inadequate perfusion and inadequate oxygenation.

Cellular respiration follows two critical pathways for the creation of energy:

- **Aerobic metabolism.** Within the cellular mitochondria, with the utilization of oxygen, glucose, and amino and fatty acids, 1 molecule of glucose converts into 34 to 36 total molecules of cellular-sustaining energy (ATP). The outcome of this process is energy, water, heat, and carbon dioxide. Energy is stored as ATP, and the carbon dioxide is eliminated from the body via the pulmonary system.
- **Anaerobic metabolism.** In the absence of oxygen, glucose refinement can progress only through the glycolysis phase, which liberates only two molecules of ATP. This process also results in pyruvate, which in the

absence of oxygen is converted into lactic acid, which is released back into the cellular fluid and body fluids, creating a detrimental and often fatal drop in blood pH. The end result of this process is insufficient energy production and harmful production of acids.

The benefit of understanding the preceding explanation is to appreciate how any disturbance in blood perfusion pressure, or the diminution of oxygen at the cellular level, results in the conversion of aerobic metabolism to anaerobic metabolism, with the consequences of inadequate energy supply and overwhelming acidosis. This in turn causes the failure of normal metabolic activities, and the cell dies. With cellular death, the walls of the cell deteriorate rapidly, and enzymes that are normally safely held within the cellular walls are liberated. These damaging enzymes start to exert their enzymatic activity on neighboring cells, causing their walls to collapse and the cells to die—leading to more enzyme release and more widespread cellular damage. In addition, capillary beds develop small permeations that allow fluid to exit the vascular system, causing more hypoperfusion.

As the blood becomes more acidic and cold, platelets start to clump together and form microemboli in the vascular system. The clotting systems of the body fail, and the cellular and vascular acidosis becomes overwhelming. The damage that started in just one capillary bed in one region of the body, given this progression of injury, now leads to tissue deterioration elsewhere in the body—it becomes a vicious circle of hypoperfusion, hypoxia, acidosis, and cellular death until the patient dies.

In summary, it is this widespread cellular death that causes tissue–organ failure, which in turn causes organ–system dysfunction, and when applied on an organism (or patient) level, death of the person results.

Stages of Shock

As stated, shock is a widespread response to inadequate perfusion and oxygenation. Cells are forced into anaerobic metabolism, which causes widespread cellular hypoxia and acidosis. Cells are injured first and die, which contributes to tissue death, organ dysfunction, system failure, and patient death. Shock has been found to be a progressive syndrome, progressing through four primary stages:

- **Initial stage.** Blood flow and oxygenation to distal capillary beds start to drop, secondary to the underlying disturbance (trauma and/or medical emergency). During the initial stage, the cells continue to extract oxygen from the adjacent bloodstream, but when this can no longer be done, the cells will enter into anaerobic metabolism. In the early stages of shock, very subtle clinical indications, if any at all, are noted. Despite the lack of clinical indications during this stage, serum lactate levels in the bloodstream start to rise and, thus, may be detected clinically at the hospital.

> Widespread cellular death causes tissue–organ failure, which in turn causes organ–system dysfunction.

- **Compensatory (nonprogressive) stage.** During this stage, the body will incorporate its own compensatory mechanisms (negative feedback mechanisms) to maintain cellular homeostasis. Be aware that during compensatory shock, however, oxygen delivery to the distal capillary beds is already markedly reduced and lactic acid levels continue to rise.

  Three compensatory mechanisms are largely initiated and regulated by the sympathetic nervous system during this stage: the chemical, neural, and hormonal mechanisms. As these compensatory mechanisms are used, they create many of the signs and symptoms seen early in the shock syndrome. The clinical problem with the use of compensatory mechanisms at this stage is that they can mask low blood volume, poor cardiac output, failing pulmonary efficiency, and other hemodynamic variances.

  Keep a high index of suspicion regarding what is going on at the cellular level based on often vague clinical findings. Be aware that by the time the most obvious clinical findings of shock are present, significant, if not irreversible, damage has already occurred at the cellular level. Table 24-1 provides a summary of these compensatory mechanisms.

- **Progressive (decompensatory) stage.** The progressive stage of shock, also referred to as the decompensatory stage, is literally the beginning of the

TABLE 24-1   Compensatory Mechanisms in Hypoperfusion

Mechanism	Effects at the Cellular and System Levels of the Body
Neural	The body has several strategically placed sensors to monitor its internal state. Baroreceptors in the aortic arch and carotid sinuses detect the drop in pressure and trigger the sympathetic nervous system. This nervous system is also triggered by the chemoreceptors in the body that detect elevating CO_2 and acid levels and faltering O_2 levels. The result of these stimuli is enhanced sympathetic tone, which results in tachycardia, narrowing pulse pressure, tachypnea, pupillary dilation, CNS excitation, and diaphoresis.
Chemical	With ongoing shock and faltering blood chemistry (diminished oxygen levels and increased levels of hydrogen and carbon dioxide), the adrenal glands will release epinephrine and norepinephrine. These hormones work together to increase cardiac output by way of elevating the heart rate, strength of contraction, and electrical conduction speed (epinephrine), and by further promoting peripheral vasoconstriction (norepinephrine) in an attempt to maintain adequate perfusion pressure.
Hormonal	Low arterial pressure causes the release of renin–angiotensin–aldosterone hormones that collectively increase thirst perception, promote vasoconstriction, and prompt reabsorption of sodium by the kidneys to preserve body fluid levels. Antidiuretic hormone release from the posterior pituitary gland further promotes vasoconstriction to nonvital tissues while enhancing reabsorption of water by the kidneys.

end of the shock syndrome. Until this point, the compensatory mechanisms have been functioning at capacity to maintain adequate perfusion and oxygenation to the body's tissues. Many of the symptoms and signs seen at that stage were the result of the body trying to maintain perfusion to essential organs, including the heart, lungs, brain, and kidneys, at the expense of the rest of the body. However, if the etiology of the hypoperfusion syndrome was not treated, was treated improperly, or worsened despite treatment, the patient will enter the third phase of shock.

The progressive stage of shock is hallmarked by the body's inability to maintain perfusion. Autoregulation of small capillary beds is lost, and the vessels dilate, which results in blood pooling in the periphery and diminished venous return. Microcirculation begins to form microemboli as platelets start clumping together, resulting in obstructed blood flow through tissues and organs and ongoing necrosis. The formation of clots depletes the body's clotting factors, and a condition known as *disseminated intravascular coagulation* (DIC) can develop, which leaves the body subject to hemorrhage.

Anaerobic metabolism is still ongoing, with progressive cellular death

and liberation of enzymes and other intracellular components. Along with increasing nearby cellular death, cardiac rhythm instability may be caused by electrolyte disorders from ruptured cells and the liberation of their contents. Digestive enzymes liberated from necrotic cells can also travel to the

lungs and start to deteriorate the alveolar surfaces, which further hampers the diffusion of gases. Although the patient has a chance for recovery with efficient and expedient treatment, the chances of recovery are rapidly diminishing. Table 24-2 summarizes the progressive effects of shock on certain body organs.

- **Refractory (irreversible) stage.** At this stage of shock, the compensatory mechanisms have failed despite treatment (or in the absence of treatment). The widespread shift from aerobic to anaerobic metabolism has now resulted in permanent cellular destruction and tissue death. Multiple organ failure occurs, and the primary body systems (cardiovascular, neurologic, and pulmonary) fail to maintain perfusion pressure and oxygenation to the body's most important organs (heart, brain, lungs, kidneys). Death will ensue regardless of the medical interventions applied at this time. A patient at this stage of shock is typically unresponsive.

The tachycardic pulse starts to become bradycardic owing to ischemia and acidosis, the respiratory rate that was once tachypneic will now start to wane, blood pressure begins to decrease (although not yet to the point of hypotension), pulse pressure narrows, pulses become weak, urinary output ceases, bowel sounds are absent, and the patient will slip into

TABLE 24-2   Effects of Shock on Body Organs and Systems

Organ or System Affected	Progressive Hypoperfusion
Brain	Ischemia, hypoxia, disrupted nerve transmission.
Heart	Tachydysrhythmias, poor coronary artery perfusion, decreased strength, low cardiac output.
Lungs	Breathing becomes rapid and shallow; diminished blood flow causes poor oxygenation, alveolar surface deterioration, pulmonary edema, acute respiratory distress syndrome (ARDS).
Pancreas	Dysfunction from ischemia, release of myocardial toxin factor from hypoperfusion.
Kidneys	Drop in urine production, elevation in blood toxins, eventual renal failure.
Integumentary	Skin pales and cools from vasoconstriction; diaphoresis occurs; eventual mottling from cardiovascular system impairment.
Gastrointestinal	Ulcerations from stress; ischemic bowel releases more toxins into bloodstream.
Hematologic	Cold, acidic, severe hypoxemia; DIC from clotting substance depletion; widespread inflammatory response.

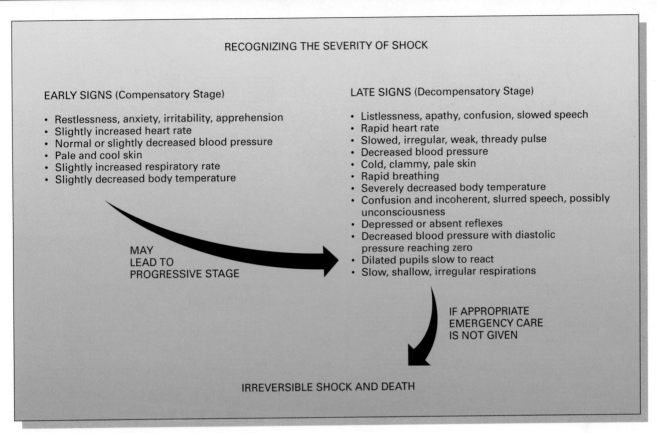

RECOGNIZING THE SEVERITY OF SHOCK

EARLY SIGNS (Compensatory Stage)

- Restlessness, anxiety, irritability, apprehension
- Slightly increased heart rate
- Normal or slightly decreased blood pressure
- Pale and cool skin
- Slightly increased respiratory rate
- Slightly decreased body temperature

MAY LEAD TO PROGRESSIVE STAGE

LATE SIGNS (Decompensatory Stage)

- Listlessness, apathy, confusion, slowed speech
- Rapid heart rate
- Slowed, irregular, weak, thready pulse
- Decreased blood pressure
- Cold, clammy, pale skin
- Rapid breathing
- Severely decreased body temperature
- Confusion and incoherent, slurred speech, possibly unconsciousness
- Depressed or absent reflexes
- Decreased blood pressure with diastolic pressure reaching zero
- Dilated pupils slow to react
- Slow, shallow, irregular respirations

IF APPROPRIATE EMERGENCY CARE IS NOT GIVEN

IRREVERSIBLE SHOCK AND DEATH

Figure 24-1 Recognizing the severity of shock.

cardiopulmonary arrest. Resuscitation at this point is often futile.

This is the "rude unhinging of the machinery of life" described as shock by early medical researchers when observing the effects of trauma. In actuality, however, this progression will occur not only from trauma but also from any etiology of hypoperfusion or hypoxia, as discussed next. ▶ Figure 24-1 discusses common findings consistent with each stage of shock.

Etiologies of Shock

As mentioned repeatedly in this topic, shock starts as a cellular syndrome of hypoxia, ischemia, and eventual death secondary to hypoperfusion and inadequate oxygen supply. These effects will occur regardless of the etiology creating this poor perfusion state. Just as stated previously, to have a sufficient supply of oxygen and other metabolic needs delivered to the cell, an adequate pump (heart), adequate blood supply (volume), and an intact vascular system (container) are necessary.

Not only must these three components exist, but they must also operate in relation to one another. For example, the container (vasculature) may be intact, but if it becomes too large (massive vasodilation), the perfusion pressure within will drop and may be insufficient to meet the metabolic needs of the body.

▶ Figure 24-2 shows the relationship among the etiologies of shock. Other etiologies of shock are discussed in Table 24-3.

ASSESSMENT FINDINGS

Shock (hypoperfusion) can be characterized as a syndrome that requires both clinical and physiologic diagnoses. More simply put, the paramedic must be able to recognize that the tissues of the body are not receiving an adequate amount of oxygen and other metabolic needs, and the dysfunction that results provides the clinical indication that shock is present.

It is also a physiologic diagnosis, as the paramedic must first recognize the clinical findings of shock and then couple this information with the patient's history to arrive at a conclusion as to which physiologic system is at fault (volume, pump, or container). Only with proper recognition of the clinical findings of shock in light of the

physiologic disturbance will the paramedic be able to provide the best care possible.

The symptoms seen in shock states are a function of the body's tissues and cells not receiving an adequate supply of oxygen and other metabolic substrates. The clinical findings are then a result of organs not receiving what they need to function. Poor kidney perfusion will result in a drop in urine production, hypoperfused muscles will become limp, poor perfusion to the brain will cause changes in mental status, and so on. Although varied by etiology, Table 24-4 identifies common characteristics of the major categories of shock.

In recent years, serum lactate monitors have also been used to identify anaerobic states. Elevated lactate levels can serve as a surrogate marker for the presence of anaerobic metabolism; for years, endurance athletes have monitored these levels to identify their aerobic threshold. In injured and ill patients, these monitors may be useful in identifying anaerobic conditions caused by hypoperfusion. Many systems are using these devices to aid in the identification of septic shock. Although the evidence is still scarce, it logically follows that lactate monitoring may be useful in identifying other shock states.

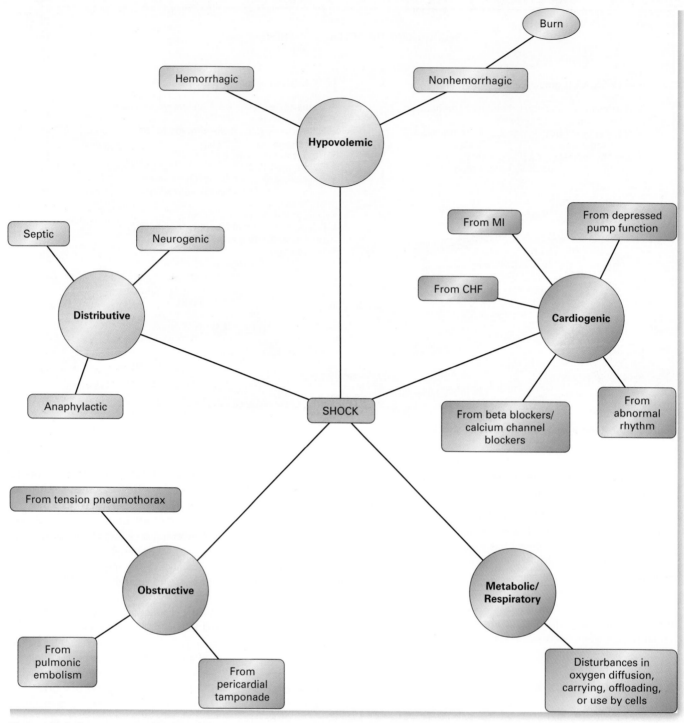

Figure 24-2 Categories and types of shock.

Shock requires immediate interventions to save the patient's life. As such, early recognition of its presence is imperative, even if the exact etiology of shock is not as readily apparent. From an overall perspective, when a patient presents with alterations in major organ function, significant disturbances in vital signs, or a history consistent with a shock state, the paramedic should initially presume that the patient is in shock or may soon go into

shock. Only through this high index of suspicion will the ill effects of the syndrome be adverted prehospitally.

EMERGENCY MEDICAL CARE

Medical direction and protocol will ultimately determine the recommended interventional steps that should be followed with the patient presenting with

shock. The shock state occurs as the result of a failure of body systems (e.g., shock could happen with traumatic bleeding, an MI, or an anaphylactic reaction).

As such, providing a specific recommendation of care in this text is difficult without first identifying the type of shock the patient is experiencing. For this reason, the following recommendations are centered around global treatment

TABLE 24-3   Etiologies of Shock

Type of Shock	Basic Pathophysiology	Causes/Etiologies
Fluid loss (▶ Figure 24-3)	Fluid in the vascular system is insufficient to carry oxygen and nutrients to the capillary beds.	External hemorrhage, internal hemorrhage, significant vomiting and/or diarrhea, excessive diaphoresis, burns
Pump failure (▶ Figure 24-4)	Heart muscle can no longer adequately maintain cardiac output needed to ensure perfusion.	Myocardial infarction, congestive heart failure, significant vasoconstriction, excessive tachycardia or bradycardia, AV valve damage, aortic valve stenosis
Container failure (▶ Figure 24-5)	Vascular system is disproportionately too large or permeable ("leaky") for volume of blood—massive vasodilation is present.	Sepsis, anaphylaxis, neurogenic, certain types of drug overdoses, spinal cord injury

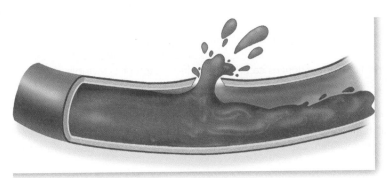

Figure 24-3 Etiology of shock: fluid loss.

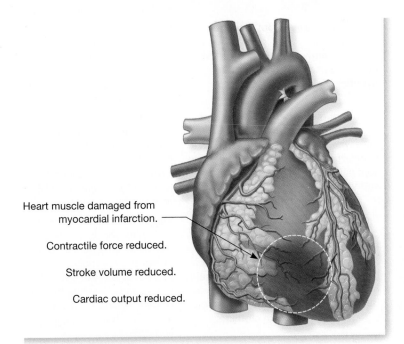

Heart muscle damaged from myocardial infarction.

Contractile force reduced.

Stroke volume reduced.

Cardiac output reduced.

Figure 24-4 Etiology of shock: pump failure.

considerations that should be undertaken for any patient displaying a shock syndrome.

Spinal Immobilization Considerations

In any patient with a known traumatic insult, especially one involving the head and neck, manual spinal stabilization should be provided. If the patient's history is unclear or the patient is unresponsive, it is best to provide manual stabilization and eventual spinal immobilization as a precautionary measure.

Airway Considerations

A patient in shock will eventually have alterations in mental status that will render him incapable of protecting his own airway. This is an important skill that must be performed correctly 100 percent of the time. Provide suctioning as necessary, and then progressively provide ongoing airway techniques starting with manual maneuvers (jaw thrust, head tilt-chin lift), then using simple mechanical adjuncts (oropharyngeal or nasopharyngeal airways), and eventually advanced mechanical adjuncts (such as blind insertion airway devices or endotracheal intubation), until the airway is clear and secure. Failure to do so will doom any future interventions to defeat.

Breathing Considerations

If the patient is breathing adequately, provide high-flow oxygen via a nonrebreather mask to ensure that adequate levels of oxygen are present to meet cellular metabolic needs. Remember that hypoperfusion states may render pulse oximetry readings inaccurate; therefore, titrating oxygen to oximetry may not be possible. In suspected shock patients, it is best to administer oxygen rather than withhold it. If the patient is apneic or breathing inadequately, ventilate with a bag-valve mask and 100 percent oxygen at a rate of 10 to 12 ventilations per minute.

Ventilate the patient carefully, being sure not to exceed the recommended ventilation rates. Recall that blood is returned to the heart via contraction of the muscles that milk the veins in conjunction with the one-way valves in the vein's lumen. Blood also returns to the heart via gravity from the head and upper torso and, finally, from the negative thoracic pressure created during spontaneous breathing (the cardiothoracic pump).

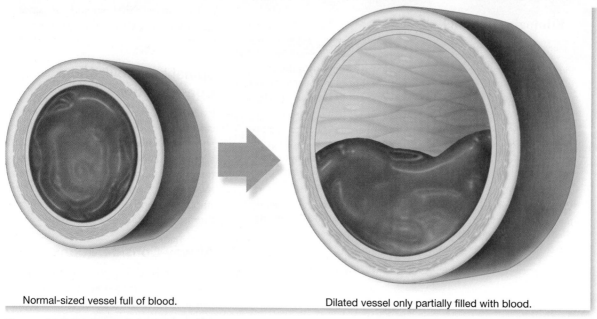

Normal-sized vessel full of blood.

Dilated vessel only partially filled with blood.

Figure 24-5 Etiology of shock: vasodilation.

Typically, a shock patient will be motionless, which eliminates venous blood flow facilitated by muscular contraction. In addition, the shock patient is commonly supine, so gravity cannot facilitate blood return to the heart. Finally, if positive pressure is being provided, there is never a moment of negative intrathoracic pressure to facilitate blood flow to the lungs.

Although the first two influences cannot realistically be mediated by the paramedic (supine position and motionless), the third influence (provision of positive pressure ventilation) and its effect on the cardiothoracic pump can be at least minimized by providing ventilations at a recommended rate, with a tidal volume just sufficient to achieve visible chest rise and produce alveolar breath sounds. It has been shown through recent research that overventilation is negatively correlated with almost all patient outcome measures and cardiac arrest survival rates.

TABLE 24-4	Characteristics of the Major Categories of Shock				
Type of Shock	Heart Rate	Respirations	Blood Pressure	Skin	General Findings
Fluid loss	Elevated initially; in final stages of shock, heart rate will abruptly slow.	Elevated initially; in later stages, respirations may become tachypneic and shallow.	Systolic maintains initially; pulse pressure narrows, eventual systolic hypotension.	Cool to the touch, diaphoretic, pallor; late stages result in mottling of the skin.	History of trauma or internal bleeding; patient may complain of thirst early. Early CNS stimulation with later confusion, disorientation, and unresponsiveness.
Pump failure	Rate most often elevated; extreme heart rates (fast or slow) may be seen. Rhythm disturbances (tachycardia or bradycardia) may be noted.	As shock ensues, respiratory rate typically increases.	Normal or elevated pressure initially; with MI, systolic pressure may drop suddenly.	Cool to the touch, diaphoretic, pallor; late stages result in mottling of the skin.	Patient may have history consistent with myocardial event (MI, ischemia). Pitting peripheral edema and inspiratory crackles may be present; jugular vein distention (JVD) may also be evident.
Container failure	Heart rate may be normal or slowed in neurogenic (spinal) shock; with other forms of massive vasodilation, heart rate is typically elevated.	Respirations may be fast and shallow with absent intercostal muscle use with spinal shock; other forms of vasodilation result in tachypnea.	Blood pressure is commonly found in the "low" range of normal, or frank systolic hypotension may be present.	In early shock from vasodilation, skin is often warm to the touch and reddened; with ensuing hypoperfusion, skin temperature cools with mottling.	May have history of trauma with spinal shock, may also display priapism. Other forms of vasodilatory shock (sepsis) may have history of general illness, and a rash may be present. Anaphylactic shock may reveal hives, redness, and itching.

Circulatory Considerations

Assess for a core pulse in any patient presenting with shock findings. Should compressions be warranted owing to cardiac arrest, start compressions immediately, recalling the "push hard, push fast" recommendation by the American Heart Association. It has been well documented in the literature that shallow compressions, slow compressions, or frequent interruptions of compressions result in reduced cardiac output, which ultimately translate into lower survival rates. Compressions that are delivered at a rapid rate (>100/min) while using a 30:2 ratio and that depress the sternum to a depth of at least 2 inches with complete recoil of the chest wall optimize the effectiveness of compression.

Another circulatory consideration is external hemorrhage. Whereas it is known that arterial bleeding can be life threatening, so can venous bleeding. The safest approach to interpreting the significance of a bleed is that if it simply looks heavy enough to cause shock and/or death of the patient, it is a significant bleed. Apply direct pressure with a pressure dressing to stop the bleed; should this fail, apply a tourniquet.

INTRAVENOUS THERAPY Do not delay transport to initiate an intravenous line. En route to the medical facility, initiate an intravenous line of normal saline. If volume expansion is needed, use a large-bore catheter (14 or 16 gauge) and a large vein. Run the fluid at a rate based on the clinical findings for the patient. Always follow your local protocol.

VOLUME LOSS ETIOLOGY If the etiology of shock is associated with volume loss (hypovolemia), the patient may benefit from the administration of fluid. The most common type of hypovolemic shock is from hemorrhage. Use the following as a guide for fluid administration. Emergency care may vary; therefore, always follow your local protocol.

Uncontrolled Hemorrhage If internal bleeding is suspected or an external hemorrhage cannot be controlled, infuse fluid at a rate to maintain a systolic blood pressure of 80 to 90 mmHg or until radial pulses are able to be palpated. Once this is achieved, back off the fluid infusion. Continue to titrate fluid to a systolic blood pressure (SBP) of 80 to 90 mmHg or presence of radial pulses.

Controlled Hemorrhage If an external hemorrhage is controlled by direct pressure or a tourniquet and continued bleeding is not present, and no internal bleeding is suspected, infuse fluid to maintain the systolic blood pressure above 90 to 100 mmHg.

In a brain-injured patient, infuse fluid to maintain the systolic blood pressure above 90 mmHg regardless of a controlled or uncontrolled hemorrhage or suspected internal injury.

VASODILATION ETIOLOGY If the etiology of shock is from massive vasodilation, two treatment recommendations to increase perfusion and blood pressure are to (1) increase vascular resistance by decreasing the vessel size and (2) fill the vessel with fluid. As a paramedic, your system may allow you to administer vasopressor medications, such as dopamine or norepinephrine, to constrict vessels. Typically, however, these medications are used after initial fluid resuscitation and, as such, are frequently impractical in the prehospital environment. That said, they can be important treatment modalities in the right circumstances. Always follow local protocol. Anaphylactic, septic, and vasogenic shock are all distributive types of shock that are typically associated with hypotension from systemic vasodilation.

CARDIOGENIC ETIOLOGY A cardiogenic etiology of shock is typically associated with left ventricular failure from an MI, congestive heart failure, or some other cause of ventricular failure, such as cardiac rhythm disturbance or cardiomyopathy. The patient is typically normovolemic and is experiencing difficulty in moving the existing volume of blood. Therefore, it is extremely important to restrict fluid administration to a keep-open rate once the intravenous line is initiated. Vasopressor medications such as dopamine are frequently used here to support perfusion but should be used with care to minimize myocardial oxygen demand in the event of acute coronary syndrome.

Other Considerations

Always attempt to maintain normothermia in the patient. In shock states, the body will cool down; this cooling worsens the effects of hypoxia and acidosis.

In the shock patient, maintaining or reestablishing perfusion to the body's capillary beds and cells in order to oxygenate and remove waste products should guide all treatment. Because the shock syndrome can rapidly cause irreversible tissue damage and death, focus only on the interventions that will have a direct and immediate impact on meeting this goal. This is perhaps best achieved by recognizing the shock state, providing high-flow oxygen, initiating ventilation as needed, and supporting the circulation while providing rapid transport to the hospital.

> **Should compressions be warranted, start them immediately, recalling the AHA's "push hard, push fast" recommendation.**

TRANSITIONING

REVIEW ITEMS

1. A patient is suspected of having suffered a spinal cord injury between C5 and C6. What impact will this injury have on the patient's ability to breathe?
   a. The patient will become apneic.
   b. The patient will be able to breathe normally.
   c. The patient will be able to breathe, but it will be labored.
   d. Spontaneous breathing will be present, but it will be slow (bradypneic).

2. During the terminal, prearrest stage of any hypoperfusion syndrome, what can be said regarding the efficiency of cellular production of ATP?
   a. Cellular efficiency increases as higher levels of ATP are created.
   b. Cellular production of ATP decreases as the cells change from aerobic to anaerobic metabolism.
   c. There is no change in cellular efficiency until all residual oxygen in the blood is used; then only nerve cells fail.
   d. Tissue cells enter into a hypermetabolic state in which energy and glucose are released to overcome the physiologic disturbance.

3. In which of the following types of hypoperfusive shock states will the heart rate be unable to increase as a negative feedback mechanism for enhancing cardiac output?

   a. neurogenic shock   b. cardiogenic shock
   c. anaphylactic shock   d. hypovolemic shock

4. A patient who presents with confusion, tachypnea, a systolic pressure of 118 mmHg, and a narrow pulse pressure is probably in what stage of shock?
   a. early   b. initial
   c. progressive   d. irreversible

5. Your female patient is experiencing a heart attack. She is borderline hypotensive, pulses are weak and rapid, and you identify other early indications of hypoperfusion. Given her history and presentation, what etiology of shock would you suspect?
   a. neurogenic   b. cardiogenic
   c. hypotensive   d. hypovolemic

APPLIED PATHOPHYSIOLOGY

A 32-year-old male patient is hit by a car while riding his bike through the park. Although he was struck at a low rate of speed, bystanders state that the patient's torso was run over by the vehicle's tires. On your arrival, the patient presents as unresponsive.

1. Given this history and basic presentation, if the patient is in shock, what cause(s) is/are most likely?

On completion of your primary assessment, you find the patient's breathing to be very shallow and tachypneic at 38/minute, the heart rate is 64/minute, blood pressure is 98/60 mmHg, and the peripheral pulses are bounding. Mental status is unchanged.

2. With this additional information, what etiology of shock is most likely the cause of this patient's presentation?

3. What clinical findings support your field impression?

4. Describe the anticipated physiologic benefit(s) for each of the interventions that may be administered to the patient hit by the car.
   a. Oxygen
   b. Positive pressure ventilation
   c. Spinal immobilization
   d. Fluid administration

CLINICAL DECISION MAKING

You are called to the scene of a collision between a compact car and an SUV. On your arrival, the fire department on scene directs you to the driver of the compact car, who is still trapped in the driver's seat. As you approach the patient, he keeps screaming, "Get me out of here—my leg is bleeding bad!" His leg, however, is pinned under the dashboard, and there is no way to apply direct pressure to the heavy bleed. His pant leg is soaked, and blood is collecting on the floor of the car. His breathing is unlabored but rapid, distal radial pulse is very weak, and he is becoming agitated.

1. Based on your primary assessment findings, identify clues that indicate the likely cause of his early shock signs.

2. What other conditions may the patient have that could cause you to identify similar findings?

About 10 minutes later, the patient is finally extricated from the car. At this point you perform a quick reassessment and find that the patient arouses to verbal stimuli, his airway is still clear, and his breathing is rapid and shallow at 36/minute with no vesicular sounds present. Peripheral pulses are now absent, and the blood pressure is 82/palpation. The neck veins are flat when positioned supine.

3. Of what life threats to the patient, if any, are you currently aware?

4. Into what stage of shock would you categorize this patient?

5. During the ongoing management of the patient, you elect to administer the following therapies. For each one, discuss in specific detail (1) the reason the intervention is warranted, (2) the expected outcome of that intervention, and (3) how you would assess to determine if that desired effect is occurring (i.e., the treatment worked):
   a. Administration of high-flow oxygen
   b. Fluid administration
   c. Maintaining normothermia

Standard Medicine

Competency Integrates assessment findings with principles of epidemiology and pathophysiology to formulate a field impression and implement a comprehensive treatment/disposition plan for a patient with a medical complaint.

TOPIC

25

SEPSIS

INTRODUCTION

The immune system attacks foreign invaders in the body with a complicated series of responses. Cell-based and humoral defenses guard against the spread of infection and protect against a variety of antigens. Normally, these defenses provide a measured response proportional to the scale of the threat. Occasionally, however, the defense against infection is exaggerated, and the responses aimed at restoring health actually begin to harm the body themselves. In general, these overwhelming steps are the basis for the syndrome defined as sepsis.

Specifically speaking, sepsis is defined as simply an infection in the bloodstream; however, the term *sepsis* has become commonly used to refer to the stages of both systemic inflammation and hypoperfusion associated with the response to infection. In this topic, we will describe sepsis in three specific stages: sepsis, severe sepsis, and septic shock.

Although defining sepsis can be tricky, every provider should clearly understand the severity of this syndrome. Septic shock has a mortality rate that is 5 times greater than that of a gunshot wound to the abdomen and 10 times greater than the mortality rate of an ST-elevation myocardial infarction. Moreover, the prevalence of patients presenting with symptoms of sepsis far exceeds that of the previous two conditions combined. EMS providers encounter these patients daily; now, more than ever, health care is recognizing the importance of time-sensitive prehospital care.

Recognition and action are the key lessons of this topic. Matching pathophysiology to outward findings will enable rapid identification, and with early identification, vital treatment can be aggressively initiated. Just as with trauma patients or with acute coronary syndrome patients, the best outcomes for sepsis patients occur with the integration of many different levels of care within the health care system. All levels of care must work together; the care that EMS provides is a vital link in this chain.

EPIDEMIOLOGY

In the United States, roughly 750,000 new sepsis cases occur each year; at least 200,000 of these cases will result in patient death. Even more startling is that the incidence of sepsis has

TRANSITION highlights

- **Overview of the epidemiology of sepsis in the United States.**
- **Review of the pathophysiology of sepsis, including systemic inflammatory response.**
- **The stages of sepsis.**
- **Recognition of sepsis, including serum lactate monitoring.**
- **Global treatment strategies and time-sensitive priorities.**
- **Review of specific prehospital treatment tactics.**

increased each year for the past five years. More and more patients undergoing invasive procedures, ranging from surgeries to catheterizations, mean more and more risk of infection. As the risk of infection increases, so does the incidence of sepsis.

Other risk factors for sepsis include the increasing prevalence of immunosuppressed patients, either from medications or as a result of disease; the extremes of age; and the recent rise of medication-resistant organisms such as methicillin-resistant *Staphylococcus aureus* (MRSA). Sepsis as a syndrome is both widespread and deadly. As a result, it is vitally important to understand how sepsis overtakes the body.

PATHOPHYSIOLOGY

Sepsis begins with an infection. In theory, this infection can be caused by bacteria, viruses, or fungi and can include almost any system. Common original infections include cutaneous (skin) infections, pneumonia, urinary tract infections, and even influenza. The immune system, sensing the infection, initially reacts with both humoral and cell-mediated defense mechanisms. These defense mechanisms include the presence of histamine and other proinflammatory chemicals that lead to inflammation. Under normal circumstances, these responses are self-limiting and over time they mitigate the offending infection.

Systemic Inflammatory Response

In some infections, however, the immune response will become systemic. A condition called *systemic inflammatory response* occurs when the specific defenses of the immune system begin to challenge and potentially harm other areas of the body.

Harmful effects result from the spread of proinflammatory chemicals as well as the proliferation of toxins released as bacteria break down. Inflammation causes capillary membrane permeability and fluid shifts out of the vascular space. This causes relative hypovolemia and hypoperfusion at a cellular level. Because cells now have a relative lack of oxygen, anaerobic metabolism begins, causing a release of lactic acid and an overall decrease in body pH. As these conditions spread, sepsis worsens.

The body compensates for these challenges in a predictable manner. The respiratory rate increases to improve oxygenation and remove excess CO_2. Heart rate and contractility increase to preserve perfusion. The sympathetic nervous system begins a neurohumoral response with the release of norepinephrine. Norepinephrine causes constriction of peripheral blood vessels in an attempt to shunt blood to vital organs.

Severe Sepsis

Severe sepsis occurs as the systemic inflammatory syndrome progresses, and organ systems begin to fail. In addition to capillary membrane permeability and the third spacing of fluids, circulating toxins can now cause vasodilation and subsequent hypotension. Serum lactate levels are now increased as a result of the widespread anaerobic metabolism and subsequent release of lactic acid.

Increasing hypoperfusion takes an immediate toll on organs that are most sensitive to a lack of oxygen. Organs such as the brain, kidneys, liver, and heart rapidly demonstrate damage under these septic conditions. Profound altered mental status and renal failure are the hallmarks of this stage of sepsis; in fact, most definitions identify severe sepsis by a combination of both hypotension and evidence of at least one organ system failure. By this point, mortality rates are high. Some estimates note the mortality rate for this stage to be as high as 35 percent.

Septic Shock

Septic shock occurs as severe sepsis progresses. Here, profound shock occurs as a result of prolonged systemic inflammatory syndrome, vasodilation, and the failure of compensatory mechanisms. Hypotension is the key marker of this stage. In fact, most definitions note that the true marker of septic shock is hypotension refractory to fluid administration. Mortality rates are exceptionally high in this stage. Some estimate rates to be as high as 50 percent to 60 percent.

PATIENT ASSESSMENT— RECOGNITION OF SEPSIS

Recognition of sepsis can be challenging, as its signs and symptoms can be vague, and it often occurs in patients with many comorbidities. That said, recognition is the most important element of caring for a patient with sepsis.

Identifying sepsis starts with recognizing the underlying infection. In fact, most early symptoms are purely related to the root infection. Recognize associated symptoms such as coughing with pneumonia, polyuria and oliguria with urinary tract infections, and swelling, redness, and pus associated with cutaneous infections.

Fever is also a very common finding, as it points to the body's response to infection. Be aware, however, that as sepsis progresses, poor perfusion and vascular tone can lead to a loss of thermoregulation. As a result, many septic patients actually present in a hypothermic state. Consider both extremes of temperature (high and low) a presumptive finding for sepsis.

When fluid is shifted out of the vascular space as a result of systemic inflammatory syndrome, edema occurs. Swelling in the face, hands, feet, and later the rest of the body is also a significant finding.

The hypoperfusion associated with progressive sepsis can also be recognized externally. Systemic inflammatory response is typically defined by at least two of the following findings:

- Temperature >38.3°C (101°F) or <36°C (97°F)
- Heart rate >90 bpm
- Altered level of consciousness
- Decreased capillary refill time
- Serum lactate levels >2 mmol/L

Serum Lactate Levels

Measuring serum lactate levels was once possible only in a hospital environment; however, recent advances in technology have enabled this test to be accomplished in the field. Lactate levels in the blood correlate to the amount of lactic acid being produced by anaerobic metabolism and can be a key indicator of the progression of sepsis. Using a device similar to a glucometer (▶ Figure 25-1), a drop of blood is rapidly analyzed for the presence of lactate. Specific measurements are attainable in seconds. Of

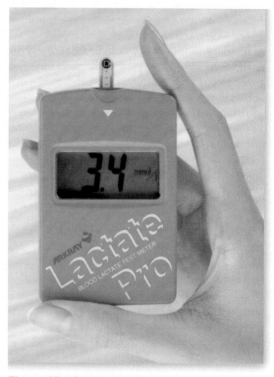

Figure 25-1 Lactate monitor.

> **Identifying sepsis starts with recognizing the underlying infection.**

TABLE 25-1   Sepsis Criteria

Severe sepsis	Signs associated with underlying infection
	Signs of systemic inflammatory response
	Hypotension (before fluid resuscitation)
	Signs of one or more organ failures
	Lactate >4 mmol/L
Septic shock	Signs of severe sepsis plus…
	Hypotension refractory to fluid administration

course, just as with glucose monitoring or any other technology, these findings are meaningful only in the context of a broader patient assessment and are subject to the failures and shortcomings of technology. Calibration and routine maintenance are important when using these monitors.

Remember that sepsis frequently occurs in patients with other underlying diseases. Patients with indwelling catheters and those who have undergone recent surgical procedures have an increased risk of sepsis. A thorough patient history is always important in identifying sepsis. Consider also that sepsis typically begins with relatively benign symptoms. Altered mental status, general complaints of not feeling well, and minor symptoms of infection are all common precursors to sepsis.

Many EMS systems have more specific criteria to define various stages of sepsis, as each stage may have particular treatment modalities. Table 25-1 provides a common set of findings used to define the latter stages of sepsis. As always, follow local protocol.

SEPSIS TREATMENT

Septic patients are not easy to treat. In fact, as previously stated, septic shock patients can have a mortality rate as high as 60 percent. However, outcomes for these patients are maximized through aggressive intervention at several levels of the health care system. Early recognition, time-sensitive antibiotic therapy, and aggressive fluid resuscitation are traditionally considered the keys to successful treatment. Medications such as pressors and antiinflammatories are also commonly used, but are generally considered secondary to more immediate priorities.

Global Strategies for Sepsis Treatment

The most important treatment for a sepsis patient is early recognition of the disorder. Appropriate care for a septic patient includes aggressive therapy at multiple levels of the health care system; recognition of the problem is the first step in activating this comprehensive care.

Many health care systems have initiated sepsis care systems similar to those of trauma systems, in which key findings activate a series of concomitant events. Consider how early identification and notification of a multisystem trauma patient may engage trauma surgeons, trigger X-rays and other tests, and initiate specific protocols. In many systems, early identification and notification of sepsis set similar events in motion. This early recognition is frequently a responsibility given to EMS providers. By using specific criteria such as those detailed in the previous section, paramedics can make a field diagnosis and activate larger, more comprehensive systems. This may include early notification and also specific destination protocols. In many cases, this provisional diagnosis may indicate particular prehospital sepsis treatment protocols.

Sepsis Treatment Priorities

Sepsis patients can have profound altered mental status; as such, airway and breathing management may be necessary. Always ensure adequate oxygenation and ventilation before moving to other treatment elements.

The relative hypovolemia of a sepsis patient must be addressed in an aggressive manner. These patients require high volume fluid resuscitation. Some system protocols allow for extraordinary fluid volumes to be administered to patients with presumptive positive findings for sepsis (usually high serum lactate levels are the key finding), but in general, restoring cardiovascular pressure is a critical goal. Common sepsis protocols call for 20 mL/kg of normal saline in the presence of high lactate, but as always, follow local protocol.

If hypotension cannot be restored with aggressive fluid resuscitation, it may be necessary to administer a pressor such as norepinephrine or dopamine. This circumstance is common, as septic shock frequently does not respond to normal volume administrations. Pressors should be used only after fluid resuscitation has been attempted.

The overall goal in the management of sepsis is to restore perfusion and attack the infection. Remember that immediate and appropriate transport of these patients can make a significant difference in their outcome. The need for volume replacement must be measured in context with the need for aggressive antibiotic therapy. Outcomes are maximized when a team-based approach is used.

> **Early recognition, time-sensitive antibiotic therapy, and aggressive fluid resuscitation are the keys to successful treatment.**

TRANSITIONING

REVIEW ITEMS

1. Which of the following has the highest mortality rate?
   a. gunshot wound to the abdomen
   b. ST elevation myocardial infarction
   c. septic shock
   d. stab wound to the abdomen

2. In systemic inflammatory syndrome, the chief cause of hypoperfusion is _____.
   a. increased membrane permeability in the capillaries

b. absolute hypovolemia

c. bradycardia causing decreased cardiac output

d. renal failure

3. Which of the following findings would be a specific indicator of sepsis?

    a. bradycardia   b. fever

    c. hypertension   d. diaphoresis

4. Which of the following findings specifically indicates the presence of anaerobic metabolism?

    a. increased blood glucose

b. decreased end-tidal CO_2

c. low oxygen saturation

d. increased serum lactate levels

5. Which of the following findings would specifically differentiate septic shock from severe sepsis?

    a. hypotension after fluid resuscitation

    b. hypotension before fluid resuscitation

    c. tachycardia

    d. delayed capillary refill time

APPLIED PATHOPHYSIOLOGY

1. Describe the root cause of sepsis. How does it begin?

2. Describe the pathophysiology of systemic inflammatory syndrome.

3. Explain how systemic inflammatory syndrome causes hypotension in severe shock.

4. Explain why pressors might be needed in septic shock.

5. Explain why a septic patient might be hypothermic despite having a massive infection.

CLINICAL DECISION MAKING

A 75-year-old female patient is found confused and somnolent. Her family says that she has been not feeling well for about a week and has complained of difficulty with her urinary catheter. You note that she is verbally responsive but very confused. She has a patent airway and is breathing rapidly. You have difficulty finding a radial pulse and note that her skin is hot to touch. The family supplies a past medical history of only hypertension and bladder control problems. They state that the patient was reasonably healthy last week.

1. Based on the scene size-up and primary assessment, provide your differential diagnosis list.

2. What further information would you need to rule in sepsis?

Although the patient does not have a radial pulse, her carotid pulse is 128. You are able to obtain a blood pressure of 72/50 mmHg. Her ECG shows a sinus tachycardia with a clear 12-lead, and you note her blood glucose to be 210.

3. Are there any immediate life threats to the patient?

4. What emergency care would you provide based on the assessment thus far?

The family states the patient takes lisinopril and a daily aspirin. They note that she has been taking acetaminophen for the fever. They say that her mental status has been in steady decline since the previous day. She has not been eating well for the past 48 hours, and she last had some crackers the preceding night. She has no known allergies.

You utilize your lactate monitor and obtain a reading of 4 mmol/L. While you are assessing her lactate, your partner obtains venous access.

5. What conditions have you ruled out in your differential diagnosis? Why?

6. What condition do you suspect? Why?

7. Does this patient require fluid resuscitation, and if so, how much?

8. What vital information would you relay to the receiving medical facility?

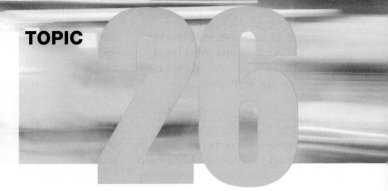

Standard Medicine

Competency Integrates assessment findings with principles of epidemiology and pathophysiology to formulate a field impression and implement a comprehensive treatment/disposition plan for a patient with a medical complaint.

TOPIC

CARDIOVASCULAR EMERGENCIES: ACUTE CORONARY SYNDROME

INTRODUCTION

Acute coronary syndrome (ACS) is a hot-button issue of modern prehospital medicine. This topic is at the forefront of discussion not only because of its sweeping mortality—cardiovascular disease is the leading cause of death in the United States—but also because it is a condition in which the swift actions of EMS providers really do have an impact on patient outcomes.

ACS is an umbrella term used to cover any cluster of clinical signs and symptoms related to diminished blood flow to the heart. In general, ACS is a supply-and-demand issue. The heart requires a constant supply of blood through the coronary arteries to deliver nutrients and oxygen to its muscle mass. When this demand cannot be met, the myocardial cells suffer damage. ACS is commonly associated with atherosclerosis and its buildup of plaque inside arterial walls, but it can also be related to other pathologies that decrease the flow of blood, such as vasospasm and aneurysm.

The spectrum of ACS can range widely, from simple chest pain with exertion (angina) to full-blown myocardial infarction (MI) with resultant muscle death and the precipitation of pulmonary edema from left heart failure. Although these disorders are grouped together, the paramedic will use specific diagnostic tools, such as 12-lead ECG, to rapidly identify and aggressively treat specific underlying disorders.

Prehospital providers can have a significant impact on patients suffering from ACS. As part of the larger health care team, paramedics represent an important link in the early identification and initial treatment of ACS. Prehospital actions are essential to maximizing patient outcome; the responsibilities of prehospital providers are likely to increase as treatment of ACS becomes more sophisticated.

This topic discusses the pathophysiology, assessment, and treatment of ACS. (Note that Topic 27 will discuss the use of diagnostic 12-lead ECG in greater detail.)

EPIDEMIOLOGY

It has been estimated that more than 62 million Americans have some form of cardiovascular disease that commonly leads to coronary artery disease (CAD). Through previous research, the

TRANSITION highlights

- Inclusion of the term acute coronary syndrome as an umbrella term for ischemic cardiac events.
- Pathophysiology of acute coronary syndrome.
- Increased emphasis on recognition of myocardial infarction and on emergency department door-to-intervention time.
- Changes in philosophy of oxygen administration to patients with acute coronary syndrome.
- Inclusion of aspirin and nitroglycerin administration for the acute care of acute coronary syndrome.
- Assessment findings indicative of cardiac arrest, as well as findings suggestive of a patient who may go into cardiac arrest.
- Importance of prehospital interventions and why they are successful in reversing cardiac arrest.

American Heart Association has found that approximately 7 to 8 million people each year will seek treatment in an emergency department in the United States for chest discomfort. Of those patients, approximately 2 million will actually suffer from a cardiac-related condition that involves the coronary arteries. About 1.5 million will suffer an actual heart attack, in which the coronary artery is occluded and a portion of the heart muscle begins to die. Of those patients, 500,000 will die from this heart attack, 250,000 of whom will die within one hour following the onset of the signs and symptoms.

In a sobering light, about every 25 seconds an American will suffer a coronary event, every 34 seconds a heart attack will occur, and about once every minute someone will die from sudden cardiac arrest. These statistics are definite indications of the significance of cardiac-related emergencies and underscore the importance of having a thorough knowledge base regarding cardiac emergencies.

PATHOPHYSIOLOGY

As stated earlier, the pathophysiology of ACS is related to a supply-and-demand problem. ACS occurs when the necessary supply of blood cannot perfuse heart tissue. This problem is most commonly associated with vascular disease. Therefore, to better understand the pathophysiology of ACS, one must first understand the basics of vascular disease.

Arteriosclerosis is a condition that causes the smallest of arterial structures to become stiff and inelastic. This is often referred to as "hardening of the arteries." A form of arteriosclerosis is *atherosclerosis*. Atherosclerosis is a systemic arterial disease that is derived from the Greek word *athere*, meaning "gruel" or "porridge," and *scleros*, which means "hard."

Atherosclerosis is an inflammatory disease that starts in the intimal (innermost) lining of the blood vessels, where endothelial cells become damaged. Common risk factors that are thought to cause this endothelial injury include smoking, diabetes, hypertension, high levels of low-density lipoproteins (LDL), and low levels of high-density lipoproteins (HDL). Once injury occurs, intimal dysfunction and inflammation progress through the following five basic pathophysiologic events (▶ Figure 26-1):

- Intimal damage allows the migration of blood platelets and other substances in the blood (serum lipoproteins) into the vascular wall. This irritates and inflames the vascular wall.

- As a result of the irritation and inflammation, different types of cells migrate to the location, as do smooth muscle cells of the tunica media layer (muscular middle layer of the blood vessel).

- As these cells proliferate, longitudinal fatty streaks develop in the lumen of the blood vessel. The blood vessel weakens as intima and media are deprived of nutrients from the expanding plaque.

- In an attempt to "close off" the fatty streaks, smooth muscle cells produce collagen and migrate over the fatty streak to form a fibrous cap.

- Fibrous caps, however, are not stable and may rupture. This causes the body's clotting mechanism to activate with development of a thrombus (clot), which may occlude the blood vessel.

The buildup of fatty deposits on the inside of the coronary arteries (atherosclerosis) is called *coronary artery disease*. The narrowing of a coronary blood vessel (also known as *remodeling*) increases the resistance to blood flow through the artery and decreases the amount of blood flow to the distal heart muscle. In addition, the fatty deposits will reduce the coronary arteries' ability to dilate (become larger) and deliver additional blood flow to the heart when needed, such as during an increase in heart rate or more forceful pumping action, as needed during stress or exercise.

Although CAD is a vascular problem in and of itself, it sets up the body for an increase risk of additional emergencies, which is the real focus of this topic: acute coronary syndrome.

Acute Coronary Syndrome

As discussed previously, ACS results from any of a variety of conditions in which the coronary arteries are narrowed or occluded by fat deposits (plaque), clots, or spasm. The word *acute* refers to a sudden onset, *coronary* refers to a condition affecting the coronary arteries, and *syndrome* indicates a group of signs and symptoms produced by the condition.

Two conditions that are part of any ACS are *angina* (stable and unstable) and *myocardial infarction* (heart attack). When the myocardial cells that make up the heart muscle do not receive an adequate amount of oxygenated blood, they become hypoxic. This condition, most commonly referred to *myocardial ischemia*, represents a state in which inadequate oxygen is delivered to the heart muscle. Ischemia can be caused by narrowing of the coronary arteries by plaque or spasms, clot formation inside the coronary artery blocking the blood flow, an increase in the work of the heart that demands more blood flow than can be supplied through the coronary arteries, or any combination of these conditions.

Angina Pectoris

Angina pectoris (literally, "pain in the chest") is a condition and a symptom commonly associated with CAD and can manifest itself as one of the ACSs (▶ Figure 26-2). Angina typically occurs when an increased workload is placed on the heart from an increase in the heart rate or the contractile function of the heart or when an increase in systemic vascular resistance causes the ventricles to work harder to keep blood moving.

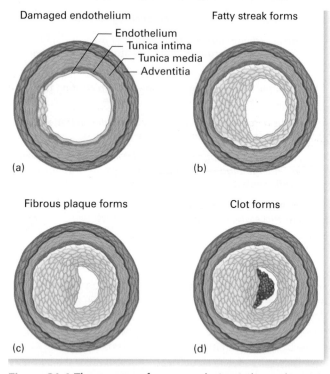

Damaged endothelium
— Endothelium
— Tunica intima
— Tunica media
— Adventitia
(a)

Fatty streak forms
(b)

Fibrous plaque forms
(c)

Clot forms
(d)

Figure 26-1 The process of artery occlusion (atherosclerosis): (a) The endothelium (inner wall) of the artery is damaged. (b) Fatty streaks begin to form in the damaged vessel walls. (c) Fibrous plaques form, causing further vessel damage and progressive resistance to blood flow. (d) The plaque deposits begin to ulcerate or rupture; platelets aggregate and adhere to the surface of the ruptured plaque, forming clots that may block the artery.

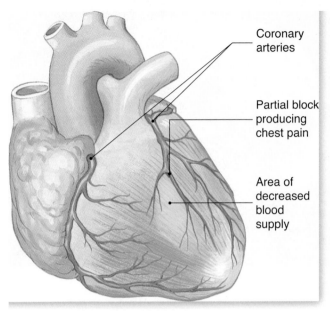

Figure 26-2 Angina pectoris, or chest pain, results when a coronary artery is blocked, depriving an area of the myocardium of oxygen.

In any instance, angina pectoris is a symptom of inadequate oxygen supply to the heart muscle, which is often caused by partial blockage of the coronary arteries that, in turn, produces cellular ischemia (reduced delivery of oxygenated blood) and tissue hypoxia (oxygen deficiency in the tissues).

Generally, angina pectoris occurs during periods of stress, either physical or emotional, at a time when the oxygen requirements of heart muscle are not met by oxygen delivery. Once the stress is relieved or the patient rests, oxygen requirements are reduced, and the pain will usually go away. Although more uncommon, angina may also occur in patients with valvular heart disease, enlarged hearts (cardiac hypertrophy), and hypertension. The pain is commonly felt under the sternum and may radiate to the jaw, or down either arm, to the back, or to the epigastrium. The pain usually lasts for about 2 to 15 minutes.

Many patients will be able to tell you that they have had angina as part of their past medical history and will have nitroglycerin prescribed for this condition. Prompt relief of the symptoms after rest and administered nitroglycerin is a key finding typical of angina.

Angina pectoris has two subcategories: *stable angina* and *unstable angina*. Stable angina patients will experience episodes of chest pain of a more or less predictable nature. Commonly, the patient will know that certain levels of physical exertion (e.g., running versus walking) or extreme emotional or mental distress will precipitate the pain. Just as stable angina has a predictable onset, its resolution with rest and/or nitroglycerin is also predictable.

Unstable angina, conversely, is a subcategory of angina pectoris in which the onset of pain cannot be predicted. Unstable angina commonly occurs unexpectedly, in patterns that are not reliable. Although the underlying pathophysiology for unstable angina is still a diminishing of blood flow to distal capillary beds of the myocardium, it may occur during sleep, in the absence of physical exertion, or concurrently with other medical conditions, such as infections or inflammations of the body. In addition, a change in the usual pattern of anginal episodes suggests unstable angina.

Variant angina (Prinzmetal angina) is a type of unstable angina in which a coronary artery spasm is the cause for diminished blood flow, but like unstable angina in general, the onset cannot be predicted. Variant angina is highly correlated with secondary lethal arrhythmias, MI, and sudden cardiac death.

Myocardial Infarction

In CAD, plaque builds up between the intimal and medial layers of the coronary vessel. Although the vessel may remodel and partially obstruct the flow of blood, the plaque is shielded from passing blood flow by the thin lining of the vessel and the fibrous cap formed over the plaque. This shielding is very important and represents a key risk factor associated with CAD, because when this shielding ruptures and plaque is exposed to flowing blood, the clotting cascade begins and a clot is formed.

The vessels of some CAD patients are well protected by a thick fibrous cap, but in other cases, this cap is thin and quite vulnerable to rupture. Why some caps rupture while others remain intact is thought to be related to dilation and constriction of the blood vessel, but is still an important question in the treatment of vascular disease. Most important, though, the rupture of a fibrous cap initiates a chain of events that can rapidly lead to the death of the patient if not recognized immediately and treated aggressively.

Topic 7, "Anatomy and Physiology: The Blood," discussed the manner in which hemostasis protects the blood vessel when a leak occurs. Specifically, in a process called the clotting cascade, platelets plug the hole in the blood vessels and coagulation forms a lasting clot. The events of an MI result from the same physiology.

When a fibrous cap ruptures, flowing blood is exposed to the plaque built up between the layers of an artery. Although the wall of the blood vessel may remain intact, the flowing blood interprets this plaque to represent a loss of blood vessel integrity and takes steps to repair the hole. Plaque, in essence, signals the start of a clotting cascade.

Just as in the creation of any clot, the first step in the creation of a coronary thrombus is platelet aggregation. Exposure of plaque and exposed collagen signals circulating platelets and other clotting factors to attach themselves and congregate in the exposed area. As platelets stick together, they "activate" and secrete their own chemical markers. Chemicals such as thromboxane enhance the attraction among platelets and further assist in gathering other circulating platelets to plug the theoretical hole.

As the clotting cascade continues, activated platelets chemically signal other distinct changes and coagulation begins. Thromboxane A_2 activates additional platelets, and glycoprotein IIb/IIIa receptors are activated to create and activate fibrin. The creation of fibrin serves to further stabilize the clot by linking platelets with a meshlike fibrin net. As the coagulation process continues, the clot grows in size.

It is important to remember that in this case, there is no actual hole in the vessel. The aggregation of platelets and the creation of a clot obstruct blood flow through the already narrowed vessel. Remember also that vasoconstriction is an important element of hemostasis and, therefore, the vessel may narrow further simply as part of the hemostatic process. In trying to defend itself from perceived blood loss,

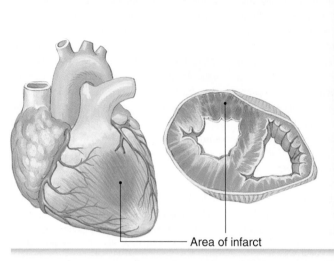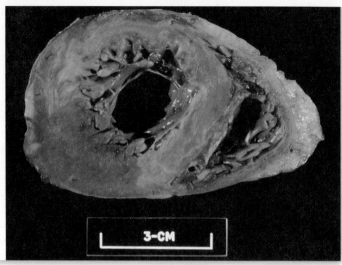

Area of infarct

Figure 26-3 (a) Cross section of a myocardial infarction. (b) A heart with normal and infarcted tissue.

the body is actually obstructing its own blood supply. If the clot grows large enough, blood flow through this diseased artery will actually stop. When this blood flow is obstructed, myocardial cells downstream from the occlusion will become ischemic and eventually die unless the clot is resolved (▶ Figure 26-3).

Tissue will die in stages. Infarcted tissue consists of a necrotic core surrounded by marginal zones that can either recover normal function or become irreversibly damaged. One of the greatest determinants of MI size is the presence of any collateral blood flow. Collateral blood flow refers to an area of the heart that is also receiving blood from a blood vessel that is not occluded. This collateral blood flow is an important determinant of infarct size and of whether the marginal zones become irreversibly damaged.

Infarcted tissue does not contribute to tension generation during systole; therefore, it can alter ventricular systolic and diastolic functions, which in turn changes stroke volume and cardiac output, often detrimentally. Infarcted tissue can also interrupt normal electrical activity within the heart, leading to potentially fatal dysrhythmias.

If the MI affects the left ventricle, which is most common, the drop in cardiac function can lead to pulmonary vascular congestion and pulmonary edema. Infarcted tissue can also precipitate abnormal cardiac rhythms and conduction blocks that further impair global cardiac functioning and may become life threatening in some cases.

Reduced cardiac output and arterial pressure can activate baroreceptor reflexes that attempt to compensate for the drop in pressure by activation of numerous neurohumoral compensatory mechanisms, such as the sympathetic nervous system, as well as fluid retention systems, such as the renin–angiotensin and aldosterone systems. Renal hypoperfusion and sympathetic nervous system stimulation promote renin release—renin is converted into angiotensin II—and aldosterone release, which enhance renal retention of sodium and water and promote vasoconstriction.

These negative feedback mechanisms cause the heart to work harder, thus increasing cardiac output. Retention of fluid by the kidneys drives up pressure by placing more fluid into the vascular system (explaining the elevated blood pressure and tachycardia seen in many MI patients). The pain and/or anxiety associated with an MI further stimulates the sympathetic nervous system and results in ongoing peripheral systemic vasoconstriction and cardiac stimulation as catecholamines (such as adrenaline, norepinephrine, and dopamine) are released from the adrenal medulla.

Although the increased sympathetic tone and fluid retention help to maintain arterial pressure, they also lead to a large increase in myocardial workload and necessitate a greater myocardial oxygen need in an environment of diminished supply. This supply–demand mismatch can lead to more myocardial hypoxia, enlargement of the infarcted region, precipitation of cardiac arrhythmias, and potentially a worsening in cardiac output. In addition, the sympathetic nervous system activation is responsible for the diaphoresis, anxiety, and nausea/vomiting commonly experienced by the patient.

After several weeks, if the patient survives the heart attack, the body remodels the infarcted tissue with a noncontractile fibrotic scar that does not contribute to ventricular strength. Long-term adaptation to the muscle loss includes development of compensatory hypertrophy or dilation, congestive heart failure, chronic dysrhythmias, and increased risk of sudden death. Table 26-1 provides an overview of the important body system

TABLE 26-1	Effects of Myocardial Infarction on Body Systems
Neurohumoral effects	• Enhanced sympathetic tone • Increased circulating catecholamines • Higher levels of angiotensin II and aldosterone • Increased arginine vasopressin
Cardiopulmonary effects	• Tachycardia • Dysrhythmias • Diminished stroke volume • Increased oxygen requirements • Pulmonary vascular congestion
Peripheral vascular effects	• Increased vascular resistance (vasoconstriction) • Elevations in blood volume • Possible systemic edema

changes secondary to an acute myocardial infarction (AMI).

ASSESSMENT FINDINGS

At any level of cardiac care, an MI is diagnosed in essentially three ways: symptoms and patient history, electrocardiogram, and cardiac enzymes. This is very important to EMS providers, for it demonstrates that even without major technological advancements, diagnosis of ACS-related syndromes is a *prehospital* capability. Although sophisticated testing will be used later to discern a more precise diagnosis, identification of at least certain types of MI is within the skill set of paramedics.

Symptoms and History

There is no such thing as a "typical" acute myocardial infarction. In fact, research has shown that there is no single symptom or historical finding that can fully rule out an AMI. As such, paramedics should "cast a wide net" and err on the side of being inclusive rather than exclusive. Some findings, though, certainly make AMI more likely.

The classic feature of an AMI is chest pain or discomfort. This discomfort is typically present in the anterior chest but can radiate to the arm (classically, the left arm), the jaw, the shoulder, and the abdomen. The pain of AMI is commonly dull in nature and is often described as squeezing or pressure.

It is important to remember that we are describing common findings—but uncommon findings do not rule out an AMI. In fact, many patients who experience an AMI do not report any chest pain. Often the patient complains of dyspnea. Shortness of breath has been found to be a very common finding after the age of 65. Nausea/vomiting is also a common symptom. Other common findings include syncope, anxiety, and diaphoresis. Interestingly, it is estimated that 10 percent of AMI patients will present with cardiac arrest as their first symptom.

The presence of risk factors for CAD also increases the likelihood of the symptoms being related to ischemia or infarction. Such risk factors include a past history of coronary or vascular disease, family history of coronary or vascular disease, smoking, hypertension, hypercholesterolemia, and diabetes mellitus.

Patients with classic angina will have a history of substernal chest pain or discomfort. The pain is usually described as a pressure or heaviness on the center of the chest; it usually occurs with activity and is relieved by rest. It may radiate to the left arm or jaw. The pain is frequently associated with dyspnea, nausea and vomiting, and diaphoresis. Depending on the significance of the myocardial ischemia, the patient may also display tachycardia and changes in blood pressure, inspiratory crackles (rales), or "cardiac asthma." ▶ Figure 26-4 lists common findings in patients with ischemic/infarction episodes.

Of special concern is the presentation of myocardial ischemia or infarction in women. Almost all common descriptions of the way ACS presents clinically have been taken from male cases. This is in part because medical literature at one time described only male patients with ACS, as they were primarily the ones who suffered cardiac events. However, as women have gained a more prominent presence in the workforce and have higher rates of smoking, poor nutrition habits, higher stress levels, and so

> **The most classic features of MI include chest discomfort that is dull in nature and typically radiates into the left arm or jaw.**

DISTINGUISHING ANGINA PECTORIS FROM MYOCARDIAL INFARCTION

	Angina Pectoris	Myocardial Infarction
Location of Discomfort	Substernal or across chest	Same
Radiation of Discomfort	Neck, jaw, arms, back, shoulders	Same
Nature of Discomfort	Dull or heavy discomfort with a pressure or squeezing sensation	Same, but maybe more intense
Duration	Usually 2 to 15 minutes, subsides after activity stops	Lasts longer than 10 minutes
Other symptoms	Usually none	Perspiration, pale gray color, nausea, weakness, dizziness, lightheadedness
Precipitating Factors	Extremes in weather, exertion, stress, meals	Often none
Factors Giving Relief	Stopping physical activity, reducing stress, nitroglycerin	Nitroglycerin may give incomplete or no relief

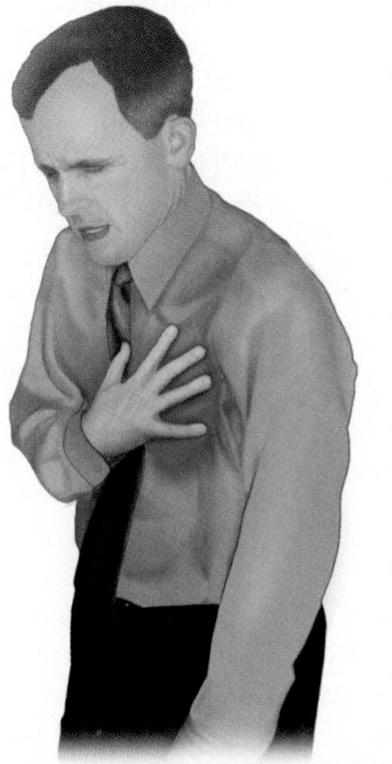

Figure 26-4 Both myocardial infarction and less serious angina can present symptoms of severe chest pain. Treat all cases of chest pain as cardiac emergencies.

forth, they are now suffering from heart attacks at rates approaching those among men. In fact, because the incidence of AMI in women is greater at older ages than in men, women are almost twice as likely to die from AMI or its complications within the first few weeks following the event.

A woman may present with different signs and symptoms from a man when she is experiencing a cardiac event; however, the event is just as dangerous and can be as deadly. Therefore, the paramedic must be sure to recognize some of the more subtle signs and symptoms that women suffering from ACS experience.

The list of symptoms in Table 26-2 is common for women suffering from cardiac ischemia or infarction. Although you will see that some descriptions are the same as for men, many others are not.

Because the death rate for women is higher than that for men when heart attack occurs, the paramedic should have a high index of suspicion of ischemia/infarction when gathering a history from the female patient. Err on the side of the patient and provide emergency care for a potential MI, despite a presentation of "atypical" signs of ischemia or infarction. Finally, note that diabetics and the elderly (Table 26-3) are also high-risk groups who may present with atypical findings.

TABLE 26-3	Special Considerations in Geriatric Cardiac Events
History of diabetes mellitus	A geriatric patient with diabetes has long-term damage to the nerve endings in the body. This causes the typical pain from an MI to be perceived poorly, if at all, by the diabetic patient. Therefore, the diabetic patient experiencing an MI may complain only of respiratory distress or dizziness when standing, or even excessive weakness and dyspnea on exertion. It is important for EMS providers to identify the patient with diabetes as potentially having an acute coronary event and to treat him appropriately.
History of trauma	If the geriatric patient is a trauma patient, there must be a high index of suspicion for cardiac involvement as well. Geriatric patients who are traumatized can slip quickly into cardiac arrest and do not respond well to typical interventions. Geriatric patients with head trauma, chest trauma, abdominal trauma, or extremity trauma with severe bleeding are especially susceptible to cardiac arrest.
History of asthma	If a patient with a history of asthma goes into cardiac arrest, the cause may be acute bronchoconstriction that led to hypoxemia, acidosis, and cardiac arrest. Until the bronchoconstriction is reversed, the patient will not regain a pulse or start to breathe again.
History of chronic obstructive pulmonary disease (COPD)	Elderly patients commonly have some form of COPD (emphysema or chronic bronchitis). The arrest may have been caused by an exacerbation of the COPD, which led to hypoxemia, acidosis, and then arrest. Remember also that COPD disorders can weaken the lung tissue and cause the development of a pneumothorax and collapse of the lung. (This too may precipitate a cardiac arrest.) Be alert for the presence or the development of a pneumothorax during positive pressure ventilation, which may cause a bleb on the lung tissue to rupture.

Electrocardiography (ECG)

AMI often causes predictable changes to cardiac conduction, and these changes are frequently noticeable through the use of 12-lead electrocardiography. Topic 27 will discuss in great detail how a 12-lead ECG is used to diagnose AMI; however, it is important that we touch on its general importance here.

A 12-lead ECG is used to rule in a specific type of AMI based on the findings of ST segment elevation. This type of MI is called an *ST elevation myocardial infarction* (STEMI). ST elevation identification is important because it has been found to be a reliable positive finding that can be used (in the proper context) at all levels of cardiac care to rule in AMI. In many cases, paramedics will combine symptoms and history with ECG findings to rapidly diagnose an AMI and initiate specific treatment strategies. Of course, ECG findings cannot be used alone to diagnose anything. As always, paramedics must assess the patient and not the monitor.

Twelve-lead ECG findings cannot not rule out an AMI. In fact, the majority of AMIs diagnosed do not initially present with ST elevation. Rather, paramedics should use 12-lead ECG to rule *in* AMI, but continue to use other assessment findings to categorize the level of ACS risk.

Cardiac Enzymes

The third way that an AMI is diagnosed is through the use of cardiac biomarkers (frequently referred to as *cardiac enzymes*). When the heart is in distress, it releases very specific biochemical markers that can be measured. In many cases, but not always, these chemicals are enzymes. In most cases, these markers are measured through a blood test with very specific diagnostic equipment. In the past, these tests were limited to the hospital setting, but with the advance of modern technology, this is no longer necessarily true. Many EMS systems use portable point-of-care tests that can enable paramedics to test for these markers in the prehospital setting.

Cardiac biomarkers can be used effectively to identify cardiac damage, but unfortunately there are limitations. Some cardiac markers do not appear until the ACS event has significantly progressed (sometimes they do not appear for as long as 12 to 24 hours) and

TABLE 26-2	Symptoms in Women with Cardiac Ischemia or Infarction

- "Classical" findings (not necessarily *common* findings)
  - Dull substernal chest pain or discomfort
  - Dyspnea or respiratory distress
  - Nausea, vomiting
  - Diaphoresis
- "Nonclassical" or "atypical" findings (not necessarily *uncommon* findings)
  - Neck ache
  - Pressure in the chest
  - Pains in the back, breast, or upper abdomen
  - Tingling of the fingers
  - Unexplained fatigue or weight gain (water weight gain)
  - Insomnia

TABLE 26-4 Cardiac Biomarkers

Marker	Description	Timing	Limitation
Troponin	Very specific and sensitive marker released as myocardial tissue is damaged.	Released after 2–4 hours but levels peak after 12 hours	Can be mimicked by severe pulmonary embolism, heart failure, and myocarditis.
Creatine kinase (CK-MB)	CK is an enzyme released when muscle is damaged. Its MB band is somewhat more specific to cardiac muscle.	Released after 3–4 hours but peaks after 10–24 hours	Also released when skeletal muscle is damaged. Can be mimicked by trauma.
Glycogen phosphorylase isoenzyme BB	Enzyme with isoform (BB) that is specific to cardiac muscle. Released as a result of ischemia. Increased levels can be diagnostic in myocardial infarction and unstable angina.	Released after 1–3 hours but peaks after 7 hours	Relatively new test. Minimal research validation.
B-natriuretic peptide (BNP)	Enzyme released from dysfunctioning myocardium. Commonly used biomarker for heart failure, but can also signal ACS.		Not specific to ACS. Can be mimicked by valvular heart disease, ventricular hypertrophy.
Myoglobin (Mb)	Protein found in skeletal and cardiac muscle. Secreted rapidly as a result of damage. Typically not specific enough to rule in an AMI, but lack of its presence can help rule out AMI.	Released after 2 hours	Low specificity for myocardial infarction. Can be mimicked by skeletal muscle damage.
Lactate dehydrogenase (LDH)	Enzyme secreted by conversion of lactate. Can be somewhat specific to heart muscle.	Released after 72 hours	High LDH levels can also be present in other conditions that cause tissue breakdown or destruction of blood cells. Mimics include cancer, meningitis, and HIV.

often they are not specific to AMI. For example, chest trauma can frequently produce many of the same chemical markers as AMI. However, when examined in context with other assessment findings, such as history and ECG, cardiac biomarkers can be a valuable diagnostic tool. Table 26-4 reviews key cardiac biomarkers.

EMERGENCY MEDICAL CARE

The treatment of ACS must be geared toward identifying and eliminating the occlusion to blood flow. Time is of the essence. Every 10 minutes of an occluded coronary artery lead to 1 percent patient mortality; therefore, rapid identification and treatment are essential. In many ways, the treatment of ACS should be approached in a manner similar to trauma care. There are very few meaningful on-scene treatments that should delay transport to definitive treatment. Rapid transport is the goal.

Definitively, AMI is generally treated in one of two ways. The first method is percutaneous coronary intervention (PCI). In this method, a catheter is inserted through a large blood vessel and is navigated to the area of the clot. The catheter can then dilate the vessel and eradicate the clot; a stent is then inserted through the catheter to keep the vessel open. This process not only is generally considered the safest alternative, but also requires extensive technology and is limited to facilities with catheterization capabilities.

The second method to treat an AMI is the use of thrombolytic or fibrinolytic therapy, in which medications such as streptokinase or tissue-type plasminogen activator (tPA) are used to chemically lyse the clot. Fibrinolytics are effective, but not specific to clots in the coronary arteries. Therefore, administration can lead to bleeding in other locations within the body and cause stroke. In some places, paramedics have been used to effectively administer fibrinolytic medications.

It is important for EMS provider to remember that both these therapies are generally available only in the hospital environment. Therefore, treatment of ACS should not interfere with rapid transport. Although prehospital administration of fibrinolytics is feasible, it is a controversial topic. As a result (and for the sake of the limited scope of this text), the treatments discussed here will focus on more universally accepted therapies.

Rapid Identification

The first element of treatment must be rapid identification. As stated previously, paramedics should cast a wide net and be inclusive when it comes to ruling out ACS. In general, there are three categories of cardiac patients. The first category is STEMI patients. This group can be rapidly and reasonably conclusively ruled in and therefore require the most aggressive treatment. The criteria for this group are positive symptomatology and history and an ST elevation on the ECG.

The second group can be categorized as ACS patients. These patients will have positive symptomatology and history, but lack ST elevation on the ECG. For the purposes of being inclusive, they fit the profile and should be treated as if they were having an MI until proven otherwise.

The final group would be non-ACS patients; this group would be populated by patients where AMI would be very unlikely. Chest pain secondary to traumatic injury would be a likely criteria for inclusion. This group should have the least number of patients, as it will be very difficult to conclusively rule out ACS given positive symptoms.

Treatment of STEMI

The treatment of STEMI patients will include the most aggressive interventions. In this group, we can reasonably conclude that an AMI is present; as such, the cost–benefit analysis shifts. In many systems, the presence of STEMI allows for bypass of the emergency department in favor of direct transport to the catheterization laboratory. By doing so, door-to-balloon time (the time from the patient entering the hospital to successful catheterization) can be decreased significantly.

The presence of STEMI may also initiate specific protocols regarding the number and placement of intravenous lines in anticipation of either PCI or thrombolytic medications. As always, follow local protocols. At a minimum, identification of STEMI should lead to immediate communication of the finding to the receiving hospital to initiate a larger team effort of cardiac care and to speed the initiation of more advanced treatment options.

Treatment Basics Revisited

Paramedics wield a wide array of medications and therapies for the treatment of their patients, but when dealing with ACS, it is vital that basic-level treatment is not forgotten. Steps as simple as calming the patient down and limiting exertion will help minimize cardiac oxygen demand and therefore limit the scope of infarction.

Position the patient. Semi- or high Fowler positioning will assist the patient in breathing and minimize the negative effects of fluid accumulating in the lungs. If positive pressure ventilation is being provided or frank hypotension is present, the patient will need to be placed supine for ongoing management.

In some cases, airway management will be necessary, but in most cases simply assuring a normal oxygenation level is most important. Provide oxygen if the patient is dyspneic, hypoxemic, has obvious signs of heart failure, or has a SpO$_2$ reading of less than 94 percent. Initiate oxygen therapy via nasal cannula at 4 lpm and titrate oxygen therapy to maintain a SpO$_2$ reading of 94 percent or greater. If the breathing is inadequate, provide positive pressure ventilation at 10 to 12/min with high-flow supplemental oxygen.

Of all the medications that are potentially available, aspirin still makes the most difference. Aspirin blocks thromboxane A$_2$ and helps prevent the activation of platelets and the further creation of a clot. The American Heart Association calls aspirin the "single most effective medication used to treat myocardial infarction." Administer 325 mg nonenteric-coated aspirin. Instruct the patient to chew the aspirin to promote a more rapid absorption. Aspirin should be administered even if the patient is on a daily regimen (unless he has taken the aspirin within the last hour).

Advanced Treatment

Immediate advanced level care may be treatment of cardiac dysrhythmias. Often ACS leads to electrical dysfunction and can cause bradycardias, tachycardias, and other arrhythmias.

Nitroglycerin is a commonly used medication to treat ACS. Nitroglycerin assists the ACS patient in two ways. First, theoretically, it dilates coronary arteries and can increase flow through otherwise obstructed vessels. Second, nitroglycerin is a primarily venous vasodilator and, as a result, increases venous pooling of blood and reduces preload. This reduction decreases the workload of the heart and reduces myocardial oxygen demand.

If the systolic blood pressure is greater than 90 mmHg or is less than 30 mmHg from the patient's baseline systolic blood pressure, administer one nitroglycerin tablet every 3 to 5 minutes. Be sure the systolic blood pressure remains above 90 mmHg following the administration. Do not administer nitroglycerin if any of the following is present:

- A systolic blood pressure <90 mmHg, or 30 mmHg or more below the patient's baseline systolic blood pressure
- Extreme bradycardia (< 50 bpm)
- Tachycardia in the absence of heart failure (>100 bpm)
- Right ventricular failure
- Erectile dysfunction medication use by the patient within the previous 72 hours

Nitroglycerin infusions have become a reliable administration route for both the treatment of ACS and the treatment of acute pulmonary edema. Infusion pumps offer an exact and controllable dose that is easily titrated to a desired effect.

Other advanced treatments can include additional medications to prevent platelet aggregation and clotting. Some EMS systems administer clopidogrel (Plavix), which works by inhibiting the glycoprotein IIb/IIIa pathway of coagulation. It is effective in minimizing clots that cause ACS, but can also cause a high risk of hemorrhage. Eptifibatide (Intergilin) is a similar medication that is less commonly used prehospitally.

Finally, analgesics may be necessary when chest pain is unrelieved by nitroglycerin. Although for many years morphine sulfate was the standard, recent studies have shown concern regarding the potentially cardiac toxic properties of narcotics. In related studies, morphine was shown to actually drop cardiac output; as a result, its utility in ACS care has, in some places, come into question. As always, follow local protocol.

Besides specific treatments, constant reassessment is essential. Remember that a frequent side effect of AMI is cardiac arrest. Paramedics must be hypervigilant and prepared for this possibility.

TRANSITIONING

REVIEW ITEMS

1. Aspirin is given in acute coronary syndrome to _____.
   a. block thromboxane A$_2$ and minimize the clotting process
   b. alleviate pain
   c. thin the blood
   d. dilate coronary vessels and increase blood flow

2. Which of the following best describes the difference between myocardial ischemia and myocardial infarction?
   a. In ischemia, the heart muscle dies.

b. In infarction, the heart muscle dies.

c. Ischemia arises from total occlusion of a coronary artery.

d. Infarction occurs when myocardial oxygen needs are not being met adequately.

3. Which of the following is a modifiable risk factor for coronary artery disease?

    a. tobacco use

    b. age and gender

    c. family history of cardiovascular disease

    d. confirmed diagnosis of diabetes mellitus

4. Your 86-year-old female patient is complaining of dyspnea, weakness, swollen ankles, and diffuse chest discomfort. She has a history of coronary bypass and hypertension. She is allergic to penicillin. Currently, her mental status is normal. Her vital signs are blood pressure 180/100 mmHg, heart rate 108 beats per minute and irregular, respiratory rate 18/minute. Given this scenario, what should your *first* action be?

    a. Administer 365 mg baby aspirin orally.

    b. Administer oxygen via a nasal cannula at 4 lpm.

    c. Assist with the administration of her prescribed nitroglycerin.

    d. Assist with the administration of her oral antihypertensive medication.

5. You arrive on scene to find a 45-year-old male patient with a chief complaint of chest pain. The patient states that the pain began while he was mowing the lawn but subsided after he sat on the couch for a few minutes. The patient has a cardiac history, and he states, "This just happened last week while mowing the lawn." Based on this information, from what do you think the patient is most likely suffering?

    a. acute myocardial infarction

    b. Prinzmetal angina

    c. stable angina

    d. congestive heart failure

APPLIED PATHOPHYSIOLOGY

A 48-year-old male patient is complaining of chest pain that he describes as dull and located substernally, with radiation to his neck. He rates the pain a 6 on a scale of 1 to 10 and complains of nausea and lightheadedness. His skin is cool and diaphoretic. His heart rate is 96 beats per minute, blood pressure is 124/82 mmHg, respiratory rate is 14, SpO$_2$ is 92 percent. He has taken two of his own nitroglycerin tablets prior to your arrival, without any relief.

1. Should you suspect that this patient is suffering from an ischemic or an infarction episode? Support your answer with the appropriate clinical findings provided.

2. Why might the administration of nitroglycerin to this patient be beneficial?

3. Describe the anticipated physiologic benefit(s) for each of the interventions that may be administered to a patient suffering from a myocardial infarction. Also list the appropriate dosage for each medication:

    a. Oxygen

    b. Aspirin

    c. Nitroglycerin

4. Discuss the differences in pathophysiology and presentation of the following acute coronary syndrome manifestations:

    a. Stable angina pectoris

    b. Unstable angina pectoris

    c. Myocardial infarction

5. Describe the pathophysiologic changes that occur to the lumen of the blood vessel resulting in atherosclerosis and occlusion of coronary blood vessels.

CLINICAL DECISION MAKING

You are summoned to a retirement community for an unknown medical emergency. On your arrival you meet a 68-year-old man sitting beside a ladder he was attempting to climb so he could clean out his gutters. On further questioning, you learn that he experienced a sensation of vertigo and nausea while climbing the ladder. A nearby family member stated that the patient was caught as he stumbled off the ladder and that no trauma occurred. The patient has also been experiencing "heartburn" for two days without relief. He last ate two hours earlier. His medical history includes hypertension, diabetes mellitus, a previous MI, and a "mini stroke" two years ago.

1. Based on the scene size-up characteristics, identify the clues that point to the field impression of either an ischemic or an infarction episode.

2. What medical condition does this patient have that could mask the common finding of an acute coronary syndrome?

The primary assessment reveals the patient to be alert and well oriented. His airway is clear; his breathing is rapid at 22/minute, respirations are slightly shallow, vesicular sounds are present, and slight inspiratory crackles (rales) are noted. Peripheral pulses are also present and noted to be rapid and slightly irregular. His blood pressure is 132/92. The neck veins are obviously engorged, and the SpO$_2$ reading on room air is 87 percent. His blood sugar is currently 142 mg/dL.

3. What are the life threats to the patient, if any, that you are currently aware of?

Further assessment reveals the patient's pupils to be equal and reactive, and the SpO$_2$ has increased to 94 percent with supplemental oxygen. Breath sounds are unchanged, and jugular venous distention is still present. His blood pressure is now 140/98, heart rate is 112 and irregular, and respirations have increased to 28/minute. The patient is starting to complain of chest "pressure" as well. During the ongoing management of the patient, you elect to administer the therapies listed below.

4. For each one, discuss in specific detail (1) the reason the intervention is warranted, (2) the expected outcome of that intervention, and (3) how you would assess to determine if the desired effect is occurring (i.e., the treatment worked).

   a. Position patient in high Fowler position

   b. Administer oxygen

   c. Administer aspirin

   d. Administer nitroglycerin

Standard Patient Assessment—Monitoring Devices and Medicine—
Cardiovascular

Competency Integrates scene and patient assessment findings with
knowledge of epidemiology and pathophysiology to form a field
impression. This includes developing a list of differential diagnoses
through clinical reasoning to modify the assessment and formulate a
treatment plan.

Integrates assessment findings with principles of epidemiology and
pathophysiology to formulate a field impression and implement
a comprehensive treatment/disposition plan for a patient with a
medical complaint.

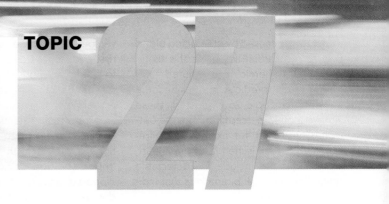

TOPIC

ACUTE CORONARY SYNDROME AND THE MULTILEAD ECG

INTRODUCTION

Every year, nearly 500,000 Americans die from acute myocardial infarction (AMI). In fact, in the acute setting of an AMI, mortality rates go up 1 percent for every 10 minutes of an occluded coronary artery. As such, treatment of these patients is truly a race against the clock. Treatment of AMI has progressed in leaps and bounds in the past 20 years, and the level of technology used to resolve this pathology is at an all-time high.

All these methodologies rely on teamwork at all levels of the health care world. To maximize outcomes, prehospital providers must pair with emergency department (ED) personnel, and hospital staff must work closely with more advanced departments, to provide the patient a smooth and rapid transition to definitive care. Few other areas of prehospital medicine rely more heavily on these partnerships.

Within this team dynamic, paramedics are used to rapidly identify and transport the AMI patient. An AMI is diagnosed using history, electrocardiograms (ECGs), and biomarkers; even though none of these elements is immediate or perfectly precise, ECG, when used correctly, can provide a reliable method to rapidly rule in at least a certain percentage of these patients. This capability has been proven to be accessible and reliable in the world of prehospital medicine.

Although the ST elevation myocardial infarction (STEMI) is present in a comparatively small minority of the overall number of patients having an AMI, it is still readily identifiable and, as such, is an important marker that can be used to initiate treatment. Moreover, this marker is used not just in the hospital, but in the prehospital environment as well. Paramedics every day combine a larger clinical picture of the patient with this key ECG finding and initiate a specific treatment standard to aggressively treat the AMI.

In some cases, paramedics will initiate thrombolytic medications, but even if definitive treatment is not administered prehospitally, the identification of an AMI and subsequent notification has been shown consistently to significantly reduce the time it takes to initiate definitive care in the hospital. Many acute coronary syndrome (ACS) systems rely on early identification of STEMI to initiate multiple levels of response to provide the highest level

TRANSITION highlights

- *Importance of acute myocardial infarction (AMI) recognition.*
- *Role of multilead monitoring in AMI recognition.*
- *Review of key monitoring steps.*
- *Findings that can indicate the AMI.*
- *Findings that mimic the AMI.*
- *The future of multilead monitoring.*

of therapy—and, in most cases, identification begins in the prehospital world. Multilead monitoring is a vital component of ACS care; every paramedic should use it to its fullest capability.

This topic reviews the role of multilead monitoring in the identification and treatment of AMI. It is not intended to be a comprehensive review of cardiac monitoring. Rather, this topic reviews the general diagnostic uses of ECG in ACS and examines key steps to make its use most beneficial. In some cases, this topic discusses specific application procedures, but it does not provide a complete step-by-step process. If you are uncomfortable with basic ECG monitoring, please refer to a paramedic textbook for more information (also see Topic 22, "Patient Monitoring Devices," for further information).

ECG AND AMI DIAGNOSIS

In ACS, ECG is only one part of a larger diagnostic picture. Paramedics must always assess and treat the patient, not just the cardiac monitor. However, ECG can be a vital tool when used in the correct context.

Paramedics must always assess and treat the patient, not just the cardiac monitor.

An AMI is caused by obstructed blood flow to myocardial tissue. As this tissue becomes ischemic and injured and begins to die, predictable signs become evident. As Topic 26 discussed, these signs are often perceptible from the outside. Chest pain, for example, is a frequent result of ischemia in the heart. Other signs can include the detectable release of chemical biomarkers that indicate cardiac injury.

Electrically speaking, ischemia, injury, and infarction also cause predictable changes in the cardiac conduction system. The pathophysiology of poor myocardial cell perfusion causes very specific changes to the depolarization and repolarization process used to initiate and transmit cardiac conduction. As blood flow (and oxygen delivery) to the myocardial cell is diminished, the cell becomes depleted of the adenosine triphosphate (ATP) that powers its sodium–potassium pump. When the pump is disrupted, the movement of sodium and potassium is delayed or stopped, resulting in a slowing or a failure of the cell to repolarize. A multilead cardiac monitor can identify the sum of these repolarization changes by looking at the ST segment of the QRS complex. ST segment depression—and, more important, ST segment elevation—signify changes in repolarization and can be used to identify ischemia and injury issues within the myocardium that are frequently caused by ACS.

Slow repolarization and infarction of cardiac cells can also cause changes in the vector of repolarization and depolarization through the heart. Depolarization of the heart occurs along a predictable pathway. Organization of pacemaker cells and the conduction pathway cause predictable deflections of the QRS complex as the heart muscle is depolarized and repolarized.

> **Most STEMI protocols are activated by the identification of ST elevation in two or more congruent leads.**

As you may recall, the direction of deflection of the various waves that make up the QRS complex represent the vector (direction) of either depolarization (as in the QRS complex itself) or repolarization (as in the T wave). When conduction in the heart is disrupted by ischemia, these vectors can change. Slowly repolarizing tissue causes the direction of conduction to be altered. For example, T waves represent the repolarization of ventricular tissue. When this tissue repolarizes slowly as a result of ischemia, T wave vectors can be found moving in opposite directions compared with the QRS complex (this condition is commonly called *flipped T waves*). Q waves can also be deepened by electrically neutral infarcted (dead) cells.

Occasionally, ischemic and infarcted cells also can cause a bundle branch block. Here, normal cardiac depolarization must bypass the area of poor conduction and typically does so by moving off the conduction pathway. Not only does this shift the axis of depolarization, but the cell-to-cell transmission also slows conduction, causing a widened QRS complex on the ECG.

Electrical Diagnostic Criteria

The pathophysiology of ACS can be represented on a multilead ECG in three ways:

- **Ischemia.** Ischemia can be seen by looking for new ST depression (an ST segment at least 1 mm depressed from the isoelectric baseline in at least two congruent leads) and flipped T waves (T waves with opposite vectors compared with the QRS complex in at least two congruent leads).

- **Injury.** Injury is identified by ST segment elevation (>1 mm in two congruent leads) (some references will note >2 mm in septal leads).

- **Infarction.** Infarction is identified by the presence of pathologic Q waves (>0.04 sec wide or 1/3 of R, with ST elevation).

Practical Application of ECG Diagnostic Criteria

Although system protocols vary, most organized STEMI protocols are activated by the identification of ST elevation in two or more congruent leads. It is also generally accepted that the presence of a new onset left bundle branch block (LBBB) is a presumptive positive finding (although differentiating new versus old in the prehospital environment may be challenging). It cannot be emphasized enough, however, that no patient is diagnosed purely on ECG criteria. Many additional clinical factors must be considered. ECG does play an essential role, however. The paramedic will use electrical findings in context with other signs and symptoms to help define a larger clinical picture.

The paramedic must further discern transient and permanent electrical findings. Pathologic Q waves identify infarcted cells but are not typically useful in the prehospital world because they are a permanent finding associated with AMI. That is, once they present, they are always there. As such, without an older ECG for comparison, it is impossible to determine whether Q waves are related to an acute event or to an older long-standing problem. Bundle branch blocks can be a permanent finding, but they can also be transient in nature.

Transient findings occur acutely, but can resolve as the dysfunction is eliminated. Transient findings are generally more important in the diagnosis of an acute event. Because transient findings are correctable, they generally symbolize new findings and are more reliable indicators of an acute problem. ST elevation is the most important finding, as it most commonly represents newly injured myocardial cells. Most ACS treatment systems use this finding (in context) to initiate specific AMI treatment. Remember also that transient changes develop (and change) over time. Initial findings may be very different from later findings. Multilead ECG is therefore an important serial finding.

There is context even within electrical findings. The importance of multilead monitoring is that it gives credibility to specific findings. Just as reporters use multiple sources to confirm a story, paramedics use multiple leads to confirm their suspicions. Multiple leads look individually at specific anatomic regions of the left ventricle (and the entire heart) and provide multiple electrical views of cardiac conduction.

Changes found in one lead are not diagnostic. For example, a singular ST elevation finding in lead II is meaningless. However, multilead ECG can confirm this finding by identifying it in other leads that look at similar regions of the heart (congruent leads). Although singular findings in just lead II are meaningless, elevations found in leads II, III, and AVF would be considered indicative of AMI. Paramedics should be familiar with the specific ECG leads and the regions of

TABLE 27-1 ECG Leads and Their View of the Heart

Region of the Heart	Leads
Inferior wall (of the left ventricle)	II, III, AVF
Septal wall (of the left ventricle)	V_1, V_2
Anterior wall (of the left ventricle)	V_3, V_4
Lateral wall (of the left ventricle)	I, AVL, V_5, V_6
Posterior wall (of the left ventricle)	V_8, V_9
Right ventricle	V_4R, V_6R

the heart to which they correspond (see Table 27-1).

Furthermore, specific findings can be reinforced by reciprocal changes. Reciprocal changes are changes that occur in a wall of the heart opposite the site of a myocardial infarction (Table 27-2). These specific changes are generally limited to the circumstances related to AMI and greatly enhance the accuracy of a diagnosis.

It is exceptionally important to remember that not every AMI presents with the electrical changes discussed previously. The development of these changes greatly depends on the depth and significance of the AMI. In many cases, these changes will develop and worsen over time. Often, a patient will present with other clinical findings and will not demonstrate electrical changes, but is indeed having a heart attack. At no time should a lack of electrical changes be used to rule out an AMI. Electrical findings, on the other hand, are used to rule in AMI. These changes—in the context of a larger clinical picture that includes chief complaint, history, and, at times, cardiac biomarkers—offer a presumptive positive for myocardial infarction.

TABLE 27-2 Reciprocal Changes

Primary Change	Reciprocal Change
II, III, AVF (inferior)	I, AVL (lateral)
I, AVL (lateral)	II, III, AVF (inferior)
V_1, V_2 (septal), V_3, V_4 (anterior)	V_7, V_8, V_9 (posterior)
V_7, V_8, V_9 (posterior)	V_1, V_2 (septal), V_3, V_4 (anterior)

ACCURACY IN DIAGNOSIS

To use the multilead ECG effectively in the diagnosis of ACS, care must be taken to use the device and interpret the results effectively. Improper use can render electrical findings meaningless. Accuracy is ensured in two ways. First, you must ensure accuracy of the setup and lead placement. These physical steps ensure the validity of the product you will next interpret. Second, you must ensure the accuracy of the interpretation to be sure your electrical diagnosis is correct.

ECG Setup and Lead Placement

The use of an electrocardiograph requires appropriate knowledge and proper utilization. As with any machine, it must be used correctly in order to obtain accurate results. ECG machines must be properly maintained, handled, stored, and calibrated according to manufacturer's recommendations in order to be reliable. ECG cables must be handled and stored with care and replaced when malfunctioning.

ECG leads rely on exact external chest placement to reliably look at specific anatomic regions of the heart. Simply put, they must be placed properly to see what they are supposed to see. A common error in ECG-related diagnosis is improper lead placement.

Proper multilead ECG placement begins with the three leads of Einthoven's triangle. These leads were designed as "limb leads" and as such, should be placed on the limbs. Movement of the hands and feet can often interfere with proper electrical tracings; if necessary, these leads can be moved closer to the body, but, by definition, they should not be placed superior to the inguinal folds of the groin or medial to the shoulder joint (▶ Figure 27-1).

Chest leads, also known as the precordial leads, also have exact placement. Table 27-3 and ▶ Figure 27-2 detail specific placement of these leads.

Accuracy of an ECG is also enhanced by obtaining a clear tracing—that is, by eliminating interference and artifacts. A paramedic can take several steps to enhance the clarity of ECG production.

- **Prepare the patient.** Paramedics should always consider preparing the skin prior to application of an ECG lead. Sweat and wetness should be wiped away. Excessive hair should be clipped or shaved. Dead skin should be gently exfoliated by using commercially available prep tape or with the simple use of gentle scrubbing with a towel. Patient preparation also includes talking to the patient about remaining still during the ECG acquisition.

- **Use appropriate leads.** Quality ECG leads are often the most important element in obtaining a quality ECG tracing. Use high-quality leads and handle them properly. Most leads use a water-based conductive gel; when left unsealed, these gels can dry out and cause poor lead contact. Keep leads in sealed containers prior to their use.

Accuracy of Interpretation

In addition to the physical elements of accuracy, accuracy of interpretation is also important. Although the scope of this topic limits a full discussion of ECG interpretation, you should consider interpretation of findings as important as any other element of diagnosis. You should take seriously this responsibility and train accordingly. ECG interpretation can be difficult even under optimal circumstances, and the only way to improve is practice. Paramedics should keep the following concepts in mind:

> A common error in ECG-related diagnosis is improper lead placement.

- **Treat the patient.** Always keep in mind that fewer than 40 percent of diagnosed AMIs occur with ST segment elevation. That means that the majority do not. Look at all the clinical findings and history that point to ACS and be inclusive, rather than exclusive. A 12-lead ECG without ST segment elevation does not rule out an AMI. Remember that, at times, diagnosis of an AMI may be a relatively low priority. Always treat immediate life threats, such as bradycardias and tachycardias, first.

- **You are not just diagnosing the ACS.** The underlying rhythm interpretation is important as well. Rhythm abnormalities, such as ventricular

Electrocardiographic Leads and Their Axes

Limb leads

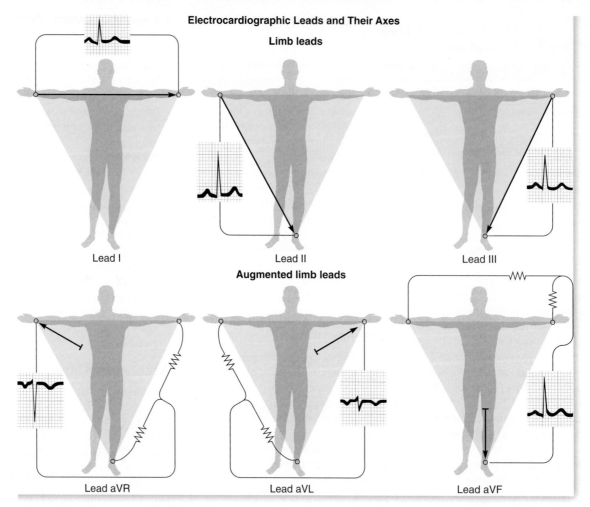

Lead I   Lead II   Lead III

Augmented limb leads

Lead aVR   Lead aVL   Lead aVF

Figure 27-1 Placement of limb leads.

rhythms and bundle branch blocks, can interfere with your ability to make ST segment judgments and identify ACS. Always start with basic ECG interpretation and then move to ST analysis.

TABLE 27-3	Precordial Lead Placement

Lead	Placement
V₁	4th intercostal (IC) space right of the sternum
V₂	4th IC space left of the sternum
V₃	Midway between V₂ and V₄
V₄	5th IC space midclavicular line
V₅	5th IC space anterior axillary line
V₆	5th IC space mid-axillary line
V₈	5th IC space mid-scapular
V₉	5th IC space between V₈ and spine
V₄R	Same as V₄ but on right chest
V₆R	Same as V₆ but on right chest

- **Look at multiple leads.** No one lead can be diagnostic in and of itself. Diagnosis of ACS requires multilead interpretation.
- **Practice and utilize quality improvement.** ECG interpretation is a skill that is acquired through practice and self-examination. Take advantage of training opportunities and always review the mistakes you made. Take time to discuss questionable findings. Discuss your thoughts with your medical director.
- **Use diagnostic software.** Although there are flaws, most modern diagnostic packages are exceptionally sensitive to recognizing STEMI. Of course, you should place that diagnosis in the context of the larger clinical picture, but think of it as a second set of eyes.

STEMI IMITATORS A variety of conditions can mimic the electrical findings of STEMI. Although there are far more conditions that can confound diagnosis, the following situations are the most commonly confused imitators:

- **Left bundle branch block (LBBB).** LBBB can cause ST elevation changes as the vector of depolarization is altered and repolarization of cells takes place more slowly outside the conduction pathway. This can cause ST elevation because of the block and not necessarily because of acute injury to cells. Unfortunately, an LBBB can actually be caused by an AMI, so it is difficult to discern whether what you are seeing is acute or chronic. As previously stated, most systems accept LBBB as a presumptive positive finding for AMI.
- **Left ventricular hypertrophy (LVH).** In this chronic condition, in which the left ventricle becomes enlarged and more massive, conduction changes (particularly axis and repolarization changes) can mimic STEMI. A key differential will be exceptionally positive or negative R and S waves. A typical diagnostic criterion is to add the depth of the S wave in V₁ or V₂ (whichever is deepest) to the

height of the R wave in V_5 or V_6 (whichever is tallest). If the total is ≥35 mm, then LVH is present.) LVH also does not present with reciprocal change, so the presence of such changes can be indicative of ACS.

- **Pericarditis.** An infection causing inflammation and the accumulation of fluid in the pericardial membrane can put pressure on the myocardium and cause resultant electrical changes in the ST segment. Pericarditis is typically differentiated by the fact that its changes are not specific to a region but are generally more global. Rather than seeing ST elevation in the inferior leads, you would see elevation among all leads. History that points to infection (fever, chronic onset, pain increased by supine position) can also guide this differential diagnosis.
- **Hyperkalemia.** Hyperkalemia, or increased potassium levels, can cause ST elevation and T wave changes that mimic STEMI. Typically, the hyperkalemic patient has a history that points toward electrolyte imbalance. Hyperkalemia is common among renal failure and dialysis patients. Hyperkalemia can typically be differentiated by looking for its signature elevated and peaked T waves, but there also may be decreasing amplitude P waves and widening QRS complexes as the condition worsens.

It is important to point out that each of these imitators has at least one element that can be identified through a thorough patient history. This fact underscores the importance of assessing the entire patient, not just the ECG finding.

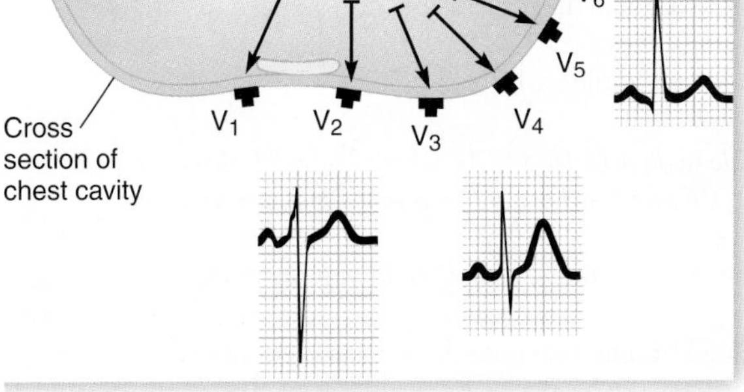

CREATING A COORDINATED RESPONSE ACROSS THE HEALTH CARE SYSTEM

In many cases, ECG is an important criterion used to activate a larger series of events. Although a lack of ST elevation does not rule out an MI, accurate interpretation of ST elevation can rule one in. As such, identifying such findings is an important start to many larger protocols. In fact, many treatment protocols identify STEMI as a separate category of care because of the relative sensitivity of the ECG finding. In other words, because ST elevation is such a reliable finding, we can be more aggressive in treating these patients. In other situations, without ECG confirmation, we may still treat ACS, but we may need to be slightly more conservative until more definitive diagnostics, such as biomarkers, are available.

Although local protocols vary, ECG findings commonly are used to guide destination choices. Many systems have developed protocols for the immediate transfer of patients to specific hospitals that are capable of percutaneous coronary intervention (PCI); typically, the most important indicator for the bypass of other facilities is ST elevation (and, in some cases, LBBB). Some systems, in the interest of decreasing door-to-open-artery time, have even allowed for bypass of the ED and transport directly to the catheterization center. Although this practice would be otherwise dangerous and create increased liability, it can be made possible by the specific finding of STEMI.

Note that ECG is not the only factor considered in any cardiac triage system; the larger clinical picture of the patient is always examined as well. ECG findings must be paired with symptomology and patient history and placed within the context of the larger system protocols. Many systems further require the use of interpretive software and some require transmission of findings. Although some paramedics consider these requirements to be a doubting of their own capabilities, these additional requirements should be viewed as enhancing the diagnostic capability and avoiding overtriage. Of course there is no way to avoid a certain number of mistakes. Most trauma systems happily accept overtriage rates as high as 10 percent to 15 percent (and, in some cases, much higher).

Even if your system does not allow for bypassing a smaller hospital or direct transport to the catheterization center, STEMI findings can still decrease door-to-open-artery time. Although you may transport to a hospital without catheterization capabilities, notifying the hospital of earlier presumptive findings can simply make all levels of care move faster. In some cases, that may mean that fibrinolytics are considered earlier; in other cases, it may mean more active steps. In any case, earlier treatment means less mortality.

THE FUTURE OF ACS CARE

Because mortality is so linked with time in ACS care, the future is surely linked to earlier and earlier identification and treatment. Most likely, the capabilities to recognize an STEMI will increase.

Paramedics should adapt their practice to include earlier acquisition of 12-lead ECG. The American Heart Association now recognizes the first 10 minutes as a target window for ECG acquisition. Paramedics should consider suspected ACS as a time-sensitive disorder. Furthermore, the criteria for 12-lead ECG should also be expanded. More patients, especially those with vague complaints, should receive a multilead ECG. Weakness, syncope, and shortness of breath should all be considered indications for a multilead ECG. Again, recognizing STEMI creates different treatment options.

In the future, technology will enhance our capabilities. Even in the past few years, interpretive software has become more sensitive and more specific. The future will likely hold advances that can assist our interpretation and rely less on

Precordial leads

Cross section of chest cavity

V_1 V_2 V_3 V_4 V_5 V_6

Figure 27-2 Precordial lead placement.

human frailties and biases. Transition capabilities have also dramatically improved. The paramedic's ability to share not only ECG data, but also the full spectrum of telemedicine findings, will enhance communication and will allow for a further extension of the health care system.

Some examples exist of paramedics initiating thrombolytic therapy in the field. In most cases, these administrations are both guided by transmission capabilities and reviewed under a rigid system of medical direction. The debate about the value of PCI and thrombolytics continues, but this area may certainly provide a boon once more information is made available.

TRANSITIONING

REVIEW ITEMS

1. New ST depression, when found in two congruent leads, would be an ECG finding that indicates _____.
   a. ischemia
   b. infarction
   c. injury
   d. normal conduction

2. New ST elevation, when found in two congruent leads, would be an ECG finding that indicates _____.
   a. ischemia
   b. infarction
   c. injury
   d. normal conduction

3. Which of the following would be the transient ECG finding most commonly used to identify injury to myocardial cells?
   a. ST depression in two congruent leads
   b. Q-waves
   c. cardiac biomarkers
   d. ST elevation in two congruent leads

4. Which of the following would be considered a presumptive positive finding that indicates AMI?
   a. left ventricular hypertrophy
   b. T-wave inversion
   c. left bundle branch block
   d. ST depression in two congruent leads

5. Which of the following would be a condition that mimicked the ECG findings associated with STEMI?
   a. asthma
   b. endocarditis
   c. hyperkalemia
   d. pulmonary embolism

APPLIED PATHOPHYSIOLOGY

1. Describe briefly why ST segment elevation occurs in some AMIs.

2. Explain the difference between transient and permanent ECG findings.

3. Why are transient ECG findings more important than permanent findings in diagnosing AMI?

4. Explain how you might differentiate pericarditis from STEMI.

5. Explain why an ECG cannot rule out an AMI.

CLINICAL DECISION MAKING

A 61-year-old woman complains of acute onset nausea, vomiting, and weakness. She states that she feels like she is going to pass out. On arrival, you find her seated on the toilet, pale, diaphoretic, and breathing rapidly.

1. Describe your initial actions and assessments.

2. Based on the initial description, do you consider ACS as a possible cause of her problems? Why or why not?

The patient's airway is patent, but she tells you she cannot catch her breath. Her respiratory rate is 30 with clear lung sounds. The patient has a weak radial pulse at 52. Her skin is wet. She is awake and alert, but notes she feels very dizzy. The patient denies chest pain and notes that the nausea and vomiting "came on out of nowhere." Initial vital signs are pulse 58, respirations 30, blood pressure 86/62 mmHg.

3. Given this primary assessment, what immediate actions do you need to take?

4. What additional diagnostic tests do you need to run?

5. Should you initiate a 12-lead ECG?

You decide to do a 12-lead ECG, which shows ST elevation in leads II, III, and AVF and T wave inversion in leads I and AVL.

6. Given these findings, what should you conclude?

7. What additional therapies does this patient need?

Standard Medicine

Competency Integrates assessment findings with principles of epidemiology and pathophysiology to formulate a field impression and implement a comprehensive treatment/disposition plan for a patient with a medical complaint.

TOPIC

28

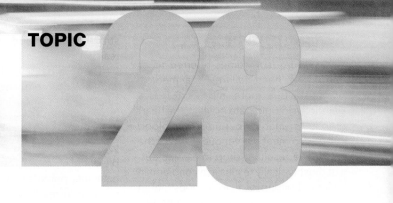

CARDIOVASCULAR EMERGENCIES: HEART FAILURE

INTRODUCTION

Diagnosing and treating a heart failure patient in acute pulmonary edema is one of the most challenging situations a paramedic can face. Although there are literally thousands of heart failure patients living in America each day, the vast majority will not need the services of EMS. However, a small percentage of those will present with life-threatening side effects, such as pulmonary edema, and will require prehospital intervention in the most desperate terms.

The acute presentation of heart failure not only can be life threatening, but also can be difficult to discern from other chronic respiratory illnesses. As a result, paramedics are faced every day with the dilemma of making important treatment decisions with only limited information at their disposal. To make matters worse, recent research has demonstrated that some commonly used therapies may be harmful if the diagnosis is wrong.

Although diagnostic technology has improved and will continue to advance, paramedics must rely on a knowledge of pathophysiology and quality assessment skills to rapidly identify this category of patient. Treatments should be goal oriented and aggressive, but must address the reality of acute pulmonary edema, not the outdated myths. Furthermore, EMS systems, in the development of protocols, should use treatment options that are forgiving and broader in scope so as to minimize the risk of misdiagnosis.

This topic provides a brief overview of the pathophysiology of acute heart failure and includes a review of both right- and left-sided failure. It also reviews key diagnostic findings and treatment, especially with regard to acute pulmonary edema.

EPIDEMIOLOGY

In the United States, heart failure is a disease state of significant concern. It has been estimated that the prevalence rate for heart failure is about 1 percent to 2 percent in the adult population. In more specific numbers, more than 400,000 patients are diagnosed yearly with heart failure, and currently about 3 million Americans have this disease state. In fact, this pathology is a

TRANSITION highlights

- *Frequency, ethnic and gender predisposition, and morbidity rates for patients with heart failure.*
- *Pathophysiologic changes that accompany this disease process:*
  - – Heart failure.
  - – Left heart failure.
  - – Right heart failure.
- *Common signs and symptoms of heart failure with specific findings that will best delineate between these emergencies.*
- *Assessment phases for a patient suffering from heart failure and the specific etiologies that accompany this disease process.*
- *Treatment interventions:*
  - – Oxygen.
  - – Pulse oximetry.
  - – Body positioning.
  - – Continuous positive airway pressure (CPAP).
  - – Medications.

common reason for hospital admittance, as up to 40 percent of heart failure patients are hospitalized every year. Heart failure has been found to be the cause of death in blacks more often than in whites (blacks are 1.5 times more likely to die from heart failure) and has a higher prevalence in men than in women (although in the population over 75 years of age, heart failure shows no gender preferences).

As to be expected, the prevalence of heart failure increases with age, affecting about 10 percent of the population older than 75 years. Finally, as a comorbid factor, patients with insulin-dependent diabetes have a significantly higher mortality rate.

PATHOPHYSIOLOGY

Heart failure (sometimes referred to as *congestive heart failure*) is a medical diagnosis, but, more important, it is a pathophysiologic state in which the heart muscle is unable to pump the blood needed to meet the venous return of the body. The resultant drop in cardiac output most typically results in a condition in which a buildup of fluid (congestion) in the body occurs as a result of pump failure. In essence, it represents the condition in which the left, right, or both ventricles fail to meet the body's needs. It may be a chronic condition that develops over a period of time (perhaps years), or it may be more acute in nature should it be associated with a large myocardial infarction (MI) or other serious disruption in the heart's ability to pump blood mechanically.

The many causes of heart failure include coronary artery disease, valvular dysfunction, and myocardial disease. Other factors that may contribute to heart failure include excessive salt or water intake, hypertension, thyrotoxicosis, pulmonary embolism, alcohol/drug abuse, and anemia.

Heart failure, as discussed, results in the reduction of cardiac output and may be caused by a decrease in stroke volume or a change in heart rate. By definition, cardiac output is the amount of blood pumped by the heart for 60 seconds. The relationship of cardiac output (CO), stroke volume (SV), and heart rate (HR) is found in the following formula:

$$CO = SV \times HR$$

A reduction in cardiac output leads to compensatory mechanisms that act to restore cardiac output. For instance, when a patient sustains an MI, dead heart muscle can prevent the heart from pumping normally, thus leading to decreased cardiac output. The body senses the decrease in cardiac output by way of baroreceptors in the aortic arch and carotid bodies and tries to compensate by increasing sympathetic tone.

Because the myocardium cannot increase stroke volume because of the damaged pump, it must compensate by increasing the heart rate. If, however, a patient has a dysrhythmia that affects only the heart rate (i.e., bradycardia), the decreased heart rate leads to a decreased cardiac output. In that case, the body tries to compensate by increasing the stroke volume and systemic vascular resistance.

The body has several other mechanisms it can use to compensate for decreased cardiac output. These include vasoconstriction of peripheral vessels and activation of the hormonal systems of the body designed to increase intravascular volume. An example of the hormonal response is brain-type natriuretic peptide (BNP). This substance is released in response to distention of the ventricles seen in heart failure. The substance, tested for as an indicator of heart failure, promotes natriuresis and tends to lower blood volume. Unfortunately, these compensatory mechanisms actually increase myocardial oxygen demand and thus are potentially detrimental to myocardial function.

Heart failure is generally divided into left ventricular (LV) failure and/or right ventricular (RV) failure, although this is somewhat arbitrary in nature, owing to the fact that the right and left ventricles perfuse different portions of the circulation. It can also be described as "backward failure" (leading to congestion) and "forward failure" (leading to diminished end-organ perfusion).

Left-Sided Failure

Left ventricular (LV) failure occurs when the left ventricle is unable to pump adequately; the heart pumps inadequately for multiple reasons. Dysfunction of the heart muscle itself, as is seen with MI, is one of the main causes of LV pump failure. Dysrhythmias also inhibit the heart's ability to pump normally.

With *backward* failure of the left ventricle, pulmonary congestion (pulmonary edema) results, leading to signs and symptoms that are primarily respiratory in nature. With *forward* failure of the left ventricle, diminished peripheral perfusion and systemic circulation result. Conditions that may be responsible for this include obstruction of outflow from the heart, as is seen in valvular disease or chronic systemic hypertension.

Right-Sided Failure

In this type of heart failure, the right side of the heart fails to function as an adequate pump to the lungs, which commonly leads to back pressure of blood into the venous and systemic circulation with *backward* failure of the right ventricle. Backward failure of the right ventricle results in excess fluid that accumulates in the body, often in dependent extremities (▶ Figure 28-1), and may cause jugular venous distention (JVD) (▶ Figure 28-2), enlargement of the liver, and possible abdominal distention in severe cases.

Right ventricular (RV) failure is most commonly caused by backward failure of the left heart muscle, which then causes an eventual backlogging of blood into the right heart circuit. Similar to the causes of LV failure, other disorders that can cause the right side to fail include dysfunction of

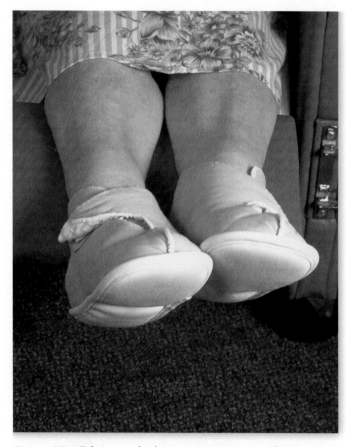

Figure 28-1 Edema to the lower extremities is a classic sign of heart failure.

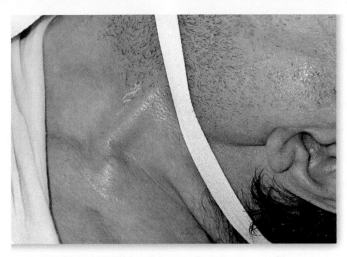

Figure 28-2 Jugular vein distention is a late sign of heart failure. (© *David Effron, M.D.*)

the heart muscle itself from chronic pulmonary hypertension or, in acute cases, right ventricular MI. Right ventricular MI is less common than LV infarctions, but it is seen. Pulmonary hypertension and stenotic pulmonary valvular disease can also result in *forward* failure of the right heart and may result in lungs being underperfused, leading to subjective respiratory distress and diminished preload to the left heart circuit.

Table 28-1 summarizes these pathophysiologic changes in right and left heart failure leading to the diagnosis of congestive heart failure. Remember, though, heart failure is the underlying problem; when the medical condition exacerbates, the presentation is often centered around dyspnea, weakness, changes in breath sounds, possible chest pain, weakness, and fluid retention.

ASSESSMENT FINDINGS

The signs and symptoms of heart failure will depend on the severity of the condition and whether it is an acute-onset or a long-term problem. During the assessment, recall that several exceptions apply to a simple left-versus-right division of heart failure symptoms. Left-sided *forward* failure overlaps with right-sided *backward* failure. Because the most common cause of right heart failure is left heart failure, patients may present with symptoms of both types (a condition known as *biventricular failure*). Regardless, the signs and symptoms of congestive heart failure include the following (▶ Figure 28-3):

- Marked or severe dyspnea (shortness of breath)
- Tachycardia (rapid heart rate, greater than 100 bpm)
- Difficulty breathing when supine (orthopnea)
- Suddenly waking at night with dyspnea (paroxysmal nocturnal dyspnea)
- Fatigue on any type of exertion

- Anxiety
- Tachypnea (rapid respiratory rate)
- Diaphoresis (sweating)
- Upright position with legs, feet, arms, and hands dangling
- Cool, clammy, pale skin
- Chest discomfort
- Cyanosis
- Agitation and restlessness from the hypoxia
- Edema (swelling) to the hands, ankles, and feet
- Crackles and possibly wheezes on auscultation
- Decreased SpO$_2$ reading
- Blood pressure normal, elevated, or low
- Distended neck veins—jugular venous distention (JVD)
- Distended and soft, spongy abdomen

Table 28-2 summarizes common findings of heart failure and discusses the pathophysiologic change that underlies them.

Medications can often help diagnose a history of heart failure. Early and mild cases of heart failure are commonly treated with beta blockers to help control rate and myocardial oxygen demand. As heart failure progresses, patients are frequently prescribed diuretics to manage fluid volume levels. Patient also frequently take angiotensin-converting enzyme (ACE) inhibitors to control afterload.

> **Medications can often help diagnose a history of heart failure.**

Diagnosing Acute Pulmonary Edema

Acute pulmonary edema is the common byproduct of left-sided failure. As pressure builds in the circuit behind the left ventricle, fluid begins to migrate out of the system. The specific challenge occurs in the acute setting when that fluid leaves the vascular space, crosses the membranes of the pulmonary capillaries, and moves into the interstitial tissue of the lungs. If the condition continues, the fluid can also occupy space in the alveoli themselves.

Pulmonary edema can be a chronic condition. As the previous section discussed, many patients describe ongoing symptoms such as dyspnea on exertion, paroxysmal nocturnal dyspnea, and orthopnea. However, pulmonary edema can also present in a life-threatening acute fashion when fluid is rapidly transferred into the lungs, causing respiratory failure.

TABLE 28-1	Pathophysiologic Changes in Right and Left Heart Failure
	Pathophysiologic Findings
Right heart failure	Right heart fails because of infarction, increased workload, valvular dysfunction, or a combination of these. It results in the congestion of blood in the vena cava, resulting in jugular venous distention, peripheral edema, enlarged liver, clear breath sounds, and probably hypotension.
Left heart failure	Left heart fails also because of infarction, increased workload (systemic hypertension), valvular dysfunction, or a combination of these. It results in the congestion of blood in the lungs, which increases pressure to a point at which fluid escapes into the alveoli, causing respiratory distress and pulmonary edema. Lung sounds often reveal crackles or "cardiac asthma," blood pressure is commonly normal to high, and peripheral congestion is absent.

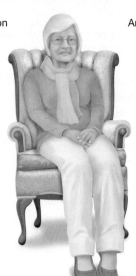

Mild to severe confusion

Cyanosis

Tachypnea

May cough up pink sputum

Low, normal, or high blood pressure

Rapid heart rate

A desire to sit upright

Anxiety

Distended neck veins (Late)

Crackles

Shortness of breath (dyspnea)

Pale, cool, clammy skin

Abdominal distention

Pedal and lower extremity edema

Figure 28-3 Signs and symptoms of heart failure.

> **The emphasis on assessment should be on the entire patient, and not just on lung sounds.**

Again, this is commonly an exacerbation of an ongoing heart failure condition, but it can also be associated with acute disorders such as MI and dysrhythmias.

Acute pulmonary edema poses a specific challenge, as paramedics are faced with both an immediate need for treatment and a disorder that can look very similar to other respiratory ailments. In many cases, acute pulmonary edema can present with wheezes, similar to those seen in asthma, and patients can exhibit other respiratory symptoms, such as those seen with exacerbation of chronic obstructive pulmonary disease (COPD). Although there are no foolproof methods of diagnosing acute pulmonary edema (particularly in the prehospital world), there are some helpful ideas that can lend accuracy to your treatment modality:

- **Listen for crackles.** Crackles (also known as rales) tell a tale of fluid in the alveoli. Although there are other causes of crackles, the most common cause in the acute setting is acute pulmonary edema. Be wary, though, of waiting for crackles. Many patients will present with other symptoms first before presenting with crackles. In fact, fluid in the alveoli is a relatively late sign of acute pulmonary edema, resulting only after nearly one liter of fluid has crossed into pulmonary tissue.

- **Check the monitor.** Often, an electrocardiogram (ECG) can demonstrate the proximal cause for acute pulmonary edema. Look for dysrhythmias and evidence of acute MI.

- **Look for history of heart failure.** Although not every patient in acute pulmonary edema will have a history of heart failure, by far the majority will. As such, inquire about previous cardiac and heart failure history. Look for medications commonly used to treat heart failure. Look for signs of undiagnosed heart failure, such as patients sleeping upright in chairs, history of dyspnea on exertion, and even physical findings such as pedal edema, weight gain, and JVD. Although physical findings such as JVD and pedal edema may not have anything to do with the acute left heart failure, they do demonstrate a prior history of failure.

- **Acute pulmonary edema tends to be acute.** Although pulmonary edema can be chronic in nature, acute episodes tend to develop rapidly with an abrupt onset. Occasionally, there will be a trigger such as exertion, stress, or other conditions that increase cardiac workload. Although onset is not definitive, it can help distinguish acute pulmonary edema from other respiratory disorders such as exacerbations of COPD and pneumonia (which tend to have far more chronic onsets).

- **Look at the whole patient.** No one fact can diagnose any patient.

Put all your findings in the context of the larger patient. Crackles are an important finding, but are even more important in the context of a patient with a history of heart failure (and even more important if that patient has had pulmonary edema in the past).

Diagnostic methods are rapidly improving and technology will help make decision making easier. Some EMS systems are now using point-of-care testing to assess for levels of BNP. It is thought that elevated levels of this biochemical marker can indicate the presence of heart failure and can be used as a surrogate marker for acute pulmonary edema.

CRACKLES AND WHEEZING Acute pulmonary edema can cause both crackles and wheezing. Crackles are heard as fluid migrates into the alveoli and small airways. Wheezes are heard as prealveolar sphincters narrow to prevent fluid from escaping the alveolar space. Both these lung sounds can be helpful in diagnosing heart failure, but can also present diagnostic challenges. Because wheezing are commonly associated with other respiratory conditions such as asthma and exacerbated COPD, paramedics can frequently be pulled down an incorrect path.

The emphasis on assessment should be on the entire patient, and not just on lung sounds. Paramedics will have to differentiate based on other findings, including those discussed previously. Unfortunately, many heart failure patients are not simple to diagnose. Many will have a variety of comorbid factors, including those that cause wheezing. Do asthma patients occasionally fall victim to acute pulmonary edema? Yes, they do. The treatment of this undifferentiated patient is very controversial. Of course, if the true etiology of wheezing is heart failure, then you should treat heart failure. Some experts would note that using bronchodilators in a patient with acute pulmonary edema causes increased myocardial oxygen demand (owing to beta$_1$ effects) and therefore can be harmful. Recently, however, the opinion has shifted slightly.

Again, if the origin is known, heart failure should be treated first, but some experts contend that measured bronchodilator use in an undifferentiated acute pulmonary edema patient is not nearly as harmful as we once imagined. These experts contend that most acute heart failure patients are already adrenergically

TABLE 28-2   Clinical Findings and Pathophysiologic Etiology of Heart Failure

Clinical Finding	Pathophysiologic Etiology
Rapid breathing (tachypnea)	Multiple reasons, such as hypoxia, carbon dioxide retention, sympathetic discharge.
Shortness of breath (dyspnea)	Changes in O_2/CO_2 diffusion across alveoli; chemoreceptors in body detect changes in gas levels and cause the perception of dyspnea.
Shortness of breath while lying down (orthopnea)	On lying down, fluid accumulation in lungs from CHF tends to increase, which diminishes gas exchange across alveoli.
Constant waking at night (paroxysmal nocturnal dyspnea)	While lying down, fluid accumulates in the lungs and causes the person to wake up. Patient may state that the dyspnea eases after sitting or standing up from sleep.
Anxiety, tremors, nausea, vomiting	Sympathetic discharge caused by the changes in blood gases and/or cardiac output.
Low pulse oximetry readings	Poor oxygenation from fluid accumulation in lungs diminishes oxygen diffusion into the bloodstream.
Cool, pale, clammy skin	Sympathetic discharge from changes in cardiac output and oxygen/carbon dioxide levels.
Sitting upright and/or tripod positioning	Sitting upright eases dyspnea because of better diaphragmatic function; it also helps to ease fluid accumulation in lungs.
Chest discomfort	Possible angina, infarction in an acute setting.
Inspiratory crackles	Fluid accumulation in the alveoli from backward failure of left ventricle.
Wheezing (cardiac asthma)	Fluid accumulation in alveoli may migrate into bronchioles from breathing, causing stimulation of "irritant receptors" in lung tissue causing bronchoconstriction.
Distended neck veins, enlarged liver, distended abdomen	Increased venous pressure from backward failure of right ventricle.
Changes in blood pressure	Hypotension often caused by failing right ventricle (thereby diminishing left-sided preload). Hypertension often caused by left-sided failure in conjunction with heightened sympathetic tone.
Objective dyspnea findings: nasal flaring, retractions, tachypnea, tripod positioning, mouth breathing, etc.	Most commonly caused by combination of right and left ventricular failure.

stimulated, and the slight increase given by inhaled bronchodilators may actually be mitigated by the increased oxygenation secondary to bronchodilation. The answer is resoundingly unclear, but strong opinions have emerged on both sides. As always, you should follow local protocol.

EMERGENCY MEDICAL CARE

The treatment for the patient with acute heart failure is geared toward improving oxygenation, diminishing fluid accumulation in the lungs, treating the patient for acute coronary syndrome should it concurrently be present, and maintaining normotension. Remember that exacerbation of acute pulmonary edema may be very scary to the patient, so good communication skills and verbal reassurance will also go a long way.

1. **Establish and maintain an open airway.** Airway management should always be goal oriented. Security of the airway may be a high priority

in these patients if hypoxia secondary to respiratory failure robs the patient of the ability to maintain an airway. Paramedics should remember that the threshold for endotracheal intubation (ETI) in this population is slightly lower than that for other respiratory disorders. In this group, ETI provides not only airway security, but also therapeutic increased positive pressure. That said, ETI should be reserved for the most serious cases when advanced airway management is necessary.

In most cases, positive pressure can be achieved noninvasively with the use of continuous positive airway pressure (CPAP). Remember also that many of these patients will be conscious; unless rapid sequence induction is available, ETI will be very difficult, with dangerous side effects associated with sympathetic discharge as a result of fighting the intubation attempt.

2. **Recognize respiratory failure.** Many acute heart failure patients will be breathing, but breathing

inadequately. When fluid occupies space in the pulmonary interstitial tissue and in the alveoli, gas exchange is interrupted. Paramedics must recognize the failure of the respiratory system to adequately meet metabolic demands. Assess aggressively for this possibility and initiate positive pressure ventilations when found. Remember again that in acute pulmonary edema patients, positive pressure can help reduce fluid from shifting into the lungs. As such, the threshold to initiate positive pressure ventilation can be slightly lower than that of other respiratory disorder patients.

3. **Provide oxygen.** If the patient is dyspneic or hypoxemic, has obvious signs of heart failure, or has a SpO_2 reading of less than 94 percent. Initiate oxygen therapy via nasal cannula at 4 lpm and titrate oxygen therapy to maintain a SpO_2 reading of 94 percent or greater. If the breathing is inadequate, provide positive pressure ventilation at 10 to 12/min with high-flow supplemental oxygen.

4. Position the patient. Semi- or high Fowler positioning will assist the patient in breathing and minimize the negative effects of fluid accumulating in the lungs. If positive pressure ventilation is being provided or frank hypotension is present, the patient may need to be placed supine for ongoing management. Many patients will wish to hang their legs off the stretcher. Surprisingly, this is not just a position of comfort, but probably a survival instinct. Although the evidence is unclear, many experts note that positioning the legs in a dependent posture can help relieve volume pressure by drawing fluid to the lower extremities. These experts suggest that if it can be done safely, patients should be allowed to hang their legs off the stretcher.

5. Use CPAP if protocol allows. CPAP can be extremely effective in the fight against acute pulmonary edema. The application of CPAP (▶ Figure 28-4) increases intra-alveolar pressure and helps prevent the movement of fluid from the pulmonary capillaries into the lungs. It is most effective when applied early and when combined with aggressive administration of nitrates to help reduce preload. CPAP devices are typically set to provide positive end expiratory pressure (PEEP) at between 5 and 10 cmH$_2$O. This pressure increases intraalveolar pressure and also pneumatically splints the small airways, preventing

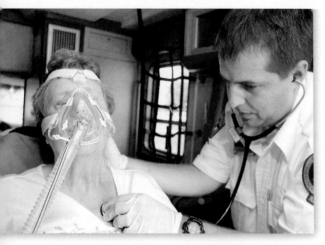

Figure 28-4 CPAP is a form of noninvasive positive pressure ventilation used in the awake and spontaneously breathing patient who needs ventilatory support. (© Ken Kerr)

atelectasis. As always, follow local protocol.

6. Initiate an intravenous line of normal saline at a to-keep-open rate. Most commonly, this access is a medication route, but some heart failure patients may require fluid. In some cases, right-sided MI can cause dramatic right heart failure and may need a measured fluid challenge to increase preload. This therapy is controversial; you should always follow local protocol.

7. Administer nitroglycerin. Nitrates are most commonly the most important medication used to treat acute heart failure. Nitroglycerine causes venous dilation and therefore venous pooling, leading to decreased cardiac preload. This reduction of preload decreases cardiac workload and can help decrease failure and backward pressure.

It is important to remember that in the event of acute heart failure, nitrates should be administered more aggressively than in the case of acute coronary syndrome (although these two conditions are frequently linked). Nitrate levels must be maintained to sustain a continued preload reduction, and as a result, dosing frequency is typically more rapid than the traditional acute coronary syndrome (ACS) regimen.

Most commonly, sublingual nitroglycerine is administered every 2 to 3 minutes as opposed to every 5 minutes in ACS. Some systems prefer nitrates to be administered intravenously to enable precise titration of blood pressure and maximum therapeutic effect. Nitrates are also administered transdermally via a paste. This can be particularly helpful in patients wearing a CPAP mask, but this route can be somewhat unpredictable in terms of onset and challenging to control in the event of hypotension. Always follow local protocol.

8. Consider additional pharmacology. If the failure is secondary to a cardiac dysrhythmia, treat the underlying cause. Both bradycardias and tachycardias can cause acute pulmonary edema. Follow

advanced cardiac life support (ACLS) guidelines to address any rhythm disturbance. Some EMS systems use ACE inhibitors such as captopril to decrease afterload and therefore diminish cardiac workload. This treatment is somewhat controversial, but can be effective if used appropriately. Furosemide, once the standard pharmacologic agent in acute pulmonary edema, is quickly losing favor.

Although diuretics can still be useful in acute heart failure, it has been found that their use should be limited only to those heart failure patients who are hypervolemic. In more than 60 percent of the cases of acute pulmonary edema, patients are not in fact hypervolemic, but rather are normovolemic and suffering only from a pump problem. When these patients are giving diuretics, they become hypovolemic, thereby adding yet another physiologic challenge to an already sick patient. Furthermore, recent studies have shown that when furosemide is given in the case of a misdiagnosis to pneumonia and exacerbated COPD patients, mortality actually increases. Of course, paramedics should always follow local protocols, but they should also keep in mind that diuresis occurs naturally as nitrates and CPAP help restore perfusion to the kidneys.

9. Ensure appropriate transport to the emergency department. Notify the receiving ED as early as possible.

Continually assess the patient and be prepared for respiratory failure and cardiac arrest. Should either of these occur, follow appropriate treatment and local protocol for supporting this lost function.

Patients suffering from exacerbation of heart failure can be among the most challenging patients encountered by the paramedic. They may present anywhere on the continuum from being alert and oriented with only minimal symptoms to being unresponsive and just moments from complete cardiopulmonary arrest. Compounding this picture is that the heart failure patient may go from one extreme to the other very quickly, without much warning. Therefore, the paramedic must always maintain a high degree of suspicion that these patients may deteriorate into arrest very suddenly.

REVIEW ITEMS

1. During your interview, your patient tells you that she has "water on the lungs." This statement most closely reflects what pathophysiologic change in heart failure?
   a. backward failure of the left ventricle
   b. frontward failure of the right ventricle
   c. biventricular failure
   d. elevation in central venous pressure

2. Of the choices below, which is most likely a determining factor causing the development of right-sided heart failure?
   a. high diastolic pressure
   b. preexisting left heart failure
   c. stenosis of the tricuspid valve
   d. history of diabetes mellitus

3. A patient presents with JVD, hypotension, clear breath sounds, and peripheral edema. These findings would be most representative of what type of heart failure?
   a. acute right ventricular failure
   b. acute left ventricular failure
   c. gradual right ventricular failure
   d. gradual left ventricular failure

4. Pulmonary edema would be a manifestation of what type of ventricular failure?
   a. acute right ventricular failure
   b. acute left ventricular failure
   c. gradual right ventricular failure
   d. gradual left ventricular failure

5. Diffusion of excessive alveolar fluid back into the perialveolar capillary bed would be best accomplished by what treatment intervention for the heart failure patient?
   a. placing the patient supine
   b. providing high-flow oxygen
   c. administration of sublingual nitroglycerin
   d. continuous positive airway pressure (CPAP)

APPLIED PATHOPHYSIOLOGY

A 76-year-old female patient has a history of hypertension, insulin-dependent diabetes, and heart failure. She summoned an ambulance because of weakness, mild chest pressure, and progressively worsening dyspnea over the past two days. The patient states that her trouble breathing got worse with physical exertion and when lying down at night to go to bed. Currently her vital signs are blood pressure 180/100, heart rate 102 beats per minute, respiratory rate 24, SpO$_2$ 92 percent on room air. During your assessment of the breath sounds, you note bilateral wheezing.

1. Identify whether you believe this patient has right or left ventricular failure. Support your answer with the appropriate clinical findings.

2. Why might the administration of nitroglycerin to this patient be beneficial to the dyspnea?

3. Identify and discuss why the patient's wheezing should *not* be treated as it would be in an asthmatic or allergic-reaction patient.

4. Discuss the differences in pathophysiology and presentation of right versus left heart failure according to the following three assessment findings:
   a. Breath sounds
   b. Systolic blood pressure
   c. Vital sign changes

5. Differentiate the pathophysiologic changes between *backward* and *forward* ventricular failure.

CLINICAL DECISION MAKING

Late one hot summer night, you are called for a patient suffering from acute respiratory distress. On arrival at the patient's home, you are escorted to an elderly female patient's bedroom on the second floor. As soon as you walk in, you see the patient lying on her back in bed with four or five pillows behind her head and shoulders, helping her to "sit up." The patient is alert and oriented; displays nasal flaring, retractions, and tachypnea; and is speaking in full sentences. On the nightstand beside the bed, you see four or five prescription bottles of medication.

1. Based on the scene size-up characteristics, identify the clues that point to the field impression of heart failure or acute pulmonary edema.

2. What would be common medications you might find on the patient's nightstand to support the field impression of heart failure?

The primary assessment reveals the patient to be alert and well oriented. Her airway is clear, her breathing is rapid at 30/minute, respirations are slightly shallow, vesicular sounds are present and diminished, and slight inspiratory crackles are noted. Peripheral pulses are also present and noted to be rapid and slightly irregular. The neck veins are obviously engorged, and the SpO_2 reading on room air is 87 percent.

3. What are the life threats, if any, to the patient of which you are currently aware?

After managing and supporting the situation described, further assessment reveals the pupils to be equal and reactive, blood glucose level is 193 mg/dL, and the SpO_2 has increased to 94 percent with high-flow oxygen. Breath sounds are unchanged; the JVD is still present. The patient's blood pressure is 100/79, heart rate is 112 and irregular, respirations are fast at 30/minute. The patient is now starting to complain of "chest pressure" as well.

4. From what etiology of heart failure is this patient likely suffering?

5. Explain the pathophysiologic cause for the following:
   a. Breath sounds
   b. Low pulse oximeter reading
   c. Jugular venous distention

6. During the management of the patient, you elect to administer the following therapies. For each one, discuss in specific detail (1) the reason the intervention is warranted, (2) the expected outcome of that intervention, and (3) how you would assess to determine whether the desired effect is occurring (i.e., the treatment worked).
   a. Position patient in high Fowler position
   b. Administer oxygen
   c. Administration nitroglycerin
   d. Application of CPAP at 10 cmH_2O pressure

Standard Medicine

Competency Integrates assessment findings with principles of epidemiology and pathophysiology to formulate a field impression and implement a comprehensive treatment/disposition plan for a patient with a medical complaint.

TOPIC

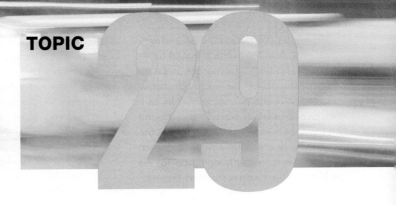

RESPIRATORY EMERGENCIES: AIRWAY RESISTANCE DISORDERS

INTRODUCTION

Calls related to respiratory distress are among the most frequent category of EMS response. Millions of patients each year seek out emergency care when they are unable to breathe normally. Airway resistance disorders, such as asthma and bronchitis, comprise a large portion of these calls and are a continued concern for modern paramedics.

Airway resistance disorders are distributed throughout a wide cross section of the patient population; the severity of their acute presentations can range from mild dyspnea to life-threatening respiratory failure. Fortunately, many of the dysfunctions that cause airway resistance are quite treatable. However, for any treatment to be effective, paramedics must accurately recognize the disorder and aggressively apply a treatment plan that accounts for the acute pathophysiology.

Differential diagnosis is not always simple with respiratory distress. A variety of very different pathologies present with similar outward findings. Paramedics will need not only a fundamental knowledge of pathophysiology, but also good judgment and an ability to use the tools of patient assessment to make appropriate treatment choices. Furthermore, our overall plan must consider the use of medication and interventions that are forgiving when applied to an inherently difficult diagnosis.

This topic reviews the pathophysiologic changes that result in detrimental resistance to airflow in the lungs. It further discusses assessment, differential diagnosis, and modern advances in treatment with regard to these disorders.

TRANSITION *highlights*

- *Frequency of airway resistance disorders in the United States.*

- *Pathophysiologic changes that occur with airway resistance disorders:*
  - Asthma (intrinsic and extrinsic).
  - Bronchitis (acute and chronic).
  - Bronchiolitis.

- *Relation of the assessment findings of respiratory distress to the pathophysiologic changes that occur due to the disease.*

- *Description of abnormal breath sounds commonly heard.*

- *Organized presentation of assessment findings to help the paramedic delineate between different restrictive airway disorders.*

- *Treatment interventions and their relationship to improving the patient's respiratory status:*
  - Oxygen administration.
  - Positive pressure ventilation.
  - Respiratory pharmacology.
  - Patient positioning.

EPIDEMIOLOGY

Between 20 and 25 million people in the United States have *asthma*. This disease accounts for more than 2 million emergency department visits per year. Asthma typically presents in childhood, but when symptoms persist into the second decade of life, patients are likely to suffer from asthma through adulthood.

Bronchitis, conversely, has been found to affect roughly 44 out of every 1,000 adults annually. More than 80 percent of these

cases occur in the fall and winter months and are often associated with an upper respiratory infection (URI). Chronic bronchitis, defined by either persistent and ongoing symptoms or a specific frequency of recurrence, has been diagnosed in more than 9.5 million people living in the United States.

Bronchiolitis is a highly contagious respiratory infection, primarily viral in etiology, which is contracted by infants during the first year or two of life. Respiratory syncytial virus (RSV) has been implicated in the majority of cases. Research has shown the incidence to peak during the fall and winter months, with the average age of those afflicted to be two to six months. Because of the maturing of the tracheobronchial tree, bronchiolitis is uncommon in children over 5 years of age. Thus, although this may not be seen as commonly by the paramedic as are adult airway resistance disorders, it is certainly common to the pediatric patient with respiratory distress.

PATHOPHYSIOLOGY

Asthma

Asthma is a chronic disease that is episodic in nature. That means that an asthma patient experiences the changes associated with asthma every day, but typically suffers severe symptoms only when an attack occurs. Asthma is characterized by three specific respiratory issues:

> **Asthma is a chronic disease that is episodic in nature.**

- **Chronic inflammation and airway remodeling.** The bronchial passages in an asthma patient are chronically inflamed and are frequently narrowed as a result of changes in the inner walls (these changes are often referred to as *remodeling*). Although the true pathophysiology of airway inflammation is still poorly understood, it is believed that immune system cells, such as T lymphocytes, play an important role in regulation of the level of inflammation and subsequent airway edema. Inflammation associated with asthma is often chronic, but can be well tolerated and managed. However, this underlying pathology frequently contributes dangerously to decompensation when combined with other more acute dysfunctions.

- **Overproduction of mucus.** Asthma patients simply secrete more mucus in the bronchial tree than nondiseased patients do. This overproduction can lead to mucus plugging of the airways and result in dangerous trapping of air in acute disorders.

- **Hyperresponsive airways.** The small bronchial passages of an asthma patient occasionally spasm in response to a particular trigger. Because of an antigen–antibody reaction, chemical mediators are released locally that promote smooth muscle constriction and restrict normal airflow. This bronchoconstriction is often stimulated by exercise, allergens, stress, and/or even cold air. These dynamic airway changes can cause significant reduction of alveolar ventilation in the acute setting (▶ **Figure 29-1**).

In general, asthma is a well-tolerated disease. With proper management, patients lead very normal lifestyles. It is the setting of the "asthma attack" in which EMS typically becomes involved. In the acute presentation, hyperresponsive airways first constrict. The initial phases of an asthma attack are almost always dominated by bronchoconstriction and spasm. Early in the progression, when mild bronchoconstriction is prevailing, the patient is able to inhale normally, owing to the active muscular contraction needed to do so. During exhalation, however, when airflow from the lungs is more passive, exhaled gases have a tendency to become trapped in the alveoli as the attack progresses. As this develops, the alveoli become distended with air; they have a tendency to collapse smaller nearby bronchioles when the lungs recoil, thereby contributing to more air trapping and making exhalation more prolonged.

The narrowing of air passages can challenge ventilation in and of itself, but is typically made worse by the other underlying issues. Spasm of the airway is bad, but it is worse when it occurs in an already inflamed or remodeled airway. Add to that an overproduction of mucus and subsequent plugging and you have conditions that are predisposed to severe decompensation. Even worse is that with time, the underlying inflammation will worsen and present a second, less treatable, level of airway obstruction.

If left unchecked, the asthma attack can interfere significantly with the exchange of oxygen and carbon dioxide and can lead to progressive respiratory failure. A severe, prolonged, and life-threatening asthma attack that produces inadequate breathing and severe signs and symptoms is called *status asthmaticus*. Status asthmaticus typically does not respond to either oxygen or medication.

If an asthma attack cannot be mitigated, respiratory failure will result. In the end, this failure comes about because of both a profound reduction in alveolar ventilation and fatigue associated with the prolonged use of compensatory muscles in a hypoxic state.

Two different etiologies of asthma can be identified. *Extrinsic* asthma, or "allergic" asthma, usually results from a reaction to dust, pollen, smoke, or other irritants in the air. It is typically seasonal, occurs most often in children and may subside after adolescence. *Intrinsic*, or "nonallergic," asthma is most common in adults and usually results from infection, emotional stress, or strenuous exercise. In either instance, paramedics should recognize an asthma attack from its presentation, not exclusively from the patient's history.

Acute Bronchitis and Chronic Bronchitis

The conducting airways of the tracheobronchial tree are lined with mucous membranes that contribute to the humidification, filtration, and warming of inspired air. At times, however, this

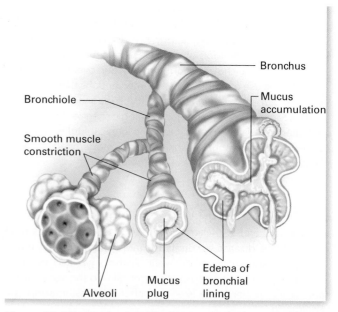

Figure 29-1 Pathophysiologic changes in the bronchioles in asthma contribute to higher airway resistance.

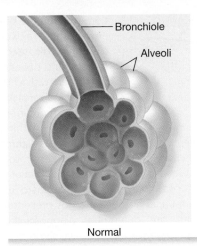
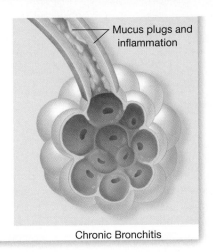

Figure 29-2 Mucus plugs and inflammation cause airway restriction in chronic bronchitis.

mucous lining can become inflamed from inhalation of an irritant, resulting in thickening of the mucosal wall and airway restriction from swelling and mucus production. These changes, when severe or when present in a patient who is susceptible to pulmonary dysfunction, can lead to respiratory distress and labored breathing. This condition is known as *bronchitis*, of which there are two categories, acute bronchitis and chronic bronchitis.

- *Acute bronchitis*, as the name implies, is a respiratory dysfunction that has a short duration, typically no more than three weeks. During an episode of bronchitis, the bronchial tubes become inflamed, and occasionally mucus production will increase to the point at which the patient also has a productive cough. Acute bronchitis can be triggered by infectious agents (viruses and bacteria) or noninfectious agents (such as dust, smoking, or other inhaled pollutants). Decreased alveolar ventilation can result from narrowed airway passages and from inflammation and increased mucus production. The bronchitis patient will typically seek EMS care as the condition worsens or as respiratory compensation fails to keep pace with the dysfunction.

- *Chronic bronchitis* is a disease process in the spectrum of chronic obstructive pulmonary disease (COPD) that involves a similar inflammation, swelling, and thickening of the lining of the bronchi and bronchioles. This in turn leads to a narrowing of the bronchial passages and a potential decrease in alveolar ventilation. In addition, there is excessive mucus production from

enlargement and multiplication of the mucus-secreting glands of the tracheobronchial tree, which leads to plugging of the smaller airways and further derangements in airflow. Distal alveoli remain unaffected by the disease. However, the inflamed and swollen bronchioles and thick mucus restrict airflow to the alveoli so they do not expand fully, causing respiratory distress and possible hypoxia. The heavy mucus that resides in the conducting airway is difficult to expel; it traps inhaled particles that, if not eliminated from the body, can manifest into recurrent respiratory infections that leave scar tissue and further narrow the airways (▶ Figure 29-2).

The major pathophysiology associated with chronic bronchitis is the swelling and thickening of the inner lining of the lower respiratory tract and an increase in mucus production. The airways become very narrow, causing a high resistance to air movement and chronic difficulty in breathing. By definition, chronic bronchitis is characterized by a productive cough that persists for at least three consecutive months a year for at least two consecutive years.

Bronchiolitis

Bronchiolitis is an umbrella diagnosis given to any number of pathologies that cause an acute onset of upper and lower airway inflammation and submucosal edema in the pediatric population. The most common etiology of bronchiolitis is infection such as that caused by RSV. The

pathophysiology of bronchiolitis is also often commonly associated with damage to the ciliated cells that transport mucus out of the lower airway, and eventual occlusion of the smaller bronchioles.

Unlike in asthma or bronchitis, in bronchiolitis, bronchial smooth muscle constriction is rare. These pathophysiologic effects result in disturbance in the ventilation/perfusion ratio and eventual presentation of subjective and objective findings consistent with labored breathing. As mentioned previously, this problem is generally confined to young infants. Bronchiolitis can affect older patients but is well tolerated because that population has larger and better developed bronchial structures that can readily compensate for additional mucus accumulation and inflamed bronchial walls.

ASSESSMENT FINDINGS

When we consider the pathophysiology of airway resistance disorders, it is logical that outward signs and symptoms are associated with poor alveolar ventilation and the steps of compensation the body takes in response to the challenge. Altered mental status, the sensation of shortness of breath (dyspnea), cyanosis, and alterations in oxygen saturation and end-tidal CO_2 ($ETCO_2$) are all related to the failed exchange of gases as a result of decreased alveolar ventilation. These findings are particularly relevant when assessing for the presence of respiratory failure.

> The hallmark of airway resistance disorders is wheezing.

The hallmark of airway resistance disorders is wheezing. As airflow is decreased through narrowed bronchial passages, the high-pitched sound of a wheeze is frequently audible. Different respiratory conditions can lead to various types of wheezes (inspiratory, expiratory, etc.), but in general this finding points to obstructed lower airways. Remember that wheezing may be noted to be of differing qualities, depending on the phase of the patient's ventilation.

Because inhalation is active and airflow enters the lungs with a higher velocity, mild bronchoconstriction may be overcome by the rush of entering air. In this phase, wheezing may not be evident. However, on passive exhalation, the airflow out of the lungs does not have the

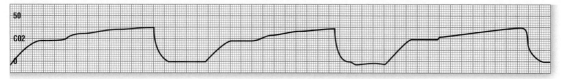

Figure 29-3 Capnographic wave form demonstrating bronchoconstriction.

same velocity, and bronchoconstriction may impede airflow in a more profound manner. As a result, expiratory wheezing will become more evident. For example, wheezing is commonly heard much earlier on exhalation during a mild (or early) asthma attack.

With worsening of the bronchoconstriction, edema, and/or mucus production, exhalation becomes a more active process as well. Here the patient is forced to use energy not only to breathe in, but also to eliminate the air from the lungs. Thus, wheezing may be present during the entire ventilation cycle.

It is also important to remember that as bronchial tubes become more and more narrow and more and more plugged with mucus, wheezing may be very difficult to auscultate, even with a stethoscope. Air is simply not moving. This silent chest is an ominous sign of severe bronchoconstriction.

Bronchoconstriction can also be seen by examining the morphology of capnographic wave forms. When lower airway obstruction is present, the classic sharp, almost vertical upstroke of the ascension phase (also known as phase 1) becomes more sloped and rises more slowly over time (▶ **Figure 29-3**). These changes are related to the difficulty bronchoconstricted patients have in expelling CO_2 from their lungs. Capnography can be a valuable tool to identify bronchoconstriction when auscultation is not available or when wheezes cannot be heard.

Assessing the patient's ability to speak is also an important element of assessment. Research has shown that the number of words a patient is able to speak without interruption by breathing can be correlated to the level of respiratory challenge. Therefore, the fewer words your patient can pro-

> **Most adult patients will present with a history that indicates the nature of the current disorder.**

duce, the worse the respiratory dysfunction.

Consider also the steps the body takes to compensate for respiratory challenges. As gas exchange is affected, sympathetic tone dominates in an attempt to normalize oxygen saturation and CO_2 levels. Increases in respiratory rates and attempted increases in tidal volume are common responses to respiratory challenges. Patients will also use positions such as the tripod position to maximize intrathoracic volume and assist ventilation. Increased sympathetic tone also causes increased heart rates and peripheral vasoconstriction. Many of these findings are assessed immediately during the primary assessment, but evaluation can be enhanced with other assessment tools.

Pulse oximetry and capnography, when used in the proper context, can deliver valuable information regarding gas exchange and should be used in any patient for whom respiratory evaluation is important. Although specific values are important, trending is probably more important as to the larger picture of respiratory distress. For example, when evaluating an asthma patient, the initial $ETCO_2$ is important, as it can identify the immediate severity of the event ($ETCO_2$ levels greater than 60 mmHg are generally considered indicative of a severe attack). However, you can also use capnography to identify trends in the current condition and response to treatment. One would expect $ETCO_2$ levels to initially decrease in response to immediate compensatory hyperventilation but then increase as alveolar ventilation is subsequently decreased.

As you look for evidence of compensation, remember to look for evidence of decompensation as well. Altered mental status, cyanosis, and unimproved poor oxygen saturation, and well as increasing $ETCO_2$ levels, paint a picture of respiratory failure. Look also for slowing or irregular respiration as a result of muscle fatigue accelerated by a hypoxic state.

Patient history is also exceptionally important. At least in the adult popula-

tion, it is rare to see new-onset airway resistance disorders. Most adult patients will present with a history that indicates the nature of the current disorder. Asthma patients typically have a history of asthma and likely have prescribed respiratory medications. Chronic bronchitis patients also commonly have similar histories. When these histories are not present in adults, our differential diagnosis frequently sways away from such chronic diseases and toward more acute-onset dysfunctions. Pediatric patients are often a challenge, as many of these disorders are seen for the first time.

Many other disorders can mimic the findings of airway resistance. Life-threatening disorders such as acute pulmonary edema, anaphylaxis, and toxic inhalations can all present with labored breathing and wheezes. Paramedics must be comprehensive in their assessment to rule out nonrespiratory causes of respiratory symptoms.

Additional Assessment Findings

The following may be found on assessment of a patient with asthma:

- Dyspnea (shortness of breath); may progressively worsen
- Nonproductive cough
- Wheezing on auscultation (typically expiratory)
- Tachypnea and tachycardia
- Anxiety and apprehension
- Possible fever
- Typical upper respiratory allergic signs and symptoms
- Chest tightness
- SpO_2 <95 percent before oxygen administration

Patients with acute bronchitis may present with the following:

- Cough, most common finding, possibly productive
- Findings of mild to severe respiratory distress
- Sore throat, usually worse with coughing or swallowing
- Edematous nasal mucosa causing runny or stuffy nose

TABLE 29-1 **Findings for Respiratory Airway Disorders**

Respiratory Airway Disorder	History Findings	Assessment Findings	Breath Sounds
Asthma	Commonly quick onset of distress. Often has a history of a known trigger.	Subjective and objective dyspnea. Respiratory distress findings may be severe.	Expiratory wheezing progressing with wheezing on inhalation and exhalation with more severe attacks. "Silent" chest is ominous.
Acute bronchitis	More gradual onset. May happen in patient with a recent URI.	Progressive but usually not debilitating dyspnea. Patient may have nonproductive cough.	Patient may display wheezing (with rhonchi in more severe cases).
Chronic bronchitis	Patient may be chronically short of breath (more typically, CO_2 retainers), may experience acute exacerbations.	Chronic respiratory distress and tachypnea, overweight, low SpO_2. Acute exacerbations may lead to inadequate breathing.	Rhonchi, diminished airflow, and wheezing should condition exacerbate.
Bronchiolitis	Gradual onset of respiratory distress, may follow URI. Common to pediatric patients under 2 years of age.	Progressively worsening cough, sore throat, stuffy nose, general malaise, muscle and joint aches.	Breath sounds may reveal crackles and diffuse wheezing.

- General malaise, fatigue, muscle aches
- Infrequently: fever, nausea, vomiting, diarrhea

The following signs are often found in patients with chronic bronchitis:

- Typically overweight
- Chronic cyanotic complexion (often called "blue bloaters")
- Difficulty in breathing, but less prominent than with emphysema
- Vigorous productive chronic cough with sputum
- Coarse rhonchi usually heard on auscultation of the lungs
- Wheezes and, possibly, crackles at the bases of the lungs

Infants with bronchiolitis often present with the following findings:

- Increasingly "fussy" during feeding (early finding)
- History of a concurrent or recent URI; findings consistent with URI
- Progressive onset of dyspnea, usually over two to five days
- Tachypnea and tachycardia

- Cough, usually nonproductive
- Possible fever
- Fine inspiratory crackles and possible diffuse wheezing
- In severe cases: tachypnea (>50/min) and low SpO_2

Table 29-1 provides a summary of the history, assessment findings, and breath sounds consistent for each of the emergencies discussed in this topic.

EMERGENCY MEDICAL CARE

Aggressive evaluation and treatment of the respiratory distress patient are very important. Time is critical because of the detrimental effects of hypoxia on all cells and organs. Paramedics must rapidly identify and treat respiratory failure and only then move on to more specific interventions.

Treating Respiratory Failure

Respiratory failure implies that the efforts being put forth by the patient are *not* meeting the patient's metabolic needs. Therefore, aggressive intervention is nec-

essary. With few exceptions, respiratory failure indicates a need for ventilatory support. Again, the patient's efforts on his own are not enough; generally speaking, this indicates the need to not only support his ongoing efforts but also add additional ventilatory intervention. Positive pressure ventilation (PPV) must at least be considered in this category, if not applied automatically. Airway management may also be necessary as mental status decreases with the onset of hypoxia and hypercapnia.

When airway management and PPV are necessary, reaching a conclusive diagnosis is relatively unimportant. Respiratory failure is almost universally treated the same way, regardless of the etiology. Once the airway and breathing are stabilized, more discrete diagnostics and therapies can be applied.

Noninvasive Positive Pressure Ventilation

Noninvasive PPV, such as continuous positive airway pressure (CPAP), is a somewhat controversial treatment for airway resistance disorders but has shown some promise in therapeutic strategies. Topic 28 discussed the use of CPAP to treat acute pulmonary edema and described its ability to pneumatically splint the lower airways and prevent atelectasis. These effects can also be beneficial in airway resistance disorders. CPAP is theorized to help prevent the collapse of the lower airways that can be common with active exhalation. It has also been shown to significantly increase oxygen saturation.

Some experts express concern with adding positive pressure to conditions such as asthma in which exhalation (ventilation) is primarily challenged. Studies are limited, and more research is necessary. As always, follow local protocol.

Oxygen

Treat hypoxia! Airway resistance can rapidly lead to inadequate oxygenation and may require supplemental oxygen to maintain normal saturation levels. Never withhold oxygen from a hypoxic patient. That said, remember that oxygen is a drug and there is such a thing as too much. In Topic 16, "Paramedic Medications," we discussed recent findings that indicate negative side effects of hyperoxia, specifically in the subcategory of COPD patients. Given this information, paramedics should use the tools of assessment (in particular

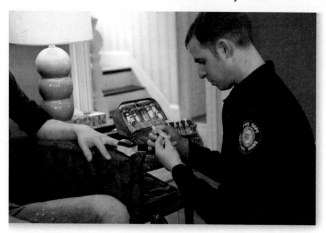

Assess the patient for need, follow your local protocol for the medication order, ensure adequate oxygenation of the patient, explain the procedure to the patient, and check for the right medication and expiration date.

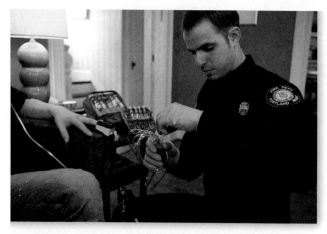

Place the medication for nebulization in the base chamber of the nebulizer. A total volume of 4 mL or greater must be used. If the drug is not already premixed, it may be necessary to dilute the medication with normal saline to a total volume of 4 mL or greater.

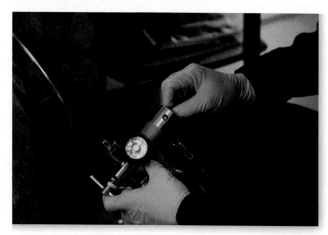

Attach the nebulizer oxygen supply tubing to the oxygen regulator. Set the flow rate at 6 to 8 L/minute to generate a fine mist.

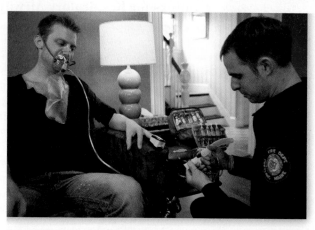

Select a mask or mouthpiece and assemble the equipment.

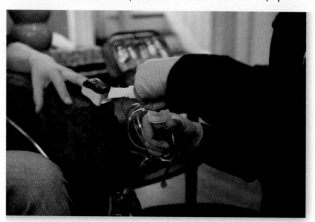

Continue with assembly by screwing the top of the device onto the medication holding chamber. Gently shake the nebulizer side to side to mix the medication.

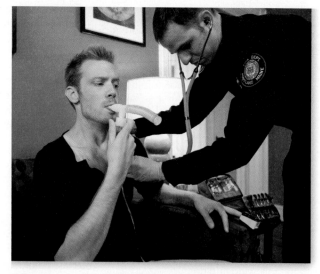

Place the patient in a sitting position. If possible, have the patient hold the nebulizer. Be careful that the patient does not invert the nebulizer and spill the medication out. Have the patient place the mouthpiece in his mouth and inhale slowly at a normal tidal volume for approximately 2 to 3 seconds, and then slowly exhale against pursed lips. Have the patient repeat this procedure until all of the medication is gone at which time the nebulizer typically begins to spurt. Reassess the patient and document the procedure.

pulse oximetry, when it can be considered reasonably accurate) to gauge the importance of oxygen and to titrate the appropriate rate of administration.

As a rule, oxygen should be delivered to restore and maintain saturations to normal levels (94 percent), but not in an uncontrolled fashion. Use the most appropriate delivery device (e.g., bag-valve mask, nasal cannula, Venturi mask) to administer an effective level of supplemental oxygen and reassess to ensure that ongoing needs are met.

Treating Bronchoconstriction

If the assessment of the patient can reasonably point to an airway restriction secondary to bronchoconstriction (especially in the context of a similar past medical history), then it is reasonable to aggressively attempt to reverse the narrowing of the bronchial tube. Paramedics have a variety of pharmacologic tools to address this disorder. Furthermore, early treatment of bronchoconstriction is important, as it can help prevent secondary inflammation that can often lead to progressive worsening of alveolar ventilation. Airway resistance disorders such as asthma should be considered time sensitive, as delays in therapy can result in worsening outcomes.

BETA$_2$ AGONISTS Beta$_2$ agonists are the stalwart treatments for lower airway resistance. These most commonly inhaled medications engage beta$_2$ receptor sites in the airway to produce bronchial smooth muscle dilation and are very effective in increasing otherwise restricted airflow. Albuterol sulfate is the most commonly distributed beta$_2$ agonist; this rapid-onset, short-acting medication can be invaluable in treating bronchospasm.

Beta$_2$ agonists are not without side effects, however, and they commonly produce beta$_1$ agonism as well. This can lead to increased heart rate and contractility and subsequent increased myocardial oxygen demand. In patients with already overtaxed hearts, this side effect can be dangerous.

Epinephrine is also a potent beta$_2$ agonist; it is traditionally used when other treatments fail. It has far more potent cardiac side effects and, in general, is reserved for only the sickest of patients, as the cost–benefit ratio is far narrower. It is valuable, however, in that it is not limited by the inhaled route, as other beta agonists can be.

Consider the need for deep ventilation to deliver and distribute inhaled respiratory medications. In a severe bronchoconstriction patient, air movement may be significantly limited. Epinephrine (most commonly delivered as an intramuscular injection in this setting) bypasses the respiratory route and can deliver therapy even when air movement is minimal.

Refer to Skill 29-1 for the procedure for administering a beta$_2$-specific agonist via a small-volume nebulizer.

PARASYMPATHOLYTICS We recognize the role of the sympathetic nervous system with regard to bronchodilation. When beta$_2$ receptor sites are engaged, bronchial passages are widened. Given that, there is at least anecdotal evidence that the parasympathetic nervous system plays a role in bronchoconstriction. It is hypothesized that muscarinic receptor sites, engaged by increased parasympathetic tone, elicit narrowing of the small airways. With this in mind, parasympatholytic medications are commonly administered to patients with bronchoconstriction to decrease the effects of parasympathetic tone and therefore cause bronchodilation.

Ipratropium bromide is the commonly used medication in this category; it has been shown to improve airflow in airway resistance disorders. Ipratropium bromide is commonly mixed with albuterol to provide a powerful "one-two punch" of bronchodilation. In this form, the medication combination is called DuoNeb and is used in a nebulized form.

MAGNESIUM SULFATE The smooth muscle relaxant properties of magnesium sulfate (MgSO$_4$) make this medication a commonly used second- and third-line treatment for lower airway obstruction. Magnesium is thought to dilate bronchial tubes to provide improved airflow. It is limited, however, by a relatively slow onset (sometimes up to 30 minutes for peak onset) and the requirement of a relatively slow administration (typically given over at least 10 minutes). This medication can be an important alternative to the inhaled route, however.

CORTICOSTEROIDS Corticosteroids are used to decrease inflammation in the bronchial tubes and can be an invaluable component in preventing long-term decompensation associated with increased bronchial edema. Medications such as prednisolone (Solu-Medrol) are administered intravenously and are an important addition to the initial bronchodilator therapy. Corticosteroids typically have a relatively slow onset, so early administration is important.

Overall, the goal of treating a patient with airway resistance is to first recognize and treat respiratory failure but then to take steps to ensure adequate ventilation and oxygenation. Remember that these patients may require aggressive intervention to maintain either one of those two goals. Frequently, airway-restricted patients will have adequate oxygenation but inadequate ventilation—and although hypercapnia is generally tolerated better than hypoxia, in the end it can be just as deadly.

TRANSITIONING • • • • • • • •

REVIEW ITEMS

1. A patient with asthma is complaining of respiratory distress. He states that his chest feels "tight." This perception of feeling "tight" is likely caused by what physiologic change?

    a. hypotension
    b. bronchoconstriction

    c. heightened ventilatory effort
    d. increased fluid accumulation in the alveoli

2. A change in "airway resistance" refers to what?

    a. impaired diaphragm excursion
    b. difficulty with achieving alveolar ventilation

c. increased opposition to airflow secondary to bronchoconstriction

d. inability for the lung tissue to ventilate because of a loss
of elasticity

3. Which of the following is a commonly cited contributor to
bronchitis and emphysema?

a. tobacco use

b. age and gender

c. family history of pulmonary disease

d. confirmed diagnosis of lung cancer or asthma

4. Corticosteroids are administered in an airway-resistance
patient to _____.

a. cause bronchodilation

b. cause bronchoconstriction

c. decrease mucus production

d. reduce inflammation

5. You arrive on the scene to find a 65-year-old man with
a chief complaint of respiratory distress. The patient
states that the dyspnea began about three days ago and
is progressively worsening. The patient says he is not a
smoker, has no known medical problems, and does not take
any medications. Vitals are stable, and the SpO$_2$ is
96 percent on room air. The patient further adds that he
has developed a nagging cough over the last day and that
his granddaughter has a "bad cold" right now. Based on this
information, from what do you think the patient is most
likely suffering?

a. asthma

b. emphysema

c. acute bronchitis

d. chronic bronchitis

APPLIED PATHOPHYSIOLOGY

*You are called to a local extended care facility for a male patient with
respiratory distress. On entering the room, you hear the "hum" of the
oxygen concentrator running beside his bed, and you note that the
patient has a nasal cannula applied. His eyes are shut, he is overweight,
and he keeps coughing. He does not respond to your verbal stimuli.*

1. Identify the most likely chronic pulmonary conditions this
patient may have.

2. What would be three assessment findings that could confirm
your suspicion?

3. Describe the anticipated physiologic benefit(s) for each of the
interventions that may be administered to a patient suffering
from an acute asthma attack:

a. Oxygen therapy

b. Metered-dose inhaler

c. Semi-Fowler positioning

4. Discuss the differences in pathophysiology and presentation of
the following airway resistance disorders:

a. Asthma

b. Chronic bronchitis

c. Bronchiolitis

5. Describe the pathophysiologic changes that occur to the lumen
of the respiratory system that contribute to the respiratory distress and altered V/Q functioning in the bronchiolitis patient.

CLINICAL DECISION MAKING

*You are called to a baseball field, where an 18-year-old boy has col-
lapsed in the outfield. His teammates state that he was complaining of
trouble breathing earlier in the game and that he said he forgot to
bring his "inhaler" with him. As you approach the patient, you find
him to be responsive to painful stimuli with purposeful motion. His
breathing looks very labored.*

1. Based on the scene size-up characteristics, identify the clues that
point to a medical history of asthma.

*The primary assessment reveals the patient to be alert to painful
stimuli. His airway is clear, and his breathing is rapid at 28/minute,
respirations are slightly shallow, vesicular sounds are markedly diminished, and coarse wheezing is present throughout the lungs. Peripheral
pulses are also present and noted to be rapid and weak. The blood
pressure is 110/68 mmHg, the neck veins are obviously engorged, and
the SpO$_2$ reading on room air is 87 percent.*

2. What are the life threats, if any, to the patient that you are aware
of currently?

3. Does this patient need oxygen by nonrebreather mask, or by
positive pressure ventilation? Why?

*Further assessment reveals the pupils to be equal and reactive, and the
pulse oximeter has increased to 94 percent with oxygen. Breath sounds
are unchanged, and jugular venous distention is still present. The blood
pressure is unchanged, heart rate is 118, and irregular, respirations have
decreased to 24/minute. The patient is starting to become more responsive and mumbles something about his "inhaler." A family member,
who has since arrived on the scene, says that she has the inhaler with her.*

4. During the ongoing management of the patient, you elect to
administer the following therapies. For each one, discuss in specific detail (1) the reason the intervention is warranted, (2) the
expected outcome of that intervention, and (3) how you would
assess to determine whether the desired effect is occurring (i.e.,
the treatment worked).

a. Positioning patient in high Fowler position

b. Administration of high-flow oxygen

c. Administration of metered-dose inhaler

Standard Medicine

Competency Integrates assessment findings with principles of epidemiology and pathophysiology to formulate a field impression and implement a comprehensive treatment/disposition plan for a patient with a medical complaint.

TOPIC

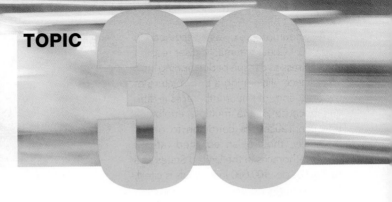

RESPIRATORY EMERGENCIES: LUNG AND GAS EXCHANGE DISORDERS

INTRODUCTION

In the preceding topic, the focus of discussion was on respiratory disorders of a restrictive nature—that is, disorders that shared a pathophysiologic change of increased bronchoconstriction that contributed to a change in pulmonary function, resulting in labored breathing. In this topic, the focus will still be on respiratory disorders, but now we will look at disorders that alter either lung compliance or the ability of gases to exchange across the alveolar surface.

Lung compliance refers to the ability of the actual lung tissue to expand when air flows in. If the lungs are "stiff," then it becomes difficult for the patient to inhale sufficiently to ventilate the alveoli and respiratory distress results. Conversely, if the oxygen in the inhaled gases cannot diffuse across the alveoli because of some disturbance, the body will not be able to adequately oxygenate the tissues—and, again, respiratory distress results. These two pathologies are the focus of this topic.

EPIDEMIOLOGY

From a frequency standpoint, respiratory disorders, in young as well as in old patients, are one of the most common prehospital emergencies the paramedic will encounter. Multiple conditions affect pulmonary function or the ability to circulate oxygenated blood, and almost all of these will lead to some degree of respiratory distress.

For example, the National Health Interview Survey has reported that emphysema occurs at an estimated rate of about 18 cases per 1,000 people in the United States. Another source estimates that 1.5 million people have been diagnosed with emphysema, and it is ranked 15th among chronic conditions that limit activities of daily living (ADL). Almost 18,000 people die annually of this disease.

Pulmonary edema, another gas exchange disorder, occurs in about 1 percent to 2 percent of the general population, most commonly between the ages of 40 and 75 years. In patients over the age of 75 years, this emergency increases to about 10 percent of the population. Although pulmonary edema has a variety of causes, this disorder is commonly encountered by the paramedic.

TRANSITION *highlights*

- *Frequency with which various lung and gas exchange disorders occur in the United States.*
- *Pathophysiologic changes that occur with pulmonary diseases that hamper either gas exchange or lung compliance:*
  - Emphysema.
  - Pulmonary embolism.
  - Spontaneous (and tension) pneumothorax.
  - Cystic fibrosis.
- *Relation of the general assessment findings of respiratory distress to the pathophysiologic changes that occur due to the various diseases.*
- *Explanation of adequate and inadequate breathing as it is affected by lung and gas exchange disorders.*
- *Differential assessment findings that relate the pathophysiology to disease onset and clinical findings to help delineate each respiratory dysfunction.*
- *Various treatment interventions and their relationship on improving the patient's pulmonary function:*
  - Oxygen administration.
  - Positive pressure ventilation.
  - Patient positioning.

Pulmonary embolism is another gas exchange etiology that causes respiratory distress. It occurs at an estimated rate of 1 per 1000 persons in the United States, with about a quarter of a million cases occurring annually. An equal number of people are diagnosed at autopsy with a massive pulmonary embolism as are diagnosed clinically; this leads to revised estimates of 650,000 to 900,000 fatal and nonfatal events of this nature in the United States annually.

A pneumothorax, as discussed in Topic 43: "Chest Trauma," causes respiratory distress as a result of diminishing lung compliance. Illustrating a clear picture of the frequency of pneumothoraces is difficult because of the multiple etiologies that can cause this condition to occur. Generally, though, an adjusted rate of pneumothoraces in the United States of 6 to 7 cases per 100,000 individuals is cited. Pneumothorax occurs more often in men than in women. The incidence peaks in the early 20s for "primary" pneumothoraces (usually less clinically severe) and peaks again in patients over age 60 for "secondary" pneumothoraces (usually more clinically severe).

Cystic fibrosis (CF) is the most common lethal hereditary disease in Caucasians. Although it can occur in other ethnicities, it does so with a much lower frequency. CF has a prevalence rate of 1 case per 3,200 persons in the United States, which may seem uncommon, but those afflicted usually die of pulmonary complications in the second or third decade of life. Although CF causes derangements in many of the body's systems, the most common pathologies leading to death revolve around pulmonary disorders.

> **Cystic fibrosis is the most common lethal hereditary disease in Caucasians.**

In conclusion, all the aforementioned conditions affect either lung compliance or the lung's ability to diffuse gases across the alveoli. Although the pathologies may not seem to occur that much individually, when one looks at the larger picture of lung compliance and gas exchange disorders, they become a common reason that a patient summons EMS.

PATHOPHYSIOLOGY

If lung compliance changes, this generally means that the ability of the lung tissue to expand and accommodate incoming airflow is hampered. If the disturbance is one that diminishes the ease by which gases diffuse across the alveolar wall and into and out of the bloodstream, then the patient will not be able to oxygenate appropriately. Recall that the key physiologic role of the lungs is to allow gas exchange, or the swapping of oxygen for carbon dioxide across the alveolar surface, thereby ensuring that adequate levels of oxygen are in the bloodstream as carbon dioxide is simultaneously removed. *External respiration*, as this is called, must occur in a sufficient manner; otherwise, the person will die.

Internal respiration is the process in which the body offloads oxygen in the capillary beds for cellular utilization, while simultaneously picking up waste carbon dioxide and returning it to the lungs for the process to repeat. Any disorder or disease that inhibits the external respiration process by way of changing lung compliance or diminishing gas exchange across the alveoli affects an individual's overall health by decreasing the oxygen saturation in the blood while carbon dioxide levels rise.

Emphysema

Emphysema is a permanent disease process that is characterized by destruction of the alveolar walls and distention of the alveolar sacs. The primary causal factor is cigarette smoking, but people who are exposed continuously to environmental toxins are also predisposed to developing emphysema.

In healthy lung tissue, certain cells (macrophages and leukocytes) use toxic enzymes to eliminate inhaled irritants. Normally, the lung produces an inhibitor substance that prevents these toxic enzymes from actually attacking the lung tissue they are trying to protect. In patients with emphysema, however, this inhibition is lacking, and the enzymes start to attack the body's normal lung tissue as well. Progressively, the lung tissue loses its elasticity, the alveoli become distended with trapped air, and the walls of the alveoli are destroyed. Loss of the alveolar wall reduces the surface area in contact with pulmonary capillaries. This results in a drastic disruption in the body's ability to adequately facilitate gas exchange, and the patient becomes hypoxic and begins to retain carbon dioxide.

The distal airways also are involved and have greatly diminished lung compliance, making the very act of breathing problematic (▶ **Figure 30-1**).

Breathing becomes extremely difficult for the emphysema patient, and exhaling progresses to an active rather than passive process, requiring muscular contraction; therefore, the patient with emphysema uses significant amounts of muscular energy to breathe. Eventually the patient will usually complain of extreme shortness of breath on exertion, which may be simply walking across a room. In addition, the loss of lung elasticity, air trapping, and exaggerated use of respiratory muscles to breathe cause the chest to increase in diameter, producing the "barrel-chest" appearance typical with this disease.

Pulmonary Edema

Acute pulmonary edema (APE) occurs when an excessive amount of fluid collects in the spaces between the alveoli and capillaries. This increase in fluid disturbs normal gas exchange and leads to hypoxia and hypercapnia, as oxygen diffusing into the bloodstream from the alveoli and carbon dioxide from the blood to the alveoli are both hampered (▶ **Figure 30-2**). The most significant problem associated with pulmonary edema is hypoxia, this being the primary reason underlying the respiratory distress complaint.

The two kinds of pulmonary edema are cardiogenic and noncardiogenic.

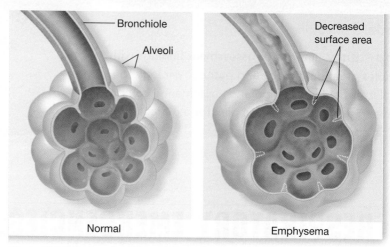

Figure 30-1 Pathophysiologic changes in emphysema include decreased surface area of the alveoli.

Normal — Bronchiole, Alveoli

Emphysema — Decreased surface area

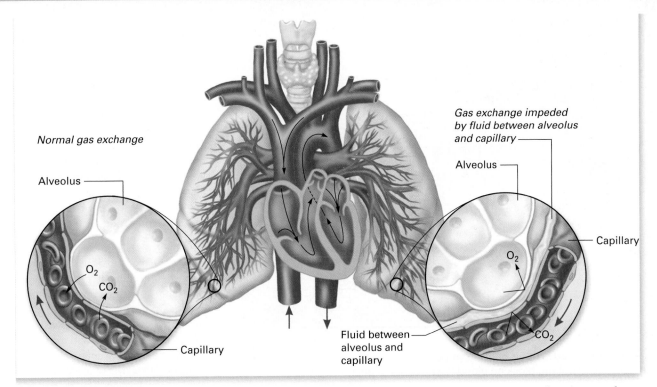

Figure 30-2 In pulmonary edema, fluid collects between the alveoli and capillaries, preventing normal exchange of oxygen and carbon dioxide. Fluid may also invade the alveolar sacs.

Cardiogenic pulmonary edema was discussed in greater detail in Topic 28, but to review, it is typically related to an inadequate pumping function of the left side of the heart that causes a backup of pressure and drastically increases the pressure in the pulmonary capillaries. This increased pressure forces fluid to leak into the space between the alveoli and capillaries and, eventually, into the alveoli themselves.

Noncardiogenic pulmonary edema, also known as *acute respiratory distress syndrome* (ARDS), results from direct destruction of the capillary bed that increases capillary permeability and allows fluid to leak out and into the interstitial spaces. Common causes of noncardiogenic pulmonary edema are severe pneumonia, aspiration of vomitus, near-drowning, narcotic overdose, inhalation of smoke or other toxic gases, ascent to a high altitude, and chest and lung trauma. Pulmonary edema is a life-threatening condition that presents with the same signs and symptoms regardless of the etiology, and in some cases, it is a dire emergency that requires immediate emergency care.

Pulmonary Embolism

A pulmonary embolism is not a disease state; rather, a pulmonary embolism is an emergency that arises from a complica-

tion of venous thromboembolism, more specifically and frequently from a deep venous thromboembolism (DVT) of the lower extremities (on rare occasions, they may originate from elsewhere in the venous system or the right side of the heart). Regardless, after the embolus breaks off, it travels through the venous system in increasingly larger blood vessels until it arrives at and is pumped through the right side of the heart.

After leaving the right ventricle, blood vessels continually get smaller and smaller as blood flows through the pulmonary system to the capillary beds of the lungs. As such, venous emboli can become trapped in one of these pulmonary blood vessels. Large emboli may lodge at the bifurcation of the main pulmonary artery (saddle embolism) or one of the smaller lobar branches. In this situation, the emboli may also cause significant hemodynamic compromise because the right ventricle will be unable to pump a sufficient amount of blood to the left side of the heart. Smaller emboli will travel more distally to smaller vessels in the lung. Occlusion here will likely cause respiratory distress in association with pleuritic (sharp, localized) chest pain by initiating an inflammatory response in the parietal pleura.

The embolism prevents blood from flowing to the lung. As a result, some

areas of the lung have oxygen in the alveoli but are not receiving any blood flow. This leads to a decrease in gas exchange and subsequent hypoxia, the severity of which depends on the size of the embolism or the number of alveoli affected. The hypoxia in this case is the result of the shunting of blood away from the oxygenated alveoli, creating a mismatch between ventilation and perfusion (▶ **Figure 30-3**).

Patients at risk for suffering a pulmonary embolism include the following:

- Patients who experience long periods of immobility (such as bedridden individuals)
- Patients who travel for a long period confined in one position
- Patients with long bone fractures or splints on extremities
- Patients with heart disease or a history of deep vein thrombosis
- Patients who have recently experienced surgery, venous pooling associated with pregnancy, cancer, or estrogen therapy

> **Pulmonary edema is a dire emergency that requires immediate emergency care.**

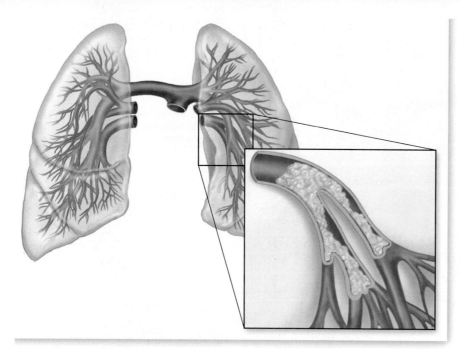

Figure 30-3 A blood clot, air bubble, fat particle, foreign body, or amniotic fluid can cause an embolism, blocking blood flow through a pulmonary artery.

- Patients with underlying coagulation disorders
- Patients who smoke

Spontaneous Pneumothorax

As you are aware, during inspiration air is drawn into the lungs as the diaphragm and intercostal muscles contract, thereby enlarging the size of the thoracic cavity. As the chest wall moves out and the diaphragm drops, the parietal pleura moves, and because of the negative pleural space pressure, the visceral pleura gets drawn out as well, which enlarges the lungs. The

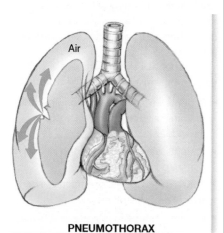

PNEUMOTHORAX

Figure 30-4 In pneumothorax, the lung collapse decreases lung tissue compliance and causes a disturbance in gas exchange that leads to hypoxia.

mechanical process of breathing cannot be damaged or deranged without some compromise on breathing adequacy, which is what happens with a pneumothorax.

If air enters the pleural cavity, either from the outside (open pneumothorax) or from air escaping through a hole in the lung and into the pleural space (closed pneumothorax), the lung may collapse; with larger pneumothoraces, it becomes mechanically impossible for the patient to breathe. The lung collapse decreases lung tissue compliance and causes a disturbance in gas exchange that leads to hypoxia (▶ Figure 30-4).

With a particular type of significant pneumothorax known as a *tension pneumothorax*, air entering the pleural cavity has nowhere to escape, so it starts to depress lung tissue; eventually it will shift the mediastinal structures toward the uninjured lung. This may lead to severe shortness of breath as well as circulatory collapse. Tension pneumothorax is a life-threatening condition that requires urgent intervention.

Men are five times more likely to suffer a spontaneous pneumothorax than are women. Most of these male patients are tall, thin, and lanky and between the ages of 20 and 40. Many also have a history of cigarette smoking or a connective tissue disorder such as Marfan syndrome or Ehlers-Danlos syndrome.

Patients with a history of chronic obstructive pulmonary disease (COPD) are more prone to spontaneous pneumothorax because of areas of weakened lung tissue called *blebs*. It is thought that the reason tall, thin, lanky men are more likely to suffer a spontaneous pneumothorax is that the visceral pleura is stretched within the chest cavity beyond its normal limit. Often the stretched and weakened area ruptures when the patient experiences an increase in intrathoracic pressure from an activity such as coughing, lifting a heavy object, or straining.

Cystic Fibrosis

Cystic fibrosis (also known as CF, mucoviscidosis, or mucovoidosis) is a hereditary disease. Although it commonly causes pulmonary dysfunction because of changes in the mucus-secreting glands of the lungs, it also affects the sweat glands, the pancreas, the liver, and the intestines.

Lining almost the entire respiratory tree in the body is a layer of tissue that is coated with a mucus lining. This mucus lining is normally watery and helps to warm and humidify inspired air, and it also serves to trap any inhaled particles. In CF, however, an abnormal gene alters the functioning of the mucus glands lining the respiratory system, and there is an overabundance of mucus, which is very thick and sticky. As this thick mucus layer develops, blockage of the airways occurs along with an increase in the incidence of lung infections, as bacteria can readily grow in the thick mucus.

Repeated lung infections, in turn, cause scarring of the lung tissue, reduce the ability of the lungs to clear the thick mucus, and promote ongoing pulmonary damage. As a result, there is progressive diminution in the efficiency of respiratory function, which leads to eventual pulmonary failure and death.

Pulmonary complications are the most common cause for a patient with this affliction to summon EMS. There is no cure yet for CF, and many individuals with this disease die at a young age (20s–30s) because of pulmonary failure. In fact, CF is cited as one of the most common life-shortening genetic diseases. Because it is possible to detect CF in a patient at a very young age, it is common for the patient experiencing a crisis to already know of this diagnosis. Fortunately, medical research and treatment are lengthening the life span of some people to as high as 50 years. In terminal states of the disease, the final medical recourse, when all other interventions have failed, is lung transplantation.

ASSESSMENT FINDINGS

A patient suffering from a lung compliance issue or gas exchange deficit, as discussed in this topic, will almost certainly present with respiratory distress. The degree of respiratory distress can vary from very minimal, subjective dyspnea to severe dyspnea with objective findings of inadequate breathing present. The most important assessment the paramedic must do when dealing with a dyspneic patient is to determine whether the patient is breathing adequately.

Recall that the patient's minute ventilation is a function of the respiratory rate and tidal volume. In almost all situations of illness or injury, the response of the respiratory rate is to increase, so identifying tachypnea is not all that uncommon or specific a finding. The tidal volume is more important to assess, however, as most all pulmonary diseases or injuries end up affecting the tidal volume (or the amount of air a patient takes with each breath).

The body must ventilate through physiologic dead space prior to the air reaching the alveoli (physiologic dead space is about 150 mL of each tidal volume). As such, if a patient's tidal volume drops from 500 mL per breath to 200 mL per breath, the body will still fill 150 mL of dead space, which means only 50 mL of air available for gas exchange in the alveoli, as compared with the normal 350 mL in a patient who is breathing adequately. The point is, however, that you cannot look at a patient and determine how many milliliters of air he is moving with each breath unless you have diagnostic pulmonary equipment. What you can do, though, is assess the clinical adequacy of the tidal volume.

Although a long list of findings may be present if the patient is breathing adequately (a different list will apply if the patient is breathing inadequately), you really need to pay close attention to two assessment findings that will illustrate the quality of the patient's breathing.

First, listen to the patient's speech patterns. A patient speaking in full sentences without discomfort is still breathing adequately.

Second, assess vesicular breath sounds over the lung's periphery. Absent vesicular (alveolar) breath sounds indicates that the patient is not breathing adequately. If the patient's mental status precludes communication with you, determine breathing adequacy by assessing the rise and fall of the chest (chest wall excursion) along with vesicular breath sounds. It is not that the actual respiratory rate is unimportant; it is just that tachypnea is commonly seen with almost all medical/traumatic emergencies (other than late brainstem/head injury or depressant drug overdose), so except in cases of *extreme* tachypnea or *extreme* bradypnea, the rate is not that all clinically relevant.

Additional monitoring may be readily available to further assess patients with compliance or gas exchange issues. Peak expiratory flow measurement, although typically more valuable with bronchoconstricted patients, may provide better insight into the movement of air than auscultation alone. Waveform capnography can also provide excellent insight into the movement of carbon dioxide. Capnography can demonstrate both the level of hypercapnia and the presence (or lack of) bronchospasm. Some systems have even integrated point-of-care blood gas capabilities to paint an accurate picture of the distribution of oxygen and carbon dioxide.

Beyond the findings of general respiratory distress and/or labored breathing, the next sections give more specific findings for conditions addressed in this topic.

Additional Assessment Findings

Patients with emphysema may present with the following:

- On home oxygen
- Thin, barrel-chest appearance
- Coughing, but with little sputum
- Prolonged exhalation with pursed-lip breathing
- Diminished breath sounds
- Wheezing and rhonchi (rattles) on auscultation with exacerbation
- Extreme difficulty of breathing with minimal exertion
- Pink complexion (Emphysema patients are often called "pink puffers.")
- Tachypnea—breathing rate usually greater than 20 per minute at rest
- Tachycardia and diaphoresis
- Tripod position
- Chronically low oxygen satuations and chronically high levels of exhaled carbon dioxide (partial pressure of end-tidal CO_2 [$PETCO_2$]) levels.

The following may be found in patients with pulmonary edema:

- Dyspnea, especially on exertion
- Difficulty in breathing when lying flat (orthopnea)
- Cough (possibly productive), frothy sputum
- Pursed-lipped breathing and grunting
- Tachycardia and tachypnea
- Anxiety, apprehension, combativeness, confusion
- Tripod position with legs dangling
- Crackles and possibly wheezing on auscultation
- Cyanosis or dusky-color skin
- Pale, moist skin
- Distended neck veins
- Swollen lower extremities
- Symptoms of cardiac compromise, including cardiac arrhythmias

Crackles (also called rales) are a sign of pulmonary edema. Be sure to auscultate the posterior lower lobes of the lungs to pick up early indications of crackles and pulmonary edema. If you are auscultating only the upper lobes, you may easily miss the condition because gravity is pulling the fluid downward into the lower portions of the lungs. Note that the signs and symptoms of APE are discussed in greater detail in Topic 28.

Patients with pulmonary embolism may present with the following:

- Sudden onset of unexplained dyspnea
- Signs of difficulty in breathing or respiratory distress; rapid breathing
- Sudden onset of sharp, stabbing chest pain
- Cough (may cough up blood)
- Tachypnea and tachycardia
- Syncope (fainting)
- Cool, moist skin
- Restlessness, anxiety, or sense of doom
- Decrease in blood pressure (late sign)
- Cyanosis (may be severe)

> The most important assessment the paramedic must do with a dyspneic patient is to determine whether the patient is breathing adequately.

TABLE 30-1 Differential Assessment Findings for Lung and Gas Exchange Disorders

Pulmonary Emergency	General Pathology	Onset of Dyspnea	Specific Differential Findings
Emphysema	Destruction of alveoli, air trapping, CO_2 retention (which is less common in emphysema)	Persistent dyspnea, acute deterioration with exacerbation	Diminished breath sounds, barrel chest, clubbing of fingers
Pulmonary edema	Fluid accumulation in alveoli from heart failure	Usually rapid onset with heart failure	Inspiratory crackles, jugular venous distention (JVD), frothy sputum
Pulmonary emboli	Occlusion of pulmonary blood vessel blocking blood flow to lung(s)	Sudden, unexplained; usually no precipitation event	Pleuritic chest pain, breath sounds possibly clear, unexplained tachycardia
Spontaneous pneumothorax	Collapse of lung tissue from air in pleural space	Sudden, may be related to straining	Pleuritic chest pain, unilateral diminishment of breath sounds
Cystic fibrosis	Excessive mucus plugging; final common pathway: respiratory failure	More gradual development, may progress to severe dyspnea	Coughing, rhonchi, history of recurrent upper respiratory infection (URI), GI distress, general malaise

- Distended neck veins (late sign)
- Inspiratory crackles
- Swollen lower extremity
- Possible fever
- SpO_2 <95 percent
- Very low $PETCO_2$ levels despite the signs and symptoms of poor gas exchange.

It is important to note that not all the signs and symptoms of pulmonary embolism will always be present. Common signs and symptoms are chest pain, dyspnea, and tachypnea (rapid breathing) with tachycardia being the most common.

Additional assessment findings for spontaneous pneumothorax include the following:

- Sudden onset of shortness of breath
- Sudden onset of sharp chest pain or shoulder pain; may be pleuritic
- Decreased breath sounds to one side of the chest (most often apical)
- Subcutaneous emphysema may be found
- Tachypnea and tachycardia
- Diaphoresis and pallor
- Cyanosis may be seen late and in a large pneumothorax
- SpO_2 <95 percent

A patient who presents with a sudden onset of shortness of breath with decreased breath sounds on one side of the chest and no evidence of trauma should be suspected of having a possible spontaneous pneumothorax.

The following may be present in patients with CF:

- Commonly, a known history of the disease
- Recurrent coughing; rhonchi may be noted with auscultation
- General malaise (weakness, fatigue, not feeling well)
- Expectoration of thick mucus during coughing
- Recurrent episodes or history of pneumonia, bronchitis, and sinusitis
- Gastrointestinal (GI) complaints, possibly including constipation or other changes in bowel movements
- Abdominal pain from intestinal gas
- Malnutrition or low weight despite a healthy appetite
- Dehydration
- Clubbing of the digits
- Trouble speaking and breathing (dyspnea) with mucus buildup

Although the most common complaint the patient with CF will have is difficulty breathing, many of the other findings are due to dysfunction of other organ systems. The abdominal findings, such as dehydration, bowel changes, and poor weight gain, are from the damage the disease inflicts on the GI tract. Pancreatitis can also cause abdominal pain, as can liver damage from the disease.

Table 30-1 summarizes the differential assessment findings for lung and gas exchange disorders.

EMERGENCY MEDICAL CARE

Treatment for lung compliance and gas exchange disorders share the same global goals as treatment for other respiratory distress patients: Ensure that the patient's airway is clear and maintained, provide positive pressure ventilation should the patient be breathing inadequately or have fatigue of respiratory muscles, reverse hypoxemia and hypercapnia, and ensure that peripheral perfusion remains intact.

Although the disorders discussed within this topic require very specific, individual treatment strategies, it is important not to lose sight of the more broad-based approaches. The following is a summary of global management considerations:

1. **Establish and maintain an open airway.**
2. **Establish and maintain adequate ventilation and oxygenation.** A patient who is having difficulty breathing but has an adequate tidal volume (as evidenced by good speech patterns, adequate chest rise, and diffuse vesicular breath sounds) and an adequate respiratory rate is in respiratory distress. Because the patient's minute and alveolar ventilation are still adequate, the patient is compensating and is in need of supplemental oxygen. Titrate the oxygen administration to achieve a SpO_2 reading of greater than 94 percent, reduce the complaint of dyspnea, and eliminate the signs and symptoms of hypoxia.

If either the tidal volume or the respiratory rate becomes (or is) inadequate, the patient's minute and alveolar ventilation will be inadequate; the patient is then said to be in *respiratory failure*, as the respiratory tidal volume or rate is no longer able to support an adequate ventilatory effort. This requires you to immediately begin ventilation with a bag-valve-mask device or other ventilation device. Supplemental oxygen must be delivered through the ventilation device. If a patient with inadequate breathing is not treated promptly, it is likely that he will deteriorate to respiratory arrest and, potentially, cardiac arrest.

3. **Position the patient.** Semi- or high Fowler positioning will assist the patient in breathing and minimize the negative effects of fluid accumulating in the lungs, especially for the patient with pulmonary edema. If positive pressure ventilation is being provided or frank hypotension is present, the patient will need to be placed supine for ongoing management.

The following sections discuss specific treatments, including a broad spectrum of therapies. As always, follow local protocols when applying any treatment plan.

Treating Emphysema

Rarely are paramedics called to specifically treat emphysema (although this may be the case in end-stage diseases). More commonly, EMS is dispatched when a secondary causes exacerbates the underlying problems associated with COPD. For example, the low oxygen levels and high CO_2 levels may be acceptable in a restricted lifestyle, but when that patient acquires a respiratory infection in addition to emphysema, standard compensation may no longer be enough. In this case, an underlying gas exchange issue is forced to the forefront, as metabolic processes are no longer capable of functioning.

Treatment strategies in exacerbated emphysema are focused on reversing the gas exchange issue and eliminating the secondary challenge, if possible. As always, find and treat respiratory failure first, but then address other respiratory concerns.

If bronchospasm is found, it is appropriate to administer bronchodilators. Beta agonists, such as albuterol, and parasympatholytics, such as ipratropium bromide, are effective choices. Corticosteroids may help reduce the inflammation associated with bronchoconstriction and improve alveolar ventilation.

Noninvasive positive pressure ventilation, such as continuous positive airway pressure (CPAP), can help improve the symptoms and help reverse gas exchange issues as well.

More global treatment strategies are very important to keep in mind when treating emphysema. This is not a problem that can be solved in the field. Often, reversing this downward course means antibiotic therapy (to resolve secondary infections) or prolonged courses on a ventilator (to relieve fatigue). Prehospital care may focus on treating symptoms and reversing gas exchange deficits.

Treating Pulmonary Edema

Topic 28 reviewed a thorough plan for treating APE. To review, the key elements were administration of nitrates to decrease preload (and workload of the heart); CPAP to increase intraalveolar pressure and reverse the pressure gradient that pulls fluid into the interstitial space and into the alveoli; administration of vasoactive medications such as angiotensin-converting enzyme (ACE) inhibitors to reduce afterload and further take the workload off the heart; and, at least theoretically, the administration of loop diuretics to remove volume, in the case of hypervolemic states.

It should be noted that diuretics remain a controversial medication in many prehospital systems. There is some evidence of an increased complication rate when diuretics are administered in incorrect settings (such as with a misdiagnosis of exacerbated COPD or pneumonia), and there is concern over the administration of diuretics to normovolemic patients.

In many cases, the specific diagnosis of pulmonary edema may be difficult to make. Many patients have an assortment of respiratory pathologies that frequently present at the same time. Is it possible for a pneumonia patient to experience pulmonary edema? Could a COPD patient have a heart attack? Of course, the answer to both these questions is yes; in these cases, a singular diagnosis may be impossible (particularly with the limited diagnostic tools of the prehospital world). In general, treatment always should address a specific disorder (nitroglycerin for APE, for example); however, with a patient with a variety of comorbid factors, treatment may have to be more global.

If the nature of the disorder is truly obscure despite thorough patient assessment, consider a broad-based approach. Start by identifying respiratory failure. If respirations are adequate, look for bronchoconstriction. Although administering bronchodilators to a patient in APE is not ideal, it is probably not as dangerous as it was once perceived to be. In undifferentiated bronchospasm, it may be appropriate to take steps to bronchodilate even if the risk of APE is present. CPAP is another viable option for the undifferentiated patient. It will be therapeutic in APE, but it will also improve gas exchange in COPD exacerbation. You should, however, avoid the nonforgiving therapies, such as diuretic administration. Here, very real damage can be done if the diagnosis is inaccurate.

Treatment of Pulmonary Emboli

Beyond treating respiratory failure, little can be done in the prehospital world to treat pulmonary emboli. As such, recognition and rapid transport to an appropriate facility are extremely important. Supplemental oxygen and proper patient positioning are really the only other steps that can be helpful in this life-threatening condition.

Treatment of Spontaneous Pneumothorax

Patients experiencing a spontaneous pneumothorax are at high risk. Not only do they have a significant impairment of lung function and potentially massive gas exchange problems, but they also have the risk of developing a tension pneumothorax. As a paramedic, your treatment will focus primarily on relieving a tension pneumothorax, but in the meantime, constant reassessment is critical. In the case of a simple pneumothorax, you will treat the underlying cause (seal open chest wounds, address other injuries, etc.) and attempt to offset gas exchange problems. Supplemental oxygen will be important, as will patient position (often an upright or high Fowler position will aid in breathing).

Assessment of breathing, circulation, and lung sounds will be essential to identify the onset of a tension pneumothorax. Look for increased dyspnea, diminishing lung sounds, and signs of shock. When a tension pneumothorax is identified, you must immediately perform a needle decompression. The technique of needle decompression will be discussed further in Topic 43, "Chest Trauma." Remember that even after a successful needle decompression, decompensation can occur. Reassessment must be ongoing and additional decompressions may be necessary. Rapid transport to an appropriate facility is also a wise option when dealing with a pneumothorax patient.

Treatment of Cystic Fibrosis

CF can present with a variety of problems, but when considering the respiratory effects, the pathophysiology generally is related to poor air movement and consequential gas exchange issues. Treatment generally focuses on those two issues. Treat respiratory failure. Supplemental oxygen can be used if the patient is hypoxic. Bronchodilator therapy may be helpful if bronchoconstriction is identified. Remember that CF patients are commonly immunosuppressed, so take care to use sterile procedures during vascular access and other invasive procedures.

CONCLUSIONS

It would be naive to imagine that it will be possible to absolutely determine the cause of respiratory distress in every patient. This is certainly not always possible. When it is, though, specific treatment plans should be used to counter individual pathophysiologies of the disorder. When a specific diagnosis cannot be made, paramedics should use global strategies and forgiving therapies to target specific symptoms and to normalize gas exchange.

TRANSITIONING

REVIEW ITEMS

1. Which pulmonary gas exchange disorder typically has a rapid onset of dyspnea, commonly associated with pleuritic chest pain?

    a. pulmonary emboli
    b. pulmonary edema
    c. cystic fibrosis
    d. emphysema

2. Which of the following disorders would most likely have unilaterally diminished breath sounds?

    a. emphysema
    b. pneumothorax
    c. pulmonary edema
    d. pulmonary emboli

3. You are assessing a patient with dyspnea whom you suspect to have emphysema. Although he says that he has not been to a doctor for years, what part of his history/presentation described below would best support your field impression?

    a. frequent use of antacids
    b. chronic use of aspirin
    c. sudden onset of dyspnea
    d. inspiratory crackles with breathing

4. Your 86-year-old female patient is complaining of dyspnea and weakness. You note that she has jugular venous distention, inspiratory crackles, and diffuse expiratory wheezing. She has a history of coronary bypass and hypertension. Her current mental status is normal. Her vital signs are blood pressure 180/100 mmHg, heart rate 108, and irregular, respiratory rate 26/minute. Given this scenario, what should your *first* drug of choice be?

    a. Administer 365 mg baby aspirin orally.
    b. Administer oxygen at 15 liters per minute (lpm) via full face mask.
    c. Assist with the administration of her prescribed metered-dose inhaler.
    d. Assist with the administration of her oral antihypertensive medication.

5. Which of these body system/organ failures results in early death of cystic fibrosis patients?

    a. cardiac failure
    b. pancreatic failure
    c. pulmonary failure
    d. gastrointestinal failure

APPLIED PATHOPHYSIOLOGY

You are caring for a patient with respiratory distress. The patient presents with an intact airway, breathing is regular at 26/minute, and vesicular breath sounds are present bilaterally but markedly diminished. The patient states that he is normally slightly dyspneic, but over the past few days his dyspnea has progressively worsened. You note a low pulse oximeter reading, tachycardia, slightly erythemic skin, and a prolonged expiratory phase. He is on home oxygen, 2 lpm via cannula, per physician's orders.

1. Should you suspect this patient is suffering from a restrictive disorder or a compliance disorder? Support your answer based on your field impression. Why might the administration of higher concentrations of oxygen be beneficial for this patient?

2. Patients with cystic fibrosis may be recipients of bilateral lung transplants to sustain life; however, patients with emphysema are commonly not considered for this surgery. Basing your answer on progressive disease pathophysiology, briefly explain why this might be.

3. Discuss the differences in pathophysiology and presentation of the following gas exchange disorders of the pulmonary system:

    a. Pulmonary embolism
    b. Pulmonary edema

CLINICAL DECISION MAKING

You are summoned to a high school basketball game. There you find an elderly male patient who came to the game to see his grandson play. Shortly after sitting down near the top of the bleachers, he started to experience chest pressure that progressed into significant respiratory distress. He states he normally takes a nitroglycerin pill when his chest feels like this, but he forgot his nitro at home. You note that his jugular veins are engorged, he is using accessory muscles to breathe, and his speech is becoming more and more choppy. His medical history includes hypertension and "a bad heart."

1. Identify clues from above that point to the field impression of pulmonary edema.

2. What medical condition does this patient have that could explain the onset of the pulmonary edema emergency?

The primary assessment reveals that the patient's airway is clear, his breathing is rapid at 28/minute, respirations are shallow, vesicular sounds are present, and inspiratory crackles are noted. Peripheral pulses are also present but are weak, rapid, and slightly irregular. His blood pressure is 182/104 mmHg. The neck veins are obviously engorged, and the SpO_2 reading on room air is 87 percent. The patient's mental status is rapidly deteriorating, and he mumbles something like "Just let me lie down to rest a bit."

3. What are the life threats, if any, to the patient that you are currently aware of?

Further assessment reveals the pupils to be equal and reactive, and the pulse oximeter has increased to 94 percent with high-flow oxygen. Breath sounds are unchanged, and JVD is still present. The blood pressure is now 180/100 mmHg, heart rate is 112, and irregular, respirations have increased to 32/minute.

4. During the ongoing management of the patient en route, you elect to administer the following therapies. For each one, discuss in specific detail (1) the reason the intervention is warranted; (2) the expected outcome of that intervention; and (3) how you would assess to determine whether that desired effect is occurring (i.e., the treatment worked).

   a. Positioning patient in high Fowler position

   b. Administration of high-flow oxygen

   c. Application of CPAP

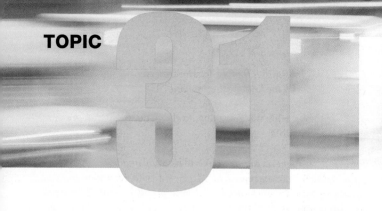
Standard Medicine

Competency Integrates assessment findings with principles of epidemiology and pathophysiology to formulate a field impression and implement a comprehensive treatment/disposition plan for a patient with a medical complaint.

RESPIRATORY EMERGENCIES: INFECTIOUS DISORDERS

TRANSITION highlights

Transition Highlights

- *Review of the frequency with which various infectious respiratory disorders occur in the United States and worldwide.*

- *Expanded discussion of common infectious disorders and how the pathophysiology is related to presenting signs and symptoms:*
  - – Pneumonia.
  - – Pertussis.
  - – Viral respiratory infections.

- *Common assessment findings as they relate to normal breathing, labored breathing, and inadequate breathing.*

- *Specific assessment findings as they relate to the aforementioned infectious disorders (beyond the general findings of respiratory distress).*

- *General emergency care for a dyspneic patient, as well as specific treatment considerations for infectious respiratory disorders.*

INTRODUCTION

As discussed in the previous two topics, respiratory distress or labored breathing is a common prehospital complaint with either medical or traumatic etiologies. Onset may be acute or gradual and can present mildly with minimal discomfort to the patient or severe enough that the patient may fear he will die if the cause is not rapidly identified and correct—and, to a large extent, that fear can be real. Breathing is an automatic process that is regulated in the brainstem and depends on functioning musculoskeletal, cardiovascular, and pulmonary systems; should one of these body systems fail, it can result in a serious condition requiring immediate intervention.

Because many findings of respiratory distress actually result from the body's attempt to improve breathing adequacy, not necessarily from the specific pulmonary condition, it is important to remember that pulmonary conditions may present very similarly. As such, many of the paramedic's treatment modalities are similar for these varied conditions. In this topic, the focus is on infectious disorders that afflict the pulmonary system and lead to respiratory distress. In any instance, however, it is important for the paramedic to recognize the signs and symptoms of respiratory emergencies, complete a thorough patient history and physical exam to determine the cause, and provide immediate intervention.

EPIDEMIOLOGY

Although cardiovascular disease is the leading cause of death in the United States and most developed nations, lower respiratory infections are the leading cause of death worldwide. Patients with immunosuppressive disorders or age extremes (very young and very old) are the ones most likely to succumb to a pulmonary infection that eventually robs them of the ability to ventilate and oxygenate adequately. With the ensuing increase in the work of breathing in an attempt to compensate for the pulmonary disturbance, the added workload to the respiratory muscles and cardiovascular system eventually leads to fatigue, acidosis, hypoxia, hypercapnia (high CO_2 levels), and death.

Pneumonia occurs more than 4.8 million times a year in the U.S. population, which can be extrapolated into more than 13,000 cases a day and 9 cases per minute. The vast majority of cases are found in nursing home and convalescent patients; pneumonia is a common cause of death in these populations. Patients infected with the human immunodeficiency virus (HIV) and others who are on immunosuppressive drugs, such as transplant patients, are also very prone to pneumonia. Additional risk factors include cigarette smoking, alcoholism, and exposure to cold temperatures.

Pertussis is a highly contagious childhood bacterial illness that is, fortunately, preventable with a vaccine. In the United States, most hospitalizations and nearly all deaths from pertussis are reported in infants aged less than 6 months (although morbidity does occur in other age groups). The Centers for Disease Control and Prevention tracks documented cases of pertussis and have found in past years that the annual incidence is about 3.3 cases per 100,000 people; however, there has been a recent outbreak in the United States. When focusing on the age of the patient, the average annual incidence rate is highest (55.2 per 100,000) in infants less than 1 year of age. In older populations, only marginal increases in pertussis have been seen.

A third common infectious respiratory condition is viral respiratory tract infections (VRIs). VRIs are the most common cause of symptomatic disease among children and adults. Each year, approximately 2 to 4 respiratory tract illnesses occur in adults, compared with 6 to 12 respiratory tract illnesses in children. These infections may cause a wide variety of diseases, from the common cold to severe pneumonia, and may result in significant morbidity and mortality within age-extreme patients and those who are already immunocompromised. Because VRIs afflict the pulmonary system, the patient often presents with some degree of respiratory distress.

PATHOPHYSIOLOGY

Pneumonia

Pneumonia is primarily an acute infectious disease, caused by bacteria, a virus, or other pathogens that affect the lower respiratory tract and cause lung inflammation and fluid- or pus-filled alveoli (▶ Figure 31-1). This leads to poor gas exchange across the alveoli and eventual hypoxia and hypercapnia. As oxygen and carbon dioxide diffusion across the alveoli becomes impaired, the patient will progress from subjective respiratory distress findings to objective findings. The progression may be slow and take days to weeks to develop, or, in the instance of bacterial pneumonia, the presentation of respiratory distress may occur more rapidly.

Often the virus or bacteria responsible for the condition initially resides in one of the lung's lobes; as it replicates itself, it migrates up the respiratory tree and can settle in other lobes or even in the opposite lung. It is possible, early in the syndrome progression, that changes in breath sounds are present in only one lung or one lobe of a lung, a condition known as *lobar pneumonia*. Although viral pneumonia does occur, respiratory viruses commonly weaken the lung tissue, which then creates an environment conducive for the development of secondary pneumonia caused by opportunistic bacteria.

Finally, a type of pneumonia called *pneumonitis* can be caused by inhalation of toxic irritants or aspiration of vomitus or other toxic substances.

Pertussis

Pertussis (also known as "whooping cough") is a respiratory disease that is characterized by uncontrolled paroxysms of coughing. It is a highly contagious disease that affects the respiratory system and is caused by bacteria residing in the upper airway of an infected person. It is spread by respiratory droplets that are discharged from the nose and mouth during coughing. Pertussis has been found to occur in patients of all ages, but it is reported most often in children. Generally speaking, the younger the patient, the more severe the clinical condition.

Pertussis typically starts out very similar to a cold or a mild upper respiratory infection. Because of this, the parents of the infant or child (or in the situation of an older patient) may try "waiting it out" before seeking medical care; thus, by the time the patient presents to EMS, the condition may be severe. Within two weeks or so of onset, the patient will develop episodes of numerous rapid coughs (15–24 episodes) as the body attempts to expel thick mucus from the airway, followed by a "crowing" or "whooping" sound made during inhalation as the patient breathes in deeply and rapidly.

Complications of pertussis include pneumonia, dehydration, seizures, brain injuries, ear infections, and even death. Most deaths occur to younger patients who have not been immunized for this disease or to patients who are exposed before finishing the vaccination series. In younger patients, the ongoing and uncontrolled coughing can severely disrupt normal breathing, diminish gas exchange in the alveoli, and promote bacterial pneumonia.

Viral Respiratory Infections

A viral respiratory infection refers to a condition in the respiratory system caused by a virus. Common VRIs include

> **VRIs are the most common cause of symptomatic disease among children and adults.**

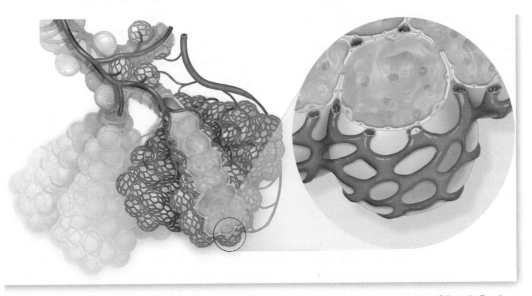

Figure 31-1 Pneumonia causes inflammation of the lungs and causes the alveoli to fill with fluid or pus, leading to poor gas exchange.

bronchiolitis, colds, and influenza ("the flu"). In most situations for adults, VRIs are fairly mild, self-limiting, and confined to the upper respiratory system. In children, however, the infection has a greater propensity to spread into the lower airways, where more significant infections can occur, resulting in patient deterioration.

Viral respiratory infections are commonly referred to by the medical community as *upper respiratory infections* (URIs) because the majority of symptoms are found in the nose and throat. In small children, however, VRIs can also cause infections of the lower airway structures, such as the trachea, bronchi or bronchioles, or lungs. When an infection involves these lower airway structures, depending on the site, the patient may be diagnosed with croup, bronchiolitis, or pneumonia. Known viruses that can cause VRIs include rhinoviruses, parainfluenza and influenza viruses, enteroviruses, respiratory syncytial virus (RSV), and some strains of the adenovirus.

> **Assess the patient's mental status and pay attention to speech patterns.**

The major pathophysiologic changes caused by these viruses on gaining entry into the body by way of patient-to-patient contact (and to a lesser extent, through inhalation of respiratory droplets) is a triggering of the inflammatory process with increased mucus production in the upper respiratory structures. Fever, coughing, runny nose, and findings of mild respiratory distress may also be associated with the infection in the majority of cases. VRIs typically run a course of about 14 days, and unless extenuating circumstances are present (i.e., a secondary respiratory infection of the lower airways or severe respiratory distress), they rarely necessitate medical attention.

In any situation, however, it is nearly impossible (nor is it practical) for the paramedic to determine whether the associated findings of respiratory distress from a VRI etiology are in fact viral in nature or not, as there is no specific treatment for viral infections that the paramedic can administer. The mainstay of treatment for respiratory distress secondary to a VRI is supportive in nature and includes patient positioning, airway and breathing maintenance, oxygen administration, and trans-port to the hospital for ongoing diagnosis and management.

ASSESSMENT FINDINGS

Normal breathing (a normal respiratory effort) requires a minimal amount of energy expenditure and is almost effortless for the patient. Normal breathing is also quiet; it does not produce abnormal sounds or noises. When assessing the patient for normal respiratory effort, first start with the respiratory (breathing) rate, which is assessed by observing the patient's chest rise and fall. The normal respiratory rate range for an adult patient at rest is typically 8 to 24 breaths per minute.

Second, assess the patient's mental status and pay attention to speech patterns. A patient who is struggling to breathe can rarely speak in normal sentences, as his need to take another breath precludes this. However, for example, if you encounter a patient with a respiratory rate of 8 breaths per minute who is alert, oriented, and able to answer your questions without gasping for a breath or showing a struggle to breathe, 8 breaths per minute may be his normal respiratory rate, and no intervention is necessary.

As an additional confirmation of breathing quality, auscultate breath sounds. You should be able to hear air exchange in the bases of the lungs bilaterally (which indicates that the alveoli are being ventilated as well).

Also assess the respiratory (or breathing) rhythm—the regularity or irregularity of respirations. Normal breathing will have a normal respiratory rhythm, but remember that the respiratory rhythm can be easily affected by speech, activity, emotions, and other factors in the conscious and alert patient.

An abnormal respiratory rhythm, however—that is, an irregular pattern of respiration—in the patient with an altered mental status is a serious concern. It may indicate a respiratory medical illness or even a chemical imbalance or brain abnormality or injury. In situations of an irregular breathing rhythm (either from conscious control in an awake patient or during periods of altered mental status or unresponsiveness), it becomes more important to assess for breathing adequacy by assessing the respiratory rate and tidal volume.

In summary, the following findings are consistent with a patient who is breathing adequately:

- A patent (open) airway
- Adequate respiratory rate
- Adequate rise and fall of the chest
- Normal respiratory rhythm
- Breath sounds present bilaterally
- Chest expansion and relaxation occurring normally
- Minimal to absent accessory muscle use to aid in breathing

The following should also occur in a patient who is breathing adequately, providing there is no disturbance to other bodily systems:

- Alert and oriented
- Normal muscle tone
- Normal pulse oximeter reading
- Normal skin condition findings

As stated, the majority of patients the paramedic will encounter will display an adequate respiratory effort (normal breathing). This does not mean, however, that the paramedic will never encounter a patient with inadequate breathing or will never find that a patient who was initially breathing adequately has deteriorated to a point at which breathing is inadequate and insufficient to sustain life. In fact, not only will failing to breathe adequately, even for short periods of time, result in hypoxia and cellular death, but all the other bodily systems will start to falter as well.

The majority of findings seen in patients with respiratory distress are caused by the body's attempt to increase ventilator exchange. As such, many respiratory conditions may have remarkably similar findings; the following sections, however, list the characteristic findings common to the infectious respiratory conditions discussed in this topic.

Assessment of the Patient with Pneumonia

The signs and symptoms of pneumonia vary with the cause and the patient's age. The patient generally appears ill and may complain of fever and severe chills. Look for the following signs and symptoms:

- Malaise and decreased appetite
- Fever (may not occur in the elderly or infants)
- Cough—may be productive or nonproductive

- Dyspnea (less frequent in the elderly)
- Tachypnea and tachycardia
- Chest pain—sharp and localized and usually made worse when breathing deeply or coughing
- Decreased chest wall movement and shallow respirations
- Possibly, patient splinting his thorax with his arm
- Possibly, crackles and rhonchi heard on auscultation
- Altered mental status, especially in the elderly
- Diaphoresis
- Cyanosis
- SpO_2 <95 percent

Assessment of the Patient with Pertussis

Pertussis actually has three stages. Stage 1 is characterized by findings consistent with a common cold or URI. Stage 2 is characterized by coughing that continues to worsen to the point that medical care is sought (EMS is summoned), and thus the suspicion for pertussis (whooping cough) is made. Stage 3 is the recovery stage; recovery is usually gradual, taking several weeks until resolution is reached. More specific findings for pertussis include the following:

- History of URI
- Sneezing, runny nose, low-grade fever
- General malaise (weakness, fatigue, "not feeling well")
- Increase in frequency and severity of coughing
- Coughing fits usually more common at night
- Vomiting from coughing hard
- Inspiratory "whoop" heard at the end of coughing burst
- Possibly, cyanosis developing during coughing burst
- Diminishing pulse oximetry finding
- Exhaustion from expending energy during coughing burst
- Trouble speaking and breathing (dyspnea) during coughing burst

Assessment of the Patient with a Viral Respiratory Infection

As stated, most people do not seek medical attention or summon EMS for a typical VRI owing to the minimal clinical findings that are easily treated with over-the-counter cold medications for symptomatic relief. However, if the patient's condition and findings of respiratory distress are severe enough to call EMS, chances are that the infection has spread into the lower airways and is starting to impinge on normal oxygenation by the lungs. Signs and symptoms of viral respiratory infections include the following:

- Nasal congestion
- Sore or scratchy throat
- Mild respiratory distress, coughing
- Fever (usually around 101–102°F)
- Malaise
- Headaches and body aches
- In infants, irritability and poor feeding habits
- Tachypnea
- Exacerbation of asthma if patient is asthmatic and contracts a VRI

Regardless of the mechanism of respiratory distress, remember the discussion in Topic 17, "Airway Assessment and Decision Making," regarding the determination of respiratory distress. If the conscious patient is unable to speak in normal sentences or does not have vesicular breath sounds, his breathing is inadequate even though other classic findings of dyspnea may not yet be present. If the patient is unresponsive, the absence of vesicular breath sounds or minimal chest wall movement is indicative of inadequate breathing. In both these situations, positive pressure ventilation and oxygen therapy are the most important intervention the paramedic can provide.

EMERGENCY MEDICAL CARE

For all the topics that have focused on different respiratory conditions, the paramedic will notice a stark similarity in the management of these symptomatically related (but pathophysiologically diverse) respiratory conditions.

Paramedics should first consider scene safety. Patients with respiratory infections can be particularly contagious, and this disease can be transmitted to health care providers. Diseases such as tuberculosis, influenza, and even the common cold pose a direct risk to people in the proximity of respiratory droplets. Although true respiratory isolation in an ambulance is difficult, providers should do their best to protect themselves from harmful pathogens. This likely includes respiratory protection (surgical or N-95 mask) for the provider and potentially for the patient as well. It may also mean actual isolation if possible.

A key point when treating patients with respiratory infections is to guard against respiratory failure. Although this is a relatively rare occurrence with most of these disorders, some patients will fail either as a result of the ongoing progression of the disease or because of fatigue in the muscles of the respiratory system. In either case, the paramedic must recognize this failure and take immediate action.

Respiratory failure patients will require positive pressure ventilation and, more than likely, advanced airway management. In most cases, the most likely clinical course will be a ventilator to relieve fatigue; as such, endotracheal intubation is a likely endpoint. This outcome may change your airway management decision process (particularly if rapid sequence intubation is available to you) or it may not, depending on your local protocols and available resources. The key, however, is to recognize the need for immediate intervention and choose a method that ensures oxygenation and ventilation.

Beyond the treatment of respiratory failure, the primary goal for any patient with difficulty breathing is to calm his apprehension with verbal reassurance, place him in a position of comfort that facilitates breathing (normally a semi- or high Fowler position), provide oxygen therapy, and, in cases of respiratory failure, provide airway support and positive pressure ventilation. En route to the medical facility, consider establishing an intravenous line of normal saline at a to-keep-open rate (follow your local protocol). The following sections offer more condition-specific interventions the paramedic may consider.

Emergency Medical Care for Pneumonia

The pneumonia patient is managed no differently from any other patient having difficulty breathing. Ensure adequate oxygenation and breathing. Some pneumonia patients will deteriorate to respiratory failure and, as such, will need positive pressure ventilation and possibly aggressive airway management. Pneumonia is an

> **Remember that pertussis is a very contagious disease.**

acute infectious disease process that is not usually associated with severe bronchoconstriction, unless it occurs as a complication of asthma or chronic obstructive pulmonary disease (COPD). Therefore, you would not expect the patient to have a metered-dose inhaler (MDI) or home nebulizer for this condition, nor would you necessarily consider its use unless indications of bronchoconstriction are present. Follow your local protocol regarding the administration of a bronchodilator via an MDI or a nebulizer (see Topic 29, "Respiratory Emergencies: Airway Resistance Disorders," for more detailed information).

Emergency Medical Care for Pertussis

Treatment of pertussis is similar to that for many other respiratory problems. It is focused on ensuring oxygenation, reversing hypoxia, and preventing airway obstruction. The patient should remain in a comfortable position. If the patient is hypoxic, the paramedic should administer high-flow oxygen at 15 liters per minute (lpm) via a nonrebreather mask. The paramedic should also encourage the patient to expectorate any mucus that is brought up with the coughing. The administration of humidified oxygen may help the mucus become less viscous and be expelled more easily. The patient will probably be anxious and/or frightened, so the paramedic should also try to ensure a quiet and calm environment.

In addition, remember that pertussis is a very contagious disease. The paramedic should take all precautions necessary to prevent cross-contamination (including putting a simple mask on the patient to catch expelled airway droplets), as long as doing so does not impinge on the patient's breathing. Following transport of a known patient with pertussis, consider totally disinfecting the patient compartment of the ambulance.

Emergency Medical Care for VRIs

The majority of VRI cases do not present to EMS because the clinical presentation is confined to nasal and pharyngeal discomfort. In the susceptible patient, however, the presence of concurrent lower-tract infections can cause some degree of respiratory distress. In all but the most severe (and uncommon) of cases, supportive treatment of positioning, oxygen therapy, emotional support, and gentle transport to the hospital are all that are necessary. If the infection is allowed to persist without medical attention, however, and it develops into a more serious viral infection (especially for the very young or very old), high-flow oxygen and, occasionally, positive pressure ventilation may become warranted.

Despite the often minimal presentation, the paramedic should always maintain a high index of suspicion for deterioration in a patient who does not respond favorably to the aforementioned supportive measures.

THE ROLE OF PUBLIC HEALTH

In the world of infectious disease, paramedics may play a role not just in the acute setting, but also in the preventive and surveillance settings. As the role of the community paramedic expands, providers will be faced with expanded responsibilities when it comes to patients such as the ones described in this topic.

Prevention plays an important part in managing respiratory infections. Simple actions such as appropriate hand washing and staying home when you are feeling sick can help stem the tide of large-scale epidemics. In recent years, EMS has played a key role in public information and awareness and will continue to do so in the future.

In the case of pertussis specifically, vaccinations play a large role in prevention of the disease. In many systems, paramedics administer these routine vaccinations as part of the public health team.

Finally, paramedics may also play a part in disease surveillance. Local public health systems may require specific reporting functions when faced with infectious diseases, and paramedics will have increasing responsibilities in this area as EMS further merges with other arms of public health.

TRANSITIONING

REVIEW ITEMS

1. A patient presents with respiratory distress with a gradual onset, has a slight fever, and has diminished breath sounds in the lower right lobe. This presentation is most consistent with what infectious disease process?
   a. pertussis
   b. pneumonia
   c. chronic bronchitis
   d. upper viral respiratory infection

2. Which of the following patients is most likely to develop pneumonia?
   a. a recent lung transplant patient
   b. a patient with a history of long bone fractures
   c. a pediatric patient with a history of Down syndrome
   d. an elderly patient with diagnosed Parkinson disease

3. What type of secondary lung infection is a patient with a recent diagnosis of VRI most likely to acquire?
   a. tuberculosis   b. pneumonia
   c. pertussis   d. asthma

4. What type of infectious lung disease would most readily spread through a day care center or kindergarten classroom?
   a. bronchiolitis   b. bronchitis
   c. pertussis   d. asthma

5. EMS is rarely summoned for patients with viral respiratory infections because _____.
   a. early respiratory distress is often mild
   b. findings are often self-limiting with use of over-the-counter medications

c. most insurance companies will not reimburse the EMS bill for VRI patients

d. the actual incidence of VRI in the United States is very rare in all age groups

6. At what stage of pertussis would EMS most likely be summoned for a patient with shortness of breath?

a. stage 1
b. stage 2
c. stage 3
d. stage 4

7. A patient with severe pneumonia is found to be tachypneic and warm to the touch, has an altered mental status, and displays absent vesicular breath sounds on auscultation. The single most important treatment for this patient is _____.

a. oxygen
b. aspirin for the fever
c. placement in a position of comfort
d. provision of positive pressure ventilation

APPLIED PATHOPHYSIOLOGY

1. Discuss the pathologic process by which a viral respiratory infection could result in the patient developing bacterial pneumonia.

2. Identify the pathogenic etiology for the following signs and symptoms given the listed infectious disease state:

a. Diminished breath sounds in the patient with pneumonia

b. Tachypnea and low pulse oximetry readings in the patient with pertussis

c. Increased mucus production and coughing in the patient with a VRI

d. Tripod positioning, nasal flaring, shallow breathing, and altered mental status in all three of the discussed infectious respiratory conditions

CLINICAL DECISION MAKING

Family members call you to the home of a bedridden patient with a known neuromuscular disease. The family states that the patient seems to be "very uncomfortable" while trying to breathe. As you approach the patient, you see an oxygen concentrator beside his bed. The patient looks at you as you approach but cannot speak due to stoma placement. You note that the stoma's inner cannula is properly placed. The skin appears "dusky," the patient has weak coughing spells that are bringing up some white phlegm through the stoma, and the conjunctivae of the eyes appear somewhat dehydrated.

1. Based on the scene size-up characteristics, identify the infectious respiratory diseases from which the patient is most likely suffering. Defend your answer.

Further assessment reveals that the 58-year-old male patient is alert and will blink his eyes as directed. The family states that he gets these "attacks" once or twice a year, and the hospital diagnoses a respiratory infection. Pulse oximetry is 97 percent on room air. Auscultation of the chest during breathing reveals clear upper lobe sounds, with diminished lower right and left breath sounds with mild inspiratory crackles.

The heart rate is 102/minute, respirations are 24, and the blood pressure is 142/82 mmHg. The patient's core is warm to the touch.

2. Does this additional information support or contradict your initial field impression? Why?

3. What immediate emergency care should you provide based on the provided assessment findings?

4. What conditions are you still considering as the possible cause? Would you add any conditions as a possible cause, and if so, which ones?

5. What are one or two possible differential diagnoses for this patient?

6. Following your treatment, what would be key indications that the patient's pulmonary function and general status are improving? What would be important indications of continued deterioration?

TOPIC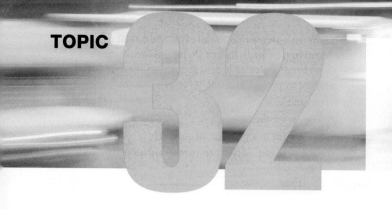

Standard Medicine

Competency Integrates assessment findings with principles of epidemiology and pathophysiology to formulate a field impression and implement a comprehensive treatment/disposition plan for a patient with a medical complaint.

NEUROLOGY: STROKE

TRANSITION *highlights*

- *Overview of the frequency with which strokes occur in the United States.*

- *Types and pathophysiology of strokes that occur that inhibit blood flow to distal brain tissue and cause permanent damage:*
  - *Ischemic.*
  - *Embolic.*

- *Types of "mini-strokes" that typically do not cause permanent damage:*
  - *Transient ischemic attack (TIA).*
  - *Reversible ischemic neurologic deficit (RIND).*

- *Type of stroke caused by hypoperfusion, rather than occlusion of blood pressure.*

- *Relating the location of the stroke with the cerebral artery.*

- *Incorporating the stroke scale assessment tools into the patient assessment format.*

- *Primary assessment and management principles for a stroke.*

INTRODUCTION

Stroke, or *acute cerebrovascular syndrome*, is an emergency involving the disruption of blood flow through a cerebral vessel within the brain. Unfortunately, it is both a dangerous and a prevalent problem for many patients seeking the help of EMS. In recent years, many advances have been made in the care and treatment of stroke patients. What used to be a devastating illness is now treatable, in many cases. This treatment, however, relies on appropriate prehospital assessment and management.

As with other time-sensitive disorders, such as trauma and myocardial infarction, stroke care is best accomplished when many elements of the medical system coordinate into a team-based approach. Disability and death associated with stroke can be reduced, but only when multiple components of the health care team work together. As a paramedic, your contribution must include early recognition and prompt and appropriate transport.

Stroke care is an emerging topic that is dynamic in nature. Care is advancing rapidly. As a paramedic, it is important that you stay current and understand your role within this vitally important topic.

EPIDEMIOLOGY

Stroke is the third leading cause of death in the United States. It is also a major cause of permanent disability and results in billions of dollars in medical costs and lost productivity. According to the American Stroke Association, 700,000 people in the United States suffer a stroke each year, which is approximately one case every 45 seconds. Every 3 minutes, a person will die from a stroke. African Americans and Hispanics/Latinos have a higher risk of suffering a stroke. Women suffer about 40,000 more strokes per year than men.

PATHOPHYSIOLOGY

A *stroke* is defined as acute impairment of neurologic function that results from an interruption of cerebral blood flow to a specific area in the brain. The two broad categories of stroke are ischemic and hemorrhagic. *Ischemic strokes* result from the occlusion of a cerebral artery by a blockage or a clot. This pathology is very similar to the causes of acute coronary syndrome and can be likened to a "heart attack in the brain." *Hemorrhagic strokes* occur from a cerebral vessel that ruptures and disrupts the blood flow and allows bleeding in and around the brain (▶ **Figure 32-1**).

Ischemic Stroke

Approximately 80 percent to 85 percent of all strokes are *ischemic strokes*. The primary etiology of these strokes is from

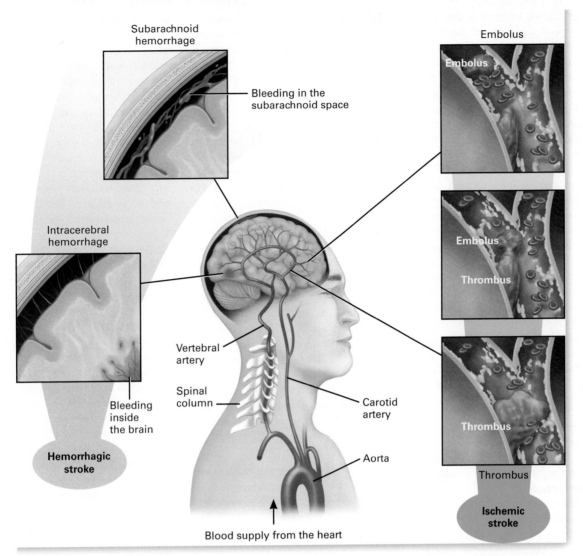

Figure 32-1 Causes of stroke. Blood is carried from the heart to the brain via the carotid and vertebral arteries, which form a ring and branches within the brain. An *ischemic stroke* occurs when a thrombus is formed on the wall of an artery or when an embolus travels from another area until it lodges in and blocks an arterial branch. A *hemorrhagic stroke* occurs when a cerebral artery ruptures and bleeds into the brain (examples shown: subarachnoid bleeding on the surface of the brain and intracerebral bleeding within the brain).

blockage of a cerebral artery that obstructs blood flow to an area of the brain. The most common underlying cause of ischemic strokes is atherosclerosis, the process in which fatty deposits collect and line the walls of vessels. This fat will continue to build up inside the vessel wall and may eventually lead to a blockage (thrombus) at the site of the buildup, or a piece of the fatty plaque can break off and travel down the bloodstream (embolus), causing a blockage in a smaller vessel distal to the fatty buildup.

Ischemic strokes are further classified as thrombotic stroke, embolic stroke, transient ischemic attack (TIA), reversible ischemic neurologic deficit (RIND), and hypoperfusion stroke.

THROMBOTIC STROKE A *thrombotic stroke* results from an acute blockage of a cerebral artery at the site of the buildup of fatty deposits, where the internal diameter (lumen) of the vessel is narrowed. This type of clot, a *cerebral thrombosis*, is often referred to as a "stationary clot" because the site of blockage is at the same site at which the clot has formed. About 60 percent of ischemic strokes are thrombotic.

The signs and symptoms of thrombotic stroke may be progressive. As clot formation progresses, blood flow is reduced to areas supplied by the affected cerebral artery, and ischemia to the brain cells worsens, producing signs and symptoms that may gradually develop and progress.

During thrombus formation, as the artery narrows, the surrounding smaller cerebral arteries may begin to dilate in an attempt to deliver more blood to the brain tissue distal to the diseased artery. This collateral circulation, which is similar to that found in the coronary vessels in the heart, may reduce the extent of brain tissue ischemia and death following the stroke.

EMBOLIC STROKE *Embolic strokes,* which account for approximately 40 percent of ischemic strokes, result from a

> **About 60 percent of ischemic strokes are thrombotic.**

cerebral embolism, which is a clot or a piece of intravascular material that commonly forms in a proximal artery or in the heart and travels through the cerebral circulation until it becomes lodged. If a piece of material breaks off a thrombus forming in a vessel and begins to travel downstream, it is referred to as a *thromboembolus*. This type of clot is often referred to as a "traveling clot," as it is not formed at the site of blockage.

Embolic strokes may present with more sudden onset of signs and symptoms, as the blockage is a sudden event, and the surrounding cerebral vessels have no chance to dilate and produce a collateral circulation effect. The most common site for thromboembolus formation is in the carotid arteries and in the heart during periods of atrial fibrillation. Atrial fibrillation causes the atria to dilate and blood to stagnate, promoting the formation of clots. An embolism does not have to be a piece of clot or plaque; it can also be an air bubble, tumor tissue, or fat tissue.

TRANSIENT ISCHEMIC ATTACK A *transient ischemic attack* (TIA) is a condition in which the patient suffers a temporary interruption of blood flow to an area of the brain from either an embolism that arises from another proximal vessel and lodges in a cerebral artery or a disruption in a plaque in an area of atherosclerosis in the vessel. The interrupted flow resolves itself after the clot is either dislodged or dissolves. Remember that the entire clotting process is in a constant state of clot formation and lysis.

TIAs produce sudden onset of the signs and symptoms of stroke; however, the signs and symptoms typically last for only a few minutes to, usually, no more than one hour. The signs and symptoms of TIA will resolve within 24 hours following onset. TIAs are often referred to by laypeople as "mini-strokes." It was once thought that no permanent neurologic damage was associated with a TIA; however, more recent evidence indicates that actual brain tissue damage occurs.

In addition to atherosclerosis and emboli, TIAs may also occur as a result of the following:

• Arterial dissection
• Inflammation of the arteries (arteritis)
• Sympathomimetic drugs such as cocaine

TIAs are highly predictive of impending stroke in patients; thus, they are also referred to as "warning strokes." Approximately 30 percent of patients who have TIAs will suffer a stroke in the future. Thus, it is imperative that EMS personnel be aggressive in assessing and managing the patient who has suffered a TIA.

Because the signs and symptoms resolve very quickly, the TIA patient may refuse emergency care and transport. Even though prehospital care for a TIA that has resolved is completely supportive, it is extremely important for paramedics to educate the patient about the high risk of suffering a true stroke in the near future that may result in permanent disability.

REVERSIBLE ISCHEMIC NEUROLOGIC DEFICIT *Reversible ischemic neurologic deficit* (RIND) is very similar to a TIA in etiology. It produces the same signs and symptoms of stroke; however, a RIND typically resolves within 24 to 72 hours after onset. Likewise, RIND is also a significant predictor of an impending stroke.

HYPOPERFUSION Hypoperfusion may cause a state in which low perfusion causes the brain to receive an inadequate flow of blood through the cerebral arteries. The entire brain becomes ischemic and is subject to brain infarction (death). Unlike thrombotic and embolic stroke, the etiology of a hypoperfusion state is not due to an isolated event of occlusion of a cerebral artery by a thrombus or embolism that produces focal ischemia and brain tissue necrosis. Instead, hypoperfusion states are associated with very poor cerebral blood flow conditions that arise from cardiac arrest, acute myocardial infarction with a decrease in cardiac output from pump dysfunction, and hemodynamically significant cardiac dysrhythmias that create poor perfusion states.

Because hypoperfusion affects the entire brain, the signs and symptoms are typically global in nature and do not result in focal neurologic deficits.

CLASSIFICATION OF ISCHEMIC STROKE BY SUPPLYING VESSEL Ischemic strokes can be further classified by the vessel and the area of the brain supplied by that respective blood vessel. The anterior portion of the brain's blood supply originates from the carotid arter-

ies. The anterior circulation is responsible for perfusing about 80 percent of the brain tissue. Occlusion of the carotid artery typically will disrupt blood flow to the cerebral hemispheres. The posterior area of the brain is supplied by the vertebrobasilar artery, which makes up the remaining 20 percent of brain perfusion. An occlusion to the vertebrobasilar artery or its branch will usually involve the brainstem. The presentation of the patient will vary based on which vessel was occluded and what area of the brain becomes ischemic and eventually infarcted.

PATHOPHYSIOLOGY OF THROMBUS FORMATION IN ISCHEMIC STROKE The concept of a ruptured plaque typical of the myocardial infarction patient leading to vessel occlusion is also true of the ischemic stroke; however, the occlusion is occurring in a cerebral vessel instead of a coronary vessel. Fatty deposits inside the cerebral vessel lead to fatty streaks. The fatty streaks promote the formation of an *atheroma* (a buildup of atherosclerotic plaque inside the vessel). The atheroma hardens and causes narrowing of the diseased artery. The atheroma becomes inflamed, and ulceration occurs. The plaque ruptures inside the vessel.

The body views the internal rupture as an injury to the vessel and begins the cascade of physiologic events to clot the injured artery. The chain starts with platelet deposits, which explains why aspirin is commonly used in this condition. This is followed by formal clot formation, which is why early administration of thrombolytic or "clot-busting" agents is effective. This chain of events is actually a protective process to stop a bleeding vessel that ends up occluding the cerebral artery and blocking the blood supply to the distal area of the brain, leading to ischemia and eventually infarction. If the occlusion occurs at the site of the thrombus formation, it becomes a thrombotic stroke.

This process explains the progressive nature of the signs and symptoms seen in thrombotic stroke. A piece of the clot can break off, travel distally in the cerebral artery or a branch until it becomes lodged, and create an embolic stroke.

Hemorrhagic Stroke

A *hemorrhagic stroke* is caused by a rupture of a cerebral vessel with resultant bleeding into brain tissue or areas surrounding the brain. Approximately 10 percent to 15 percent of all strokes are hemorrhagic in nature. When a vessel ruptures, the blood leaks from the vessel, accumulates in the brain, and causes the brain tissue to become compressed. Brain damage from a ruptured vessel may result from direct trauma to the brain cells, the compression of the brain from increasing intracranial pressure, release of chemical mediators, spasm of local blood vessels, loss of blood flow distal to the ruptured cerebral vessel, and edema formation from the expanding blood and its compressive effects.

Two common causes of a ruptured vessel leading to hemorrhagic stroke are aneurysms and arteriovenous malformations (AVMs). An *aneurysm* is a weakened area in a blood vessel that balloons out. It may continue to weaken and eventually rupture and bleed into the brain or its surrounding tissue.

An *arteriovenous malformation* is an abnormal formation of blood vessels that diverts blood away from the brain tissue and connects the arteries directly to the veins. The abnormal vessels of AVMs are weakened and dilate over a period of time. The vessels are prone to rupture from the high pressure contained within the arteries. AVMs are most often caused by congenital defects and are not easily detected prior to rupture. AVMs may be found within brain tissue or within the subarachnoid space in the meningeal layers above the brain tissue.

TYPES OF HEMORRHAGIC STROKE
The two major types of hemorrhagic stroke are intracerebral hemorrhage and subarachnoid hemorrhage. An *intracerebral hemorrhage* (ICH) is caused by a cerebral vessel that ruptures and bleeds directly into the brain tissue. The ruptured vessels are usually small arterioles that have been damaged over time by chronic hypertension.

In a *subarachnoid hemorrhage* (SAH), the vessel ruptures into the subarachnoid space located above the actual brain tissue. Aneurysms are more often the cause of SAH, whereas AVMs are less likely the etiology. When an aneurysm ruptures, it bleeds into the subarachnoid space at the systemic arterial pressure. This produces the sudden onset of severe and dramatic signs and symptoms.

ICH is more common than SAH. Both ICH and SAH carry a higher acute mortality rate than does ischemic stroke. Remember that the vast majority of ICH is caused by spontaneous hemorrhage in vessels damaged by chronic hypertension.

Pathophysiology of Neurologic Dysfunction and Damage in Stroke

Brain cells need two critical elements for normal function: oxygen and glucose. Without these two elements, brain cells begin to dysfunction and will eventually die. When an artery becomes occluded from thrombus formation, collateral circulation will assist with the maintenance of blood flow to the areas of the brain distal to the occluded artery. This may prevent a larger area of brain tissue death; however, the area surrounding the dead tissue will continue to receive some blood flow but may become ischemic from a low blood flow state.

When cerebral blood flow to an area of brain tissue drops below its normal level, it may cause the cells to become "electrically silent." The brain cells are still intact and retain the ability to function; however, they cease the transmission of electrical impulses. Thus, the cells are not dead but act as if they are and will not transmit electrical impulses. This causes the patient to present with neurologic deficits such as motor, sensory, or cognitive dysfunction.

If the blood flow is restored to these ischemic cells, they will become electrically active, continue to function, and once again transmit electrical impulses. This may be evident in the patient who initially presents with what seems to be a severe stroke with significant neurologic dysfunction but who then later regains function in many of the previously dysfunctional areas.

If the cerebral blood flow drops drastically, the brain cells begin to fail. Brain cells are particularly vulnerable owing to the fact that, unlike many other cells in the body, they do not store glucose and rely completely on glucose delivered via the bloodstream. Calcium levels within the cells and potassium levels outside the cells increase. Because of a reduction of glucose delivery to the cells, the production of energy (adenosine triphosphate [ATP]) is severely depleted. With the loss of ATP, the sodium–potassium pump fails and allows potassium to remain outside the cell, whereas sodium is no longer pumped out of the cell. Because sodium attracts water, the cells begin to swell and will eventually rupture and die. This process is known as *cytotoxic edema*.

The area of the brain surrounding the primary stroke site that continues to receive cerebral blood flow from collateral circulation is termed the *ischemic penumbra* or *ischemic shadow*. Because the tissue is receiving a lower cerebral blood flow than normal, the brain cells become "electrically silent." Irreversible brain cell damage in this area has not yet occurred, though, and the function of these brain cells can be reversed. This is the area of brain that can possibly be salvaged and the extent of the brain injury limited. Neuroprotective agents are being researched that can protect the ischemic penumbra and preserve the brain cells.

> **An aneurysm may continue to weaken and eventually rupture and bleed into the brain or its surrounding tissue.**

ASSESSMENT OF THE STROKE PATIENT

Time is paramount in the management of a stroke patient. It may mean the difference between a patient who suffers significant permanent disability and one who recovers completely or with only minor deficits. A very narrow window of 3 to 4.5 hours is available for the administration of thrombolytic drugs that can destroy a clot and restore circulation to the ischemic brain tissue. (Mechanical methods of clot removal may increase this window.) It is imperative that EMS personnel be able to recognize even the most subtle signs and symptoms of stroke so that rapid and aggressive stroke treatment can be provided.

Signs and Symptoms of Stroke

The signs and symptoms of stroke may be subtle and unrecognized as significant by the patient, relatives, or bystanders. Simple numbness of the arm may be downplayed as insignificant by the

> **There is a very narrow window within which thrombolytic drugs can be used to dissolve a clot and restore circulation to the brain tissue.**

patient for a long period of time until the signs and symptoms progress to a more severe condition. The patient may then seek EMS assistance; however, several hours may have passed, during which the chance for reversal of the stroke may have been eliminated.

It is imperative that in your history taking you attempt to determine the precise time of onset of the first sign or symptom of stroke, no matter how subtle. This is vital information that must be reported to the receiving medical facility. It is often referred to by the American Stroke Association as time "last normal." That is, what was the specific time the patient was last seen as "normal" with no neurologic deficits? This is extremely important information for the paramedic to collect and report to the receiving medical facility.

General signs and symptoms of stroke include the following:

- Facial droop (▶ Figure 32-2)
- Slurred speech
- Difficulty in speaking (dysphasia) or inability to speak (aphasia)
- Numbness to the face, arm, or leg, especially on one side of the body
- Headache (may not be severe in ischemic stroke)
- Weakness (paresis) or paralysis (plegia), especially to one side of the body (hemiparesis and hemiplegia) (▶ Figure 32-3)
- Confusion, agitation, or other severe altered mental status

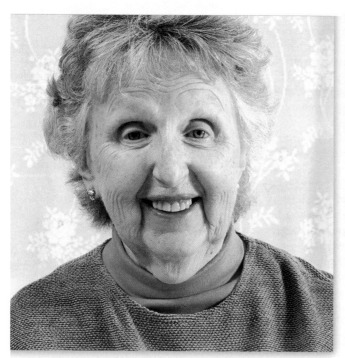
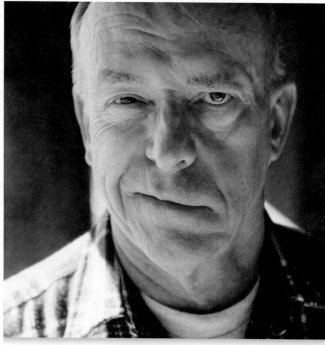

Figure 32-2 (a) The face of a nonstroke patient has normal symmetry. (b) The face of a stroke patient often has an abnormal, drooped appearance on one side. (© *Michal Heron*)

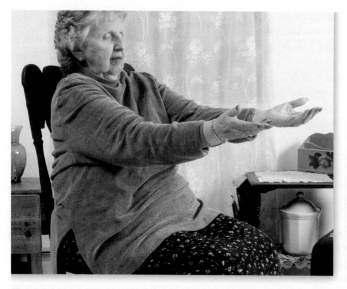
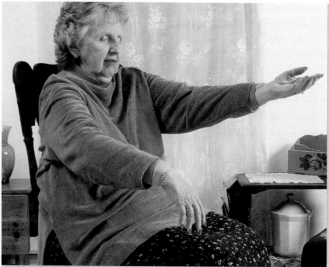

Figure 32-3 (a) A patient who has not suffered a stroke can generally hold the arms in an extended position with eyes closed. (b) A stroke patient will often display "arm drift" or "pronator drift"—one arm will remain extended when held outward with eyes closed, but the other arm will drift or drop downward and pronate (palm turned downward).

- Gait disturbance, noted by trouble walking
- Dizziness associated with vomiting
- Loss of balance or coordination
- Loss of vision or disturbed vision in one or both eyes
- Inability to understand
- Incontinence

Patients who experience an ICH or SAH may present with many of the aforementioned signs and symptoms. However, ICH and SAH patients typically complain of a sudden onset of the "worst headache they have ever experienced" with pain that may radiate to the face and neck. The headache may be accompanied by nausea, vomiting, intolerance to light and noise, and an altered mental status. These signs and symptoms, especially deterioration in the mental status, may continue to progress as the bleeding continues within the brain. Patients with ICH and SAH will typically present with more severe depressed mental status and headache as compared with ischemic stroke patients.

Stroke Assessment Scales

Two common stroke assessment scales with high predictive value used in the prehospital setting are the Cincinnati Prehospital Stroke Scale (CPSS) (Table 32-1) and the Los Angeles Prehospital Stroke Screen (LAPSS) (Table 32-2). Either of these scales should be included in your assessment of the stroke patient and reported to the medical facility. A Glasgow Coma Scale score should also be obtained on the suspected stroke patient. It is imperative for EMS personnel to collect and report this information to ensure adequate and aggressive assessment and management of the stroke patient.

EMERGENCY MEDICAL CARE

The emergency care provided to a stroke patient is primarily supportive; however, it must be geared to reverse any hypoxemia and hypoperfusion. It is vital to ensure an adequate airway, adequate ventilation, adequate oxygenation, and adequate circulation in the primary assessment. Provide the following emergency care:

- **Airway.** Stroke patients are at an increased risk of loss of airway control and aspiration. Ensure that an adequate airway is established and maintained. To prevent aspiration, place the patient in a lateral recumbent position. If vomiting is severe and the airway is severely compromised, it may be necessary to use an advanced airway device to protect the patient from aspiration.

TABLE 32-1	Cincinnati Prehospital Stroke Scale (CPSS)	
Sign of Stroke	**Patient Activity**	**Interpretation**
Facial droop	Ask the patient to (a) look at you; (b) smile; (c) show his teeth.	*Normal*: Both sides of face are symmetrical. *Abnormal*: One side of face droops, or both sides do not move symmetrically.
Arm drift	Have the patient (a) lift his arms up and (b) hold them out, palms facing up, for 10 seconds with his eyes closed.	*Normal*: Both arms move symmetrically. *Abnormal*: One arm drifts downward, or both arms do not move symmetrically.
Speech abnormalities	Have the patient repeat the sentence, "You can lead a horse to water, but you can't make it drink."	*Normal*: The patient repeats the sentence using the correct words, without slurring. *Abnormal*: The patient slurs his words, uses the wrong words, or exhibits aphasia.

Note: Any abnormality is consistent with a possible stroke.

TABLE 32-2	Los Angeles Prehospital Stroke Screen (LAPSS)			
Considerations*	**Yes**	**Unknown**	**No**	
Age >45 years				
No history of seizures or epilepsy				
Duration of symptoms <24 hours				
Patient able to walk prior to onset of symptoms				
Blood glucose level 60–400 mg/dL				
Physical Exam to Determine Unilateral Asymmetry	**Equal**	**Right Side Weakness/ Deficit**	**Left Side Weakness/ Deficit**	
Have patient look up, smile, show teeth		Droop	Droop	
Compare grip strength of upper extremities		Weakness in or inability to grip	Weakness in or inability to grip	
Examine arm strength for drift or weakness		Inability to maintain position—arm drifts or falls	Inability to maintain position—arm drifts or falls	

*If answer is "Yes" or "Unknown" to these considerations, patient should be considered as having an acute stroke.

- **Ventilation.** Assess the tidal volume and rate of ventilation. If either the tidal volume or rate is inadequate, immediately begin ventilation at a rate of 10 to 12 per minute.
- **Oxygenation.** Apply a pulse oximeter to monitor the oxygen saturation levels. If the patient exhibits signs of hypoxia, shock, or heart failure; complains of dyspnea; or has a SpO_2 reading of <94 percent, or if no SpO_2 reading is available, provide supplemental oxygen via a nasal cannula at 2 to 4 liters per minute (lpm). Titrate the oxygen to the signs and symptoms and SpO_2 reading.

  Be sure to respond immediately to declines in oxygen saturation by reassessing the adequacy of the airway or ventilation, managing the airway or ventilating if necessary, or increasing the oxygen concentration. If the SpO_2 reading continues to decline, does not increase above 94 percent, or the signs of hypoxia are not subsiding, place the patient on a nonrebreather mask at 15 lpm. If the tidal volume or respiratory rate becomes inadequate, immediately begin bag-valve-mask ventilation.
- **Circulation.** Initiate an intravenous line of normal saline. Obtain a blood sample if your protocol allows. Run the IV at a to-keep-open rate. If the systolic blood pressure drops below 90 mmHg, increase the rate of fluid administration. It is important to keep the systolic blood pressure at a level that is normal for the patient, as the brain develops very specific ranges in which it autoregulates cerebral perfusion. Be careful not to provide excessive amounts of fluid. Hypertension in the stroke patient is not treated in the prehospital setting.
- **Blood glucose level.** Obtain a blood glucose level (BGL), as hypoglycemia can mimic stroke. If the BGL is <50 mg/dL, administer 25 grams of 50% dextrose in water. *Do not* administer glucose or glucose containing solutions if the patient has a normal or high BGL reading.
- **Transport.** Protect and rapidly transport an acute stroke patient to the most appropriate medical facility for proper medical management.

TRANSITIONING

REVIEW ITEMS

1. A 58-year-old male patient presents with a sudden onset of left facial droop, slurred speech, and hemiparesis to the left arm. The patient states he has a headache when questioned during the history. You should suspect _____.
   a. an embolic stroke
   b. a subarachnoid hemorrhage
   c. an intracerebral hemorrhage
   d. a reversible ischemic neurologic deficit

2. You are assessing a patient who presents with confusion and is drooling. The family states that she was watching television and began to act confused. Her blood pressure is 298/132 mmHg, radial pulse is 112 beats per minute (bpm), and respirations are 19 with adequate chest rise. The skin is warm and dry to touch. The SpO_2 reads 98 percent on room air. You should _____.
   a. apply a nonrebreather mask at 15 lpm
   b. administer a tube of oral glucose
   c. suction the airway
   d. place the patient in a lateral recumbent position

3. What assessment finding would indicate that the neurons have become "electrically silent" from a decrease in cerebral perfusion and subsequent cerebral ischemia?

   a. an SpO_2 reading that is less than 94 percent
   b. loss of motor and sensory function
   c. an increase in systolic blood pressure
   d. an irregular heart rate

4. One of the most vital pieces of information for EMS to pass on to the receiving facility when managing a suspected ischemic stroke patient is _____.
   a. the last oral intake
   b. the event prior to the stroke
   c. the exact time of onset of signs or symptoms
   d. whether the patient is complaining of a headache

5. An ominous sign that the patient is experiencing a hemorrhagic stroke is _____.
   a. severe systolic hypertension
   b. a continuous deterioration in mental status
   c. an irregular heart rate with a weak radial pulse
   d. facial droop and slurred speech

APPLIED PATHOPHYSIOLOGY

1. List and describe the pathophysiology of the two general types of stroke.

2. Explain how to differentiate between a transient ischemic attack and a thrombotic stroke.

3. Explain why neurons become "electrically silent" and the associated clinical patient presentation.

4. Explain the pathophysiology associated with an acute clot formation within a cerebral artery, leading to an ischemic stroke.

5. Describe what type of stroke would typically cause a presentation in which the patient appears sicker and continues to deteriorate.

CLINICAL DECISION MAKING

You find a 68-year-old female patient who is awake and alert but is not responding appropriately to your questions or commands. Her husband states that the patient was in the kitchen cooking dinner and suddenly began to pour water into the oven. When questioned, she responded inappropriately. She is seated on a chair in the kitchen.

1. Based on the scene size-up, list the possible conditions you should suspect.

The primary assessment reveals that that patient is alert but not responding appropriately to your questions and commands. Her respiratory rate is 16/minute with adequate chest rise. Her radial pulse is irregular, at a rate of 80 bpm. Her skin is warm and dry. Her SpO$_2$ reading is 97 percent on room air.

2. Are there any immediate life threats to the patient?

3. What emergency care would you provide based on the primary assessment?

Following the secondary assessment, you note that the patient's pupils are equal and reactive to light, there is no evidence of trauma to the head, and the oral mucosa is pink and moist. There is no jugular venous distention, the breath sounds are equal and clear bilaterally, and the abdomen is soft. When assessing the extremities, you note that the patient is not moving her left arm or leg. She freely moves the right side of the body. She does not respond appropriately when you attempt to perform a neurologic exam of the extremities.

The blood pressure is 188/108 mmHg, the heart rate is 82/minute, and the respirations are 16/minute with adequate chest rise. The blood glucose is 114 mg/dL. She takes warfarin (Coumadin) and atenolol (Tenormin) and has a history of an "irregular heartbeat," according to her husband. She last ate at lunch, approximately three hours earlier. She has no known allergies.

4. What conditions have you ruled out in your differential diagnosis? Why?

5. What condition do you suspect? Why?

6. Why is the heart rhythm significant in this patient?

7. What further emergency care would you provide?

8. What vital information would you relay to the receiving medical facility?

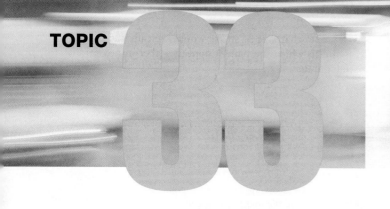
Standard Medicine

Competency Integrates assessment findings with principles of epidemiology and pathophysiology to formulate a field impression and implement a comprehensive treatment/disposition plan for a patient with a medical complaint.

ABDOMINAL EMERGENCIES AND GASTROINTESTINAL BLEEDING

TRANSITION *highlights*

- *Overview of the frequency of abdominal and gastrointestinal bleeding emergencies.*

- *Types of organs present in the abdominal cavity to help illustrate how they may present with pain:*
  – Solid organs.
  – Hollow organs.
  – Vascular organs.

- *Types of pain the patient with an abdominal emergency may be experiencing:*
  – Visceral pain.
  – Parietal pain.
  – Referred pain.

- *How to relate the type of pain with the organ affected:*
  – Distention.
  – Inflammation.
  – Ischemia.

- *Common abdominal emergencies causing pain:*
  – Mesenteric ischemia.
  – Rectal foreign body obstructions.
  – Rectal abscess.

- *Primary assessment and management principles for a patient experiencing abdominal pain or gastrointestinal bleeding.*

INTRODUCTION

The abdomen and pelvis house many of the body's most vital organs. Therefore, injuries and illnesses that affect these areas can be rapidly life threatening. The anatomy of this region spans multiple different organ systems, and the physiology combines a variety of different vital functions. Because of

these complexities, diagnosis of abdominopelvic disorders is often challenging—and frequently impossible—in the limited prehospital setting. Nonetheless, it is extremely important to recognize the critical nature of the organs housed within this vault. Although a specific diagnosis may be out of the reach of most paramedics, recognizing potential life threats is not.

When managing a patient with abdominal or pelvic complaints, your assessment must first attempt to identify the frequently life-threatening conditions associated with this area of the body. More specific diagnosis may be made by using your knowledge of anatomy and pathophysiology, but it should never take the place of immediate life support. In many cases, the most appropriate care for a person with an abdominopelvic complaint will be to make the patient as comfortable as possible, administer oxygen, initiate an intravenous line, and transport.

EPIDEMIOLOGY

Acute abdominal pain is a very common condition, accounting for 10 percent of all emergency department visits. Gastrointestinal bleeding is also very common and has an incidence of 100 per 100,000 in the population. Not only are these problems frequent, but abdominal pain and GI bleeding are also complex diagnostic challenges. Medical texts cite approximately 100 different causes of abdominal pain.

The abdomen is truly an intersection of many vastly different systems. Acute abdominal pain may arise from the cardiac, pulmonary, gastrointestinal, genital, urinary, reproductive systems, or a combination of them. Moreover, many of these systems represent serious and life-threatening problems.

PATHOPHYSIOLOGY

The abdominal cavity contains three types of structures that may contribute to a patient's pain (▶ Figure 33-1):

- **Hollow organs.** The appendix, bladder, common bile duct, fallopian tubes, gallbladder, intestines, stomach, and uterus are all hollow organs located within the abdominal cavity.

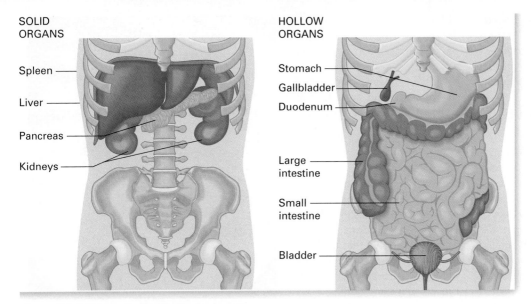

SOLID ORGANS

- Spleen
- Liver
- Pancreas
- Kidneys

HOLLOW ORGANS

- Stomach
- Gallbladder
- Duodenum
- Large intestine
- Small intestine
- Bladder

Figure 33-1 Organs in the abdominal cavity.

Causes of Abdominal Pain

Abdominal pain usually results from one of the following three mechanisms: distention, inflammation, or ischemia.

- **Distention.** If an organ is stretched out or inflated, it can result in pain. If the distention of the organ occurs rapidly, the patient's pain will be acute; if the onset is gradual, the patient may experience little or no pain. When a solid organ is stretched, it usually results in a steady pain. The peritoneum may also be stretched and result in pain if an organ tugs on it, if there are adhesions from surgery, or if a forceful movement of the small intestine associated with a bowel obstruction occurs. Pregnant women in their third trimester usually do not experience this type of pain because their peritoneum is stretched so far that it is no longer sensitive.
- **Inflammation.** Inflammation of a hollow organ may irritate the lining of the walls of the organ, causing a crampy type of pain.
- **Ischemia.** Pain associated with ischemia to an abdominal organ will be steady and severe and will continue to worsen as the organ becomes more hypoxic.

Each of these organs contains some type of substance that may leak out into the abdominal cavity if it is perforated or injured. This may cause chemical or bacterial peritonitis.

- **Solid organs.** The kidneys, liver, ovaries, pancreas, and spleen are solid abdominal organs. These organs are very vascular and tend to bleed more than hollow organs if they are injured or ruptured. Some of them are covered by a thick fibrous capsule that, when stretched, can cause abdominal pain.
- **Vascular structures.** Portions of the descending aorta and the inferior vena cava are located in the abdominal cavity. Rupture or injury to either vessel will result in major bleeding, rapid blood loss, and death.

Types of Abdominal Pain

Abdominal pain can be classified as visceral pain, parietal pain, or referred pain.

- *Visceral pain* occurs when the organ itself is involved. Most organs do not have a large number of highly sensitive nerve fibers; therefore, the pain is usually less severe, poorly localized, dull, or aching, and may be constant or intermittent. Visceral pain is commonly associated with nausea, vomiting, diaphoresis, and tachycardia. Even if the pain may not appear to be severe, this does not mean that the patient is not suffering from a severe condition.
- *Parietal pain*, also called *somatic pain*, is associated with irritation of the peritoneal lining. The peritoneum has a larger amount of highly sensitized nerve endings than abdominal organs do; therefore, the pain is more localized, intense, sharp, and typically constant.
- *Referred pain* is actually visceral pain that is felt elsewhere in the body. It is usually poorly localized but is felt consistently in the part of the body to which it is referred. Referred pain occurs when organs share a nerve pathway with a skin sensory nerve. The brain becomes confused in the interpretation of the impulse and causes the patient to feel pain at a location that may be totally unrelated to the organ involved (▸ **Figure 33-2**).

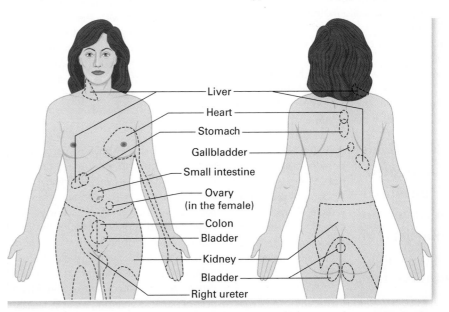

- Liver
- Heart
- Stomach
- Gallbladder
- Small intestine
- Ovary (in the female)
- Colon
- Bladder
- Kidney
- Bladder
- Right ureter

Figure 33-2 Sites of referred pain. The lines point to locations where pain may be felt when there is disease of or injury to the named organ.

Abdominal pain usually does not create a perception of cutting or tearing, except with certain aortic complications. If an organ is torn, the pain usually results from the blood irritating the peritoneum.

Conditions Causing Acute Abdominal Pain

The following are some common conditions that may cause abdominal pain. Definitive care for almost all these conditions is hospitalization and, possibly, surgical intervention. It is not necessary to try to isolate the exact cause of the pain or distress in the field; however, it is imperative that you accurately assess and manage your patient with an abdominal emergency.

GASTROINTESTINAL BLEEDING *Gastrointestinal (GI) bleeding* can occur anywhere within the gastrointestinal tract and can be attributed to numerous causes. Most bleeds are classified by their location, in either the upper tract or lower tract. The most common causes of upper GI bleeding are ulcers and esophageal varices. Lower GI bleeds are frequently caused by diverticulosis and tumors. Other conditions that may cause lower GI bleeding are polyps and tumors, hemorrhoids, Crohn disease, arteriovenous malformations, and colitis.

Signs and symptoms of gastrointestinal bleeding vary and may include hematemesis (vomiting blood), melena (dark foulsmelling tarry stools), and hematochezia (bright red blood in the stools). The color of the blood is important to note. If the blood is bright red, it may signify a rapid onset; if it is dark, it can indicate that the blood has been partially decomposed and digested. Abdominal pain, tachycardia, altered mental status, and signs of shock may occur if gastrointestinal bleeding exists.

> **Signs and symptoms of gastrointestinal bleeding vary and may include hematemesis, melena, and hematochezia.**

PERITONITIS Irritation and inflammation of the peritoneum is called *peritonitis*. Peritonitis occurs when blood, pus, bacteria, or chemical substances leak into the peritoneal cavity. The severity of the pain depends on the quantity and type of substance that is leaked. Because of their pain, patients with peritonitis usually resist any movement.

APPENDICITIS *Appendicitis* is the inflammation of the appendix. It is usually caused by a blockage in the intestines. Pain is initially felt as poorly localized periumbilical pain that becomes more distinct and localized to the right lower quadrant. Unusual presentations are more common in the young and the elderly. If left untreated, the tissue may die and rupture, which could result in abscess formation, peritonitis, or shock.

PANCREATITIS *Pancreatitis* is the inflammation of the pancreas. It may cause severe pain in the middle of the upper quadrants of the abdomen, which may radiate to the mid- to lower back. Pancreatitis may be triggered by a variety of causes, including ingestion of alcohol, gallstones, or infection. Complications that may result from pancreatitis include abscesses, sepsis, hemorrhage, tissue death, hypoglycemia or hyperglycemia, and organ failure.

CHOLECYSTITIS *Cholecystitis* is the inflammation of the gallbladder. It is commonly associated with the presence of gallstones that may actually block the opening of the gallbladder to the small intestine. This blockage causes an increase in pressure inside the gallbladder that can cause severe pain and, if left untreated, may cause tissue death, perforation, or pancreatitis.

ESOPHAGEAL VARICES *Esophageal varices* are bulging, engorged, or weakened blood vessels in the lining of the lower part of the esophagus. They are caused by increased pressure in the venous blood supply system of the liver, stomach, and esophagus. The most common cause is chronic heavy alcohol use, although any cause of cirrhosis can also cause varices. Varices are usually identified by painless bleeding that can be profuse, which can make managing a patient's airway and breathing difficult.

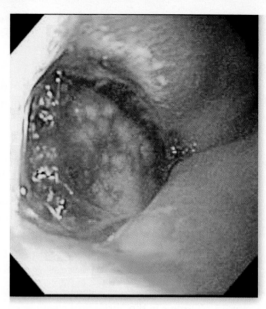

Figure 33-3 Endoscopic view of a duodenal ulcer.

GASTROENTERITIS *Gastroenteritis* is the inflammation of the stomach and small intestines. It is commonly associated with a sudden onset of vomiting and diarrhea. Chronic gastroenteritis is most commonly a result of an infection. Acute gastroenteritis is normally caused by a viral or bacterial infection and is commonly diagnosed in children. If left untreated, it may result in the breakdown of the mucosal layers in the gastrointestinal tract and can lead to dehydration, hemorrhage, ulceration, and perforation.

ULCERS *Ulcers* are open wounds or sores within the digestive tract that are associated with a breakdown of the protective lining of the gastrointestinal tract (▶ Figure 33-3). The type of abdominal pain associated with an ulcer is affected by its location and severity. Most ulcers are located in the stomach or the beginning of the small intestines. If left untreated, bleeding, peritonitis, perforation, hemorrhage, or shock may occur.

INTESTINAL OBSTRUCTION An *intestinal obstruction* is a blockage that interrupts the normal flow of the intestinal contents within the intestines. Blockages occurring in the small intestines are usually the result of an adhesion or a hernia. Blockages of the large intestines are commonly caused by a tumor, fecal impaction, or volvulus (a twisting of the intestine). If left untreated, intestinal obstruction may lead to sepsis, perforation, infarction, or peritonitis.

> **If left untreated, intestinal obstruction may lead to sepsis, perforation, infarction, or peritonitis.**

HERNIA A *hernia* is a protrusion or thrusting forward of a portion of the intestine through an opening or weakness in the abdominal wall. Hernias are most commonly associated with increased pressure in the abdominal cavity during heavy lifting or straining, causing the peritoneum to be pushed into the weakness or opening. Most are not life threatening but, if left untreated, may lead to tissue death or perforation.

ABDOMINAL AORTIC ANEURYSM An *abdominal aortic aneurysm* is a weakened, ballooned, and enlarged area of the wall of the abdominal aorta. Pain from an aneurysm may be felt in the abdomen, back, and groin. The aneurysm may eventually rupture and is one of the most lethal causes of abdominal pain. Death may occur from massive blood loss into the abdominal cavity or retroperitoneum.

VOMITING, DIARRHEA, CONSTIPATION *Vomiting, diarrhea,* and *constipation* can all cause abdominal pain. Rarely are they emergencies by themselves; however, if the vomiting has persisted for hours or if diarrhea has persisted for days, the patient may become dehydrated. Significant fluid loss, electrolyte imbalances, shock, cardiac arrhythmias, or other conditions may occur if these conditions are left untreated.

RECTAL OBSTRUCTION A rectal obstruction is a blockage that obstructs the normal excretion of feces from the GI system. Most commonly, rectal obstructions occur because of foreign bodies that have been inserted through the anus (usually during sexual activity). Rectal obstruction can occur naturally, however, typically as a result of gallstones or even fecal impaction. Far less commonly, ingested foreign bodies can cause rectal obstruction as they pass through the GI system and become lodged in the rectal space.

In many cases of rectal obstruction, particularly when dealing with foreign bodies, the patient seeks medical attention when difficulty removing the object is encountered. Care for rectal obstruction is often delayed because of the patient's embarrassment; as a result, more serious secondary issues can arise. Perforations and trauma are possible, as are infections related to the foreign body.

Patients will frequently complain of abdominal pain and may present with symptoms of infection. Obtaining an accurate history may be challenging, as patients may be unwilling to discuss the true nature of their disorder. Providing a professional and private atmosphere will likely aid your assessment.

Major life threats include hemorrhage for perforations and lacerations. Infection and sepsis are also possible. Remember also that hiding of illicit drugs can also cause rectal obstructions; as a result, you may also be faced with the threat of overdose.

In most cases, resolution of a rectal obstruction will occur in the emergency department or in the operating room. Assessment and transport are important prehospital strategies.

RECTAL/ANAL ABSCESS Rectal and anal abscesses occur most commonly as a result of infections in and around the glands surrounding the anus. Bacterial infection causes a buildup of pus that can accumulate in the rectum and in the space surrounding the anus. These abscesses can obstruct the excretion of feces and cause severe pain and fever. Patients who are immunosuppressed, such as transplant and acquired immunodeficiency syndrome (AIDS) patients, are more likely to develop these disorders, but other patients, including those who have Crohn disease, diabetes, and sexually transmitted diseases, also have high risk for developing abscesses. Foreign bodies can also cause abscesses.

MESENTERIC ISCHEMIA Mesenteric ischemia occurs as a result of interrupted blood flow to the intestine. Although it can occur chronically, its acute presentation has the highest mortality rate. Embolism, thrombus, and prolonged vasoconstriction (typically from shock states) are the three most common etiologies of this disorder. In each case, blood flow is disrupted, resulting in ischemia and infarction (if left uncorrected). The presentation of a patient with mesenteric ischemia typically includes intense, visceral abdominal pain. Occasionally, nausea and vomiting will be present. Prior episodes of pain are also common. In cases of thrombus and embolism, patient history will usually include atherosclerosis or other similar risk factors.

Very little can be done for these patients in the field. Awareness can help narrow the diagnosis, however.

ASSESSMENT FINDINGS

All patients with abdominal pain should be considered to have a life-threatening condition until proven otherwise. This is especially true if the pain lasts for six hours or longer, regardless of its intensity. Priority transport should be provided if the patient has a poor general appearance, is unresponsive, or has an altered mental status, severe pain, or signs of shock.

Begin your assessment by securing a safe scene. Face and eye protection should be used if the patient is vomiting. Look for any mechanism of injury to rule out trauma. Note any distinct smells, emesis in wastebaskets or garbage cans, and over-the-counter medications that may have been used to help alleviate the abdominal pain before your arrival.

As you approach the patient, form a general impression. Stabilize the spine if injury is suspected. A person with an acute abdomen generally appears very ill and will assume a guarded position (▶ Figure 33-4). You may find a patient experiencing parietal pain lying supine with the knees flexed up toward the chest. This position limits the stretch of the abdominal muscles and puts less pressure on the peritoneum. The patient in this position is usually very still and breathing shallowly so the diaphragm does not push on the peritoneum and abdominal organs and cause more pain.

Ensure a patent airway and suction if needed. Titrate oxygen to maintain a saturation greater than 95 percent; assist the patient's ventilations if necessary. Assess circulation by checking the pulse for rate and regularity, identifying and controlling major bleeding, and noting skin color, temperature, and condition. Look for signs of shock.

In addition to SAMPLE and OPQRST questions, you should ask whether the patient has a history of abdominal pain, surgeries, appetite changes, nausea or vomiting, color and type of stools or emesis, difficulty urinating, or other any other associated complaints.

The physical exam will focus on the abdomen; however, you should still assess the rest of the body for associated signs and symptoms. Begin by inspecting the abdomen. Palpate each quadrant, beginning with the area of the abdomen that is the least painful and farthest from the site of pain. The abdomen should be soft and nontender. Note any rigidity, guarding, or

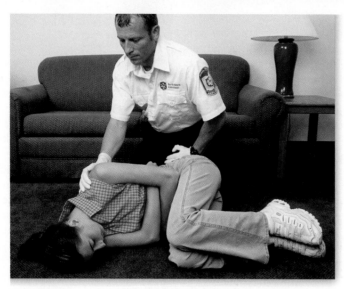

Figure 33-4 A patient with acute abdominal pain may be found in a guarded position.

masses. Obtain and document the patient's baseline vital signs.

Signs and Symptoms

The following signs and symptoms may be associated with acute abdominal pain:

- Pain or tenderness—can be diffuse or localized; crampy, sharp, aching, or knifelike
- Rapid and shallow breathing and tachycardia
- Pulsating masses
- Nausea, vomiting, and/or diarrhea
- Rigid abdomen (involuntary reflex that produces a boardlike abdomen) or guarding (voluntary contraction of the abdominal muscles)
- Distended abdomen
- Fever or chills
- Belching or flatulence

- Changes in bowel habits or urination
- Other signs and symptoms associated with shock

EMERGENCY MEDICAL CARE

The following procedures should be following when caring for a patient with an abdominal emergency:

1. **Keep the airway patent.** Be prepared to suction. Consider airway management if necessary.

2. **Place the patient in the position of comfort if no spinal injury is suspected.** If the patient is vomiting or has an altered mental status, place him in a lateral recumbent position to protect the airway. If hypovolemic shock is suspected or evident, place the patient in a supine position.

3. **If breathing is adequate, administer oxygen based on the SpO$_2$**

reading and patient signs and symptoms. If the SpO$_2$ reading is greater than 95 percent and no signs or symptoms of hypoxia, shock, or respiratory distress are present, you may choose to apply oxygen via a nasal cannula at 2 to 4 liters per minute (lpm). If signs of hypoxia, shock, or respiratory distress are present, or if the SpO$_2$ reading is less than 95 percent, place the patient on a nonrebreather mask at 15 lpm.

4. **Never give anything by mouth.**

5. **Calm and reassure the patient.** Provide emotional support.

6. **Initiate an intravenous line of normal saline or lactated Ringer's with a large-bore catheter.** Draw blood according to your local protocol. If signs of shock are present or the patient is hypotensive, administer fluid to maintain a radial pulse or the systolic blood pressure above 90 to 100 mmHg. Be sure to monitor the patient's breath sounds for an indication of fluid overload, especially in the elderly and those with heart disease. If the patient begins to complain of dyspnea and crackles (rales) are heard in the posterior lower lobes, reduce the amount and rate of fluid being infused.

7. **Consider antiemetics if your protocols allow.** Medications such as ondansetron or promethazine can suppress nausea and vomiting and provide comfort to the patient. Always follow local protocol.

8. **Initiate efficient transport.**

Perform reassessment during transport. Document and record all vital signs. Communicate all findings to the receiving facility. Reassess the patient every 5 minutes.

TRANSITIONING ● ● ● ● ● ● ● ●

REVIEW ITEMS

1. A patient presents with copious amounts of bright red hematemesis. Based on that initial finding, you suspect the patient may have _____.
   a. ruptured esophageal varices b. acute appendicitis
   c. cholecystitis   d. a bowel obstruction

2. Which of the following is a common cause of lower gastrointestinal bleeding?
   a. appendicitis   b. hepatitis
   c. diverticulosis   d. pancreatitis

3. Abdominal pain lasting more than _____ hours should be considered an emergency.

   a. 4   b. 6

   c. 8   d. 12

4. Patients complaining of severe abdominal pain are commonly found in what position?

   a. supine   b. prone

   c. guarded   d. high Fowler

5. The presence of melena indicates _____.

   a. partially digested blood in the vomit

   b. undigested blood in the vomit

   c. partially digested blood in the stool

   d. undigested blood in the stool

APPLIED PATHOPHYSIOLOGY

1. Explain the difference between visceral and somatic pain.

2. Explain why referred pain is felt in other areas of the body.

3. Explain why palpation of the most painful abdominal quadrant should be performed last.

4. List five illnesses that can cause a patient to present with gastrointestinal bleeding.

CLINICAL DECISION MAKING

You are dispatched to the residence of a 33-year-old female patient complaining of abdominal pain. On arrival, you ensure that the scene is safe. You are escorted into the residence by a teenage boy who identifies himself as the patient's son. As you approach the patient, you notice that she appears to be in severe pain and is lying in a fetal position on the living room floor. She has a wastebasket on the floor next to her with greenish-colored vomit in it.

1. Based on the scene size-up characteristics, list the possible conditions you suspect the patient is experiencing.

The primary assessment reveals that the patient is anxious, alert, and disoriented, and she is complaining that her stomach hurts; she denies any trauma. She is breathing adequately with a respiratory rate of 20/minute. Her heart rate is 114 beats/minute, and her radial pulses are rapid and strong. Her skin is pale, cool, and diaphoretic. The SpO₂ reading is 94 percent.

2. What are the life threats to this patient?

3. What immediate emergency care should you provide based on the primary assessment?

4. What conditions have you ruled out from your initial consideration in the scene size-up?

5. What conditions are you still considering as the possible cause?

During the secondary assessment, your patient states that she has been in pain for the past three hours. She says the pain, which is severe and colicky, began about 30 minutes after eating spicy fajitas at a Mexican restaurant. She states that she is nauseated and vomited three times after she took Tums and Pepto-Bismol. She denies any allergies, past medical problems, or taking any other medications. Her abdomen is soft, and tenderness is noted to the upper right side and under the right costal margin. Her pelvis is stable, and no deformities or trauma are evident. Her blood pressure is 106/68 mmHg.

6. What conditions have you ruled out in your differential field diagnosis? Why?

7. What conditions are you considering as a probable cause? Why?

8. Based on your differential diagnosis, what are the next steps in emergency care? Why?

9. Explain how you came to a differential field diagnosis based on specific history and physical assessment findings.

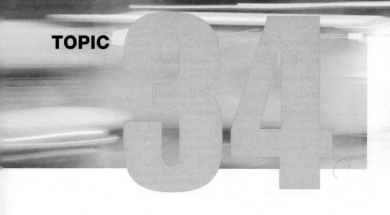

Standard Medicine

Competency Integrates assessment findings with principles of epidemiology and pathophysiology to formulate a field impression and implement a comprehensive treatment/disposition plan for a patient with a medical complaint.

IMMUNOLOGY: ANAPHYLACTIC AND ANAPHYLACTOID REACTIONS

TRANSITION *highlights*

- *Overview of the frequency of immunologic emergencies to include frequency, types, and death rates.*

- *Pathology underlying important types of immunologic emergencies:*
  - Anaphylactic reaction.
  - Anaphylactoid reaction.
  - Vascular organs.

- *Chemical mediators that result in detrimental changes to body physiology during anaphylactic and anaphylactoid reactions:*
  - Increased capillary permeability.
  - Decreased vascular smooth muscle tone.
  - Increased bronchial smooth muscle tone.
  - Enhanced mucus secretion in the respiratory tree.

- *Illustration of the relationship between pathophysiologic changes by body system and the types of signs or symptoms that would be present.*

- *Review of how to distinguish between a mild and severe anaphylactic or anaphylactoid reaction.*

- *Why epinephrine is the drug of choice with a moderate to severe anaphylactic or anaphylactoid reaction.*

INTRODUCTION

An *allergic reaction* is an immunologic or nonimmunologic response to an allergen or antigen resulting in the release of chemical mediators from specific cells within the body. Allergic reactions can occur on a continuum from mild to severe. Anaphylaxis, in the simplest sense, is an allergic reaction on the severe end of the continuum. However, it is important to understand that the condition of anaphylaxis can present

with a multitude of clinical manifestations. Thus, anaphylaxis itself has its own continuum of criticality, from mild to severe, which is not well agreed on in the medical literature.

EPIDEMIOLOGY

Anaphylaxis is not a reportable disease; therefore, the morbidity and mortality rates are not well established. Studies suggest that the lifetime risk of an individual experiencing an anaphylactic reaction is between 1 percent and 3 percent, with a mortality rate of 1 percent. It is estimated that 20,000 to 50,000 persons suffer an anaphylactic reaction in the United States each year. The incidence rate has been reported to be increasing, especially in individuals under 20 years of age.

Penicillin (0.7% to 10%), insect stings (0.5% to 5%), radiocontrast media (0.22% to 1%), and food (0.0004%) remain the most common triggers. Food is the most common trigger in children, adolescents, and young adults, whereas medications, insect venom, and idiopathic (unknown) causes are more often seen in middle-aged and older individuals.

PATHOPHYSIOLOGY

Classically, *anaphylaxis* can be best defined as a systemic, misdirected, immune-mediated hypersensitivity reaction resulting in the release of chemical mediators from mast cells and basophils, affecting multiple organ systems. Historically, anaphylaxis was thought to occur only in patients who were previously sensitized and subsequently reexposed to an allergen.

Anaphylactic Reaction

In an anaphylactic reaction, the patient must be sensitized. Sensitization occurs when an antigen is introduced into the body and viewed as a foreign substance. Antigens may include venom, foods, pollen, medications, latex, and other substances (see Table 34-1). The body responds by producing antibodies, specifically immunoglobulin E (IgE), to fight off the antigen.

The IgE antibodies attach to mast cells, which are found in connective tissue, and basophils, which are immature mast cells

TABLE 34-1 Common Causes of Anaphylactic Reactions

Venom	Wasps, hornets, yellow jackets, fire ants, deer flies, gnats, horseflies, mosquitoes, cockroaches, miller moths, snakes, spiders
Foods	Peanuts, Brazil nuts, macadamia nuts, other nuts, milk, eggs, shellfish, white fish, food additives, chocolate, cottonseed oil, berries
Pollen	Plants, ragweed, grass
Medications	Antibiotics, local anesthetics, vitamins, seizure medication, muscle relaxants, insulin, tetanus and diphtheria toxoids
Other substances	Latex, glue

found circulating in the blood. These antibodies could remain attached to the mast cells and basophils for seconds, minutes, days, weeks, months, or years.

As long as the antibodies remain attached, the patient is considered to be sensitized and primed for an allergic reaction if the antigen is reintroduced in the body. On reexposure, the antigen physically attaches itself to the antibodies on the mast cells and basophils and creates a condition that is often referred to as the classic antigen–antibody induced reaction. This reaction causes the mast cells and basophils to degranulate (break down), releasing chemical mediators into the interstitial fluid surrounding the cells.

Common chemical mediators that are released are histamine, leukotriene, prostaglandin, and tryptase. These mediators are absorbed by capillaries, enter the blood, and begin to circulate throughout the body, producing systemic multiorgan effects. Thus, for this type of classic anaphylactic reaction to occur, the patient must have been exposed to the antigen previously, antibodies must have been produced, and the antibodies must attach to the mast cells and basophils and remain attached. On reexposure to the antigen, the antigen must attach to the antibodies, the mast cells and basophils must break down, and chemical mediators must be released.

For the patient to experience the systemic and multiple-organ pathologic response and exhibit the typical signs and symptoms, a large enough quantity of mediators must be released from the mast cells and basophils. If the reaction remains localized or only a small amount of mediators are released, the patient may present with minor signs and symptoms. Likewise, if the organs and vascular structures do not respond to the chemical mediators, the signs and symptoms will not likely be significant.

Anaphylactoid Reaction

Previously, EMS education materials addressed only the classic type of anaphylactic reaction. Thus, when EMS providers arrived on scene to treat a patient suspected of having an anaphylactic reaction, the history gathering focused on an attempt to identify what the potential antigen was and when the reexposure occurred. If the patient presented with signs and symptoms of a classic anaphylactic reaction but had never been exposed previously to the substance that was thought to be the antigen, the question arose as to whether the patient was truly experiencing an anaphylactic reaction.

Consider this example: A patient has received a prescription for a narcotic to treat pain. He has never taken any narcotic in any form. After taking the narcotic for the first time, he develops typical signs and symptoms of an anaphylactic reaction. Based on the classic antigen–antibody reaction, he could not be experiencing a true anaphylactic reaction because he never took the narcotic previously, and his body would not have produced the antibodies to fight off the introduced antigen (narcotic). He would not be sensitized, and no antibodies would be attached to the mast cells and basophils to initiate the reaction.

Such a situation could cause conflicting and confusing information for the EMS provider, and in some cases treatment might be altered or withheld because of the lack of evidence of sensitization and reexposure. In this example, the patient was experiencing what is known as an *anaphylactoid reaction*. The patient undergoes basically the same pathologic processes and exhibits the same signs and symptoms of the classic anaphylactic reaction.

The anaphylactoid reaction is not the typical immunologic antigen–antibody reaction, however. The anaphylactoid substance that the patient ingests, injects, absorbs, or inhales causes the mast cells and basophils to break down and release chemical mediators. Because the anaphylactoid substances are "direct" chemical mediator-releasing agents, antibodies do not have to be produced or attached to mast cells and basophils, the patient does not have to be sensitized, and reexposure to the substance does not have to occur (see Table 34-2).

> The anaphylactoid reaction presents with the same pathologic conditions and signs and symptoms as the classic anaphylactic reaction.

The first-time exposure may cause a direct release of a mass of chemical mediators and create a life-threatening condition, with signs and symptoms that appear to be a full-blown anaphylactic reaction. Thus, even though the patient in our example has never ingested a narcotic before in his life, this first-time ingestion has stimulated the direct release of chemical mediators and produced a life-threatening anaphylactoid reaction.

The anaphylactoid reaction presents with the same pathologic conditions and signs and symptoms as the classic anaphylactic reaction. Thus, other than history of exposure and the underlying mechanism, the conditions are indistinguishable and are treated exactly the same.

TABLE 34-2 Common Causes of Anaphylactoid Reactions

- Radiopaque contrast media
- Nonsteroidal antiinflammatory drugs (NSAIDs)
- Aspirin
- Opiates
- Thiamine

EFFECTS OF CHEMICAL MEDIATORS

The antigen or substance triggering the anaphylactic reaction itself is harmless and does not have any real effect on the tissues or organs; however, it does cause the release of chemical mediators from mast cells and basophils. Histamine, the primary chemical mediator, along with leukotriene, prostaglandin, and tryptase, is released when the mast cell or basophil membrane breaks down in response to the antigen in an anaphylactic (or direct chemical-releasing substance in an anaphylactoid) reaction. The chemical mediators circulate and produce the abnormal cell, tissue, organ, and organ system response.

Almost all fatal episodes, signs displayed, and symptoms experienced by the patient experiencing an anaphylactoid reaction are related to one of the following more common effects of the chemical mediators (▶ Figure 34-1):

- Increased capillary permeability
- Decreased vascular smooth muscle tone (vasodilation)
- Increased bronchial smooth muscle tone (bronchoconstriction)
- Increased mucus secretion in the tracheobronchial tract

Increased Capillary Permeability

An increase in capillary permeability allows fluid to leak from the capillary bed and collect in the interstitial space around the cells. This is commonly seen as edema in the patient. Often the edema is noted around the face, tongue, and neck, because of the large number of vessels in that area of the body, and in the hands, feet, and ankles, caused by gravity pulling the fluid downward (▶ Figure 34-2).

The increased capillary permeability in the mucous membranes can lead to edema in the airway structures, including the oropharynx, hypopharynx, larynx, and tracheobronchial tract. The swelling occurs inward, reducing the internal diameter of the airway structures; this leads to an increase in resistance to airflow, making it difficult for the patient to move air in and out of the lungs. The swelling could lead to complete airway closure, a common cause of death in severe allergic reactions.

The fluid loss creates a decrease in plasma volume, thereby reducing the overall blood volume in the vascular space. This loss could produce hypotension from a decrease in cardiac preload, leading to poor perfusion. When hypotension and poor perfusion are present, the patient is categorized as being in *anaphylactic shock.*

Decreased Vascular Smooth Muscle Tone (Vasodilation)

A decrease in vascular smooth muscle tone causes vessels to dilate. This creates an increase in the internal diameter of the vessel. When the vessel size increases, the resistance to blood flow inside the vessel decreases. A decrease in vascular resistance leads to a decrease in blood pressure, which may result in poor perfusion. As the vessel dilates, more blood volume is needed to fill the vascular space. If the space is not filled, the pressure inside drops, leading to hypotension. In anaphylaxis, both vasodilation and fluid loss from an increase in capillary permeability can produce severe hypotension and extremely poor tissue and organ perfusion.

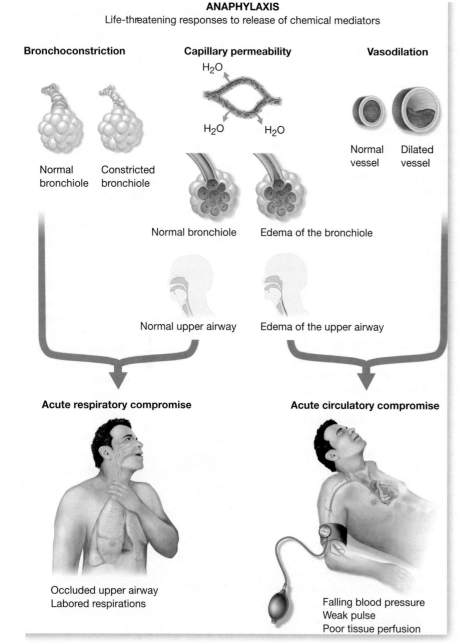

ANAPHYLAXIS
Life-threatening responses to release of chemical mediators

Bronchoconstriction

Normal bronchiole   Constricted bronchiole

Capillary permeability

H_2O H_2O H_2O

Normal bronchiole   Edema of the bronchiole

Normal upper airway   Edema of the upper airway

Vasodilation

Normal vessel   Dilated vessel

Acute respiratory compromise

Occluded upper airway
Labored respirations

Acute circulatory compromise

Falling blood pressure
Weak pulse
Poor tissue perfusion

Figure 34-1 Life-threatening responses in anaphylactic reaction: bronchoconstriction, capillary permeability, vasodilation, and an increase in mucus production.

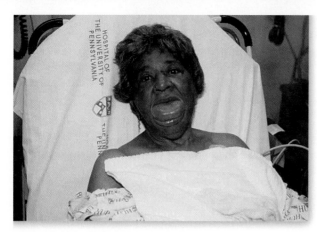

Figure 34-2 Localized angioedema to the tongue from an anaphylactic reaction. (© *Edward T. Dickinson, MD*)

Increased Bronchial Smooth Muscle Tone (Bronchoconstriction)

The chemical mediators may cause the bronchial smooth muscle to constrict, leading to an increase in airway pressure. The higher airway pressure makes it more difficult for the patient to move air in and out of the alveoli. The lower airway could be further narrowed by swollen mucous membranes from an increase in capillary permeability. This may cause a reduction in the amount of air moved in and out of the lungs (tidal volume) and alveoli (alveolar ventilation), leading to severe hypoxia and the retention of carbon dioxide.

Patients with bronchoconstriction will likely present with wheezing and signs of respiratory distress. Signs of hypoxia, such as a poor SpO$_2$ reading and anxiety, may also be present.

Increased Mucus Secretion in the Tracheobronchial Tract

An increase in mucus secretion can lead to plugging of the smaller airways. The mucus is thick and sticky and difficult for the patient to expectorate. The patient often presents with an unproductive cough that is an attempt to expel the mucus.

These pathophysiologic responses related to chemical mediator effects on cells, tissue, organs, and organ systems produce the signs and symptoms seen in the patient. Hemodynamic instability and airway and ventilatory compromise are also a result of the mediators. If the chemical mediator effects can be reversed, the signs, symptoms, airway and ventilatory compromise, and hemodynamic instability will be eliminated. Thus, emergency care is geared toward reversing the pathophysiologic effects of the chemical mediators.

ASSESSMENT FINDINGS

During the scene size-up, you may find evidence of the actual antigen or direct chemical mediator-releasing substance or route of introduction into the body. As with poisoning, the route may include injection, ingestion, inhalation, or absorption. Injection is the route most often associated with anaphylactic reactions.

Fatal episodes of anaphylaxis are associated with airway occlusion, respiratory failure, severe hypoxia, and circulatory collapse. Thus, it is imperative to pay particular attention to the airway, ventilation, oxygenation, and circulatory status during the primary assessment. It may be necessary to be very aggressive with airway management if stridor or other evidence of airway occlusion is present.

Carefully assess for an adequate tidal volume and respiratory rate. If either respiratory rate or tidal volume is inadequate, immediately initiate positive pressure ventilation. In the spontaneously breathing patient, deliver a high concentration of oxygenation via a nonrebreather mask, or deliver it via the ventilation device in a patient with inadequate breathing.

Assess the circulatory status by checking peripheral and central pulses and skin color, temperature, and condition. Weak or absent peripheral pulses are an indication of poor perfusion. Warm, flushed skin is an indication of vasodilation, whereas edema and urticaria (hives) (▶ Figure 34-3) indicate an increase in capillary permeability. Both contribute to hypotension and poor perfusion.

When gathering a history, in addition to the standard information collected, be sure to inquire about the following:

- Are the signs and symptoms getting worse?
- Does the patient have a history of allergic reaction or anaphylaxis? If so, how severe was the reaction? Was the patient hospitalized?
- Has the patient ever been exposed to the suspected triggering substance previously?
- Has the patient taken any medications in an attempt to relieve the signs and symptoms?
- How quick was the onset of the signs and symptoms?

The signs and symptoms of the reaction typically involve the skin, respiratory tract, cardiovascular system, gastrointestinal system, central nervous system, and genitourinary system. Common signs and symptoms of anaphylactic reactions by body system are listed in Table 34-3.

> Patients with bronchoconstriction will likely present with wheezing and signs of respiratory distress.

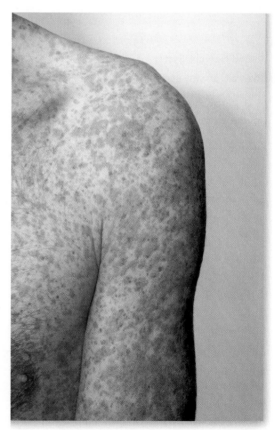

Figure 34-3 Urticaria (hives) from an allergic reaction to a penicillin-derivative drug.

TABLE 34-3 Common Signs and Symptoms of Anaphylactic Reactions

Sign or System	Pathophysiology
Integumentary System (Skin)	
Warm, tingling feeling in the face, mouth, chest, feet, and hands	Vasodilation and increased capillary permeability
Intense itching (pruritus), especially of the hands and feet	Increased capillary permeability
Urticaria (hives)	Increased capillary permeability
Flushed or red skin	Vasodilation causing blood to pool in peripheral vessels
Swelling of the face, lips, neck, hands, feet, and tongue	Increased capillary permeability causing fluid to leak into interstitial spaces
Cyanosis	Bronchoconstriction and increased capillary permeability reducing alveolar ventilation and gas exchange
Respiratory System	
Complaint of "lump," "tightness," or obstructed feeling in throat	Increased capillary permeability causing swelling of laryngeal tissue
Cough	Increased mucus production producing a cough in an attempt to expel mucus
Tachypnea	Bronchoconstriction and increased capillary permeability reducing alveolar oxygenation
Labored breathing and other evidence of respiratory distress or failure	Bronchoconstriction and increased capillary permeability reducing alveolar oxygenation
Wheezing	Bronchoconstriction and increased capillary permeability narrowing the internal diameter of the bronchiole
Stridor	Increased capillary permeability causing swelling of the laryngeal tissue
Hoarseness or inability to talk	Increased capillary permeability causing swelling of the laryngeal tissue
Difficulty in breathing	Bronchoconstriction and increased capillary permeability reducing alveolar oxygenation
Cardiovascular System	
Tachycardia	Increased capillary permeability, vasodilation, and hypoxia from bronchoconstriction
Hypotension	Increased capillary permeability and vasodilation
Absent or weak peripheral pulses	Increased capillary permeability and vasodilation
Central Nervous System	
Increased anxiety and restlessness	Hypoxia associated with bronchoconstriction and hypotension from increased capillary permeability and vasodilation
Confusion to unresponsiveness	Hypercarbia associated with bronchoconstriction
Lightheadedness	Hypoxia associated with bronchoconstriction and hypotension from increased capillary permeability and vasodilation
Headache	Vasodilation
Seizure	Hypoxia associated with bronchoconstriction and hypotension from increased capillary permeability and vasodilation
Gastrointestinal System	
Nausea and vomiting	Increased capillary permeability and smooth muscle contraction
Diarrhea	Increased capillary permeability
Abdominal cramping	Increase in smooth muscle contraction
Difficulty in swallowing	Increase in smooth muscle contraction and increase in capillary permeability, causing swelling of the opening to the esophagus
Genitourinary System	
Urgent need to urinate	Increase in smooth muscle contraction
Uterine cramping	Increase in smooth muscle contraction
Generalized Signs and Symptoms	
Itchy, watery, red eyes	Increased capillary permeability
Runny and stuffy nose	Increased capillary permeability and vasodilation

When assessing the vital signs, the respiratory rate is likely to be elevated with evidence of respiratory distress. As the condition progresses and the patient tires, the respiratory distress may deteriorate to respiratory failure. The respiratory rate may begin to decrease as the patient continues to fail. Tachycardia is typical with weak pulses. In severe cases, the peripheral pulses may be absent. Unlike other types of shock, the skin is red, warm, and dry with urticaria (hives) and pruritus (itching). Hypotension is common in a severe reaction.

The following are other notable characteristics associated with assessment:

- Parenteral (injection) introduction of the antigen or direct chemical-releasing substance typically produces the most severe reactions.
- The faster the onset of signs and symptoms, the more severe the reaction. Most reactions occur within minutes; however, reactions usually occur within 30 minutes. In rare occasions, the reaction may take hours to days to occur.
- Signs and symptoms often peak within 15 to 30 minutes.
- Skin and respiratory signs and symptoms are the most common and earliest to appear.
- Mild signs and symptoms could progress to a severe reaction within minutes and without warning.

- Most fatalities occur within 30 minutes of exposure.
- A biphasic or multiphasic reaction may occur. The patient may respond effectively to the emergency care and appear to be recovering when the signs and symptoms of the reaction recurs.

EMERGENCY MEDICAL CARE

One of the initial keys to emergency care is to recognize whether the reaction is mild, moderate, or severe (see Table 34-4).

A mild reaction typically requires only minimal care—most often, only oxygen administration—and close reassessment for deterioration to a moderate to severe reaction. Patients experiencing a moderate to severe reaction require much more aggressive emergency medical care. The emergency care should include the following:

- Establish and maintain a patent airway. Early signs indicating that the patient might require aggressive airway management, including insertion of an advanced endotracheal tube, are hoarseness, edema to the oropharynx, stridor, and edema to the tongue (lingual edema).
- Suction secretions.

- Administer a high concentration of oxygen via a nonrebreather mask to the patient with an adequate tidal volume and respiratory rate. Titrate the oxygen to maintain a SpO_2 reading of greater than 94 percent. If the tidal volume or respiratory rate is inadequate, immediately initiate positive pressure ventilation with a bag-valve-mask device while maximizing supplemental oxygen administration. It may be difficult to ventilate the patient because of the high airway resistance created by the upper and lower airway edema and bronchoconstriction.
- Initiate an intravenous infusion of normal saline or lactated Ringer's with a large-bore (14- to 16-gauge) catheter in a large vein. Infuse the fluid wide open until a minimum systolic blood pressure of 90 mmHg is obtained. Maintain the systolic blood pressure above 90 mmHg. This may require the infusion of large amounts of fluid; therefore, a second intravenous line may be required.
- Epinephrine should be administered to patients with an anaphylactic reaction who present with systemic signs and symptoms, especially those with hypotension, poor perfusion, airway swelling, or difficulty in breathing. Administer epinephrine by auto-injector or intramuscular (IM) injection in the

TABLE 34-4	Differentiating Between a Mild and a Moderate to Severe Reaction	
Sign or Symptom	Mild Reaction	Moderate to Severe Reaction
Pruritus (itching)	Present	Present and usually widespread
Urticaria (hives)	Present, localized	Present and usually widespread
Flushed skin	If present, localized	Widespread
Cyanosis	Not present	Present around lips, oral mucosa, and nail beds
Edema	Present but mild to moderate	Severe in face, lips, tongue, neck, and distal extremities
Heart rate	Normal to slight tachycardia	Moderate to severe tachycardia
Blood pressure	Normal	Moderately to severely decreased with signs of poor perfusion
Peripheral pulses	Present and normal amplitude	Weak or absent
Mental status	Anxious but alert and oriented	Decreases to unresponsive
Respirations	Normal or slightly tachypneic; normal tidal volume	Severely tachypneic with evidence of respiratory distress or failure; tidal volume likely decreased
Wheezing	None or slight with good breath sounds	Present in all lung fields to very poor lung sounds with little air movement
Stridor	None	May be present

anterolateral aspect of the middle third of the thigh. This location provides the fastest absorption. Epinephrine can be administered subcutaneously (SQ); however, when this route is used, the absorption is much slower, and epinephrine delivery to the core circulation might be delayed significantly when the anaphylaxis is associated with poor perfusion or hypotension.

The recommended adult dose is 0.2 to 0.5 mg of a 1:1000 dilution administered intramuscularly. The adult epinephrine auto-injector typically delivers a 0.3 mg dose. The pediatric dose is 0.1 mg/kg, not to exceed the adult dose (0.2 to 0.5 mg). The pediatric epinephrine auto-injector delivers a dose of 0.15 mg. The pediatric auto-injector should be used in children less than 66 lbs or 30 kg. If the child is larger than 66 lbs or 30 kg, use the adult epinephrine auto-injector.

Epinephrine can be repeated every 5 to 15 minutes if the patient continues to exhibit evidence of hypotension, airway swelling, and severe respiratory distress or failure. Patients who are taking beta blockers present a unique challenge in anaphylaxis. Their routine beta blockade can impair epinephrine's most important effects. In this case, paramedics should consider the concurrent administration of glucagon to counteract the beta blockers while administering epinephrine. These patients may require additional or higher dosing of epinephrine. Consult on-line medical direction for more specific dosing and always follow local protocols.

- Administer diphenhydramine (Benadryl). Diphenhydramine is a histamine blocker and negates the ongoing effects of circulating histamine.

Although it is very effective at controlling long-term effects, its slower onset and relatively delayed mechanism of action require it to be administered only after epinephrine in the case of a moderate to severe reaction. A typical dose is 25 to 50 mg IV or IM.

- Administer corticosteroids. Although the effects of corticosteroids are not usually seen in the prehospital time frame, these medications are very important to the overall treatment of anaphylaxis. Corticosteroids help stabilize capillary membrane permeability and prevent subsequent swelling. The antiinflammatory property of these medications can also help prevent ongoing (posttreatment) recurrences.

- Initiate rapid transport.

- If the reaction is associated with a sting or an injection of the antigen to an extremity, apply a loose tourniquet proximal to the site and place the extremity in a dependent position.

- If the patient continues to present with respiratory distress and diffuse wheezing after the administration of epinephrine and no signs of hypotension or poor perfusion are present, consider the administration of an aerosolized beta$_2$ agonist delivered via nebulizer or metered-dose inhaler. Albuterol is commonly nebulized at a dose of 2.5 mg diluted to 3 mL of normal saline in both adult and pediatric patients or levalbuterol at 0.625 to 1.25 mg diluted to 3 mL of normal saline in the adult and 0.31 to 0.625 mg diluted to 3 mL of normal saline in the pediatric patient.

- If no signs of respiratory distress or failure are present, and the airway is not compromised by edema and the patient continues to present with hypotension, continue to infuse large amounts of normal saline or lactated Ringer's at a wide-open rate. It may be necessary to establish a second intravenous line.

Why Epinephrine?—The Drug of Choice

Recall that the etiology of almost all the signs and symptoms and fatal events—such as airway compromise, respiratory failure, hypoxia, and cardiovascular collapse—associated with an anaphylactic or anaphylactoid reaction are related to an increase in capillary permeability, bronchoconstriction, vasodilation, and an increase in mucus production. If these can be reversed, the signs and symptoms and chance of a fatal episode also will be reversed. Thus, a focus in the emergency care of the patient is to decrease the permeability of the capillaries, dilate the bronchioles, and constrict the vessels.

Epinephrine becomes the drug of choice because of its ability to stimulate alpha and beta receptors. Alpha stimulation causes vascular smooth muscle contraction, leading to vasoconstriction. Vasoconstriction decreases the vessel diameter and increases resistance to blood flow, leading to an increase in blood pressure and perfusion. The vasoconstriction also tightens the capillaries. This will also reverse hypotension by reducing the leakage of plasma volume to the interstitial space. The beta$_2$ stimulation dilates the bronchiole smooth muscle and reverses the bronchoconstriction. Thus, epinephrine administration eliminates the capillary permeability, vasodilation, and bronchoconstriction associated with anaphylaxis.

TRANSITIONING

REVIEW ITEMS

1. A patient presents with widespread urticaria covering the majority of his body. Based on that initial finding, you should suspect the patient is also likely to present with _____.
   - a. cardiac dysrhythmias
   - b. bradycardia
   - c. pale cool skin
   - d. hypotension

2. An anaphylactic patient presents with stridor, hoarseness, and an increased effort to breathe. Which property of epinephrine would likely reverse these signs?
   - a. alpha stimulation
   - b. beta$_1$ stimulation
   - c. beta$_2$ stimulation
   - d. delta stimulation

3. The pathophysiologic response that creates a life-threatening upper airway compromise is related to _____.
   a. an increase in mucus secretion
   b. an increase in capillary permeability
   c. a decrease in vascular tone
   d. an increase in smooth muscle contraction

4. Immediately following the administration of epinephrine, the patient appears to be responding effectively. Which of the following should you suspect may present as a direct result of the emergency care?
   a. an increase in heart rate
   b. an increase in flushing of the skin
   c. a decrease in peripheral pulse amplitude
   d. a widened pulse pressure

5. Following the administration of epinephrine, the hypotension, poor perfusion, stridor, and severe respiratory distress are reversed. However, the patient continues to present with diffuse bilateral wheezing and mild respiratory distress. You should _____.
   a. begin to assist the patient's spontaneous respirations with a bag-valve-mask device
   b. administer a second dose of epinephrine by deep intramuscular injection
   c. continue with oxygen therapy and reassess the respiratory status in 5 minutes
   d. contact medical direction for an order to administer a beta$_2$ agonist by inhalation

APPLIED PATHOPHYSIOLOGY

1. List the four primary pathophysiologic responses to the release of chemical mediators that produce the life-threatening condition and signs and symptoms in anaphylaxis.

2. Explain the difference in the patient presentation between an anaphylactic and anaphylactoid reaction.

3. Explain the process of sensitization in the IgE-mediated anaphylactic reaction.

4. What triggers the release of the chemical mediators from mast cells and basophils in the IgE-mediated reaction?

5. List the properties of epinephrine and their specific effects on reversing the pathophysiologic responses to the chemical mediators.

6. What property of epinephrine would be considered a side effect? Why?

CLINICAL DECISION MAKING

You encounter a 23-year-old male patient sitting on the front porch of his residence. You note a lawn mower out in the front yard, and the grass is partially cut. As you have determined that the scene is safe, you approach the patient. He is sitting upright in a tripod position and appears to be in significant respiratory distress.

1. Based on the scene size-up characteristics, list the possible conditions you suspect the patient is experiencing.

The primary assessment reveals that the patient is anxious, confused, and disoriented and has stridorous sounds on respiration, a respiratory rate of 28 per minute with chest rise and fall, circumoral cyanosis, absent peripheral pulses, and a heart rate of 128 beats per minute. The skin is warm and flushed. The SpO$_2$ reading is 74 percent.

2. What are the life threats to this patient?

3. What immediate emergency care should you provide based on the primary assessment?

4. Explain the pathophysiologic causes for the following:
   a. Anxiousness
   b. Confusion and disorientation
   c. Stridorous sounds
   d. Warm flushed skin

5. What conditions have you ruled out from your initial consideration in the scene size-up?

6. What conditions are you still considering as the possible cause? Are there any conditions that you would add as a possible cause?

During the secondary assessment, you note an edematous tongue and swollen oral mucosa; urticaria to the face, neck, and upper chest; and diffuse bilateral wheezing. The patient has a new-onset cough that is nonproductive. He also complains of a headache and severe dizziness. His respiratory distress is worsening. The abdomen is soft and nontender, the pelvis is stable, and no deformities or evidence of trauma to the extremities are present. The extremities are warm, flushed, and dry. The peripheral pulses are all absent. The patient has no known allergies, has a history of mild asthma, and takes no prescription medication. He had a diet cola about 20 minutes prior to your arrival. He was cutting the grass when he suddenly began to experience shortness of breath and lightheadedness. He admits to taking 800 mg of ibuprofen for a bad headache with the diet cola. His blood pressure is 76/42 mmHg, his heart rate is now 142 beats per minute, and his respirations are 32 per minute and more labored.

7. What conditions have you ruled out in your differential field diagnosis? Why?

8. What conditions are you considering as the probable cause? Why?

9. Based on your differential diagnosis, what are the next steps in emergency care? Why?

10. Explain how you came to a differential field diagnosis based on specific history and physical assessment findings.

11. What was the trigger for the condition the patient is experiencing?

12. Based on the history, what type of reaction is this patient experiencing?

13. If his circulation is not improved, what skin signs will begin to appear? Why?

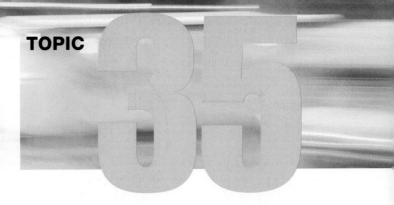

Standard Medicine

Competency Integrates assessment findings with principles of epidemiology and pathophysiology to formulate a field impression and implement a comprehensive treatment/disposition plan for a patient with a medical complaint.

TOPIC

35

ENDOCRINE EMERGENCIES: HYPOGLYCEMIA

INTRODUCTION

*D*iabetes mellitus (DM) is a condition in which the patient experiences a chronically elevated blood glucose level (BGL). Most DM patients struggle on a daily basis to decrease their BGLs to within a normal range, but EMS frequently responds for those with a low BGL (hypoglycemia). The occasional acute hypoglycemic event carries a high risk of morbidity and mortality. Thus, it is imperative that paramedics quickly recognize the signs and symptoms of hypoglycemia and manage the patient accordingly to prevent any long-term effects from the episode.

EPIDEMIOLOGY

DM is the most common endocrine disorder, with approximately 6 percent of the population afflicted with the disease. Whites are much more likely to have the disease than nonwhites.

Types of Diabetes Mellitus

DM is typically characterized as type 1 or type 2. Type 2 is much more prevalent and makes up approximately 90 percent to 95 percent of cases of DM. Type 1 accounts for the remaining 5 percent to 10 percent of cases.

TYPE 1 DIABETES MELLITUS Type 1 DM results from a chronic autoimmune process that destroys the insulin-producing cells (beta cells) in the pancreas. Interestingly, the cells responsible for secreting other hormones in the pancreas are typically preserved and continue to function. The exact cause of the disorder is not clearly understood; however, theories link genetics, environment, and viruses to the etiology.

Characteristics of type 1 diabetes patients are:

- Typically younger than 40 years of age (peak age is 10 to 14 years of age)
- Lean body mass
- May have rapid weight loss
- Polyuria (excessive urination)

TRANSITION *highlights*

- Frequency of diabetes mellitus and the ethnic predisposition of the disease.
- Etiologies of diabetes mellitus (type 1 and type 2).
- Roles that the hormones insulin and glucagon play in glucose metabolism.
- Cellular metabolism of glucose.
- Discussion of how low blood sugar (hypoglycemia) can result from the presence in the body of either too much or too little insulin or from insufficient levels of glucose.
- Signs and symptoms seen in hypoglycemia from either the hyperadrenergic or neuroglycopenic pathophysiology.
- Emergency medical care for the hypoglycemic patient and the role of oral glucose administration during patient management.

- Polydipsia (excessive thirst)
- Polyphagia (excessive eating)

Insulin levels in the blood are low to absent; however, glucagon levels are high. (Both hormones are explained in more detail later in this topic.) Because the pancreas is secreting little to no insulin, type 1 patients must take supplemental insulin to manage their BGLs. Such patients are more prone to hypoglycemia and diabetic ketoacidosis (DKA).

TYPE 2 DIABETES MELLITUS The pancreas in the patient with type 2 diabetes continues to secrete insulin; however, the BGL is elevated despite the insulin. This is caused by impaired insulin function, an inadequate amount of insulin being released

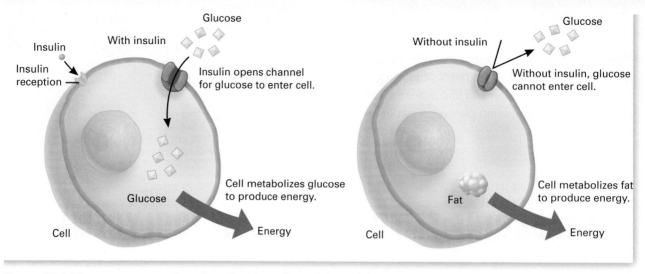

Figure 35-1 Glucose movement into the cell with insulin and the inability of glucose to get into the cell without insulin.

by the pancreas, inability of the insulin to reach the receptor sites on the cells, or failure of the organ to respond to the circulating insulin.

Characteristics of type 2 diabetes patients are:

- Onset usually in middle-age or older adults (however, more children and adolescents are being diagnosed with type 2)
- Obese body mass (however, 20 percent are not obese)
- More gradual onset of signs and symptoms

Type 2 diabetes is usually controlled through diet, exercise, and oral hypoglycemic medications. In some severe cases, the patient may require insulin supplementation. These patients are more prone to developing hyperglycemic hyperosmolar nonketotic syndrome (HHNS).

PATHOPHYSIOLOGY

Hypoglycemia results from a sudden decrease in the amount of glucose circulating in the blood. It is more common in type 1 diabetics who are taking insulin; type 2 diabetics taking oral hypoglycemic drugs can experience a hypoglycemic episode, but it is much more uncommon. Although hypoglycemic episodes are less common in the type 2 diabetic taking oral medications for blood sugar regulation, the longer half-life of the oral medications makes hospitalization necessary—and refusals of care risky, owing to the poten-

tial for additional blood glucose derangements hours later.

To understand the signs and symptoms of hypoglycemia, one must comprehend some basic normal physiology and pathophysiology. The primary energy fuel for cells is glucose, a simple sugar that accounts for approximately 95 percent of the sugar in the blood after gastrointestinal absorption. Thus, it is the BGL that paramedics and other health care practitioners are most interested in determining.

Insulin and Glucagon

Insulin is a hormone secreted by the beta cells in the pancreas. The primary function of insulin is to move glucose from the blood and into the cells, where it can be used for energy. Insulin does not directly carry glucose into the cell; however, it triggers a receptor on the plasma membrane to open a channel allowing a protein helper, through the process of facilitated diffusion, to carry the glucose molecule into the cell (▶ Figure 35-1).

As long as insulin is available in the blood and it is active, effective, and able to stimulate the receptor, it will continue to move glucose into cells, even if the BGL falls below the lower level of normal. When this occurs, a large amount of glucose is moved out of the blood, leaving an inadequate supply for the brain cells, which do not store glucose. If the pancreas is functioning normally, insulin secretion will decrease as the BGL drops.

Approximately 60 percent of the blood glucose after a meal will be sent to the liver to be stored in the form of glycogen.

Glycogen is a complex carbohydrate molecule that will be broken down through a process known as *glycogenolysis* and returned back to the blood as free glucose. This will allow a person to maintain a near-normal BGL between meals. *Glucagon* is a hormone released by the alpha cells in the pancreas that stimulates glycogenolysis and the conversion of non-carbohydrate substances into glucose (*gluconeogenesis*), subsequently raising the BGL. As the BGL decreases to approximately 70 mg/dL, insulin secretion will cease, whereas glucagon will be released to maintain a normal level of glucose and constant supply to the brain cells (▶ Figure 35-2).

Cell Metabolism of Glucose

Once in the cell, glucose is metabolized and produces energy in the form of adenosine triphosphate (ATP). ATP is necessary for cells to maintain a normal function. Without an adequate BGL, alternative energy sources must be used by the cells. As a result, ATP production and cellular function may be altered.

The brain cells, unlike many other cells in the body, cannot effectively use any other energy source but glucose for ATP production. Interestingly, the blood–brain barrier does not require the presence of insulin to move glucose across the brain cell membrane. The brain cannot synthesize glucose, store it for extended periods of time, or concentrate it from the blood. Thus, a decrease in the BGL to below normal may result in brain cell dysfunction from a lack of ATP production, a decrease

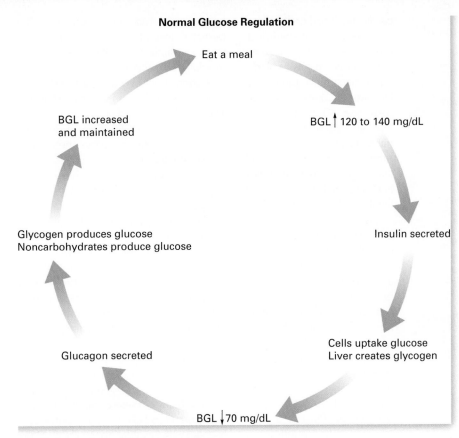

Normal Glucose Regulation

Eat a meal

BGL ↑ 120 to 140 mg/dL

Insulin secreted

Cells uptake glucose
Liver creates glycogen

BGL ↓ 70 mg/dL

Glucagon secreted

Glycogen produces glucose
Noncarbohydrates produce glucose

BGL increased
and maintained

Figure 35-2 Normal glucose regulation.

in oxygen uptake, and a decrease in cerebral blood flow. A prolonged and severe decrease in the BGL could result in brain cell death.

HYPOGLYCEMIA

A decrease in the BGL below a normal range is known as *hypoglycemia*. Hypoglycemia is precipitated by having either too much insulin or not enough glucose in the blood. This may result from taking too much insulin, missing a meal or not eating enough calories to match the insulin dose, increasing energy output through exercise or work-related activities and not increasing caloric intake, an increased dose of oral hypoglycemic agents (sulphonylureas or meglitinides), or unknown causes. Alcohol ingestion inhibits the gluconeogenesis and glycogenolysis, which may predispose the patient to hypoglycemia.

Most DM patients become symptomatic when the BGL decreases to 40 to 50 mg/dL; however, this varies among patients. Patients have different thresholds and may present with severe signs and symptoms with reported BGLs that are higher or lower than 50 mg/dL, which may also vary within the same individual

on repeated episodes of hypoglycemia. The onset and severity of signs and symptoms also depend on how quickly the glucose level falls, how low it falls, and the typical level for the patient.

When the BGL decreases beyond the normal range, the body will secrete counterregulatory hormones in an attempt to increase it. Glucagon is secreted from the alpha cells, and epinephrine is released from the adrenal medulla. Both glucagon and epinephrine stimulate gluconeogenesis and glycogenolysis in the liver. Epinephrine will also cause the breakdown of proteins into amino acids for conversion to glucose and will decrease the secretion of insulin from the pancreas. Growth hormone, cortisol, and vasopressin are also secreted as counterregulatory hormones; however, they do not have as significant an effect.

ASSESSMENT FINDINGS

The signs and symptoms exhibited by the hypoglycemic patient are caused by an activated sympathetic nervous system, epinephrine circulating throughout the

body in an attempt to increase the BGL, and brain cells that are not functioning properly as a result of the lack of glucose.

Hypoglycemia was once referred to as "insulin shock" because of the similarities of the signs exhibited by both hypovolemic shock and hypoglycemic patients. The primary hormone that produces tachycardia and pale, cool, and clammy skin in the shock patient is epinephrine, which is also released in the hypoglycemic patient, producing similar signs. Because of the stimulation of the sympathetic nervous system and circulating epinephrine, the signs of shock appear in the hypoglycemic patient.

The signs and symptoms of hypoglycemia can be categorized as being either hyperadrenergic, which is associated with an increase in the sympathetic nervous system activity or circulating epinephrine, or neuroglycopenic, which is a result of direct brain cell dysfunction from the lack of glucose (see **Table 35-1**).

Severe episodes of hypoglycemia may cause hemiplegia, making the patient present as if having a potential stroke. Thus, be sure to assess the BGL in a suspected stroke patient; however, never administer glucose without a confirmed low BGL, typically less than 60 mg/dL.

EMERGENCY MEDICAL CARE

The hypoglycemic patient needs sugar to raise the BGL as quickly as possible to prevent brain cell death. However, EMS providers may be faced with several priorities when managing this type of patient. First and foremost, provider safety may be a concern. The altered mental status that results from hypoglycemia can often make patients violent. Paramedics should always consider safety before approaching the patient.

On the other end of the spectrum, hypoglycemia can cause airway compromise due to decreasing mental status; this

> **Most DM patients become symptomatic when the blood glucose level decreases to 40 to 50 mg/dL; however, this varies among patients.**

TABLE 35-1 — Signs and Symptoms of Hypoglycemia

Hyperadrenergic (epinephrine release and activation of the sympathetic nervous system)	Sign or Symptom
	Tachycardia
	Pale, cool, clammy skin
	Sweating
	Tremors
	Weakness
	Palpitations
	Irritability
	Nervousness
	Tingling or warm sensation
	Hunger
	Nausea
	Vomiting
Neuroglycopenic (inadequate glucose available to brain cells)	**Sign or Symptom**
	Confusion
	Drowsiness
	Amnesia
	Impaired cognitive function
	Incoordination
	Headache
	Visual disturbance
	Irritation
	Aggressive behavior
	Depressed motor function
	Seizures
	Coma
	Strokelike symptoms

issue must be addressed immediately. Paramedics should keep in mind that hypoglycemia is commonly easily reversible and choose advanced airway measures with that in mind. Although the patient's mental status may indicate endotracheal intubation, as you restore mental status, this intubation may become very complicated. In most cases, basic life support (BLS) maneuvers are the far better choice.

If breathing is adequate, administer oxygen based on the SpO$_2$ reading and patient signs and symptoms. If the SpO$_2$ reading is greater than 95 percent and no signs or symptoms of hypoxia or respiratory distress are present, oxygen may not be necessary. If signs of hypoxia or respiratory distress are present, or the SpO$_2$ reading is less than 95 percent, apply a nasal cannula at 2 to 4 liters per minute (lpm). If breathing is inadequate (inadequate tidal volume or respiratory rate), immediately provide positive pressure ventilation with supplemental oxygen attached to the ventilation device.

After addressing primary assessment issues such as airway and breathing, the paramedic's next priority is to deliver glucose to the cells. In many cases, sugar

can be replaced orally. Many patients, although confused, are capable of following commands and will gladly eat a snack of simple carbohydrates or drink a sugared beverage. Oral glucose is also an option in this scenario. When possible, these methods are the safest and least complicated remedies and should be used by all levels of EMS providers.

As the saying goes, "Just because you *can* start an IV doesn't mean you *should*." More invasive therapies such as intravenous medications bring with them faster results, but far higher complication rates. That said, the oral route is not always safe. Administration of oral glucose may pose a problem if the patient is unable to understand or obey your commands. Placing a substance in the mouth of a patient who has an altered mental status can lead to aspiration, which would complicate the condition.

If oral remedies are not possible, glucose can be administered intravenously. Dextrose 50% is the most common medication used in this situation. The typical dose is 25 g and can be repeated if necessary to restore mental status and normalize blood glucose. Paramedics should take care with the administration of glucose, however. Dextrose 50% is extremely viscous and can be difficult to push through a small IV or through an intraosseous (IO). It is also extremely necrotic if allowed to extravasate into surrounding tissue. Paramedics should routinely assure patency of the IV line before and during administration of this medication. Many providers now are choosing to dilute this medication before administration to aid infusion and to help prevent secondary complications. Both the dextrose 25% and dextrose 10% concentrations are suitable for administration to adults and children; dilution should always be used if administering dextrose through the IO route. As always, follow local protocol.

If an intravenous line cannot be established rapidly, 1 to 2 mg of glucagon can

be administered intramuscularly. The pediatric dose of glucagon is 0.025 to 0.1 mg/kg intramuscularly. It can be repeated in adults and children every 20 minutes. Glucagon should be administered only if an intravenous line cannot be established. The onset of action of glucagon is 10 to 20 minutes, with a peak effect of 30 to 60 minutes. Because the sympathetic nervous system also releases glycogen stores, there is no guarantee that there will be any glycogen left upon the administration of glucagon. Liver glycogen must be available for glucagon to be effective. Therefore, if glucagon was administered and then an intravenous line was established, proceed with the administration of intravenous dextrose. The IO route may be considered in severe cases when IV access is not available and glucagon is not effective, but it should be limited to only these patients.

Hypoglycemia is easily reversible; many patients will regain a normal mental status following administration of medications. Many of these patients will refuse transport. Good clinical judgment should be used when evaluating the ability of the patient to sign off, but in a few situations, even greater concern should be expressed and transport should be initiated if possible:

- Patients who are alone or unable to take care of themselves.
- Patients taking oral antidiabetics—the effects of these types of medications are ongoing and will likely result in another bout of hypoglycemia if not treated properly.
- Patients with infections or other underlying illnesses—higher metabolic rates associated with fever and infection can cause sugar to be metabolized at a faster than normal rate. Correction to insulin dosing may be necessary. Remember also that hypoglycemia can also cause injuries associated with altered mental status. Be sure to complete a thorough patient assessment.
- New-onset diabetics—patients with recently diagnosed diabetes often struggle to find their appropriate insulin dose and are highly likely to experience additional hypoglycemia. These patients should be evaluated.
- Patients who have had multiple episodes of hypoglycemia in recent history.

REVIEW ITEMS

1. Your patient's blood glucose level is 180 mg/dL; however, there is a decrease in the amount of insulin being released from the pancreas and circulating in the blood. This will result in _____.
   a. an inadequate uptake of glucose by the brain cells
   b. an immediate decrease in the blood glucose level
   c. a reduction in the amount of glucose entering the cell
   d. an increase in the metabolism of glucose by the cell

2. Tachycardia associated with hypoglycemia occurs because of _____.
   a. a reduction in the insulin level in the blood
   b. secretion of epinephrine from the adrenal gland
   c. a reduction in the amount of blood volume
   d. cardiac failure from a low glucose state

3. In a nondiabetic patient, an increase in the blood glucose level will cause _____.
   a. the pancreas to secrete insulin
   b. the sympathetic nervous system to discharge
   c. a decrease in the heart rate
   d. an increase in the amount of circulating glucagon

4. Glucagon secretion will result in _____.
   a. a decrease in the uptake of glucose by the brain
   b. a reduction in the amount of circulating glucose
   c. the cessation of metabolism of glucose by the cell
   d. an increase in the circulating blood glucose level

5. The signs and symptoms exhibited by the hypoglycemic patient are a direct result of _____.
   a. an attempt by the pancreas to increase the insulin secretion
   b. brain cell dysfunction and the release of epinephrine
   c. an increase in the amount of glucagon circulating in the blood
   d. a reduction in the insulin level and release of glucagon

6. The adult dose of $D_{50}W$ is _____.
   a. 2–4 mL/kg
   b. 0.5–1 g/kg
   c. 10 g
   d. 25 g

APPLIED PATHOPHYSIOLOGY

1. Explain the difference between type 1 and type 2 diabetes.

2. Explain the function of insulin and its effect on the blood glucose level.

3. Explain the function of glucagon and its effect on the blood glucose level.

4. Explain how a low blood glucose level affects the brain cells.

5. Explain the difference in the requirement for transport of glucose into a regular cell as compared with the brain cells.

6. Explain the two categories of signs and symptoms of hypoglycemia. List the signs and symptoms based on each category.

CLINICAL DECISION MAKING

You arrive on the scene and find a 23-year-old female patient in the bathroom of a bar. The patrons called 911 because the patient suddenly began to act strangely and became aggressive. She then fled to the bathroom, where she remains. As you approach the patient, she is sitting on the bathroom floor, slumped to her right side and talking incomprehensibly.

1. Based on the scene size-up, list the possible conditions you suspect.

2. What is your major concern when approaching this patient?

As you conduct the primary assessment, you note the patient is making incomprehensible sounds in an attempt to talk. Her airway is clear, and her respirations are 18/minute with good chest rise. Her radial pulse is 128 beats per minute (bpm), and her skin is pale, cool, and clammy. Her SpO_2 reading is 98 percent on room air.

3. Are there any immediate life threats?

4. What emergency care should you provide based on the primary assessment findings?

5. Explain possible causes for the incomprehensible sounds.

6. Explain possible causes for the pale, cool, and clammy skin.

7. Have you ruled out any conditions? What conditions are you still considering?

During the secondary assessment, you note no evidence of trauma to the head, the pupils are equal and reactive to light, and the mouth and nose are clear of any blood, vomitus, or secretions. The oral mucosa is pink. There is no evidence that the patient bit her tongue or oral cavity. There is no jugular vein distention, tracheal deviation, or subcutaneous emphysema. The breath sounds are equal and clear bilaterally, and the chest rise and fall are symmetrical. The abdomen is soft and nontender. You note multiple bruises to the abdomen in different areas. The peripheral pulses are present, and the patient moves all four extremities. The patient does not comply with a sensory test to the extremities. There is no evidence of trauma to the chest, abdomen, posterior thorax, or extremities. The blood pressure is 128/74 mmHg, heart rate is 132 bpm, and respirations are 18/minute with adequate chest rise. Her skin is more pale and cool. The patient is very diaphoretic. The blood glucose is 42 mg/dL. None of the bar patrons knows the patient well enough to provide any history.

8. Based on the assessment findings, what condition do you suspect?

9. Explain the reason for the following findings:
   a. Tachycardia
   b. Pale cool skin
   c. Diaphoresis
   d. Initial aggression
   e. Decrease in mental status
   f. Blood glucose level

10. What cells are getting glucose, and what cells are being deprived of glucose?

11. What emergency care should you provide?

Standard Medicine

Competency Integrates assessment findings with principles of epidemiology and pathophysiology to formulate a field impression and implement a comprehensive treatment/disposition plan for a patient with a medical complaint.

TOPIC

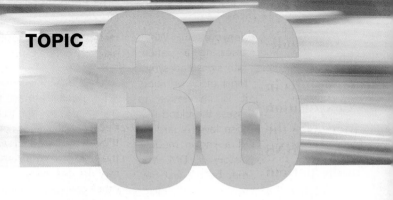

ENDOCRINE EMERGENCIES: HYPERGLYCEMIC DISORDERS

INTRODUCTION

Hyperglycemia refers to conditions in which the blood glucose is excessively elevated beyond a normal level. It is on the opposite end of the continuum of diabetic emergencies as compared with hypoglycemia. Two acute hyperglycemic conditions that paramedics will encounter in the prehospital environment are diabetic ketoacidosis (DKA) and hyperglycemic hyperosmolar nonketotic syndrome (HHNS). HHNS is also frequently referred to as hyperglycemic hyperosmolar nonketotic *coma* (HHNC).

DKA and HHNS must be considered while forming a differential diagnosis when assessing and managing a patient with an altered mental status. This is especially true if the patient has a history of diabetes mellitus (DM). However, be aware that the onset of DKA or HHNS may be the first sign of DM in a patient with no known history. Thus, it is imperative to obtain a blood glucose reading on any patient with an altered mental status, especially if the patient appears to be dehydrated, regardless of a positive or negative history of DM.

In addition to the blood glucose reading, the history—particularly the onset—and physical assessment findings will contribute to the formulation of a differential diagnosis and the appropriate emergency management of the patient.

EPIDEMIOLOGY

DKA most often occurs in type 1 DM. The onset is typically associated with some type of stressor to the body, such as trauma, infection, myocardial infarction, or stroke. Although it is not as common, DKA can occur in type 2 diabetes patients. In approximately 25 percent of cases of DKA, the patient has no known history of DM.

HHNS is most commonly found in elderly patients in their 70s who have type 2 DM; however, it has also been reported in pediatric patients as young as 18 months and in some with type 1 DM. The incidence of HHNS is higher than that of DKA, with 17.5 cases occurring for every 100,000 people. HHNS is slightly more prevalent in female patients than in male patients.

TRANSITION *highlights*

- *Frequency, age and gender distribution, and contributory causes of hyperglycemic episodes.*
- *The major pathophysiologic changes in a hyperglycemic patient with diabetic ketoacidosis:*
  - *Metabolic acidosis.*
  - *Osmotic diuresis.*
  - *Electrolyte disturbances.*
- *Symptomatology of diabetic ketoacidosis (DKA).*
- *Major pathophysiologic changes in a hyperglycemic patient with hyperglycemic hyperosmolar nonketotic syndrome (HHNS).*
- *Signs and symptoms associated with DKA and HHNS.*
- *Common emergency care steps for the hyperglycemic patient suffering from either DKA or hyperglycemic hyperosmolar nonketotic coma (HHNC).*

Elderly residents of nursing homes who have preexisting disease or an acute onset of illness—especially if associated with an infection, poor fluid intake, or an increase in urine output—and who are demented are at the highest risk for experiencing HHNS. The dementia typically causes poor fluid intake from a lack of recognition of dehydration. Any condition or illness that results in dehydration increases the risk of HHNS in the patient with type 2 DM, especially in the elderly. The mortality has been reported as high as 10 percent to 20 percent.

Approximately 20 percent to 33 percent of the patients who suffer an acute onset of HHNS have no previous history of DM. These patients are at the highest risk, as they often do not recognize the early warning signs and symptoms of the ensuing severe

> **Diabetic ketoacidosis most often occurs in type 1 DM.**

> **Any condition or illness that results in dehydration increases the risk of HHNS in the patient with type 2 DM.**

dehydration. When assessing a patient with signs and symptoms of dehydration, it is imperative to assess the blood glucose level regardless of a known medical history of DM. You may be the first person to initially diagnose the DM condition in the prehospital setting.

DIABETIC KETOACIDOSIS

Because of the variation in the pathology of the condition, the patient experiencing DKA presents significantly differently from one who is hypoglycemic. As with hypoglycemia, by understanding the basic pathophysiology of DKA, there is no need to memorize signs and symptoms in order to recognize and differentiate between the various conditions.

Pathophysiology of DKA

Unlike hypoglycemia, in which the insulin level is excessive and the blood glucose level is extremely low, DKA is associated with a relative or absolute insulin deficiency and a severely elevated blood glucose level, typically greater than 300 mg/dL. Because of the lack of insulin, tissues such as muscle, fat, and liver are unable to take up glucose. Even though the blood has an extremely elevated amount of circulating glucose, the cells are starving. Because the blood–brain barrier does not require insulin for glucose to diffuse across it, the brain cells are receiving more than an adequate amount of glucose.

Basically, the general body tissue is starving, whereas the brain has more than an adequate supply of glucose. Thus, the patient does not experience the sudden onset of mental status changes, cognitive and behavioral disturbances, or other brain cell dysfunction (neuroglucopenic) signs and symptoms associated with hypoglycemia.

Three major pathophysiologic syndromes associated with an excessively elevated blood glucose level in DKA contribute to the delay in onset and produce the majority of the signs and symptoms:

metabolic acidosis, osmotic diuresis, and electrolyte disturbance.

METABOLIC ACIDOSIS In *metabolic acidosis*, cells are not receiving an adequate fuel source to produce energy because of the lack of insulin. Even though the blood is loaded with glucose, the cells go into a starvation mode. This triggers the release of glucagon and other counterregulatory hormones that promote the breakdown of triglycerides into free fatty acids and initiate gluconeogenesis to produce more glucose for the starving cells. This further elevates the blood glucose level, as the body begins to metabolize protein and fat to produce a source of energy.

Because of the insulin deficiency and release of large amounts of glucagon, free fatty acids circulate in abundance in the blood and are metabolized into acetoacetic acid and B-hydroxybutric acid, both of which are strong organic acids and are referred to as *ketones*. Acetone, produced as acetoacetic acid, is metabolized and begins to accumulate in the blood. Small amounts of acetone are released in the respiration and produce the characteristic fruity breath odor.

In normal metabolism, ketones would be used as fuel in the peripheral tissue; however, because of the starvation state of the cells the ketones are not used. An increase in ketone production and a decrease in peripheral cell use lead to a metabolic acidosis that is referred to as *ketoacidosis*. This is reflected in a decreasing pH value, typically less than 7.40. The patient will also begin to eliminate large amounts of ketones through excretion in the urine.

OSMOTIC DIURESIS *Osmosis* refers to the movement of water (solvent) across a semipermeable membrane from a low particle concentration to a high particle concentration. *Diuresis* refers to urination, which is typically excessive. When the blood glucose level reaches approximately 225 mg/dL, a significant amount of glucose spills over into the urine. A glucose molecule (particle) produces an osmotic effect by drawing water across a semipermeable membrane. As an excessive amount of glucose enters the renal tubules, it draws a large amount of water, which ends up producing a significant amount of urine. This is known as *osmotic diuresis* and

leads to volume depletion and dehydration in the patient.

ELECTROLYTE DISTURBANCE Also collecting in the urine is a large amount of ketones. Because ketones are strong organic acids, they must be buffered in order to be excreted. Sodium is typically used as the buffer. Where sodium goes, water follows. Therefore, the sodium used to buffer the ketones also draws a large amount of water into the renal tubules, producing excessive urine and leading to further volume depletion and dehydration. The loss of large amounts of fluid because of osmotic diuresis leads to further *electrolyte disturbance* and the excretion of other electrolytes, such as potassium, calcium, magnesium, and phosphorus. This produces electrolyte imbalance and disturbances.

The term *diabetic ketoacidosis* literally explains what the patient is experiencing. The term *diabetes* is often thought of as dealing with a glucose derangement or imbalance. However, that is not true. *Diabetes* simply means an increase in urine output. Thus, the *diabetic* in DKA implies an increase in urine output that occurs from osmotic diuresis. The term *ketoacidosis* is fairly self-explanatory. It refers to the metabolic acidosis resulting from ketone production from fat metabolism.

The DKA patient is therefore prone to metabolic acidosis from ketone production, severe dehydration from osmotic diuresis, and electrolyte disturbances. These pathophysiologic syndromes produce the signs and symptoms exhibited by the patient.

Assessment Findings Associated with DKA

Unlike the hypoglycemic patient who experiences a sudden onset (within minutes) of signs and symptoms when the supply of glucose to the brain is severely depleted, the DKA patient's brain has a very large and abundant supply of glucose. The slow and gradual onset of signs and symptoms associated with DKA is related to the accumulating effect of the dehydration from osmotic diuresis and buildup of acid from ketone production. As the cells slowly become dehydrated and acidotic, the signs and symptoms begin to appear. As the brain cells slowly dehydrate and are affected by the increasing acidic state over hours to days, the mental status slowly begins to become altered.

Osmotic diuresis typically produces the classic signs and symptoms of hyperglycemia:

- Polyuria (excessive urination)
- Polydipsia (excessive drinking of fluids)
- Constant thirst
- Frequent urination at night

Osmotic diuresis leads to dehydration and a potential hypovolemic state from fluid loss, producing the following signs:

- Dry and warm skin
- Poor skin turgor
- Dry mucous membranes
- Tachycardia
- Hypotension
- Decreased sweating
- Orthostatic vital signs

Other signs and symptoms include the following:

- Nausea and vomiting
- Abdominal pain (especially in children, caused by gastric distention or stretching of the liver capsule)
- Fatigue
- Weakness
- Lethargy
- Confusion

Kussmaul respirations are deep and rapid respirations that are an attempt to compensate for the increasing ketoacidosis (▶ **Figure 36-1**). The deep and rapid respiratory rate blows off carbon dioxide. Carbon dioxide is necessary for the production of carbonic acid. With the decreased availability of carbon dioxide, less carbonic acid is produced, thereby increasing the pH value and allowing more ketoacids to accumulate.

Another common sign is a fruity or acetone odor on the breath. This is a direct result of small amounts of acetone being disposed of through respiration.

ECG changes and dysrhythmias may also result from the electrolyte disturbance.

HYPERGLYCEMIC HYPEROSMOLAR NONKETOTIC SYNDROME

HHNS is another emergency that the DM patient may experience. Although the condition is also commonly referred to as hyperglycemic hyperosmolar nonketotic coma (HHNC), fewer than 10 percent of patients with HHNS truly become comatose. As the name implies, this condition is associated with an excessively elevated blood glucose level and hyperosmolar extracellular fluid (ECF) without the production and accumulation of a mass amount of ketones in the blood. The primary pathophysiology associated with the condition produces severe dehydration and electrolyte disturbances.

Pathophysiology of HHNS

HHNS is associated with severe elevations in the blood glucose level, often exceeding 600 mg/dL, from an absolute or relative insulin deficiency or from a decreased response of the tissue to the circulating insulin (insulin resistance). This results in glycogenolysis, gluconeogenesis, and a decreased uptake of glucose by the peripheral tissue. A decline in renal function, which is typically found in elderly patients or in patients with renal disease, also contributes to a decrease in glucose clearance. Glycogenolysis may have a limited contribution to the hyperglycemic state, as many of the patients are debilitated or suffering from an acute illness and have a poor diet

for several days, causing the glycogen stores in the liver to be depleted over time.

The elevated blood glucose level creates a hyperosmolar extracellular space that begins to pull fluid and dehydrate the intracellular space. Initially, this influx of fluid into the intravascular space will maintain the blood pressure and perfusion. Once the blood glucose level exceeds 180 to 250 mg/dL, a significant amount of glucose spills off into the urine. As the osmotic diuresis continues, the intravascular volume is profoundly depleted, which further decreases renal perfusion and the ability of the kidneys to remove glucose from the blood. The average fluid loss is typically 9 to 10 liters in a 70-kg patient. A common cause of death is circulatory collapse.

Because of a change in the serum osmotic pressure, potassium, sodium, chloride, phosphate, magnesium, and bicarbonate may be depleted from the tissues, even though the serum electrolyte levels may appear to be normal or elevated. Sodium, potassium, phosphate, and magnesium are typically lost during the osmotic diuresis, leading to electrolyte imbalances.

Unlike a patient with DKA, the patient with HHNS does not develop ketoacidosis. There are many theories as to why there is a lack of ketogenesis; however, the exact cause is not well understood. It is thought that the continued secretion and availability of small amounts of insulin decrease the mass release of counterregulatory hormones and reduce the availability of free fatty acids needed to produce ketones. With no ketoacidosis, the patient will not present with Kussmaul respirations or a fruity (acetone) odor on the breath.

Pneumonia, chronic renal insufficiency, gastrointestinal bleeding, urinary tract infection, and sepsis are common precipitating factors of HHNS. Factors that stress the body, such as trauma and burns, will trigger a stress response, releasing a number of hormones (epinephrine, cortisol, and glucagon) that have a tendency to counter the effects of insulin and raise the blood glucose level. Other common underlying causes are:

- Stroke
- Myocardial infarction

> **Unlike a patient with DKA, the patient with HHNS does not develop ketoacidosis.**

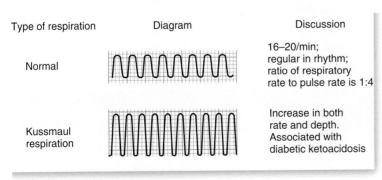

Type of respiration	Diagram	Discussion
Normal		16–20/min; regular in rhythm; ratio of respiratory rate to pulse rate is 1:4
Kussmaul respiration		Increase in both rate and depth. Associated with diabetic ketoacidosis

Figure 36-1 Kussmaul respirations.

- Intracranial hemorrhage
- Cushing syndrome
- Poor compliance with oral hypoglycemics or insulin therapy
- Hemorrhage
- Elder abuse or neglect, leading to underhydration
- Renal disease
- Dialysis
- Diuretics
- Beta blockers
- Histamine-2 (H_2) blockers
- Glucocorticoids
- Phenytoin
- Immunosuppressants

Assessment Findings Associated with HHNS

The clinical presentation of HHNS is related to volume depletion and dehydration with a slow onset of the signs and symptoms, usually progressing over a few days. In the early phase of HHNS, the signs and symptoms may be vague, such as leg cramps, weakness, and visual disturbances. As the blood glucose level continues to increase and the patient dehydrates further, the signs and symptoms usually progress in severity to include an alteration in the mental status. Other signs and symptoms include the following:

- Thirst
- Fever (may suggest sepsis or infection as the predisposing factor)
- Polyuria (early)
- Oliguria (often a late sign of a severe dehydrated state)
- Drowsiness, confusion, lethargy, or coma
- Focal seizures that may be continuous (epilepsia partialis continua) or intermittent
- Generalized seizures
- Hemiparesis or sensory deficits
- Tachycardia
- Orthostatic hypotension
- Hypotension (late signs of profound dehydration)
- Poor skin turgor (not a reliable sign in the elderly)
- Dry skin and mucous membranes
- Sunken eyes
- Excessively elevated blood glucose level

EMERGENCY MEDICAL CARE

The signs and symptoms of DKA and HHNS are much more similar to each other than to those of hypoglycemia (see Table 36-1). The focus in emergency care for hypoglycemia is administration of glucose, whereas in DKA and HHNS, the prehospital focus is on rehydrating the patient. Emergency care for both DKA and HHNS may include the following:

1. **Establish and maintain a patent airway.** If the patient presents with an altered mental status or is comatose, it may be necessary to establish an airway by a manual maneuver and, in patients with severely altered mental states, potentially with a mechanical device. Altered mental states may lead to aspiration of secretions and warrant the use of an advanced airway.

2. **Establish and maintain adequate ventilation.** If the patient's respiratory rate or tidal volume is inadequate, it is necessary to provide positive pressure ventilation.

3. **Establish and maintain adequate oxygenation.** Assess the patient for evidence of hypoxia. Apply a pulse oximeter and determine the SpO_2 reading. If either clinical evidence of hypoxia exists, the patient complains of dyspnea or exhibits signs or respiratory distress, or a SpO_2 reading of less than 95 percent on room air is present, administer oxygen via a nasal cannula at 2 to 4 lpm. Titrate the oxygen by increasing the liter flow and possibly changing the delivery device to maintain a SpO_2 greater than 95 percent, and abolish the signs of respiratory distress or complaint of dyspnea.

4. **Assess the blood glucose level.** In any patient with preexisting disease who presents with signs and symptoms of dehydration or an altered mental status, especially the elderly, the blood glucose must be checked, regardless of a positive history of DM. DKA and HHNS may be the first indication that the patient has DM. Even though the major complication of the disease

| TABLE 36-1 | Signs and Symptoms of Diabetic Emergency Conditions | | |

Sign or Symptom	DKA	HHNS	Hypoglycemia
Onset	Slow, over days	Slow, over days	Sudden, over minutes
Heart rate	Tachycardia	Tachycardia	Tachycardia
Blood pressure	Low	Low	Normal
Respirations	Kussmaul	Normal	Normal or shallow
Breath odor	Sweet and fruity	None	None
Mental status	Coma (very late)	Confusion	Bizarre behavior, agitated, aggressive, altered, unresponsive
Oral mucosa	Dry	Dry	Salivation
Thirst	Intense	Intense	Absent
Vomiting	Common	Common	Uncommon
Abdominal pain	Common	Uncommon	Absent
Insulin level	Low	Low	High
Blood glucose level	High	Very high	Very low

Emergency care and patient needs	DKA	HHNS	Hypoglycemia
Basic care	Oxygen	Oxygen	Oxygen, oral glucose
ALS care	Fluids	Fluids	IV glucose
Patient needs	More insulin	More insulin	Glucose

is severe dehydration, HHNS carries the highest mortality rate of the diabetic emergencies.

5. **Initiate an intravenous line of normal saline.** Draw blood according to your local protocol. If the patient is hypotensive, administer fluid to maintain the systolic blood pressure above 100 mmHg; otherwise, infuse fluid at a rate of 1 to 2 liters over 1 to 3 hours. In pediatric patients, administer a 20 mL/kg fluid bolus over 1 hour. Be sure to monitor the patient's breath sounds for an indication of fluid overload, especially in the elderly and those with heart disease. If the patient begins to complain of dyspnea, and crackles (rales) are heard in the posterior lower lobes, reduce the amount and rate of fluid being infused.

TRANSITIONING

REVIEW ITEMS

1. A sign that is common to both DKA and HHNS is _____.
   a. a fruity odor on the breath
   b. warm, flushed skin
   c. Kussmaul respirations
   d. dry oral mucosa

2. Orthostatic hypotension found in both the DKA and HHNS patient is caused by _____.
   a. vasodilation
   b. osmotic diuresis
   c. hyperventilation
   d. cellular hypoxia

3. A large amount of glucose in the vascular space will cause _____.
   a. interstitial fluid to be drawn into the vessel
   b. intravascular fluid to leave the vessel
   c. the vessel to constrict
   d. the vessel to dilate

4. The excessive blood glucose level seen in DKA is typically a result of _____.
   a. too little glucagon production
   b. an excessive amount of insulin
   c. an excessive amount of glucagon
   d. an inadequate amount of insulin

5. Why is metabolic acidosis not typically found in the HHNS patient?
   a. The blood glucose level is not as high as in DKA.
   b. The patient is still producing and secreting some insulin.
   c. Fat cannot be metabolized without insulin available to the cells.
   d. No fat is available for the liver to metabolize.

APPLIED PATHOPHYSIOLOGY

1. Explain the three major pathophysiologic conditions that occur in DKA.

2. Why is glucagon secreted from the pancreas in DKA when the blood glucose level is already significantly elevated?

3. Explain why the onset of the signs and symptoms of DKA occur over days, as compared with minutes in hypoglycemia.

4. Differentiate between the pathophysiology of DKA and HHNS.

5. What causes excessive dehydration in both DKA and HHNS?

6. Why doesn't the HHNS patient experience a severe metabolic acidosis as in the DKA patient?

CLINICAL DECISION MAKING

You are called to a residence and find a 14-year-old male patient lying supine in bed. The parents state that he has not been feeling well for the past week or so. He has gotten much worse over the past two days. The parents thought it was a virus their son picked up from school. As you approach the patient, he is not alert. His breathing appears to be extremely fast and deep.

1. Based on the scene size-up, list the conditions that are possible.

During the primary assessment, you find that the patient responds to verbal stimuli with incomprehensible words, has an intact airway, and has a respiratory rate of 32/minute. His breathing is very deep and full. His radial pulse is weak and rapid. His skin is warm, dry, and flushed. The SpO$_2$ reading is 99 percent on room air.

2. Are there any immediate life threats?

3. What emergency care should you provide based on the primary assessment findings?

4. Explain possible causes for the respiratory rate and tidal volume.

5. What do the skin signs indicate?

6. Have you ruled out any conditions? What conditions are you still considering?

As you perform the secondary assessment, you note no evidence of trauma to the head; the pupils are midsize, equal, and reactive to light; and the mouth and nose are clear of any blood, vomitus, or secretions. The oral mucosa is pink but excessively dry. The tongue is furrowed. You note a peculiar odor on the breath that smells like fruity gum. The jugular veins are flat with the patient in a supine position. There is no tracheal deviation or subcutaneous emphysema. The breath sounds are equal and clear bilaterally, and the chest rise and fall are symmetrical. The abdomen is soft; however, the patient makes a facial grimace when you palpate the right upper quadrant. The peripheral pulses are barely palpable, and the patient moves all four extremities to a painful stimulus. There is no evidence of trauma to the chest, abdomen, posterior thorax, or extremities. The blood pressure is 82/64 mmHg, heart rate is 136 bpm, and respirations are 34/minute with a deep and full tidal volume. The skin is warm, dry, and appears flushed.

The blood glucose is 482 mg/dL. The parents indicate that the patient has no known medical history and takes no medications. He has not been feeling good for the past week or so and has felt worse over the past few days.

7. Based on the assessment findings, what condition do you suspect?

8. Explain the reason for the following findings:
   a. Tachycardia
   b. Warm, flushed skin
   c. Decrease in mental status
   d. Blood glucose level
   e. Rapid deep respirations
   f. Hypotension
   g. Dry oral mucosa and furrowed tongue
   h. Right upper quadrant pain

9. Which cells are getting glucose, and which cells are being deprived of glucose?

10. What emergency care should you provide?

Standard Medicine

Competency Integrates assessment findings with principles of epidemiology and pathophysiology to formulate a field impression and implement a comprehensive treatment/disposition plan for a patient with a medical complaint.

TOPIC

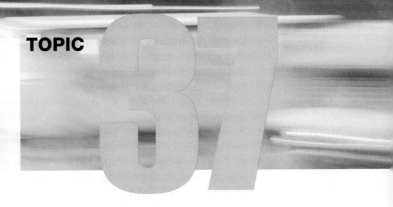

PSYCHIATRIC DISORDERS

INTRODUCTION

It is difficult to separate a person's physical and mental health into two categories because they are so interdependent. To make things even more complex, a physiological problem will often mimic the signs and symptoms of a behavioral emergency, and vice versa. The prevalence of psychological disorders in society is surprisingly high—but a history of a mental illness does not mean that someone is actively suffering from symptoms or will suffer from symptoms in the future. Many people with a psychological diagnosis function very well, both in society and in their own lives. The treatments available allow for many psychological disorders to be controlled, and they therefore often go undetected even to health care providers.

When health care providers are dealing with psychological emergencies, the patient is actively suffering from symptoms or in acute crisis. An important first step in dealing with a behavioral emergency is to quickly and safely identify life threats. These include identifying nonbehavioral causes that could create a change in someone's behavior and mentation. Once a field impression has been made that the person is having a behavioral emergency, a treatment can be devised that best fits the patient's needs and medical personnel's safety.

Legal and safety concerns are common with the treatment and transportation of this population. Determining when a behavioral patient has lost his autonomy is determined by individual state protocols and regulations. These often take into account whether the person in crisis is an *immediate* threat to themselves or others. Law enforcement is a resource often used for both safety and the transportation of persons nonvoluntarily.

PATHOPHYSIOLOGY

The brain is a complex system of neurons that communicate by releasing chemicals called *neurotransmitters*. Outside of having a proper level of neurotransmitters, the brain needs a constant supply of two vital substances to function properly: glucose and oxygen. Biological concerns that can create a shortage of glucose or oxygen can affect a patient's mentation. Stroke, hypoglycemia, hypoxia, traumatic brain injuries, and respiratory

emergencies all affect how oxygen and glucose reach the brain. Temperature can also affect the offloading of oxygen, so consider hypothermia and hyperthermia as possible causes of altered mental status as well.

People respond to their environment and to the events that transpire in their lives. Having an emotional response to a traumatic event is normal, and coping skills vary for each individual. Cultural differences can also contribute to misunderstandings between communicating parties. Some cultural differences may include a difference in body language or eye contact. In some cultures, genders may communicate or behave differently around one another. A female patient acting shy, for example, may be not an inappropriate response to a social setting, but more of a cultural norm. Some of the interactions in a social setting can include a person's affect, body language, and ability to communicate.

Injury or illness can create very different behaviors. Whether the injury is to the patient or to a person's loved one, events such as these can cause dramatic changes in a person's emotional state. The key to behavior being normal is that it is appropriate for the circumstances. It would be understandable, then, to have emotional behavior associated with illness and injuries. With injuries and some illnesses, expect that the person or loved one will be experiencing a physiologic response that increases sympathetic response from the nervous system. This increase of sympathetic tone in conjunction with an increase in stress could cause the person to show signs of anger, sadness, anxiety, or several other manifestations of behavioral emergencies. Expect unusual behaviors surrounding diagnoses of terminal illnesses from both the patient and his loved ones.

Substance abuse has been a long-standing problem and is often associated with patients with a history of mental illness. In the past, there had been a drive to see which came first, the mental illness or the substance abuse. Currently, they are typically treated simultaneously. Some substance abuse can also cause mental illness, such as inducing a psychosis or long-term changes in brain chemistry that result in depression or schizophrenia.

Substance abuse can include abuse of prescription or recreational substances. Defining when a substance use becomes an abuse is difficult, especially with substances such as alcohol that are widely used in society. Often definitions of substance abuse look at societal norms and how the use affects someone's physical and social well-being.

Dependence on a substance often has both a physiologic and a psychological base. Some psychological symptoms are due to a permanent or temporary change in the brain chemistry that the substance has caused. Dependence can be psychological as well, including a need for a particular substance in order to feel normal and/or function in life.

When a person is under the influence of a chemical substance, the ability to make appropriate decisions can be compromised. Motor skills can also be influenced, possibly affecting the way a person ambulates or is able to operate machinery. Patients under the influence of a chemical substance should be evaluated for their ability to make sound and responsible decisions surrounding their health care.

Keep in mind that some chemicals take more time than others to begin affecting the brain and body. Someone may seem fine and be able to answer questions, but 5 minutes later the effects of the chemicals may begin to impair the person. An example of this is would be a person who drinks several shots of hard alcohol. The liquor can be consumed rapidly but it will likely take time to enter the bloodstream before the effects begin to show. The amount of a chemical used and the route of entry of the drug can also affect the intoxication of a person.

Many people do not comply with their prescribed medications, whether they are blood pressure medications, antidepressants, or others. Aside from forgetfulness, people do not take their medications for a number of reasons, including an inability to afford medications or trying to avoid side effects. Not taking psychiatric medications as prescribed can have profound effects on a person's behavior, mentation, and mood. Physiologic withdrawals and effects may also ensue from stopping several of these medications.

The side effects of several psychiatric medications can influence a person's feelings, including decreasing sexual desires, decreasing the "high" feeling of manic periods, and sometimes creating a flat affect. Even though the benefits of most of these medications outweigh the side effects, this fact can be difficult for some patients to see while they are taking the medications. Some patients also feel that they have become better while using psychiatric medications, and go off them at that point.

EVALUATING ABNORMAL BEHAVIOR

Who gets to decide what normal behavior is and is not? The typical definitions for "normal" behavior look at whether behavior is acceptable to the people who know the patient and to the society in which the patient lives. They also look at whether the patient is a threat to himself or to others. Abnormal behavior must be placed in context, looking at the surrounding situation and events that the person is experiencing in his life. A grown woman who is inconsolable after the death of a child, for example, is likely experiencing a normal emotional response to the loss of a loved one. If the same woman is experiencing the same amount of distress at a coffee shop because it ran out of her favorite food item, she is having an abnormal response to a stimulus. Special considerations must also be given to someone's age, maturity, and culture. A three-year-old boy who begins crying over the same donut being sold out is acting appropriately for his age group and coping skills.

Psychiatric Disorders

Abnormal psychology encompasses a wide spectrum of disorders, each with specific criteria for being diagnosed. The *Diagnostic and Statistical Manual of Mental Disorders* (DSM; APA, 2000) is a reference used by the psychological field to diagnose behavioral and psychological disorders. Prehospital personnel do not diagnose psychological disorders, but should be aware of the symptoms associated with common diagnoses and categories of disorders. Background knowledge of this topic can help you understand the processes of certain mental illnesses.

COGNITIVE DISORDERS Cognitive disorders affect the way people think and process information. Cognitive disorders can include delirium, dementia, and memory-related disorders. The way that people think and process information is very complex. The specific category of thought disorders includes schizophrenia and psychosis. Schizophrenia tends to have an onset in late teenage years to early adulthood and has a large genetic component. Several types of schizophrenia exist, categorized by the symptoms present for each person. Symptoms can include positive (added) symptoms, such as visual or auditory hallucinations. Remember that hallucinations feel as real to the patient at the reality that we see and hear around us. Schizophrenia can also include changes in affect or behavior and can include paranoid or bizarre thought processes. Keep in mind that substance abuse and some medical conditions can create the same symptoms of both cognitive and thought disorders, which are especially important in an acute onset of symptoms.

MOOD DISORDERS Mood disorders are very common in the United States.

Some mood disorders, such as depression, have a genetic predisposition. A genetic predisposition means that the genetics for a disease process are present, but events in life may or may not trigger the disease process. Depression is categorized by a wide range of symptoms and the duration of the symptoms. Some of the symptoms can include decreased appetite, decreased enjoyment in activities that typically brought happiness, hypersomnia or insomnia, or a decrease in sexual activity. Some of these symptoms are natural grieving emotions after the loss of a loved one or a tragedy in one's life. Take into account whether the patient's behavior seems normal for the environment and the events of his life.

DELIRIUM   Delirium is defined as "the disturbance of consciousness and a change in cognition or perceptual disturbance, caused by substance-induced, substance withdrawal, multiple etiologies or other non-specified causes" (APA, 2000, p. 83). Risk factors for agitated delirium include a medical history or diagnosis of a cognitive disease, substance abuse, or withdrawing from a substance. Symptoms can include "reduced clarity of awareness of the environment, reduced ability to focus, disorientation, memory deficits, language disturbances and aggression" (APA, 2000).

BIPOLAR DISORDER   Bipolar disorder includes periods of depression and mania. Mania is a period of extreme energy. People often feel as though they need less sleep, and may act similarly to patients on a stimulant. Some manic patients will behave in risky manners, examples being sexual promiscuity or spending excessive amounts of money. These are often behaviors that are out of character for the person.

ANXIETY DISORDERS   Neurotic, or anxiety, disorders have a large environmental component. This means that the percentage of different populations with anxiety vary from area to area. Anxiety disorders include panic attacks, phobias, obsessive-compulsive disorder, and post-traumatic stress disorder, among others. Patients with anxiety-related symptoms often have the physiologic effects of activation of the sympathetic nervous system, including tachycardia, tachypnea, dilated pupils, and so on. Many of the symptoms are similar to those of a respiratory or cardiac emergency. Even a history of anxiety disorders or panic attacks does not rule out a respiratory or cardiac emergency in these patients.

Many anxiety disorders have a stimulus that triggers the anxious response. There is a wide range of stimuli for phobias, for instance, ranging from animals to inanimate objects to situations. Anxiety disorders look at a reaction being abnormal for a given situation. Normal behavior may include being anxious when a child is late for curfew. An abnormal situation for extreme fear or anxiety would be seeing a normally harmless animal or simply leaving one's home.

SUBSTANCE ABUSE   Substance-related disorders are divided into two groups according to the DSM: substance-induced disorders and substance use disorders. A wide range of legal and illegal chemicals are used. People can begin using at different ages and different times in their lives. People who begin using at a young age may develop this as a constant defense mechanism. Substance abuse is often seen as a dual diagnosis with a mental illness. The addiction or substance abuse is treated along with any mental illness diagnosis.

Substance use can induce delirium; persisting dementia; persistent amnesia; psychotic, mood, anxiety, sexual, and sleep disturbances; and persistent hallucinations. A provider does not need to recognize whether a mood disorder was caused by a history of substance abuse or other causes. It is important, though, to understand that the substances that enter the body can change the brain for a long-term or permanent duration and can cause some mental illnesses.

SOMATOFORM DISORDERS   Somatoform disorders deal with the body, or soma. Symptoms can include "pain in different parts of the body, physical complaints such as fatigue, hypochondriac behavior or a pre-occupation with a body image" (APA, 2000, p. 229). Realize that these patients' symptoms feel real to them. (Although it is not the job of prehospital personnel to diagnose a "real" or "fake" complaint, it is important to understand that some medical complaints are created by patients. The intention of the patient with a fictitious disorder is not isolated to looking for pain medications.)

IMPULSE CONTROL DISORDERS   Impulse control disorders involve a patient not being able to resist the urge to "start a fire, steal objects, gamble, assault someone, pull out one's hair, etc." (APA, 2000, p. 281). Typically, the impulsive act itself, if nonviolent, will not result in EMS being needed.

PERSONALITY DISORDERS   Personality disorders are very complex and wide-ranging. The general basis surrounding a personality disorder diagnosis is, "beginning in early adulthood or adolescence, the person's inner experience and behavior differ greatly from the expectations of their culture in ways of cognition, emotional response, interpersonal functioning, or impulse control" (APA, 2000, p. 287). These disorders range greatly in their symptomatology. Examples of personality disorders include paranoid, schizoid, antisocial, dependent, and obsessive-compulsive disorders.

SUICIDE AND SUICIDAL IDEATION   An important topic in prehospital involvement with behavioral emergencies is suicide and suicidal ideation (or suicidal thoughts). The patient may also have thoughts of worthlessness and a feeling of being helpless with no escape. Some patients will give away their possessions to loved ones when preparing for the act. Some patients have a feeling of peace once a suicide plan has been made. All patients who have attempted suicide should be taken seriously; the attempt should never be regarded as merely a cry for attention.

Be sure on all calls, including those for nonbehavioral emergencies, to document all comments made that resemble a suicidal ideation or an expression of giving up on life. It can be important to identify behavior and things said by these patients.

ABUSE AND NEGLECT   Some behavior, including violence, abuse, and neglect, has a learned component. This can explain some patterns in generations of families showing abusive tendencies. Just because children or family members are raised in these conditions, though, this does not mean that they will act in a similar way in life. When a patient has

> Many anxiety disorders have a stimulus that triggers the anxious response.

> **No assessment should be done that cannot ensure the safety of EMS crew.**

been a victim of abuse, several factors must be taken into account. As a health care worker, you are required to report abuse in certain patient populations. The victim's age is an important piece. Children and older adults fall into the mandatory reporting category for abuse, which includes neglect. It is important to be a strong patient advocate. The prehospital setting is unique in the ability to enter and see patient's living areas. This may be the only chance for someone to see a child's or elderly person's home and living conditions.

In the patient population for domestic abuse, the victims are often protected by privacy acts and seldom fall into the group of mandatory reporting. These patients can be difficult to assist, but all efforts should be made to advocate for them as well. One way is to offer a potential victim or domestic abuse the phone numbers for a local domestic abuse help center or hotline. Be sure to never confront an aggressor about any abuse and avoid making accusations or implications. Agitating an aggressor will not help the victim, and may place the person in more danger. Also consider law enforcement for all abuse calls.

Scene safety is imperative for health care providers and patients in these settings. Understand that domestic abuse is a very complex process, and quite often adult victims of domestic violence will not leave the perpetrator. Signs of abuse can include bruising, fractures, and other physical symptoms. Also look for nonverbal cues, such as a patient not wanting to answer questions or looking to a partner/parent for answers.

PSYCHOTIC BEHAVIOR Behaviors that are considered in the diagnosis of psychotic disorders include "delusions, hallucinations, disorganized speech and/or grossly disorganized or catatonic behavior" (APA, 2000, p. 153). If it is possible, determine whether the symptoms are chronic or acute. If the symptoms are acute, try to rule out possible organic causes while maintaining the safety of personnel. Substance abuse, as well as substance withdrawal, should be considered in these patients. Consider medical

causes, such as dementia, sepsis, hypoglycemia, and the like. Mental illness is another cause for psychosis. Mental illnesses can include psychotic symptoms as well. Various types of schizophrenia, for instance, include psychotic symptoms in their diagnosis. Other nonspecific mental illnesses have psychotic symptomatology associated with them.

In the prehospital setting, managing a patient with psychotic behavior can be difficult for the providers involved. These patients require extreme caution with regard to provider and patient safety. Auditory and visual hallucinations feel as real to the patient as the things other people normally see and hear. Never argue with the patient about his symptoms or play along in delusions. Include law enforcement in the management of these patients, and consider acceptable restraint devices for safety. (Always follow local guidelines for restraining patients.)

When interacting with patient's exhibiting psychotic symptoms, try to modify behavior in a similar way to approaching a patient with violent behavior. Modifications can include using nonaggressive body language and explaining all interventions to the patient before trying to complete them. Be cautious when approaching the patient. Consider the use of sedatives or antipsychotic medications as allowed by local protocols. Sedation can provide a safe transport for both the patient and providers.

This section has given a basic overview of both psychiatric and substance abuse diagnoses. Remember that there are very specific criteria that are used for each diagnosis of a psychiatric illness, and patients cannot be diagnosed definitively in the prehospital setting.

ASSESSMENT

When assessing a psychiatric patient, remember that abnormal psychology encompasses a huge variety of symptomatology and disease processes. The patient with panic attacks will require a very different assessment from the patient with paranoid schizophrenia. A general approach can be used to assess psychiatric patients, though, to help and maintain a safe environment and rule out some pertinent negatives. Each patient's individual needs should be assessed.

First and foremost, the safety of the EMS crew must be maintained from the start of the call to the end. No assessment should be done that cannot ensure the safety of EMS crew. If a patient presents a safety hazard, law enforcement should be requested before the assessment continues. The secondary consideration is the safety of the patient and the bystanders.

Once all safety considerations have been made, the patient should be assessed for biological and psychiatric causes for the change in behavior. Biological causes of an altered mental status and cognitive impairment must be ruled out. These impairments include any chemical or physical process that causes oxygen or glucose deprivation to the brain, or that changes the natural chemistry of the brain and body. Some of these include hemorrhagic and ischemic strokes, traumatic brain injuries, hypoglycemia, hyperglycemia, hypothermia, hyperthermia, respiratory emergencies, cardiovascular emergencies, hypoxia, substance abuse, and seizures. The assessment should include mental status, cognitive exams, oxygen saturation, vital signs, ECG, pupillary response, and temperature. Do not forget to tell your patient when you are physically assessing and touching him, even for things as simple as taking his blood pressure.

Assessing mental status is very important in a psychiatric patient. The first thing to assess is whether the patient is conscious. The mnemonic AVPU (alert, verbal, painful, and unresponsive) is a good tool for initially assessing consciousness. The Glasgow Coma Scale can also be used as a tool when assessing mental status. Next, assess whether the patient is oriented. Orientation can be assessed by evaluating whether the patient knows himself, his location, the events surrounding the incident, and the relative time.

Patients have varying energy and activity levels. Assessing a patient's activity can be done by asking both the patient and any bystanders or family members if the patient's activity levels have been normal. Is the patient more hyperactive than usual, or does he have less energy? For patients with an increase in activity and energy, assess whether they are physically sitting still or moving all around an area.

Assess the patient's speech. Part of the speech assessment will include whether or not the patient is slurring his words or unable to repeat phrases. (Remember that strokes can present with similar symptoms to those of a behavioral emergency.) Second, assess whether the speech is organized and understandable. If the speech appears to be very disorganized or the topics become disconnected, record and present this finding. Disorganized thoughts may present through disorganized speech. The patient's ability to process thoughts and maintain a continuous thought process is important in distinguishing which type of mental illness is present.

Memory impairment is an important cognitive finding. To assess a patient's memory, ask about recent events in his life, as well as past events. Questions can include asking what month it is or having the patient recall what he had for breakfast. If someone familiar with the patient is available, ask what the patient's baseline for remembering events is. If the patient is not oriented, ask whether the patient has a history of any illnesses that affect memory, such as dementia or Alzheimer disease.

A patient's affect and mood are also very important assessment points. Some types of schizophrenia are categorized by a flat affect, or no reaction and emotion. A patient in distress or showing signs of violence is an important finding. A patient who talks about feeling hopeless and worthless may have the symptoms of clinical depression.

People's perceptions of the events in their lives will be different. Some clinical findings for perceptions include whether people helping the patient are being perceived as a threat. Something as simple as a patient perceiving that everything is going wrong in life is a clue to the patient's thought process.

Physiologic changes will be different for individual illnesses. For a manic patient, expect tachycardia, high energy, and high levels of alertness. For a patient experiencing depression, ask about weight gain or loss in the past few weeks or months, changes in sleep patterns, or a decrease in energy.

Recognizing that patients come from different social backgrounds is important. Some patients have a large support network of family and friends, whereas others are very much alone. Some patients are also very introverted and may normally be shy to answer questions. Obtain a social and medical history of the patient if the patient, or someone familiar with the patient, is able to provide one.

Even though some patients are dishonest in medicine, it is a good start to ask the patient if he has feelings of wanting to hurt himself or others. You will be surprised at the honesty of patients when they are asked questions in a compassionate way. Take into account whether a patient has made comments to others about wanting to hurt themselves. If a patient is an immediate threat to himself or others, he must be evaluated at a hospital.

Approaching Aggressive Psychiatric Patients

People have a natural startle reflex that causes them to tighten their muscles and prepare to fight when startled. This reflex is a great example of how violence is, in some ways, inherent to one's natural need to defend oneself. When some people feel, scared, sad, or extremely emotional, they can show signs of violence. When assessing a patient with a behavioral emergency, keep in mind that several psychiatric disorders alter a patient's emotions, and sometimes his physical senses as well. For this patient population, anticipate that the patient may be scared or angry, or may have hallucinations, even when there is no trigger that can be identified by medical personnel.

When approaching any patient, especially the patient in an acute behavioral emergency, be aware of behaviors that can indicate violence. These can include increasing the volume when speaking, body language and stance that appear aggressive, tachycardia, tachypnea, and verbal threats of violence. If someone appears to be violent or if his behavior seems to be leading to violence, confrontation can make things worse. Safety is the number one concern for EMS personnel. Always maintain safety of the medical crew; leave the scene if necessary until adequate resources can be allocated to maintain safety. Never stay at a scene that becomes unsafe.

Resource Fatigue

Providers deal with many psychiatric patients who are "regulars." This can be understandably exhausting for health care resources. It is acceptable to recognize the frustration surrounding this small subset of patients who require more assistance on a regular basis. Remember, though, that there is an enormous population of people diagnosed with psychiatric disorders who will never require an ambulance or hospitalization. It can also be helpful to think of psychological diseases as largely chemically based, and not the choice of the patient.

In the population that requires more help, even at two o'clock in the morning, an empathetic response is imperative. The patient's experience in the prehospital setting can affect whether he will ask for help again, especially when dealing with suicidal ideations. The old idea that a person who wants to kill himself will not ask for help is both ridiculous and inaccurate. A warm smile from someone wanting to help can be the difference in the experience for these patients. It is also important to let them know that resources are available to them when they do not feel safe.

MANAGEMENT

For patients with any signs of violent behavior, communicate in a nonaggressive manner. Crisis intervention skills can help with deescalating a patient. Realize, though, that all patients react differently. Be conscious of body language that appears annoyed or impatient. Many patients may just need someone compassionate and willing to speak with them. Try to turn down portable radios and pagers, to decrease background noise. Never tell a patient you know how he feels. Even if you have been through exactly the same circumstance, this does not mean that you know how that individual patient feels. Consider providing crisis numbers for patients, especially those who have recently lost a loved one.

Transportation decisions can be difficult in nonvoluntary patients. The typical criteria for a mandatory transport assess whether the patient is an immediate threat to himself or to others. If a patient appears to need transport and is refusing, contact local medical direction and law enforcement. Under these criteria, law enforcement can take a patient into protective custody. Typically, patients in protective custody do not have a right to refuse treatment or transport. Always follow local protocols.

Restraints

If it is determined that force or restraints will be needed to maintain crew and patient safety, a plan should be devised on how to restrain this particular patient. A few different restraint methods are available; each has its purpose. It is important to understand the gravity of restraining a person and taking away his autonomy. During any restraint process, talk to your patient and explain what you are doing and why you are doing it. Follow state protocols for restraining a patient, which may include obtaining permission from a physician or law enforcement for using restraints.

When physically restraining someone, use additional resources, including law enforcement and multiple people, to assist. It is not safe for only two providers to try to restrain a patient. Once a decision has been made to restrain a person, discuss with one another how you are going to approach the patient. Use soft restraints or manufactured restraints if they are available. If using any restraint that affects the chest, use multiple straps to prevent restriction of the patient's chest wall. Never restrain your patient face down, and constantly reassess your patient's airway. Being restrained inappropriately can cause positional asphyxiation.

Even if physical restraints are needed, consider the addition of chemical restraints such as benzodiazepines. These medications can be an effective way to maintain patient and provider safety. Sedation can often be given in conjunction with physical restraints and may be administered as an intramuscular injection.

Tasers are another restraint option for those trained in using them. Some patients are too out of control to be safely restrained by any other means. Other restraint devices should be used after other methods have been exhausted, though.

Medication

Some patients receive pharmacologic treatments for mental disorders. These include several classes of medication and are used for a variety of different symptoms. Antidepressants are used to treat depression and related disorders. Several types of antidepressants are

available, but almost all of them increase the levels of serotonin and norepinephrine in the brain. These two chemicals in the brain are what produce happy feelings in the body.

Amphetamines, antipsychotics, and phenothiazine are also used to treat psychiatric disorders. Amphetamines are stimulants that can be used to treat hyperactive disorders such as attention deficit hyperactivity disorder (ADHD). Antipsychotics and phenothiazines can be used for people experiencing psychotic symptoms or extreme distress.

As previously discussed, noncompliance with medications is a large problem in this population. Even though the benefits outweigh the side effects with most medications, that can be difficult for psychiatric patients to understand. Side effects can affect people's personality, mood, sexual desire, and the like. It is sometimes difficult for patients to understand the benefits of being on a medication when they no longer have the symptoms of the illness and are left only with the side effects. The problem is that when medications are stopped, the symptoms often return from the disorder; the patient can also undergo withdrawals from the medication.

Schizophrenia can also be a difficult disorder for medication compliance. If someone with schizophrenia does not want to be on medications and he is not an immediate threat to himself or to others, there is no way to force treatment. This can be hard on families who want to have a loved one to be in treatment, but legally have no right to force him into treatment. Antipsychotics, sedatives, and some other medications can be used in an emergency setting. Antidepressant medications often take weeks to begin taking effect, however.

Documentation

In behavioral emergencies and mental illness calls, documentation is imperative. Document in quotes things that the patient said. Document your full assessment, including the patient's presentation and affect. If the patient's behavior seems abnormal, even on a nonbehavioral call, document it and report it to the receiving staff. Give an oral report to the receiving medical facility, as well as a

written copy of any findings. What happened in the prehospital setting can be important in deciding the patient's treatment plan. If any restraints or nonvoluntary transportation were implemented, document all resources used and the reasons for doing so. Poor documentation in these cases can create legal implications for the providers involved.

Communicating abuse in mandatory reporting populations must be done in accordance with state protocols. It is not enough to document and/or give an oral report of the abuse to a receiving facility. A mandatory report must go to the local department of human services personnel as well. This must be done by every person who believes there is abuse. Often, a hotline or phone number is available in the hospital. Be sure to personally call if abuse is suspected in children, older adults, mentally handicapped patients, and other special populations. There is a moral and legal obligation to do so.

SPECIAL POPULATIONS
Pediatrics

The use of psychiatric medications in pediatric patients up through age 18 is difficult. Many medications work differently in children and teenagers and can actually make some disorders worse. Antidepressants can cause suicidal ideation in patients under the age of 18. This can be a difficult struggle for psychiatrists in this population. Pediatric patients typically have fewer coping skills than most adults for events in their lives. Some disorders begin in childhood and continue through adulthood, so document any findings in your assessment that may appear as abnormal behavior.

Geriatrics

It is important to pay careful attention to the tone and affect of older adults. These patients are at risk for suicidal ideations and depression, but this can often be overlooked. Ask these patients about their social lives and support networks. Convey and document any signs of hopelessness, depression, or other psychiatric findings to the hospital receiving staff.

REVIEW ITEMS

1. Which of the following best describes the definition of "normal" behavior?

    a. appropriate for the circumstances

    b. calm and quiet

    c. matching those around the patient

    d. matching expectations of the evaluating providers

2. Which of the following is a reference used by the psychological field to diagnose behavioral and psychological disorders?

    a. The *Diagnostic and Statistical Manual of Mental Disorders*

    b. The *Manual of Acute Psychiatric Crisis*

    c. The *Registry of American Mental Disorders*

    d. The *Psychiatric Digest*

3. Which of the following is considered a cognitive disorder?

    a. acute anxiety

    b. depression

    c. delirium

    d. bipolar disorder

4. A patient who complains of unexplained pain in different parts of the body, physical fatigue, or hypochondriac behavior would most likely be suffering from _____.

    a. a cognitive disorder

    b. an anxiety disorder

    c. a somatoform disorder

    d. delirium

5. When evaluating a patient with psychiatric hallucinations, the most important aspect of the assessment would be _____.

    a. ensuring the safety of the EMS crew

    b. identifying organic causes of the hallucinations

    c. informing the patient that the hallucinations are not real

    d. differentiating the specific psychiatric cause

APPLIED PATHOPHYSIOLOGY

1. Psychological disorders are not physiological diseases—true or false? Explain your answer.

2. What treatment methods are used for clinical depression?

3. What substances used by a patient can mimic manic behavior?

CLINICAL DECISION MAKING

A 44-year-old male patient has been found by his family to be acting abnormally. The family states that he has been abusive and has hallucinations and "garbled" speech. On arrival, you see patient pacing back and forth on his porch and shouting curses.

1. Does this situation present a safety threat to the approaching EMS providers?

2. What clues can be identified from the scene assessment that this situation is potentially unsafe?

As you await law enforcement arrival, the patient's family members approach you and provides some background on the situation. They note that the patient has been acting strangely for about 12 hours. They tell you that he is significantly worse tonight. They also note that the patient has a long history of schizophrenia and may not be taking his medications.

3. Are there medical conditions that could account for this presentation? If so, what are some of the most important concerns?

4. Does the history provided by the family point to a behavioral issue? If so, why?

RESOURCES

American Psychological Association (APA). *Diagnostic and Statistical Manual of Mental Disorders.* 4th ed., Text Revision. Washington, DC: American Psychiatric Association, 2000.

Deglin, J., and A. Vallerand. *Davis's Drug Guide for Nurses.* Philadelphia: E. A. Davis Co., 2000.

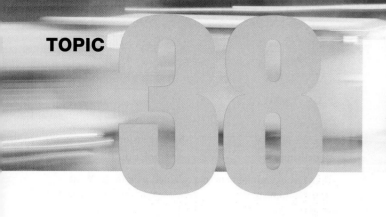

TOPIC

Standard Medicine

Competency Integrates assessment findings with principles of epidemiology and pathophysiology to formulate a field impression and implement a comprehensive treatment/disposition plan for a patient with a medical complaint.

HEMATOLOGY

TRANSITION *highlights*

- *The ethnic predisposition and frequency in which blood disorders occur in the United States.*

- *Types of cells found in the blood (red and white), and the role of platelets.*

- *Disorders and disease processes that can afflict the blood:*
  - Red blood cell diseases:
    - ◆ Anemia.
    - ◆ Sickle cell disease.
    - ◆ Polycythemia.
    - ◆ Thalassemia.
  - White blood cell diseases:
    - ◆ Leukopenia/neutropenia.
    - ◆ Leukocytosis.
    - ◆ Leukemia.
    - ◆ Lymphoma.
  - Platelet diseases/clotting disorders:
    - ◆ Thrombocytopenia.
    - ◆ Thrombocytosis.
    - ◆ Hemophilia.
    - ◆ Von Willebrand disease.
    - ◆ Disseminated intravascular coagulation.
    - ◆ Multiple myelomas.

- *Brief overview of basic assessment findings.*

- *General treatment interventions for a patient suffering from a hematologic disorder.*

INTRODUCTION

Hematology is the study of the blood and blood products. Blood consists of plasma, red blood cells, white blood cells, and platelets. Various medical conditions result from changes associated with these components. Lab tests, combined with history and physical exams by physicians, are needed to accurately diagnose hematologic conditions.

EPIDEMIOLOGY

Hematologic conditions are common but do not often present as the primary complaint of patients in the prehospital environment. Some conditions are not very common in the overall population but are more prevalent in a specific population. For example, one of the more common hematologic conditions encountered by the paramedic in the prehospital environment is sickle cell disease, also known as sickle cell anemia. Sickle cell anemia occurs in about 1 in every 400 African Americans in the United States. The sickle cell trait is found in 8 percent to 10 percent of African Americans in the United States.

PATHOPHYSIOLOGY

The composition of the blood is a primary factor associated with hematologic conditions. It is necessary to understand the basic functions of each of the blood components to gain a better understanding of hematologic disorders.

Blood is composed primarily of plasma, red blood cells, white blood cells, and platelets. *Plasma* is the pale yellow liquid portion of blood; it is composed primarily of water but also contains proteins, chemical messengers, gases, salts, and other nutrients. Plasma transports the cellular components throughout the body and conveys the cellular waste products to the kidneys, lungs, and liver to be removed.

Red blood cells, or *erythrocytes*, are disk-shaped cells responsible for the transport of oxygen from the lungs to the tissues and carbon dioxide transport in the reverse direction. Red blood cells contain *hemoglobin*, a protein chemical that contains iron, which is bright red in color. Oxygen transport is influenced by the amount of hemoglobin, its oxygen affinity, and blood flow (▶ Figure 38-1).

White blood cells, or *leukocytes*, are the body's primary defense against infections. They are capable of moving outside the bloodstream to reach tissues being invaded by microbes.

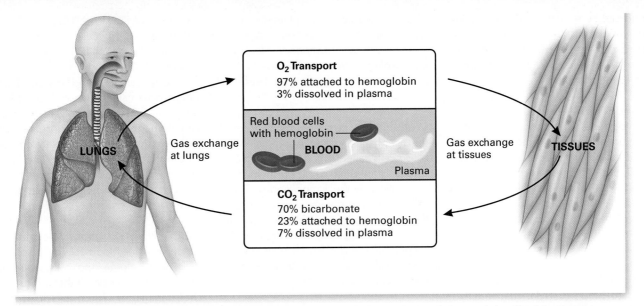

Figure 38-1 Oxygen is transported in the blood in two ways: attached to hemoglobin and dissolved in plasma. Carbon dioxide is transported in the blood in three ways: as bicarbonate, attached to hemoglobin, and dissolved in plasma.

The five major types of white blood cells are basophils, eosinophils, lymphocytes, monocytes, and neutrophils. When an infection occurs, the number of white blood cells within the body will significantly increase.

Platelets, or *thrombocytes*, are cell-like particles that help in the clotting process. They gather at a bleeding site and clump together to form a hemostatic plug. They also release substances that help promote further clotting.

Red Blood Cell Diseases

ANEMIA *Anemia* is a condition defined by a reduced number of red blood cells that results in a decreased ability to carry oxygen effectively in the blood. The types of anemia are listed in Table 38-1. Blood loss, lack of red blood cell production, or high rates of red blood cell destruction are the three main causes of anemia. These causes may stem from a number of disorders, such as vitamin deficiencies or other factors.

Mechanisms that help maintain tissue oxygenation in patients with gradual onset of anemia include peripheral vasodilation, increased cardiac output, change in the oxygen–hemoglobin dissociation curve, and the shunting of blood away from circulation-rich organs to critical organs. With severe or long-lasting anemia, the lack of oxygen in the blood can damage the heart, brain, and other organs of the body.

SICKLE CELL DISEASE *Sickle cell disease* is an inherited blood disorder that results in the production of abnormal hemoglobin. The hemoglobin deoxygenates and clumps together, causing the red blood cells to become stiff and develop a crescent or C shape or sickle form. These sickle-shaped cells can block blood vessels and can prevent adequate oxygenation of the tissues, contributing to severe pain and organ damage.

Sickle cell crises, or *vaso-occlusive crises*, are episodes of pain resulting from the blockages that are usually followed by periods of remission. Illness, physical stress, cold temperature, or being at high altitudes may increase the risk of a crisis. The most serious dangers associated with a sickle cell crisis are acute chest syndrome, long-term damage to major organs, stroke, and complications during pregnancy, such as high

TABLE 38-1	Types of Anemia	
Cause	**Type**	**Pathophysiology**
Inadequate production of red blood cells	Aplastic	Failure to produce red blood cells.
	Iron deficiency	Iron is the primary component of hemoglobin.
	Pernicious	Vitamin B_{12} is necessary for correct blood cell division during its development.
	Sickle cell	A genetic alteration, in low oxygen states, causes production of a hemoglobin that changes the shape of red blood cells to a C, or sickle.
Increased red blood cell destruction	Hemolytic	Body destroys red blood cells at a rate greater than production; red blood cell parts interfere with blood flow.
Blood cell loss or dilution	Chronic disease	Hemorrhage leads to cell loss; excessive fluid leads to a dilution of red blood cell concentration.

blood pressure in the mother and low birth weight in the infant. The mean life expectancy for people diagnosed with sickle cell anemia is 48 years for women and 42 years for men.

POLYCYTHEMIA *Polycythemia*, or *erythrocytosis*, is a condition resulting from an abnormally high level of red blood cells in the blood. The increase is usually due to an excess production of red blood cells. Pseudoerythrocytosis may appear secondary to dehydration. The higher the red blood cell levels, the greater is the risk of thrombosis in the individual.

THALASSEMIA *Thalassemia* is an inherited blood disorder that results in the decreased production of hemoglobin and red blood cells. It usually affects people of Mediterranean or Asian ancestry. Severe thalassemia is normally identified by the age of 2 years. Signs and symptoms include pallor, anorexia, listlessness, and jaundice.

White Blood Cell Diseases

LEUKOPENIA/NEUTROPENIA *Leukopenia* is the condition involving too few white blood cells. This indicates a problem with either production of white blood cells in the marrow or the destruction of white blood cells. *Neutropenia* is said to exist when a patient's peripheral neutrophil count is lower than usual. Yemenite Jews and black individuals have an increased risk of developing neutropenia. Neutropenia is most commonly induced by chemotherapeutic agents.

LEUKOCYTOSIS *Leukocytosis* is the condition involving too many white blood cells. Leukocytosis is usually caused by a bacterial infection or arises when the body is particularly stressed—for example, because of rheumatoid arthritis, diabetic ketoacidosis, pain, or exercise.

LEUKEMIA *Leukemia* is a cancer of the bone marrow and blood that results from the rapid production of abnormal white blood cells. These cells are unable to fight infection and impair the production

> **Most of the symptoms of blood disorders are vague and nonspecific.**

of red blood cells and platelets in the bone marrow. The two main types of leukemia are called *lymphocytic leukemia* and *myelogenous leukemia* based on the predominant blood cell type. Leukemia can be acute or chronic.

LYMPHOMA *Lymphoma* is a cancer of the lymphatic system. Abnormal white blood cells called *lymphocytes* form cancerous lymphoma cells, which multiply and collect in the lymph nodes. These cells can impair the immune system and the body's ability to fight infection. The two main types of lymphoma are Hodgkin lymphoma and non-Hodgkin lymphoma. About half the blood cancers that occur each year are lymphomas.

Platelet Diseases/Clotting Disorders

THROMBOCYTOPENIA *Thrombocytopenia* is an abnormal decrease in the number of platelets. It can be caused by a decrease in the number of platelets produced in the blood marrow, sequestration of platelets in the spleen, or destruction of the platelets. Some medications, including heparin, contribute to thrombocytopenia.

THROMBOCYTOSIS *Thrombocytosis* is an increase in the number of platelets. This is usually caused by an increase in the production of platelets. This condition is often seen with leukemias, autoimmune disorders, and acute hemorrhage.

HEMOPHILIA *Hemophilia* is a blood disorder in which one of the proteins necessary for blood clotting is missing or defective. This results in the blood not clotting properly and increases the risk of severe hemorrhage from what would appear to be a minor injury. Males are affected more than females. Patients with hemophilia may suffer from damage to their joints, tissues, and organs caused by internal bleeding and typically present with acute painful swelling in the joint (hemarthrosis).

VON WILLEBRAND DISEASE *Von Willebrand disease* is an inherited disease that results from a deficiency or defect in the body's ability to make von Willebrand factor, a protein that helps blood clot. Von Willebrand disease is usually milder than hemophilia and can affect both males and females.

DISSEMINATED INTRAVASCULAR COAGULATION *Disseminated intravascular coagulation* (DIC) is a condition in which blood clots form throughout the body's small blood vessels. These blood clots can reduce or block blood flow through the blood vessels, which can damage the body's organs. This reduces the number of platelets and clotting factors in the blood needed to control bleeding, and excessive bleeding occurs. DIC is typically seen late in severe infections.

MULTIPLE MYELOMA *Myeloma* is a cancer of white blood cells called plasma cells. In myeloma, the cells overgrow, forming a mass or tumor that is located in the bone marrow. These cells may spread to other bones in the body. These abnormal cells interfere with the production of normal blood cells and the body's ability to fight infection. Kidney damage, bone destruction, and fractures can result from myelomas.

ASSESSMENT FINDINGS

Patients who have hematologic problems often present with various signs and symptoms. Most of the symptoms of blood disorders are vague and nonspecific. Symptoms that may suggest an underlying blood disorder include fatigue, weakness, shortness of breath, bleeding or bruising easily, headache, dizziness, confusion, jaundice, and many others. Obtaining a good history and anticipating complications from a hematologic condition is very important.

EMERGENCY MEDICAL CARE

Emergency medical care for patients with hematological emergencies is primarily supportive. Patients may present with a wide variety of signs and symptoms, based on their underlying condition, that require emergency medical care. The emergency care may include the following:

- **Establishing and maintaining a patent airway.** This may require the insertion of a mechanical airway device or suction if necessary.
- **Administration of oxygen based on the patient's presentation.**

Maximize oxygenation in a patient suspected of having a vaso-occlusive crisis. If the patient is breathing adequately, use a nasal cannula or nonrebreather mask. Use a ventilation device in the patient who requires ventilation.

- **Provide positive pressure ventilation** if the tidal volume or respiratory rate is inadequate.
- **Control external hemorrhage.** Anticipate complications from these disorders, and treat the patient for shock if indicated.

- **Consider analgesia.** Patients in sickle cell crisis will be in extreme pain. When local protocol allows, consider analgesics such as fentanyl to reduce acute pain.
- **Initiate transport** and provide comfort measures.

TRANSITIONING

REVIEW ITEMS

1. A patient presents with excessive bleeding from a small laceration on the forearm, which has not been easily controlled by direct pressure. Based on that initial finding, you should suspect _____.
   a. anemia
   b. hemophilia
   c. leukemia
   d. lymphoma

2. Which of the following blood components contains hemoglobin?
   a. plasma
   b. red blood cells
   c. white blood cells
   d. platelets

3. Leukocytes respond to infection by _____.
   a. increasing hemoglobin production
   b. decreasing clotting factors
   c. decreasing in number
   d. increasing in number

4. Which of the following conditions results when excessive clotting is followed by excessive hemorrhage?
   a. disseminated intravascular coagulation
   b. von Willebrand disease
   c. non-Hodgkin lymphoma
   d. myelogenous leukemia

5. Clotting is primarily a function of which blood component?
   a. erythrocytes
   b. thrombocytes
   c. leukocytes
   d. plasma

APPLIED PATHOPHYSIOLOGY

1. List four compensatory mechanisms used to help maintain tissue oxygenation in patients with gradual anemia.

2. What are the two major classifications of lymphoma?

3. Explain the difference between thrombocytopenia and thrombocytosis.

4. Explain how a vaso-occlusive crisis occurs in a patient with sickle cell anemia.

CLINICAL DECISION MAKING

You are dispatched to a residence for a patient complaining of severe pain in his legs. After determining the scene to be safe, you approach the patient, a 19-year-old African American male, who is sitting in bed and appears to be in significant pain. No apparent mechanisms of injury are present, and the patient denies any trauma.

The primary assessment reveals that the patient is anxious, alert, and oriented. He has a respiratory rate of 24/minute with adequate chest rise and fall. The patient has a strong radial pulse of 120 beats per minute. The skin is pale, very warm, and dry. The SpO$_2$ reading is 90 percent.

1. What are the life threats to this patient?

2. What immediate emergency care should you provide based on the primary assessment?

The patient states he is having severe pain in his legs. He says that the pain began two days ago and has continued to get worse. He reluctantly admits that he called now because he has had a painful erection for the past four hours that has not gone away.

3. List the possible conditions you suspect the patient may be experiencing.

4. What cultural considerations might influence your care for this patient? Why?

During the secondary assessment, the patient also complains of dizziness, fatigue, and weakness. You note jaundice in the sclera of his eyes. The abdomen is soft and nontender, pelvis is stable, and there are ulcers on the lower extremities. No deformities are noted to the extremities. The patient does have a priapism. His peripheral pulses are present. The patient has no known allergies, has a history of sickle cell disease, and states he used to take prescribed medication for the pain but has not been able to afford it for the past couple of months. He has been drinking a lot of water and ate some cereal for breakfast about five hours ago. He admits to taking 800 mg of Motrin for the pain after breakfast. His blood pressure is 160/92 mmHg, heart rate is now 112 beats per minute, and his respirations are 20 per minute.

5. What conditions are you considering as a probable cause? Why?

6. Based on your differential diagnosis, what are the next steps in emergency care? Why?

Standard Medicine

Competency Integrates assessment findings with principles of epidemiology and pathophysiology to formulate a field impression and implement a comprehensive treatment/disposition plan for a patient with a medical complaint.

TOPIC

39

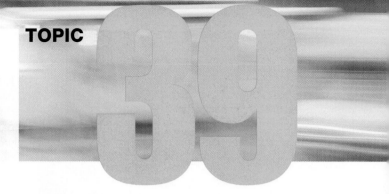

GENITOURINARY AND RENAL DISORDERS

INTRODUCTION

Normal function of the renal and genitourinary system plays a vital role in supporting life. The ability of these systems to do their job affects a variety of other body systems and plays an important role in maintaining homeostasis. The circulatory system is affected by fluid balance and the ability of the kidneys to excrete excess water. The nervous system is affected by the adrenal glands, which are housed on the kidneys, and the blood itself benefits from the renal and genitourinary systems' ability to filter toxins and excrete waste products. Injuries and illness to the renal and/or the genitourinary system therefore pose a major threat to the body. This topic discusses the role of the renal and genitourinary systems and disorders that threaten their vital function.

EPIDEMIOLOGY

Kidney disease affects about 20 million people in the United States. An estimated 11.5 percent of adults over the age of 20 have physiologic evidence of chronic kidney disease. Approximately 350,000 Americans receive dialysis for end-stage renal disease every year. More than 33 billion dollars in public and private spending has been used in the treatment of kidney failure. More than 50,000 Americans die each year from kidney disease.

A variety of other genitourinary disorders affect patients each year, but by far the most common is the urinary tract infection (UTI). UTIs account for more than 7 million hospital visits in the United States each year. These infections are more common in women than in men and more common in adults than in children, but their effects are widespread. It is estimated that roughly 40 percent of women will contract a UTI in their lifetime. Although most of these infections are benign, UTIs are currently the leading cause of sepsis.

PATHOPHYSIOLOGY

The major functions of the kidneys and the genitourinary system include the production and elimination of urine from the body. The kidneys also play a role in homeostasis by regulating the body's pH (acid–base levels) and electrolytes, controlling the

TRANSITION *highlights*

- *Frequency and mortality rates for renal diseases in the United States.*
- *Overview of normal renal function and its role on homeostasis.*
- *Pathophysiologic changes that can occur with renal disease and overview of common renal conditions:*
  - *Kidney stones.*
  - *Renal failure (acute and chronic).*
- *Role of dialysis as therapy for renal patients:*
  - *Hemodialysis (done in a medical facility).*
  - *Peritoneal dialysis (done in the home).*
- *Important assessment findings when caring for a patient with kidney stones or renal disease.*
- *Treatment strategies the paramedic can employ when caring for a patient with a renal emergency.*

blood volume, eliminating waste products, and regulating the blood pressure.

Traumatic and nontraumatic causes can damage the kidneys and affect their ability to function properly. Inflammation, infection, physical obstruction, and hemorrhage can cause renal emergencies. Many toxins, such as overdoses of aspirin, can destroy kidney function. The kidneys are also quite sensitive to changes in perfusion. In a state of peripheral vasoconstriction, as occurs in prolonged compensated shock, the lack of blood flow to the renal system can cause organ death and system failure.

In general, renal disorders can be subdivided into categories that describe the nature of their dysfunction. Prerenal conditions include decreased blood flow to the kidneys (as in shock or occlusion). Intrarenal conditions include disease or damage within the kidneys themselves (as in trauma or cancers). Postrenal problems occur when there is a blockage to the urine-collecting

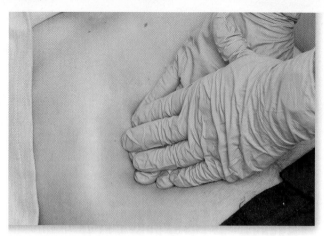

Figure 39-1 Patients who experience a renal emergency may complain of abdominal, flank, or lower back pain, or tenderness on palpation.

system. An example of this type of condition would be kidney stones.

> **Many patients who experience renal or genitourinary emergencies will complain of abdominal or flank pain.**

Disorders of the genitourinary system include problems affecting the ureters, the bladder, the urethra, and the external genitalia. Just as with the kidneys' obstruction, infection, inflammation, and trauma can lead to a disruption of function.

Initially, many patients who experience renal or genitourinary emergencies will complain of abdominal or flank pain (▶ **Figure 39-1**). It is not necessary to try to pinpoint the exact cause of the pain, but it is necessary to assess and manage the patient properly based on the presentation.

Renal Conditions

Three of the most common renal emergencies that will be seen in the prehospital environment involve kidney stones, renal (kidney) failure, and dialysis-related emergencies. Dialysis and kidney transplantation may be necessary for patients who have kidney failure.

KIDNEY STONES *Kidney stones*, or *renal calculi*, are crystals of substances such as calcium, uric acid, struvite, and cystine that are formed from metabolic abnormalities (▶ **Figure 39-2**). Renal calculi are believed to originate in the kidneys and must pass through the rest of the urinary system to be eliminated from the body.

Visceral pain noted unilaterally in the flank is normally followed by severe pain as the stone is dislodged and passes through the ureter into the bladder. Hematuria is a common finding when the stone is being passed, although this is commonly seen only by testing the urine.

Lithotripsy or other surgical interventions may be necessary if the patient is unable to pass the stones on his own. If left untreated, renal calculi can lead to loss of kidney function, obstruction of the urinary tract, or kidney damage.

RENAL (KIDNEY) FAILURE *Renal failure*, or *kidney failure*, occurs when the kidneys fail to function adequately. The two main types of kidney failure are acute renal failure and chronic renal failure.

- *Acute renal failure (ARF)* normally occurs over a period of days and often results from a significant decrease in urine elimination. Causes of ARF include decreased blood flow to the kidneys, trauma, cardiac failure, surgery, shock, sepsis, and urinary tract obstruction. It is imperative that this condition be identified as soon as possible because, depending on the cause and extent of the damage, it is sometimes reversible. Some patients with ARF will require dialysis. If left untreated, ARF can lead to life-threatening metabolic derangements.

- *Chronic renal failure (CRF)* normally occurs over a period of years and results from a permanent loss of nephrons (the functional units of the kidneys). The causes of CRF are numerous; however, diabetes and hypertension are linked to a majority of the cases. CRF leads to an accumulation of waste products and fluids that cannot be removed from the

body properly. These uremic changes can affect every organ system in the body. CRF is a permanent and life-threatening condition. Symptoms of CRF range from mild at first to severe when end-stage renal failure develops. Patients ultimately will require dialysis or a kidney transplant for survival.

Dialysis *Dialysis* is an artificial process used to remove water and waste substances from the blood when the kidneys fail to function properly. It generally works through osmosis and filtration of fluid across a semipermeable membrane. In general, the blood containing waste products passes on one side of the membrane while a dialysate (special fluid used for dialysis) passes on the other side. When this occurs, the water and waste products travel from the blood across the membrane and into the dialysate, thus removing the waste from the patient.

The two major types of dialysis are hemodialysis and peritoneal dialysis.

- **Hemodialysis.** In hemodialysis, a machine containing the dialysate is connected to an access site on the patient. The access site may be a shunt, fistula, port, or graft. The patient's heparinized blood is then pumped through the access site and

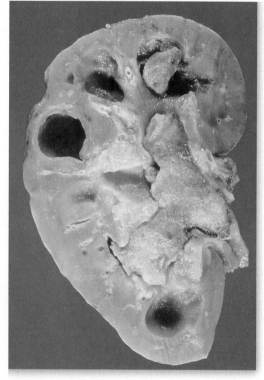

Figure 39-2 Sectioned kidney with kidney stones. (© *SIU/Photo Researchers, Inc.*)

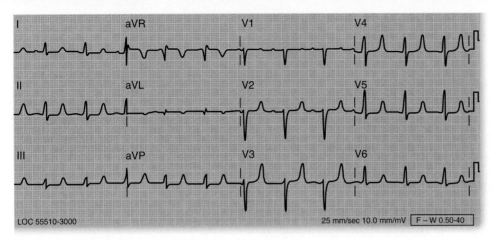

LOC 55510-3000   25 mm/sec 10.0 mm/mV F – W 0.50-40

Figure 39-3 Peaked T waves associated with hyperkalemia.

into the machine, where the waste is removed. The paramedic should *not* take the blood pressure of a dialysis patient on the side of the patient's access site. In general, care must be taken not to occlude the access site.

- **Peritoneal dialysis.** In peritoneal dialysis, the dialysate is run through a tube into the patient's abdomen. The peritoneal membrane functions as the semipermeable membrane. The fluid remains in the abdomen for several hours so it can absorb the wastes, and then it is drained out of the body through a different tube.

Although dialysis provides a necessary treatment for patients with kidney failure, it has risks that can result in life-threatening complications such as hypotension, muscle cramps, peritonitis, hemorrhage, infection, or cardiac arrest. If they miss their dialysis treatments, patients who require dialysis also may experience life-threatening problems, such as elevations in potassium or pulmonary edema.

HYPERKALEMIA The chief cause of hyperkalemia (increased potassium in the body) is renal failure. This condition is life threatening because of the important role potassium plays in the heart. Hyperkalemia can occur chronically or acutely, but typically occurs in the context of kidney damage or disease. Severe mental status changes are common, as are peaked T waves on an electrocardiogram (ECG) (▶ Figure 39-3). In end stages, widened QRS complexes can also occur. Hyperkalemia patients are at high risk for cardiac arrhythmias and should be constantly reassessed to identify these issues.

Genitourinary Conditions

Many conditions impair genitourinary function but are not related to the kidneys. When we think of these types of disorders, we typically consider problems that interfere with the movement of urine from the kidneys to the outside world. As stated, problems can involve trauma obstruction, inflammation, or infection.

URINARY TRACT INFECTIONS Urinary tract infection (UTI) is the most common genitourinary disorder. An infection can occur high in the system and affect the kidneys themselves (pyelonephritis) or occur lower in the system and affect the bladder (cystitis) or the ureters (urethritis). Generally speaking, the higher the infection, the more serious the condition.

Indwelling catheters are the leading cause of UTI. In this case, bacteria from the catheter are introduced into an otherwise sterile environment and causes infection. Other common causes include sexual activity (especially in women) and incomplete emptying of the bladder, such as occurs in men with enlarged prostate glands.

The specific symptoms of a UTI include difficulty with urination. Some patients report frequent urination (polyuria), whereas others complain of difficult or painful urination. UTIs in children (especially infants) are often difficult to diagnose, as they frequently lead to generalized discomfort and restlessness. Other symptoms include signs of infection such as fever, chills, and altered mental status.

Most UTIs will be handled easily by the immune system. Antibiotic administration is commonly effective in treating the root cause of a UTI, but immunosuppressed patients and patients with increased resistance to antibiotic therapy are at high risk. As a UTI initiates a systemic inflammatory response to fight the ongoing infection, sepsis can progress rapidly.

ASSESSMENT FINDINGS

After ensuring a safe scene, it is important to determine whether the patient has been injured or is suffering from a medical illness. Some patients may become dizzy or weak and may fall as a result of their medical condition. Remember that dialysis patients may be on heparin, a blood thinner.

Form a general impression of your patient and determine whether the patient is alert and oriented. An altered mental status may reflect changes occurring as a result of the disease process. Renal failure can cause altered mental status through a variety of mechanisms. Acid–base balance problems, rising uric acid levels, dehydration, and infection can all play a role in an unusual mental status. Pay attention to the airway, ventilation, oxygenation, and circulation as well.

Kidney failure and metabolic derangements can affect every organ system in the body and may precipitate shock or other life threats. Because of this, aggressive management of any potential life threats is necessary. Priority transport should be provided if the patient has a poor general appearance, has an altered mental status, shows signs of shock, or is in severe pain.

When gathering a history, in addition to the standard information collected, be sure to inquire about the following:

- How long has the patient been sick or suffering from these signs and symptoms?
- What is the patient's medical history? When was the last time he saw a doctor for his medical condition? Has he had any surgeries?
- Is there any genital pain or discharge? If so, what are the color, consistency, and odor like?
- Is there a change in urine? If so, what are the color and odor like?
- Does the patient receive dialysis? If so, when was the last treatment received? When is the next treatment due?

- Does the patient have any abdominal, pelvic, or flank pain?
- Has the patient had any nausea or vomiting? If so, when and how much?
- Does the patient have any pain associated with urination, defecation, or sexual intercourse?

The physical exam will focus primarily on genitourinary complaints and will normally involve the abdominal and pelvic area. Because renal conditions can affect other body systems, though, you must assess them all. Perform the physical examination of the abdomen carefully and gently. Begin by inspecting and palpating the abdomen. Determine whether there is any bleeding, pain, or tenderness. You should also note whether a urinary catheter is in place.

Obtain and document the patient's vital signs. Hypertension or hypotension may exist based on the underlying cause. Remember that hemodialysis patients are commonly slightly hypotensive as a baseline. Make sure that you do not obtain a blood pressure in the arm with the fistula or shunt. Decreased blood pressure, tachycardia, and pale, cool, moist skin are indicators of shock.

> **Do not obtain a blood pressure in an arm with a fistula or shunt.**

When performing your physical exam, you may find a variety of signs and symptoms, depending on the cause of the emergency. Some common signs and symptoms of renal emergencies include the following:

- Urine with an abnormal color, consistency, or odor
- Abdominal, pelvic, or flank pain or tenderness
- Malaise, nausea, and vomiting
- Fever or chills
- Syncope or altered mental status
- Pain or burning during sexual intercourse, urination, or bowel movement
- Frequent or urgent need to urinate or decreased urine output
- Blood in the urine (hematuria)
- Edema of the feet, ankles, and/or legs

- Hypertension or hypotension
- Anorexia
- Tachycardia

EMERGENCY MEDICAL CARE

Do not try to isolate the exact cause of abdominal or pelvic pain or a renal condition. Correctly assess and identify the signs and symptoms and provide the proper emergency medical care.

1. **Maintain manual spinal stabilization** if trauma is suspected.
2. **Keep the airway patent.** Always be alert for vomiting and the potential for aspiration. It may be necessary to place the patient in the left lateral recumbent position to protect the airway if the patient has an altered mental status. Be prepared to suction.
3. **If breathing is adequate, administer oxygen based on the SpO$_2$ reading and patient signs and symptoms.** If the SpO$_2$ reading is greater than 95 percent and no signs or symptoms of hypoxia or respiratory distress are present, oxygen may not be necessary. If signs of hypoxia or respiratory distress are present, or the SpO$_2$ reading is less than 95 percent, place the patient on a nonrebreather mask at 15 liters per minute (lpm).
4. **Control any major bleeding if present;** recheck the access site for bleeding in a dialysis patient.
5. **Place the patient in the position of comfort if no trauma is suspected.** If spinal stabilization is required, fully immobilize the patient on a backboard. If signs or symptoms of shock are present, place the patient in a supine position. If pulmonary edema is suspected, place the patient in an upright position.
6. **Calm and reassure the patient.** Be supportive and nonjudgmental.
7. **Initiate a quick and efficient transport.**
8. **If an IV is initiated, do so en route to the hospital.** Do not use an arm that has a shunt for IV access. Use caution with IV fluid administration. Administer fluid boluses cautiously

to patients with renal failure and to those on dialysis.

9. **Continuously monitor and reassess your patient.**
10. **Prevent renal failure**—aggressively manage shock patients and prevent hypotension. Remember that poor perfusion associated with compensated shock is a leading cause of renal failure.

Care for Kidney Stones

Kidney stones are often described as one of the most painful disorders a patient can experience; unfortunately, EMS can do little to resolve the issue. In most cases, kidney stones will pass through the system and resolve on their own, but until they do, they can cause knee-buckling pain.

Occasionally, judicious fluid administration can help ease pain, but there is little more than anecdotal evidence to support its use. Analgesia is very important in this group, and, in fact, is probably the most important treatment a paramedic can provide. Consider fentanyl, morphine, or other medications to ease pain.

In severe cases, kidney stones can lead to infection and even sepsis. Be on guard for the signs of shock that can occur in such disorders.

Care for Urinary Tract Infections

UTIs in and of themselves are typically not an acute or emergent problem. Most patients simply need antibiotics and supportive care to resolve the infection. However, as previously stated, UTI is the leading cause of sepsis; as such, providers should be particularly on watch to recognize the systemic effects of an ongoing infection. Signs of systemic inflammatory response, such as tachycardia, altered mental status, increased temperature, increased blood glucose, and increased respiratory rate, can point to systemic infections and severe sepsis. Consider also the use of lactate monitors to identify underlying anaerobic metabolism and shock associated with sepsis.

These patients will need emergent treatment and high quantities of isotonic fluids. See Topic 25, "Sepsis," for more information.

REVIEW ITEMS

1. A patient presents with severe unilateral flank pain. Based on that initial finding, you should suspect the patient most likely will also present with _____.
   a. warm and dry skin
   b. tachycardia
   c. bradycardia
   d. hypotension

2. Which of the following is commonly associated with chronic renal failure?
   a. hypotension
   b. Graves disease
   c. diabetes mellitus
   d. Crohn disease

3. About how many Americans are affected by kidney disease?
   a. 5 million
   b. 10 million
   c. 15 million
   d. 20 million

4. Kidney stones can usually be composed of all of the following *except* _____.
   a. calcium
   b. potassium
   c. uric acid
   d. cystine

5. Severe pain from renal calculi is most commonly experienced as the stone passes through the _____.
   a. kidney
   b. ureter
   c. urinary bladder
   d. urethra

APPLIED PATHOPHYSIOLOGY

1. List the primary functions of the kidney.

2. Explain the difference between acute renal failure and chronic renal failure.

3. Differentiate between hemodialysis and peritoneal dialysis.

4. What complications could occur if chronic renal failure is left untreated?

5. Explain why dialysis or kidney transplantation is necessary if a patient has end-stage renal failure.

CLINICAL DECISION MAKING

You are called to a residence for a 28-year-old male patient with abdominal pain. On arrival, you encounter the patient pacing on the front porch of his residence with his hands on his back. You note that he appears to be in significant distress and there is no sign of trauma. As you determine the scene is safe, you approach the patient, who states that he is in severe pain.

1. Based on the scene size-up characteristics, list the possible conditions you suspect the patient is experiencing.

The primary assessment reveals that the patient is anxious, restless, alert, and oriented. He has adequate respirations at a rate of 22/ minute with good chest rise and fall. His radial pulses are strong and regular at a rate of 112 beats per minute. His skin is pale, cool, and clammy. The SpO2 reading is 95 percent.

2. What are the life threats to this patient?

3. What immediate emergency care should you provide based on the primary assessment?

4. What conditions are you still considering as the possible cause? Would you add any conditions as a possible cause?

During the secondary assessment, you note no signs of any traumatic injuries. The patient states that he was playing basketball when he suddenly had a severe pain in his lower back. He said the pain started about 15 minutes earlier and that he has vomited because of the pain. He describes the pain as the worst in his life and says it feels like it is moving down into his groin. He denies any head, neck, or chest pain. His abdomen is soft and tender on palpation. He says that when he urinated it was bloody and painful. His pelvis is stable, and no deformities or trauma to the extremities are evident. The patient has no known allergies or past medical problems, and he takes no prescription medication. He states that he had eaten a sandwich and drank bottled water about an hour prior to your arrival. His blood pressure is 134/72 mmHg, heart rate is now 106 beats per minute, and his respirations are 16/minute.

5. What conditions have you ruled out in your differential field diagnosis? Why?

6. What conditions are you considering as a probable cause? Why?

7. Based on your differential diagnosis, what are the next steps in emergency care? Why?

TOPIC
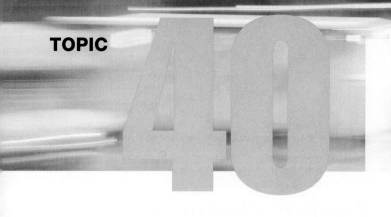

Standard Medicine

Competency Integrates assessment findings with principles of epidemiology and pathophysiology to formulate a field impression and implement a comprehensive treatment/disposition plan for a patient with a medical complaint.

GYNECOLOGIC EMERGENCIES

TRANSITION highlights

- *Frequency and types of gynecologic emergencies encountered in the United States.*

- *Pathophysiologic changes that occur with select gynecologic emergencies likely to be encountered in the prehospital environment:*
  - Vaginal bleeding (traumatic and nontraumatic).
  - Pelvic inflammatory disease.
  - Pregnancy.
  - Sexual assault.

- *Review of important physical assessment findings when caring for a patient with a gynecologic emergency.*

- *Treatment strategies the paramedic can employ when caring for a patient with a gynecologic emergency.*

INTRODUCTION

Gynecology refers to the study of female health and the female reproductive system. A variety of gynecologic emergencies may cause abdominal pain, vaginal bleeding, or discharge. These emergencies can be both medical and traumatic in nature. If left untreated, gynecologic conditions can deteriorate into life-threatening complications. Knowledge of the female reproductive system and its function is pertinent for accurate assessment, differential diagnosis, and treatment of these conditions. Take time to review the anatomy of the female reproductive system (▶ Figure 40-1).

EPIDEMIOLOGY

More women every year are taking steps to improve their overall health. Each year an estimated 19.4 million women receive a preventive gynecologic examination. Even with routine preventive screenings, though, gynecologic emergencies can arise. Pathophysiology specific to vaginal bleeding, traumatic vaginal bleeding, pelvic inflammatory disease, pregnancy, and sexual assault is discussed in the next section.

PATHOPHYSIOLOGY

Vaginal Bleeding

Vaginal bleeding is a common chief complaint among women requesting emergency medical care. Normal vaginal bleeding occurs cyclically in women who have achieved menarche. This typically starts at approximately 12 to 13 years of age and continues until the onset of menopause, around the age of 51. The regularity of the menstrual cycle is dependent on a complex feedback mechanism involving the hypothalamus, pituitary gland, uterus, and ovaries. Duration of the normal menstrual cycle is an average of four days, with a blood loss of approximately 50 mL.

Abnormal vaginal bleeding occurs in women of all ages and can result from a variety of causes, such as anatomic abnormalities, complications of pregnancy, malignancies, infection, systemic diseases, and endocrine imbalances.

Approximately 5 percent of women 30 to 45 years of age will seek medical attention for abnormal non-pregnancy-related vaginal bleeding, also known as *dysfunctional uterine bleeding*. Thirty percent of all women report having prolonged or excessive uterine bleeding occurring at regular intervals.

Dysfunctional uterine bleeding is more prevalent in extremes of age during the reproductive years. It also affects 50 percent of premenopausal women. There is no distinction among races; however, black women have a higher incidence of uterine fibroids, which inherently cause vaginal bleeding.

Obtain an accurate history of the chief complaint to establish the extent of the emergency at hand. Question the patient as to when the bleeding started. Ascertain whether the bleeding started at the scheduled onset of a menstrual period. Ask the patient about the volume and duration of the bleeding. Useful information includes the number of tampons or pads changed over the preceding 12 to 24 hours.

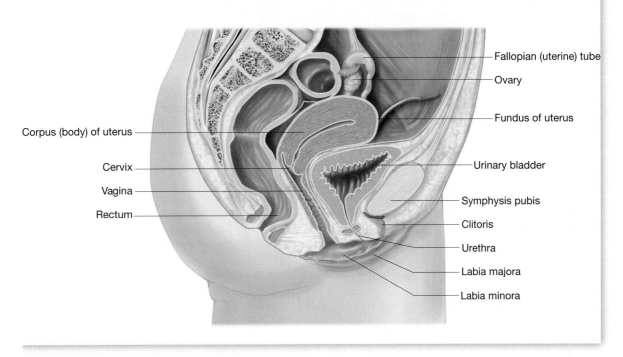

Figure 40-1 Anatomy of the female reproductive system.

A tampon or pad holds an average of 20 to 30 mL of vaginal effluent. Women with heavy bleeding typically change pads or tampons a minimum of every three hours. Determine whether the pads are saturated and whether blood clots are present. Clots with a diameter of greater than 1 cm are associated with menstrual blood loss of at least 80 mL.

Do not discount the possibility of the patient being pregnant. Has the patient missed a period? Some bleeding may actually occur during implantation of the embryo, making the patient believe that the bloody vaginal discharge is her normal period. Does she have unprotected sex? Has she had sexual intercourse since her last menstrual cycle? Obtain a menstrual history in the premenopausal patient to include the date of the last period, any change in the frequency of periods, whether the flow is usually heavy or prolonged, and whether the patient has had similar episodes of bleeding. A gynecologic and obstetric history should include methods of contraception, the outcome of all prior pregnancies (miscarriages, abortions, and deliveries), pregnancy complications, and previous pelvic infections.

The physical exam is aimed at determining the amount of blood loss and attempting to identify the underlying etiology of the bleeding. Inspect the abdomen for a mass or distention and palpate to localize the area of abdominal tenderness. Baseline vital signs are obtained to assess hemodynamic stability. Postural changes in vital signs can be indicative of the patient's volume status. Hypotension and tachycardia, as well as pale skin and conjunctiva, are indicative of hypovolemic shock and require aggressive management.

Traumatic Vaginal Bleeding

Although obstetric-related trauma is the most common cause of injury to the female genital tract, nonobstetric trauma is also common. Vaginal lacerations and traumatic vaginal bleeding occur more often than recognized. These lacerations can result in significant blood loss and life-threatening hypovolemic shock if not properly managed.

Vaginal lacerations not related to childbirth vary greatly in comparison with obstetric lacerations. Nonobstetric vaginal lacerations are generally classified into two groups. The first group is associated with the first encounter of sexual intercourse, or even with normal sexual intercourse. This results in a relatively minor laceration to the vagina and resolves with minimal or no treatment. The second group of vaginal lacerations is deeper, more extensive, and causes copious vaginal bleeding. These lacerations can lead to significant blood loss and require rapid intervention.

Seventy-five percent of the vaginal lacerations reported by women who are requesting emergency medical care require repair. These patients present with marked vaginal bleeding. In addition, an average of 15 percent of these patients have perineal and/or lower abdominal pain. Hemorrhagic shock manifests in 15 percent of these cases.

The most common mechanism of injury for nonobstetric vaginal lacerations is sexual intercourse. Predisposing factors that can account for this injury are virginity, disproportion of male and female genitalia, insertion of foreign bodies, previous surgery, stenosis or scarring of the vagina from congenital abnormalities, and vaginal atrophy in postmenopausal women. Be certain not to discount the possibility of sexual assault in these patients. Many women with these injuries are embarrassed and do not seek help until self-treatment is unsuccessful. These patients then present late with significant blood loss and impending hypovolemic shock.

Noncoital reproductive tract injuries can include blunt and penetrating trauma. Traumatic vaginal bleeding can be the consequence of trauma to the abdomen, especially trauma involving pelvic fractures.

> **Do not discount the possibility of the patient being pregnant.**

Straddle injuries are also known to cause substantial vaginal laceration and bleeding. Although straddle injuries are more commonly seen in children with bicycle injuries, these injuries can be seen in adults involved with activities such as water or jet skiing.

Physical exam and emergency care of traumatic vaginal bleeding should focus on accurate assessment and treatment of clinical presentation. Swiftly determine the cause and amount of hemorrhage. Place a pad to help absorb the hemorrhage, but do not pack the vagina. Obtain baseline vital signs, and establish the effects of blood loss to the patient. Expeditiously transport the patient, and frequently reevaluate for signs and symptoms of shock.

Pelvic Inflammatory Disease

Pelvic inflammatory disease (PID) is a community-acquired infection of the upper female reproductive system, which includes the uterus, fallopian tubes, and neighboring pelvic structures. PID is a serious condition initiated by an infectious process that ascends from the vagina and cervix. The inflammatory response and infectious process can result in endometritis, salpingitis, oophoritis, peritonitis, or tubo-ovarian abscess. A delay in diagnosis and treatment of PID can lead to chronic pelvic pain, adhesions, and even infertility (▶ Figure 40-2).

PID is the most common serious infection reported among women 16 to 25 years of age. In the United States, 1 million women are estimated to experience an episode of PID per year. It has a higher incidence in white females of a lower socioeconomic status. An estimated 10 percent to 20 percent of untreated gonorrheal and chlamydial infections turn into PID. More than 100,000 women are estimated to become infertile each year because of this condition. However, only 0.29 of every 100,000 women 15 to 44 years of age succumb to PID. The most common cause of death in these cases is secondary to rupture of a tubo-ovarian abscess.

Evaluation of risk factors for sexually transmitted disease (STD) and risk factors that increase the probability for PID can be helpful in the diagnosis of this condition. Risk factors for STD include age less than 25 years, nonbarrier contraception or oral contraception, multiple or symptomatic sexual partners, and first intercourse at a young age. Factors that potentially facilitate PID include a history of the disease, sex during menses, vaginal douching, bacterial vaginosis, and the use of an intrauterine device.

This community-acquired infection is typically caused by an STD. *Neisseria gonorrhoeae* and *Chlamydia trachomatis* are usually identified in women with PID. Gonococcal disease tends to have a rapid onset of symptoms, whereas chlamydial disease has a more insidious onset. Lower abdominal pain is the cardinal presenting symptom in patients with PID, experienced by 90 percent of patients. Pain that worsens with coitus and jarring movement or after menses is also suggestive of PID.

On exam, abdominal pain is usually diffuse in the lower quadrants and may or may not be symmetrical. Rebound tenderness and decreased bowel sounds are also common findings. In addition to abdominal pain, abnormal uterine bleeding occurs in one-third of patients with PID. Other associated signs and symptoms that are not specific to PID but are typically present include purulent vaginal discharge, fever, and chills. Purulent vaginal drainage is seen in approximately 75 percent of patients.

Pregnancy

A woman's reproductive years start at the onset of menstruation and end at the cessation of menstruation, or menopause. When evaluating a female patient in her reproductive years, it is important to remember the possibility of her being pregnant. In some cases, the patient's current complaint is the first sign that she is pregnant. In the United States each year, more than 6 million women are clinically recognized as being pregnant.

Most women experience signs and symptoms of pregnancy as early as three weeks after conception. The cardinal sign of pregnancy is amenorrhea or absence of menstrual flow. Pregnancy should be suspected whenever a woman of childbearing age has a cessation of menstruation or delay of menstruation greater than one week. In addition to amenorrhea, sexual activity without contraception or misuse of contraception should also increase your suspicion of pregnancy.

Other signs and symptoms of early pregnancy include nausea, vomiting, breast tenderness, increased urinary frequency, and fatigue. The

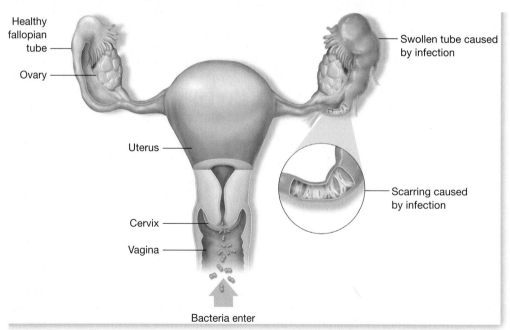

Healthy fallopian tube

Ovary

Swollen tube caused by infection

Uterus

Scarring caused by infection

Cervix

Vagina

Bacteria enter

Figure 40-2 Illustration of the way in which pelvic inflammatory disease (PID) affects the reproductive organs.

term *morning sickness* refers to the tendency for most pregnant women to develop nausea, and in some cases vomiting, between 6 and 12 weeks of gestation. The nausea is typically worse in the mornings and improves as the day progresses. If nausea and vomiting are accompanied by fever, dizziness, headache, or abdominal pain, however, then a cause other than pregnancy should be considered. Pregnant women often notice an enlargement in their breasts with a strong sensation of soreness. This is due to estrogen and progesterone fluctuations. Pregnancy causes an increased total urinary output, which leads to an increase in urinary frequency. Finally, profound fatigue is frequently seen in pregnancy. It is most common in the first trimester and becomes less prominent in the second and third trimesters.

You can ask specific questions to help verify your suspicion of pregnancy. Inquire as to when the patient's last menstrual period occurred and whether it was normal. Ask whether the patient has been sexually active since her last menstrual cycle. If she has been sexually active, did she use a form of contraception, and did she use it properly? It is unlikely that you will be able to determine early pregnancy by physical exam. However, your assessment of the signs and symptoms, as well as the patient's history, can help you determine the likelihood of pregnancy. Maintain a high index of suspicion in women of childbearing age even if the history is not consistent with the diagnosis.

Sexual Assault

Sexual assault refers to an act of violence in which sexual intercourse and/or sexual activities are performed without consent. Although anyone can be a victim of sexual assault, victims of such crimes are typically women and often know their assailant. It is not uncommon for victims who know their assailant not to report the crime to the proper authorities. However, as a paramedic, you are required to report sexual assault cases to law enforcement and the proper authorities. Make sure you follow your local protocol when caring for these patients.

On arrival at the scene of a sexual assault, ensure scene safety. Law enforcement is often dispatched to these calls for service; however, they are not always on scene at the time you arrive. Be cautious as to the possibility that the assailant may

still be present. Once the scene is secure for you to enter, address the safety needs of the patient and others at the scene.

Once the scene is safe, you can assess the patient for life-threatening injuries and provide the appropriate emergency care. Make certain that you provide emergency care that addresses both the physical and emotional needs of the patient. In addition, you want to emphasize the need for the patient to seek medical evaluation and collection of evidence at the hospital.

If the patient agrees to emergency care and evidence collection, explain how to preserve the evidence until it can be collected. Do not allow her to bathe, brush her teeth or hair, change her clothes, urinate or defecate, smoke, eat, or drink. If possible, do not cut or touch the patient's clothing unless it interferes with emergency care.

Let the patient know that most of her clothing will be taken for evidence. Offer to bring a clean change of clothes with her or have someone bring clothing to the hospital. If the patient has already changed her clothing, collect the original clothing in a separate bag and handle the evidence as little as necessary. Initiate transport to the hospital and, when applicable, transport the patient to a facility other than the one to which the suspect has been taken.

En route to the hospital, provide physical as well as emotional care as appropriate. Provide a safe environment for the patient. Remain nonjudgmental and protect confidentiality by asking only questions that are pertinent to the assessment and emergency care of the patient. Do not touch the patient unnecessarily, and ask for consent before performing procedures. Obtain a baseline set of vital signs, and evaluate for any other associated injuries. Be certain to document all your findings objectively and accurately. Be familiar with the hospitals in your area that have specialized personnel and facilities for sexual assault victims; it is preferable to transport the patient to those facilities.

ASSESSMENT

As always, use your dispatch information to help you determine what is taking place at the scene. This information should trigger you to think of possible causes for the chief complaint. Dispatch information can also lead you toward whether the patient is suffering from a traumatic injury or a medical condition. If sexual assault is a possibility, ensure that law enforcement

has been notified. Remember that it is always possible that the assailant may still be at the scene. Once you arrive, ensure that the scene is safe for you to enter and use Standard Precautions before you approach the patient.

As you approach the patient, look around the scene to obtain a general impression. Assess the situation to determine whether a traumatic injury is involved. If you suspect an injury, establish manual stabilization of the spine. Ensure that the patient's airway is open and clear of any potential obstruction. Evaluate the rate, rhythm, and quality of the patient's respirations. In addition to clinical assessment findings, use a pulse oximeter to determine whether the patient requires oxygen administration.

Pay particular attention to the patient's circulatory status. Bleeding can be both external and internal. Avoid missing internal bleeding by evaluating the patient's pulses, skin color, and temperature. A patient who presents in shock needs to be treated aggressively and transported rapidly to an appropriate medical facility. Patients who require expeditious transport include those presenting with poor general appearance, altered mental status, severe pain, uncontrolled bleeding, and shock.

Obtain a baseline set of vital signs, including blood pressure, and begin your physical exam. Typically, the physical exam focuses on the gynecologic complaint; however, be sure to examine the rest of the body for other associated signs and symptoms. Remember that it is not necessary to diagnose the exact cause of the gynecologic complaint, but it is necessary to rule out the cause as stemming from another body system.

During your secondary assessment, continue to protect the patient's privacy and modesty. Be mindful that it is necessary to ask the patient personal questions and that she may

> As a paramedic, you are required to report sexual assault cases to law enforcement and the proper authorities.

> During your secondary assessment, continue to protect the patient's privacy and modesty.

be hesitant to answer, especially in the presence of many people. Be compassionate and professional when obtaining a history and physical exam from patients who have been sexually assaulted.

EMERGENCY MEDICAL CARE

As mentioned previously, it is not imperative that you diagnose the exact cause of the patient's abdominal pain and/or vaginal bleeding. However, it is imperative that you accurately assess and identify the patient's signs and symptoms. Then you can provide appropriate emergency care based on the patient's clinical presentation. Emergency care should include the following:

- **Maintain manual spinal stabilization.** If you suspect trauma, take precautions to maintain spinal immobilization.
- **Maintain a patent airway.** Be prepared for the possibility that the patient may vomit. If no trauma is suspected, transport the patient in a left lateral recumbent position to protect the airway.
- **Determine the patient's respiratory status.** Administer oxygen based on the patient's signs and symptoms and the SpO_2 reading. If the SpO_2 reading is greater than 95 percent and the patient is asymptomatic, oxygen administration may not be necessary. However, you can apply a nasal cannula with 2 to 4 liters per minute (lpm) of oxygen if you

feel it is appropriate. If the SpO_2 reading is less than 95 percent and the respirations are adequate, place the patient on a nonrebreather mask at 15 lpm. Inadequate respirations require positive pressure ventilation with a bag-valve mask and high-concentration oxygen.
- **Control any major bleeding.** If vaginal bleeding is present, place a pad to absorb the flow. Do not pack the vagina.
- **Initiate transport.**
- **IV access and fluid administration may be warranted en route.** Follow local protocol for guidelines on IV fluid boluses.
- **Calm and reassure the patient.** Be supportive and nonjudgmental, especially in cases of sexual assault.

TRANSITIONING

REVIEW ITEMS

1. What is the best indicator of blood loss in a patient presenting with vaginal bleeding?
    a. "This is more bleeding than normal for my period."
    b. "I noticed a small blood clot on my sanitary napkin."
    c. "My tampons are saturated, and I have changed them four times in the last hour."
    d. "I have had a period for the past seven days."

2. What is the most common nonobstetric cause for traumatic vaginal bleeding?
    a. vaginal delivery of a baby   b. straddle injuries
    c. sexual intercourse   d. none of the above

3. Which of the following is not a risk factor for PID?
    a. sexual intercourse during menstruation

    b. multiple sex partners
    c. age less than 25 years
    d. consistent condom use

4. Which is the most common sign of pregnancy?
    a. amenorrhea
    b. breast tenderness
    c. increased urinary frequency
    d. morning sickness

5. Who is most likely to be a victim of a sexual assault?
    a. 4-year-old girl   b. 10-year-old boy
    c. 25-year-old woman   d. 35-year-old man

APPLIED PATHOPHYSIOLOGY

1. List three common causes of vaginal bleeding.

2. Describe the signs and symptoms associated with pelvic inflammatory disease.

3. If pregnancy was suspected in a woman of childbearing years, what signs indicating pregnancy would you expect you find?

CLINICAL DECISION MAKING

You are called to the scene of an 11-year-old girl suffering from what appears to be a straddle injury from a bicycle accident. The child is lying supine on the ground next to the bicycle, with blood saturating her pants. As you approach the child, her eyes are closed, and she is not crying.

1. Would you manually stabilize the spine in this patient? Why or why not?

2. What technique would you use to open the patient's airway? Why?

The SpO₂ reading is 90 percent with a respiratory rate of 16 and adequate respirations.

3. What oxygen therapy would you provide to this patient?

When assessing the circulation you observe pale skin, weak pulses and a heart rate of 180. After exposing the patient, you observe a heavy flow of blood from the vagina.

4. How would you treat the vaginal bleeding?

5. Why does the patient have weak pulses, tachycardia, and pale skin?

6. Would you expect the blood pressure to be normotensive, hypotensive, or hypertensive?

7. Would you begin an IV for fluid administration? If so, what would you use to determine the amount of intravenous fluids you should administer?

TOPIC

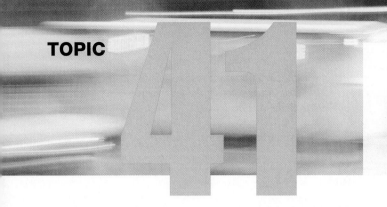

Standard Medicine

Competency Integrates assessment findings with principles of epidemiology and pathophysiology to formulate a field impression and implement a comprehensive treatment/disposition plan for a patient with a medical complaint.

EMERGENCIES INVOLVING THE EYES, EARS, NOSE, AND THROAT

TRANSITION *highlights*

- *Frequency, types, mortality, and morbidity of facial injuries.*

- *Overview of how kinetic energy produces the forces causing the various types of facial injuries.*

- *Pathophysiologic changes that occur with facial emergencies likely to be encountered in the prehospital environment:*
  - *– Eye injuries.*
  - *– Epistaxis.*

- *Specific questions to ask and assessment findings pertinent to these types of emergencies.*

- *How to use a Morgan Lens kit for eye irrigation.*

- *General treatment parameters the paramedic can employ when caring for a patient in an emergency involving the eyes, ears, nose, and throat.*

INTRODUCTION

Trauma to the eye, face, or neck can cause a patient not only significant injury, but emotional stress as well. Patients often experience fear and panic when they think of the possible outcomes from their injury. In some situations, these injuries can bring about loss of vision, scarring, and permanent disfigurement. As a paramedic, you will have to care for both physical and emotional trauma.

Moreover, an injury to the face or neck can pose significant airway and circulatory compromise. With eye, face, and neck injuries, the likelihood for airway compromise, severe bleeding, and shock is high. In addition, trauma to the face and neck has the potential to cause spinal column or cord injury. You must anticipate the complications that accompany these injuries. Always

maintain a high level of awareness, and give priority to caring for life-threatening airway, ventilatory, and circulatory compromise.

Knowledge of the anatomy of the eyes, face, and neck is imperative when treating these emergencies. Attentiveness to the location of structures and major blood vessels can allow you to predict the complications that often arise with these injuries (▶ Figure 41-1 and ▶ Figure 41-2).

EPIDEMIOLOGY

More than 3 million facial injuries occur in the United States each year. In urban communities, facial trauma is most commonly secondary to assaults, motor vehicle crashes, and industrial accidents. The number one cause of facial injuries in the rural setting is motor vehicle crashes, followed by assaults and recreational activities. Injuries to the midface, such as LeFort fractures, occur most commonly in motor vehicle crashes with patients who were not wearing a seatbelt. In assaults, zygomatic and mandible fractures are commonly seen. Other important causes of facial injuries include penetrating trauma, domestic violence, and abuse in children and the elderly.

The incidence of major injury accompanying high-impact facial fractures is as high as 50 percent, as compared with 21 percent in low-impact fractures. Associated cervical spine injury varies between 0.2 percent and 6 percent. Mortality is as high as 12 percent in high-impact fractures; however, this is rarely due to the maxillofacial injury. Mortality typically arises from a secondary injury associated with impact, such as head injury. Maintain a high index of suspicion for other injuries when caring for these patients.

Pathophysiology

The dispersion of kinetic energy during deceleration produces the force that results in injury. Kinetic energy, defined as the energy possessed by an object because of its motion, equals mass (weight in pounds), times the velocity (feet per second) squared, divided by two:

$$\frac{\text{Mass} \times \text{Velocity}^2}{2}$$

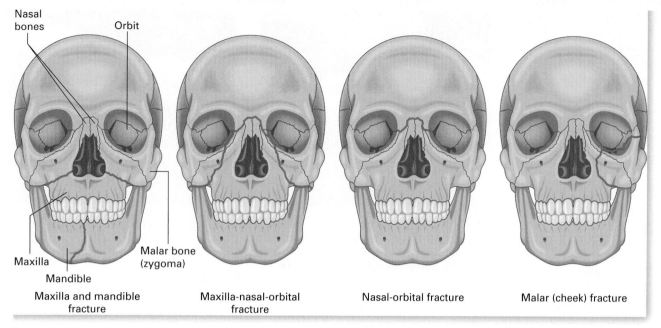

Figure 41-1 Types of facial fractures.

Nasal bones

Orbit

Maxilla

Mandible

Malar bone (zygoma)

Maxilla and mandible fracture

Maxilla-nasal-orbital fracture

Nasal-orbital fracture

Malar (cheek) fracture

High-impact force is defined as a force greater than 50 times the force of gravity. Low-impact force is less than 50 times the force of gravity. The zygoma (cheek) and nasal bone need only a low-impact force to cause damage. The supraorbital rim of the eye, mandible (jaw), and frontal bones require a high-impact force to cause injury.

Finally, the most common of all facial fractures are simple nasal fractures.

ASSESSMENT

Primary assessment in a patient with an injury to the eye, face, or neck should include inline manual stabilization of the spine as you approach the patient. These injuries are traumatic in nature and have the potential to cause injury to the cervical spine. Use a jaw-thrust maneuver to open the airway. Suction blood and any other secretions or potential obstructions from the airway.

If breathing is inadequate, provide positive pressure ventilation and high-concentration oxygen via the ventilation device at a rate of 10 to 12 ventilations per minute in the adult patient. Infants and children should be ventilated at a rate of 12 to 20 ventilations per minute. Your patient may require advanced airway maneuvers but beware of the difficulties if there is trauma to the airway. Often, landmarks may have been displaced or obscured by blood and trauma. As a paramedic, you must weigh the benefit of procedures such as endotracheal intubation against the risks of a difficult procedure.

Control any major bleeding with direct pressure. Consider an appropriate transport destination, and include early notification of the hospital so that specialty resources can be put in motion.

Once life-threatening conditions are managed, obtain a history. Important questions to ask include:

- Did the patient lose consciousness? If so, for how long was the patient unconscious?
- Does the patient have any vision problems, such as blurred vision, diplopia, or photophobia?

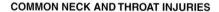

COMMON NECK AND THROAT INJURIES

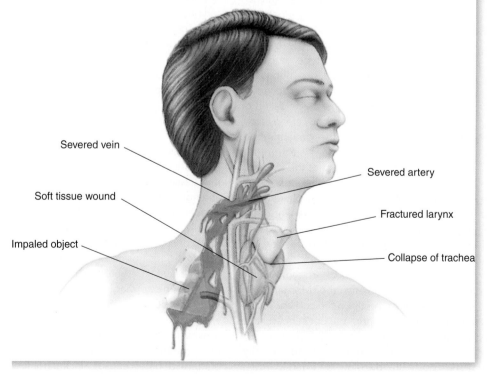

Severed vein

Soft tissue wound

Impaled object

Severed artery

Fractured larynx

Collapse of trachea

Figure 41-2 Common neck and throat injuries.

- Does the patient have any hearing problems, such as muffled tones or ringing in the ear?
- Does the patient have any clear-fluid drainage from the nose or ears that may be indicative of cerebrospinal fluid?
- Does the patient have malocclusion or misalignment of the teeth?
- Does the patient have numbness or tingling in the face?
- Is the mechanism of injury secondary to abuse or domestic violence?

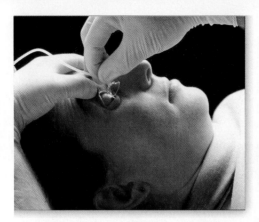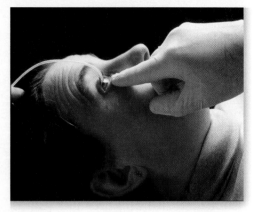

Figure 41-3 Inserting the Morgan Lens: (A) Have the patient look downward; set the lens on the upper aspect of the eye and allow the lid to sit over the lens. (B) Have the patient look upward to facilitate placement of the lens on the lower aspect of the eye. Allow the eyelid to cover the bottom aspect of the lens.

EMERGENCY CARE

Whether you are treating an injury to the eye, face, or neck, emergency care focuses on airway, breathing, and circulation. Emergency care may include the following:

- Establish manual inline stabilization of the spine, followed by complete immobilization.
- Open the airway, using a jaw-thrust maneuver.
- Suction the airway.
- Consider the need for more aggressive airway management (airway protection).
- If there are signs of hypoxia, provide oxygen. Administer positive pressure ventilation and supplemental oxygen to the patient with inadequate respiratory function.
- Control major bleeding with direct pressure.
- Provide emotional support.

SPECIFIC EMERGENCIES AND MANAGEMENT

Eye Injuries

In some eye injuries, irrigation of the eye may be necessary. These instances include chemical burns and attempting to remove foreign particles from the eye such as dirt, sand, or other particles that tears may not wash away naturally.

Should it be determined that eye irrigation is necessary, you may flush the eye with clear, clean water. The water does not necessarily have to be sterile, but it should be clean. Hold the eyelids apart, and flush the water from the inner canthus of the eye downward to the outer edge of the eye. Position the patient's head to facilitate drainage of the water as it passes over the eye into a basin and not to contaminate the uninjured eye.

In cases of chemical burns, flush the eye continuously for 20 minutes. If the chemical involves alkali, flush the eye for at least an hour or until arrival at the hospital.

MORGAN LENS Use of the Morgan Lens® is beneficial in flushing a patient's eye, especially during the prolonged irrigation of chemical burns. The Morgan Lens is a contact-lens-type irrigation device that provides slow, continuous eye irrigation. The lens itself is attached to intravenous tubing primed with saline or Ringer's lactate. With a slow, steady flow, place the lens onto the patient's eye. Have the patient look downward, set the lens on the upper aspect of the eye, and allow the lid to sit over the lens (▶ Figure 41-3A). Then have the patient look upward to facilitate the placement of the lens on the lower aspect of the eye. Allow the eyelid to cover the bottom aspect of the lens (▶ Figure 41-3B).

The steady flow of irrigant during placement prevents the Morgan Lens from sitting directly on the cornea. Secure the tubing to the patient's head, and adjust the flow accordingly. Take caution to not allow the solution to run dry. Absorb the overflow of irrigant into a towel. To discontinue the use of the Morgan Lens, continue the flow. Retract the lower eyelid, and hold it in position. Then remove the lens downward, and terminate the flow of the solution. Pat the excess solution dry while instructing the patient not to rub the eyes.

Epistaxis

Epistaxis, or nosebleed, is a common problem, occurring in 60 percent of the general population. Epistaxis is more likely to affect children before the age of 10 and adults between 45 and 65 years of age. There is a male predominance for epistaxis prior to the age of 49, but the sex distribution equalizes thereafter. This can be attributed to the protective effects of estrogen in women through relief of capillary permeability. There is a higher proportion of epistaxis in the winter months, caused by the increased incidence of upper respiratory tract infections, allergic rhinitis, and mucosal changes associated with fluctuations in the temperature and humidity during the winter months.

Epistaxis is often self-limiting in nature. It is classified by the source of bleeding: anterior and posterior. Anterior epistaxis frequently originates from the nasal septum. It is the most common, accounting for 90 percent of all nosebleeds. Posterior epistaxis does not occur as regularly, but it can result in significant hemorrhage, and even hemorrhagic shock, if not controlled properly.

Epistaxis often results from mucosal trauma or irritation. Nose picking is the most common cause; however, there are numerous other causes, including low moisture content in the ambient air,

> Epistaxis is a common problem, occurring in 60 percent of the population.

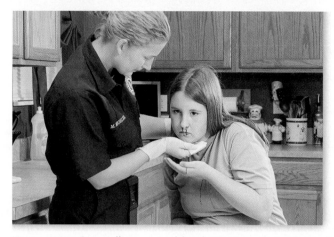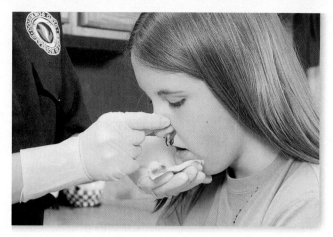

Figure 41-4 Controlling a nosebleed: (A) Have the patient sit and lean forward. (B) Pinch the fleshy part of the nostrils together.

mucosal hyperemia secondary to allergic or viral rhinitis, nasal steroid use for seasonal allergies, presence of a foreign body, chronic excoriation from intranasal drug use, and facial trauma. Epistaxis can also be secondary to several medical conditions, such as hemophilia, platelet disorders, conditions requiring the use of anticoagulants or blood thinners, and nasal neoplasms.

The primary assessment of epistaxis should focus on evaluation of airway management, respiratory function, and cardiovascular stability. Ensure that the patient's airway is clear of blood and secretions. If necessary, suction the airway so it is free of any potential obstruction. If your patient is awake and alert, you can provide him with a hard suction catheter so he may clear any secretions as often as he prefers.

Assess the patient's respiratory rate and adequacy of ventilation. Provide high-concentration oxygen as needed (although bleeding control has priority, which may prevent the use of a mask or nasal cannula). Evaluate the patient's circulatory status by palpating central and peripheral pulses for rate and quality. Also, use a skin assessment to help determine the patient's circulatory status. Cool, clammy skin with a weak pulse could indicate hypovolemic shock.

Once it is determined that the patient's airway, breathing, and circulatory function are adequate, the next step is to achieve hemostasis (▶ Figure 41-4). Properly instructed patients may achieve this by holding direct pressure and pinching the fleshy portion of their nostrils together. Instruct the patient to exert pressure by grasping the nostrils distally and pinching them tightly against the septum.

The patient must maintain direct pressure for 10 consecutive minutes. Ensure that the patient does not check to see whether the bleeding has stopped prior to holding direct pressure for 10 minutes. In addition, you may have the patient sit down and bend forward at the waist. This will help the patient expectorate blood accumulation in the pharynx and prevent him from swallowing excess blood. If possible, apply ice or a cold pack to the bridge of the nose to facilitate vasoconstriction.

Once hemostasis is achieved, the timing, frequency, and severity of the epistaxis should be determined. Is this an isolated episode or one of many? Are there any medical conditions that can be exacerbated by blood loss? Examples of these conditions include coronary artery disease and chronic obstructive pulmonary disease. Is the patient experiencing any signs or symptoms associated with these conditions, such as chest pain, dyspnea, weakness, or dizziness?

TRANSITIONING

REVIEW ITEMS

1. Which method is the simplest, most effective way of managing anterior epistaxis?
   a. direct pressure
   b. nasal packing
   c. cauterization
   d. ice application

2. In which situation would you consider irrigation of the eye with a Morgan Lens?
   a. chemical burn to the eye
   b. ruptured globe
   c. corneal abrasion
   d. impaled metal object into the cornea

3. Which solution should you use with a Morgan Lens?
   a. normal saline
   b. 5% dextrose in water
   c. 50% dextrose in water
   d. hypertonic saline

4. *Diplopia* is a term that refers to:
   a. Ringing in the ears
   b. Loss of vision in one eye
   c. Vertigo
   d. Double vision

APPLIED PATHOPHYSIOLOGY

1. List five causes of epistaxis.

2. Which epistaxis poses the biggest threat of significant hemorrhage—anterior or posterior?

3. Describe the process of inserting a Morgan Lens.

4. List five injuries you expect to see in a patient with high-impact trauma to the face.

CLINICAL DECISION MAKING

You are dispatched to the local bike trail for a male patient who crashed his bicycle. When you arrive on scene, you observe a man lying prone on the cement approximately five feet away from his bicycle. Bystanders state he struck an object in the roadway and flipped over the handlebars.

1. What is your first step in rendering care and positioning of this patient for adequate assessment?

Once the patient is supine, you observe multiple abrasions and contusions about his face. There is a large hematoma to the right eye, causing the eyelid to be swollen shut. There are bloody secretions flowing out of his mouth, and a broken tooth on the ground near his head. There is auditory gurgling with the patient's respirations. His respirations are shallow and slow. Aside from the bleeding in the oral cavity, there does not appear to be any other major bleeding.

2. Summarize the steps you will take to care for the patient's ABCs.

3. Would you consider requesting ALS backup for this patient? Why or why not?

Standard Trauma

Competency Integrates assessment findings with principles of epidemiology and pathophysiology to formulate a field impression to implement a comprehensive treatment/disposition plan for an acutely injured patient.

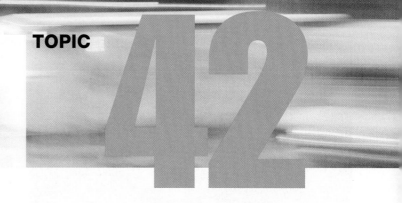

BLEEDING AND BLEEDING CONTROL

INTRODUCTION

Experience from recent military conflicts has consistently shown that bleeding from extremities is among the leading causes of preventable battlefield deaths. Although it is always difficult to compare military and civilian medicine, avoiding preventable death by controlling external hemorrhage is an important lesson EMS should learn from the experience of military medics.

Every paramedic should understand the importance of hemorrhage control and be competent in the basic procedures involved in controlling external bleeding. Although the paramedic brings to the table a wide array of advanced capabilities, the basic skills of hemorrhage control are among the most important treatments for any trauma patient. Paramedics must correctly prioritize these basic procedures as they formulate their treatment plans. This topic focuses on recognizing and treating external hemorrhage.

EPIDEMIOLOGY

According to the National Safety Council, unintentional injury is the fifth leading cause of death in the United States and the leading cause of death in patients 1 to 44 years of age. It is difficult to pinpoint how many of those deaths are related purely to bleeding, but some studies point to exsanguination (bleeding to death) as accounting for more than 40 percent of trauma-related deaths. Although the vast majority of these deaths are related to internal bleeding, external hemorrhage still accounts for a significant number of preventable trauma deaths each year.

PATHOPHYSIOLOGY

Blood is the supply system for the cells. Oxygen binds to red blood cells, dissolves in plasma, and is pumped to cells by the heart. Carbon dioxide and other waste products are removed and transported back to the alveoli for elimination. This perfusion of the cells is essential for life; when it fails, shock sets in. A leading cause of shock is hypovolemia, which occurs when perfusion fails owing to a lack of blood. Although there are other causes of hypovolemia, actual blood loss is most common.

TRANSITION highlights

- **Rates of unintentional trauma and victim death from exsanguination (bleeding to death).**

- **Types of hemorrhage:**
  - External hemorrhage.
  - Internal hemorrhage.
  - Exsanguinating hemorrhage.

- **Types of assessment findings the paramedic will identify in a patient with internal or external bleeding.**

- **The currently recommended procedure for progressively managing external bleeding.**

Always remember that bleeding can be external or internal. A patient can rapidly bleed to death internally without any evidence on the outside.

External bleeding, however, depends greatly on the extent and location of the injury. The volume of hemorrhage generally can be correlated directly to size of the damaged vessel, pressure within that vessel, and the amount of blood contained within the circulatory system. Damage to large vessels will typically create larger volumes of blood loss; damage to the higher-pressure arteries will result in a more rapid loss of blood. However, as pressure and volume fall within with circulatory system, the volume and rate of bleeding will decrease.

Besides trauma, bleeding may be associated with fractured bones, gastrointestinal tract disorders, abdominal or chest trauma, and problems in the reproductive system.

Exsanguinating Hemorrhage

Exsanguinating hemorrhage is a very specific and very rare classification of bleeding. In this case, an artery or series of blood vessels has been damaged significantly enough to allow massive,

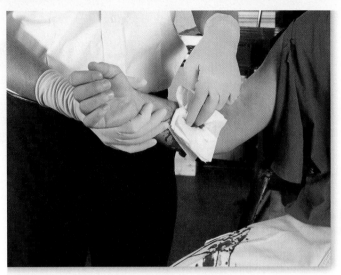

Figure 42-1 When treating external bleeding with direct pressure, apply gloved fingertip pressure over a dressing directly on the point of bleeding.

life-threatening blood loss. This type of bleeding is typically associated with trauma to the large blood vessels, such as the femoral and brachial arteries, and the hemorrhage exceeds what we normally consider "severe bleeding." In this case, the patient may bleed to death in less than 1 minute. When this type of bleeding is identified, it must become the most important treatment priority.

> **Not all bleeding can be seen externally.**

ASSESSMENT FINDINGS

Your primary assessment will give you a rapid opportunity to identify blood loss. At this point, you will visually inspect the patient for bleeding. Remember to check void spaces and bulky clothing with your hands if you cannot see all areas of the patient. You will also assess for basic shock findings such as mental status, the presence (or lack) of a radial pulse, and skin condition. Pale skin, rapid pulse and respirations, and delayed capillary refill time can all indicate the presence of internal hemorrhage and shock.

> **If resources must be delegated, treatment of exsanguinating hemorrhage must come first.**

Remember that not all bleeding can be seen externally. Often the most severe bleeding is occurring internally and must be assumed based on other signs and symptoms.

External hemorrhage must be evaluated rapidly. *If you identify exsanguinating hemorrhage, you must act immediately.* In cases of exsanguinating hemorrhage, the traditional ABC model of the primary assessment now becomes XABC, with *X* standing for "exsanguinating hemorrhage." In these rare instances, treating the massive bleeding is more important than even addressing airway concerns (although it would be best if both could be addressed simultaneously).

Other, less severe, hemorrhage will need to be evaluated and treated using good clinical judgment. Typically, even serious external bleeding will be less of a priority than airway and breathing concerns. When identified in the primary assessment, take steps to control the external blood loss. Your immediate decision-making process will focus on how fast the patient is bleeding and how much volume he is losing. Keep in mind that exsanguinating hemorrhage is exceptionally rare.

EMERGENCY MEDICAL CARE

The urgency of bleeding control will vary depending on decisions you make during your primary assessment. Your assessment will help you define how severe the bleeding is and, in turn, how urgent is the need for bleeding control.

Your assessment will also help you identify the importance of bleeding control within the list of immediate priorities. For example, if you identify a moderate external hemorrhage on a trauma patient without a viable airway, you should open the airway before controlling the bleeding. In this case, the airway is certainly more important than the bleeding. On the other hand, if the bleeding were exsanguinating, then your priorities would have to change (unless you had enough resources to treat both issues simultaneously). With assessment questions answered, you will then select the most appropriate treatment options.

Bleeding Control Progression

Unless the injury is known to be purely isolated (e.g., a limited extremity laceration), you should always assume that the worst bleeding is occurring internally. The true treatment for internal bleeding is rapid transport and delivery to an appropriate trauma facility. Remember the urgency of definitive treatment and focus most of your on-scene priorities on rapid evacuation.

DIRECT PRESSURE Most external bleeding control begins with direct pressure. Direct pressure forces blood from the small surface vessels and aids in clot formation. For an overwhelming number of external hemorrhage cases, direct pressure is the only necessary treatment. Direct pressure is accomplished by placing a clean—preferably sterile—dressing over the wound and applying force to the wound area and proximal surrounding tissue (▶ Figure 42-1). It is best if this pressure can be distributed over a wide area to avoid pinpoint "poking" force. The exception to this rule is when a wound is wide, or gaping, and a bleeding point can be identified. In this case, it is appropriate to place pinpoint pressure directly on the bleeding vessel.

Direct pressure is best when applied over bone so that soft tissue is compressed between the force and a rigid surface. Consider the angle you are using to apply force to ideally compress the wound against a bony backstop.

Direct pressure must be a constant force. A common mistake in bleeding control is frequent checking of the wound. Direct pressure must be applied for a minimum of 5 minutes (longer in more severe bleeding) to be effective. Frequent checking often destroys newly formed clots and is counterproductive to stopping the bleeding. Direct pressure needs steady, firm pressure. For severe arterial bleeding, you may need to use heavy force, such as leaning onto the wound with body weight. Always use good clinical judgment to determine the appropriate amount of force.

DRESSINGS A dressing is used to protect and cover a wound, not to hide bleeding. Beware of using too many absorbent dressings only to hide severe bleeding. Direct pressure is still necessary as long as bleeding continues.

Pressure dressings—dressings combined with a tight (nonoccluding) bandage—are helpful in simple bleeding control. Although they should not take the place of direct pressure in the cases of severe bleeding, these types of dressings can often be substituted for direct pressure in moderate bleeding to allow the provider to move on to other important tasks. Consider using a bandage that allows for tight application of the dressing without cutting off blood flow to the distal extremity. The pressure of these dressings will diminish distal circulation, but the dressings should not occlude circulation to the point of losing a distal pulse.

Commercial pressure dressings are widely available, but simple alternatives include ACE® type bandages and Coban® wrap. Keep in mind that direct pressure may still be necessary for more severe bleeding.

HEMOSTATIC AGENTS   A number of commercially available hemostatic agents are designed to aid in the control of external hemorrhage. Be sure to check local protocol before using these products. Hemostatic agents come in powders, pouches, and impregnated dressings, and are designed to be placed into and around wounds to aid the clotting process (▶ Figure 42-2). In general, they work as drying

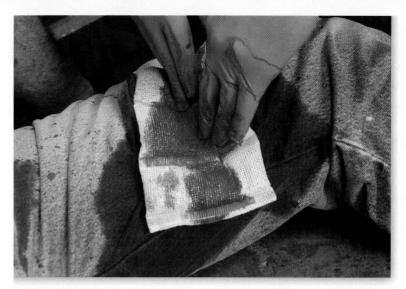

Figure 42-3 Application of a hemostatic dressing.

agents to help remove the liquid portion of the blood and promote clot formation. In general, these agents are safe and very effective, but some do have specific side effects. Early agents produced an exothermic reaction that caused heat when applied. Although most agents have been redesigned to avoid this reaction, some still have this effect. Always follow the manufacturer's recommendations for use.

Hemostatic agents are typically applied directly against or into the wound. When possible, avoid applying the agent into a puddle of blood. First wipe the wound clean, and then apply the agent (▶ Figure 42-3). Direct pressure should immediately follow application.

SPLINTING AND POSITION   The splinting of fractures can often assist in bleeding control. Proper positioning and the application of a splint often are effective methods of slowing and stopping bleeding. Elevation can sometimes aid in bleeding control. When possible, elevate the extremity above the heart. Keep in mind, however, that elevation of potentially fractured extremities may increase blood loss if done prior to appropriate splinting. Always follow local protocol.

Tourniquets

Tourniquets were once thought to be dangerous, "life or limb" treatments to be used only when we were willing to trade loss of a limb to keep our patient alive. Recent experiences in the operating room and anecdotal evidence from battlefield medicine, however, have shown us that tourniquets may be safer than we once assumed. In many cases, early tourniquet application is an important element of treating severe bleeding.

It is important to remember that tourniquets are still a last resort. All other bleeding control options should be exhausted prior to their application. That said, it is important to move to this step rapidly when other treatments fail.

There are many commercially available tourniquets (▶ Figure 42-4). Tourniquets can also be created from improvised

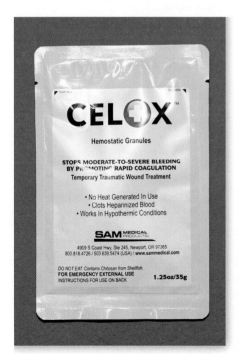

Figure 42-2 Topical hemostatic agents, such as Celox™, are a recent development in wound care.

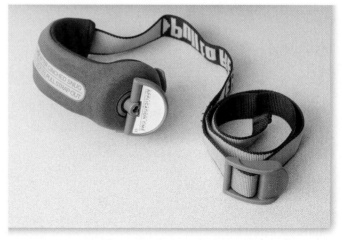

Figure 42-4 Example of a commercially available tourniquet.

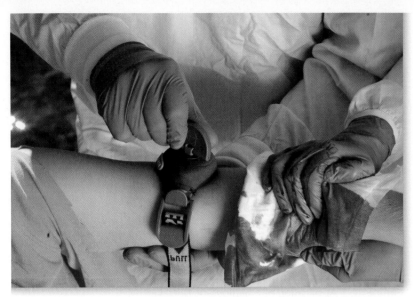

Figure 42-5 Proper placement of a tourniquet is proximal to the wound, between the wound and the heart.

extremities, such as the tibia/fibula and radius/ulna, the major arteries run between the bones. As a result, occlusion of these arteries by a tourniquet is difficult. For this reason, some experts recommend that tourniquets should never be used distal to the elbow or the knee. Always follow local protocol as to tourniquet location.

In general, tourniquets should be tightened until the bleeding stops and a distal pulse is lost in the extremity.

Tourniquet application is a painful process. Many patients who need a tourniquet may be conscious; in these cases, you should anticipate a reaction to the pain. Take steps to address the emotional component and provide a clear understanding that although it is a painful treatment, it is absolutely necessary. As a paramedic, you should also consider analgesic agents such as fentanyl to help manage the pain of a tourniquet application.

Putting It All Together

Bleeding control is a linear process. It starts simply and adds steps when initial treatments fail. Direct pressure is the most important element and forms the foundation for many other treatments. Concentrate on the proper application of direct pressure, and escalate to more aggressive treatments when necessary.

materials, such as the windlass method. Regardless of where a tourniquet is obtained, all tourniquets must have these common elements:

- Tourniquets must be a wide band (most references state at least 1 to 2 inches wide). More narrow bands must be avoided, as they can cut into soft tissue as they tighten.
- Tourniquets must have a method of applying mechanical force to tighten. That is, there should be a way to twist or ratchet the tourniquet to tighten it, as opposed to simply pulling it tight. Hand tightening may not provide enough force to stop the bleeding of a major artery.

APPLYING A TOURNIQUET Tourniquets are used in extremity injuries only. They should be applied proximal to the wound, between the wound itself and the heart (▶ Figure 42-5). Remember that the idea of a tourniquet is to compress and occlude an artery. In lower

TRANSITIONING

REVIEW ITEMS

1. Which of the following signs of bleeding would you consider the most life threatening?
    a. delayed capillary refill time and pale skin
    b. oozing blood from an abrasion
    c. venous bleeding from a hand laceration
    d. vomiting with warm, pink skin

2. You are assessing a patient following a motor vehicle crash. He complains of abdominal pain, and you note that he has a rapid heart rate and is a bit pale. He has no obvious bleeding. You should suspect _____.
    a. internal hemorrhage
    b. external hemorrhage

    c. the patient has no injury
    d. the patient is simply upset

3. Massive, life-threatening bleeding from a major blood vessel can be otherwise defined as _____.
    a. exsanguinating hemorrhage
    b. venous hemorrhage
    c. capillary hemorrhage
    d. extracorporeal hemorrhage

4. Direct pressure should be applied for a minimum of _____.
    a. 5 minutes   b. 5 seconds
    c. 30 minutes   d. 30 seconds

5. Proper placement of a tourniquet includes which of the following elements?
   a. application proximal to the wound
   b. application distal to the wound
   c. application between the wound and the end of the extremity
   d. application directly over the wound

APPLIED PATHOPHYSIOLOGY

1. List three signs of exsanguinating hemorrhage.

2. Explain how exsanguinating hemorrhage might differ from another "severe" hemorrhage.

3. Discuss how exsanguinating hemorrhage might change the normal progression of the primary assessment.

4. Describe the components of proper direct pressure when used for bleeding control.

CLINICAL DECISION MAKING

An 18-year-old man has been shot in the upper thigh. On arrival, you find the patient lying on the ground. You note a massive, spurting hemorrhage coming from the leg wound and a large amount of blood already on the ground.

1. Assuming the scene is safe, and given your general impression, what immediate actions are necessary?

2. Would you classify this bleeding as exsanguinating hemorrhage? If so, why?

To control the bleeding you apply a bulky dressing and apply direct pressure. Bleeding immediately soaks through the dressing.

3. What is the next step in the progression of bleeding control?

4. At what point should you consider the use of a tourniquet?

5. Please describe the following components of proper tourniquet application:
   a. Location (where it should be placed)
   b. Width of band
   c. Tightness

You arrive by yourself to treat this gunshot wound patient. Bystanders note that they do not think he is breathing.

6. How might this fact affect your immediate treatment? Please discuss which primary assessment problem (bleeding or breathing) you would treat first, and why.

7. During which part of the call would you start an IV? At what rate would you run the IV?

TOPIC

43

Standard Trauma

Competency Applies fundamental knowledge to provide basic and selected advanced emergency care and transportation based on assessment findings for an acutely injured patient.

CHEST TRAUMA

TRANSITION highlights

- *Annual injury and death rates for patients who are victims of chest trauma.*

- *Importance of mechanism of injury in determining presence of chest trauma.*

- *Pathophysiologic changes that occur with chest trauma and their effect on normal physiology:*
  – Tension pneumothorax.
  – Open pneumothorax.
  – Flail chest.
  – Hemothorax.
  – Acute pericardial tamponade.

- *Identification and differentiation of clinical findings of chest trauma with the altered physiology creating them.*

The amount of external bleeding is not an indicator of the potential or severity of internal bleeding associated with an underlying trauma.

INTRODUCTION

Injuries to the chest can affect a variety of vital organs and are a leading cause of death in trauma patients. Chest injuries can range from relatively minor contusions and broken ribs to immediately life-threatening penetrations of the chest wall and tension pneumothoraces. As a paramedic, it is important to have a high index of suspicion with regard to chest injuries because of the vital nature of the underlying organs. Even minor injuries can have a significant impact on the mechanism of breathing and disturb the ever-important exchange of gases at the alveolar level. Furthermore, some life-threatening chest injuries can present with subtle signs and symptoms. The assessment of the chest must be comprehensive in order to find all injuries, not just those that are visually dramatic.

In most systems, paramedics provide a level of intervention in response to chest injuries that can, in fact, be lifesaving when applied correctly. Recognition and resolution of the tension pneumothorax is an important paramedic skill but recent research has pointed out that it may be frequently used incorrectly. Paramedics must take care to both utilize the skill in the appropriate circumstances and perform the technique correctly, using appropriate equipment.

In many systems, paramedics are also charged with monitoring patients with chest drainage systems. These situations present unique challenges to ALS providers; a basic understanding of the physiology of chest drainage is essential.

EPIDEMIOLOGY

Approximately 20 percent to 25 percent of trauma deaths each year in the United States are caused by thoracic trauma. The deaths are most often associated with motor vehicle crashes in which severe blunt trauma ruptures the myocardial wall or thoracic aorta. Those deaths are usually immediate and occur at the scene. Other early deaths from thoracic trauma are associated with a tension pneumothorax, pericardial tamponade, flail segment, open pneumothorax, and hemothorax.

MECHANISM OF INJURY

Thoracic injury may result from both penetrating and blunt trauma. Penetrating trauma has a tendency to be more obvious in the initial phases of assessment because of the presence of an open wound to the thoracic wall. External bleeding may or may not be present. The amount of external bleeding is not an indicator of the potential or severity of internal bleeding associated with an underlying trauma.

High-velocity gunshot wounds and bullets that enter the thoracic cavity and ricochet can produce multiple organ, vascular, and structural damage. The physical location of the gunshot entrance or exit wound does increase one's index of suspicion of underlying internal organ and structural damage; however, it does not provide a precise prediction of the complete scope of the internal injury. Low-velocity wounds to the chest, such as those produced by a knife, produce more predictable underlying organ and structural damage because of the kinematics associated with the injury.

Blunt trauma may produce gross physical findings such as large contusions, tenderness, fractured ribs, and flail segments, or relatively little external evidence of injury. The chest wall may be severely compressed during the application of the blunt force, causing the internal organs to be stretched, torn, or sheared. After the blunt force is removed, the chest may recoil, leaving significant, moderate, or minor evidence of the temporary cavitation that occurred during the impact.

If little external injury is evident, one may suspect minor or no internal thoracic damage, whereas the patient may be suffering from multiple and severe organ, vascular, and structural injury. In both cases, rely on patient complaints and physical exam findings to increase your index of suspicion of internal organ and structural injury.

Blunt and penetrating trauma may produce injury to several structures within the thoracic cavity. Some injuries have a much higher incidence when associated with a specific mechanism, such as acute pericardial tamponade related to penetrating injury to the chest and upper abdomen, and esophageal injury associated with penetrating trauma to the neck and upper chest. Anatomic structures that have the potential to be injured in thoracic trauma are the chest wall, lung tissue, pulmonary tract, myocardium, great vessels (inferior and superior vena cava, and aorta), esophagus, and diaphragm. Thus, the injury may involve muscles, bones, organs, and vessels.

PATHOPHYSIOLOGY

A compromise in ventilation, oxygenation, and circulation may occur because of the anatomic structures typically involved in thoracic trauma. Injuries such as rib fractures and flail segment may interfere with the "bellows" action of the chest and lead to inadequate mechanical ventilation. Oxygenation may be impaired by a large pulmonary contusion that is restricting gas exchange through the collection of blood within the alveoli and the alveolar–capillary interface, or from a large area of collapsed lung tissue resulting from a pneumothorax. Hypotension from blood loss from a hemothorax or a reduction in cardiac output from a mechanically compressed myocardium associated with an acute pericardial tamponade can produce significant circulation and tissue perfusion disturbances.

Some injuries, such as a tension pneumothorax, may lead to ventilatory, oxygenation, and circulation compromise, which can produce lethal results quickly if not rapidly identified and managed. Some injuries, such as simple rib fractures, may produce such excruciating pain that the patient intentionally hypoventilates to reduce chest wall movement and becomes secondarily hypoxic.

As with any patient, the focus in the treatment of thoracic trauma is to establish and maintain an adequate airway, ventilation, oxygenation, and circulation. This may involve emergency management aimed at preventing further organ or structural involvement, reducing the existing life threat, or minimizing the progression of the pathophysiologic compromise.

ASSESSMENT

The basic principles of assessment apply to thoracic trauma. A systematic approach is critical to ensure that all potential life-threatening injuries are identified and managed rapidly. Thoracic injury is also associated with a relatively high incidence of extrathoracic trauma, especially when a blunt mechanism of injury is involved.

A shotgun approach to assessment may lead to missed or late identification of life-threatening injuries, potentially resulting in a poor patient outcome as a result of lack of immediate emergency intervention, or failure to identify the severity of the patient's condition, producing unnecessarily long on-scene times, lack of proper notification of the receiving medical facility, or an improper destination decision. Developing tunnel vision in the assessment approach and focusing just on the thoracic injury may cause the EMS practitioner to miss injuries to other body systems and cavities. Similarly, continued reassessment is required, especially if the patient's condition deteriorates.

The primary assessment is designed to identify and manage life threats to the airway, ventilation, oxygenation, and circulation. As previously noted, these may all be compromised in thoracic trauma. Airway obstruction, hypoventilation, hypoxia, and severe hypotension are often the primary reasons for deterioration and death in the trauma patient.

Once the scene is secured, and as you approach the patient, get a general impression. Identify, through a quick body scan, any obvious life-threatening injuries or conditions that may require immediate management, such as an obvious open chest wound, especially if it is producing a sucking sound; blood, vomitus, or other substances in the oral cavity that may result in aspiration; major bleeding (arterial or venous); and a flail segment, although the early signs are often subtle.

Provide manual spinal stabilization if a spinal injury is suspected. Establish and maintain an open airway, inspect inside the oral cavity, and suction or remove any substance that can be aspirated or lead to an airway obstruction.

As you assess breathing as part of the primary assessment, consider a "look, listen, feel" approach. Ensure that the patient is breathing. Look at the chest, exposing it if necessary. Look for signs of injury and any unusual findings. Use a stethoscope and briefly listen for lung sounds bilaterally. Although you will perform a much more thorough assessment of lung sounds in the secondary assessment, listening to the chest here allows for the rapid identification of a pneumothorax that may require immediate intervention.

Consider also the adequacy of breathing. Many chest injuries can affect the body's ability to adequately exchange gases. Assess both the tidal volume and respiratory rate and consider how dysfunction may affect alveolar ventilation. If breathing is inadequate, consider immediate corrective action, such as needle decompression and/or positive pressure ventilation. If the patient is breathing adequately, assess the need for supplemental oxygen, especially if signs of hypoxia or shock are present.

If positive pressure ventilation is used, be sure to provide very controlled ventilation rates and

Overventilation may lead to exacerbation of a pneumothorax and the conversion to a tension pneumothorax.

volumes. Do not overventilate the patient. Overventilation may lead to exacerbation of a pneumothorax and the conversion to a tension pneumothorax; reduction of preload, cardiac output, blood pressure and perfusion, especially in patients with significantly increased intrathoracic pressure; and other secondary barotrauma.

Feel the chest to identify crepitus, tenderness, or any deformity or inequality of expansion. Palpation can often rapidly identify the presence of a chest injury and can help point out "red flags" when often other more subtle visual findings may be difficult to identify.

Assess the status of circulation by comparing the amplitude of peripheral and central pulses, obtaining a heart rate, and observing skin temperature, color, and condition. If the thoracic trauma patient presents with pale, cool, and clammy skin; tachycardia; and weak or absent peripheral pulses, you should suspect the possibility of bleeding in the thoracic cavity, mechanical compression of the heart and great vessels, or bleeding in another area of the body.

> **Do not rule out the possibility of pericardial tamponade or tension pneumothorax when JVD is not found.**

Following the primary assessment, a rapid secondary assessment will be conducted to identify all other potentially life-threatening injuries. Immediately life-threatening thoracic injuries include tension pneumothorax, open pneumothorax, pericardial tamponade, severe hemothorax, and a flail chest.

The vital signs, including a systolic and diastolic blood pressure, heart rate, respiratory rate, and skin findings, along with a pulse oximeter and end-tidal carbon dioxide reading, will provide valuable information in the recognition and differentiation of thoracic injuries. It is necessary to understand and link thoracic injury to possible findings in other areas of the body when conducting your rapid trauma assessment. For example, inspecting the pupils is not only necessary to assess for the possibility of a brain injury, but sluggish pupillary reaction may also indicate significant hypoxia related to a chest injury.

Likewise, jugular venous distention (JVD), especially if associated with the inspiratory phase of respiration (referred to as the Kussmaul sign) may be an indication of a thoracic injury that has resulted in a high intrathoracic pressure (i.e., tension pneumothorax) or interference with ventricular filling and cardiac output (i.e., pericardial tamponade). This may be a subtle finding; however, a patient with tension pneumothorax and pericardial tamponade may present with signs that mimic those of a hypovolemic patient. One would not suspect JVD in hypovolemia, however, because of the low venous pressure. Recognizing the JVD, even though it may be very subtle or late, may be one sign that gets the paramedic thinking about a condition other than hypovolemia.

Also, do not rule out the possibility of pericardial tamponade or tension pneumothorax when JVD is not found, as a large percentage of patients with chest injury may also be hypovolemic, resulting in a low venous pressure that will preclude the jugular veins from engorging. It is necessary to think critically and consider and process all the assessment information during the exam.

Signs of other chest injuries that may be identified during the secondary assessment may include rib fractures, simple pneumothorax, simple hemothorax, pulmonary contusion, and cardiac contusion. The specific signs, symptoms, and emergency care of the most immediately life-threatening conditions will be discussed in the following section.

EMERGENCY MEDICAL CARE

The most immediately life-threatening thoracic injuries that require rapid recognition and intervention and expeditious transport are tension pneumothorax, open pneumothorax, flail chest, massive hemothorax, and acute pericardial tamponade. Focus on establishing and maintaining an airway, and on adequate ventilation and oxygenation. As with any other trauma patient, an intravenous line of normal saline or lactated Ringer's should be initiated once the patient is en route to the medical facility.

Do not delay transport to start an IV line. Use a large-bore catheter (14 or 16 gauge) and run the fluids to maintain a systolic blood pressure of 80 to 90 mmHg or until radial pulses are regained. Once this is achieved, reduce the fluid infusion and titrate to maintain the systolic blood pressure at 80 to 90 mmHg or to maintain radial pulses. Some protocols require that the systolic blood pressure be maintained at 70 mmHg to reduce the incidence of hemodilution and increased bleeding associated with aggressive fluid administration in the trauma patient with uncontrolled bleeding. Follow your local protocol.

Tension Pneumothorax

A tension pneumothorax occurs from the disruption of the parietal pleura, visceral pleura, or tracheobronchial tree associated with blunt or penetrating trauma, or iatrogenically from certain medical procedures, such as the use of positive end-expiratory pressure (PEEP) with ventilation or central venous catheter insertion. Also, excessively aggressive ventilation with high pressure and excessive tidal volumes may convert a simple pneumothorax to a tension pneumothorax.

The disruption allows air to escape into the pleural space. Typically, the injury to the pleural lining creates a one-way valve that allows air to enter the pleural space during periods of negative intrathoracic pressure associated with inhalation; however, when air attempts to escape with the increase in intrathoracic pressure, the one-way valve is forced closed, trapping the air in the pleural space. With each inhalation, more air enters the pleural space and becomes trapped. The air begins to build rapidly, collapsing the involved lung.

Because of the nature of lung tissue, the lung has a natural tendency to recoil and collapse, similar to a rubber band when stretched and released. When the water seal is broken between the visceral and parietal pleura, the lung will continue to exert a pulling effect inward and recoil while continuing to create a relative negative pressure inside the pleural space that promotes air entry.

As the air collects in the pleural space on the injured side, the volume and pressure continue to build. This will eventually cause the mediastinum to shift away from the injured hemithorax and contralaterally toward the uninjured hemithorax, resulting in compression of the uninjured lung, right atrium, and vena cava (▶ Figure 43-1). Because the injured lung has already collapsed, compression of the uninjured lung will lead to severe ventilatory and oxygenation compromise. The patient will exhibit signs of severe respiratory distress and hypoxia.

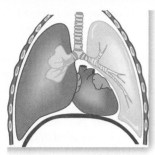

Figure 43-1 In a tension pneumothorax, air continuously fills the pleural space, the lung collapses, pressure rises, and the trapped air compresses the heart and the other lung.

Compression of the vena cava and right atrium will lead to reductions in preload, left ventricular end-diastolic filling volume, and cardiac output. Hypotension, tachycardia, and other signs of poor perfusion will become evident. A tension pneumothorax causes both significant respiratory and circulation compromise, making it an immediate life-threatening condition that requires rapid identification and intervention.

The following are the early signs and symptoms associated with a tension pneumothorax:

- Dyspnea
- Tachypnea
- Tachycardia
- Chest pain
- Anxiety
- Fatigue
- Decreased breath sounds on the injured side

The following are the late findings in a tension pneumothorax:

- Altered mental status
- Hyperexpanded chest wall from hyperinflation of the pleura on the injured side (asymmetrical chest wall)
- Severe respiratory distress to respiratory failure
- Hypotension
- Severely decreased or absent breath sounds on the injured side
- Decreased breath sounds on the uninjured side
- Cyanosis
- Increased resistance to bag-valve ventilation
- Bradypnea (ominous sign of impending respiratory or cardiac arrest)

- Pulsus paradoxus (decrease in systolic blood pressure by >10 mmHg during inhalation)
- A reduction in peripheral pulse amplitude during inspiration
- JVD (may be seen early during inspiration, or not at all if the patient is hypovolemic)
- Displacement of the apical pulse
- Tracheal deviation away from the injured side (late, inconsistent, and very difficult to accurately assess and find)
- Hyperresonance on the injured side
- Subcutaneous emphysema

The first priority of management upon identification of a tension pneumothorax is to reduce the pressure of the affected pleural space. If an occlusive dressing has been applied to an open pneumothorax, it is necessary to remove the dressing and allow any air that has been built up to escape. Be sure to leave the dressing off for a few exhalations. If this is ineffective or if the patient does not have an open pneumothorax, needle decompression of the affected pleural space is necessary.

NEEDLE THORACOSTOMY Needle thoracostomy can be an effective and life-saving intervention in a patient with a tension pneumothorax. However, the skill must be performed correctly and used only on an appropriate patient.

Indications for needle decompression are truly the signs of a tension pneumothorax. It is important to differentiate a tension pneumothorax from a simple pneumothorax, as the latter does *not* indicate needle decompression. As such, the true indicator for needle thoracostomy is the identification of a pneumothorax with hemodynamic side effects—all the potential signs and symptoms of a collapsed lung (e.g., respiratory distress, pain, unequal breath sounds) *plus* signs of hemodynamic dysfunction (low blood pressure, poor perfusion).

Needle thoracostomy is performed with a large-bore chest decompression needle. Recent research has found that standard intravenous needles are likely ill suited for needle decompression. Large-bore IV needles traditionally are not long enough and the "flashback" chamber may actually interfere with the removal of air from the chest cavity once the pleural space is reached. A 2007 study in the *Journal of Military Medicine* found an

average chest wall thickness of 4.5 cm (1.8 inches), meaning that 1.5-inch standard trauma IV catheters would not be long enough to penetrate the pleural space on many patients. Many EMS systems have now moved to utilizing specifically designed chest decompression needles as a result; if one is not available, though, be sure to use a needle long enough to complete the task at hand.

The traditional sites for needle decompression include the second intercostal space, midclavicular line, and the fourth or fifth intercostal space, mid- or anterior axillary line. Some recent information indicates that paramedics frequently are too medial when using the midclavicular site. Remember that the clavicle extends from the suprasternal notch all the way to the acromioclavicular joint in the shoulder. That typically translates to a midclavicular landmark at or lateral to the position of the nipple. Of course every patient is slightly different, but beware of performing a decompression too medially, as this enhances the risk of accidentally penetrating other organs or vital structures.

Controversy exists regarding how to handle the catheter once pressure has been relieved. Some systems suggest using a three-way valve to enable continued release of pressure. There is little evidence supporting this; however, there is also little evidence opposing it. As always, follow local protocol.

After the needle thoracostomy has been performed, ensure that you have established and are maintaining an adequate airway, ventilation, and oxygenation. If ventilating the patient, use minimal rates and tidal volumes. Rapidly transport the patient to an appropriate medical facility capable of managing thoracic trauma. If the tension pneumothorax was relieved in the field, continuously reassess the patient and be cognizant of the redevelopment of a tension pneumothorax.

Open (Communicating) Pneumothorax

When air enters the pleural space through an open wound in the chest wall and parietal pleura, it is termed an *open pneumothorax* or *communicating pneumothorax*. As the air enters the pleural space, it collapses the lung, as in a simple pneumothorax. The difference between the two is that in an open pneumothorax the air enters the thoracic cavity from a wound to the chest wall and not from the

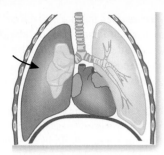

Figure 43-2 In an open pneumothorax, air enters the chest cavity through an open chest wound or leaks from a lacerated lung. The lung then cannot expand.

trachea, as in normal ventilation (▶ Figure 43-2). The wound creates an alternative conduit for air to enter the chest when the intrathoracic pressure becomes negative during inhalation.

If the opening in the chest is large enough, a majority of the air will follow the pathway of least resistance and enter the pleural space directly through the open wound, bypassing the respiratory tract and lungs. A large or significant wound is thought to be two-thirds of the internal diameter of the trachea. In an average-size adult, this means that the wound may need to be only the size of a nickel to be significant.

If a majority of the airflow is into the pleural space and not the lungs, the patient will develop hypoxia rapidly from lack of effective ventilation and oxygenation. The patient will appear to be breathing while the chest wall moves during inspiration and expiration; however, with each chest wall expansion, the negative pressure that is created inside the thorax will draw more air into the open wound, causing the lung to collapse further.

If not impeded by skin, muscle, bone, or other tissue, the open wound may allow air to escape during exhalation. One might think that this would then pose no real danger for the patient, as the air is escaping with each breath. However, remember that the significant wound will draw the majority of air into the pleural space and not the lung, drastically reducing lung ventilation and oxygenation. Even with the escape of air during exhalation, the patient will deteriorate rapidly from the loss of effective alveolar ventilation.

If the air is prevented from escaping during exhalation, the condition may quickly develop into a tension pneumothorax. If the patient is initially assessed in a quiet environment and the open wound is large enough, it may be possible to hear a sucking sound with inhalation and possibly with exhalation. This rare episode is referred to as a *sucking chest wound*.

The following are the signs and symptoms of an open pneumothorax:

- Open wound to the thorax
- Decreased breath sounds on the affected hemithorax
- Tachypnea
- Tachycardia
- Dyspnea
- Subcutaneous emphysema
- Deteriorating SpO_2 reading
- Frothy blood at open wound
- Other signs of respiratory distress

The priority in management of an open pneumothorax is to occlude the open wound to the thorax. This should be done immediately upon its identification. You can initially occlude it with a gloved hand as soon as it is found and, as rapidly as possible, apply an occlusive dressing taped on three sides. Plastic wrap, Vaseline™ gauze, plastic covering from an oxygen mask, or a commercial device such as an Asherman chest seal can be used.

When the wound is sealed, proceed with the standard trauma care to include establishing and maintaining an airway and ventilation, maximizing oxygenation, maintaining circulation, and providing rapid transport to the medical facility. Carefully reassess the patient because the open pneumothorax can develop into a tension pneumothorax, especially if the visceral pleura is injured, allowing air to escape internally into the pleural space from the injured lung.

Flail Chest

Flail chest is defined differently by various sources. Most define it as two or three adjacent ribs fractured in two or more places, which creates a free-floating segment within the chest wall (▶ Figure 43-3). The flail could be anterior or posterior, or it could involve the sternum with ribs on both sides fractured. It typically takes a significant blunt force applied to the thorax to produce a flail segment. In patients with some type of pathology that causes the ribs to weaken, such as osteoporosis, less force may be required to create a flail chest. When such significant force is applied to the chest, the lung has a tendency to become contused. Thus, pulmonary contusion is a second injury common to this type of injury, which may be more lethal than the flail chest.

When a true flail segment is present, it has the ability to move independently of the remainder of the chest wall. Thus, when the chest wall is expanding, the negative intrathoracic pressure will draw the free-floating flail segment inward as the remainder of the chest is moving outward. As the chest wall begins to reduce its size during exhalation, the positive intrathoracic pressure will cause the free-floating flail segment to move outward (▶ Figure 43-4). This abnormal chest wall movement may interfere with effective generation of intrathoracic pressure and lung inflation.

The pulmonary contusion allows blood to seep into the alveolar–capillary interface and within the alveoli. This interferes with the ability of oxygen and carbon dioxide to cross the alveolar membrane

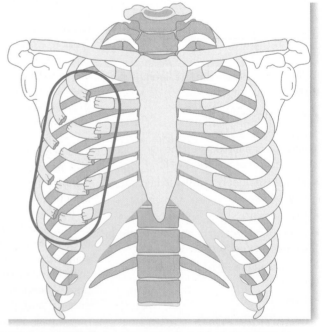

Figure 43-3 Flail chest occurs when blunt trauma causes the fracture of two or more ribs, each in two or more places.

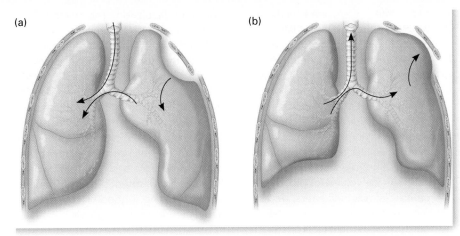

(a)

(b)

Figure 43-4 With a flail chest, (a) the flail segment is drawn inward as the rest of the lung expands with inhalation; (b) the flail segment is pushed outward as the rest of the lung contracts with exhalation.

and alveolar–capillary interface and enter into the capillary, impeding effective gas exchange.

The flail segment and pulmonary contusion will cause respiratory compromise. Both conditions may lead to severe hypoxia and hypercarbia.

Pain associated with the rib fractures is typically a predominant complaint, along with signs and symptoms of respiratory distress. The severe pain may cause the patient to intentionally hypoventilate, leading to hypoxia and hypercarbia. The respiratory distress, hypoxia, and hypercarbia may also be associated with a large pulmonary contusion. A poor SpO₂ reading; pale, cool, and clammy skin; and cyanosis may be present.

Paradoxical movement is often thought to be the predominant sign of a flail segment. When the ribs fracture, however, the intercostal muscles may spasm, and the patient may intentionally limit his breathing, causing the flail segment initially to be stabilized. Thus, the paradoxical movement may be missed on initial inspection of the chest; however, palpation will reveal the unstable segment. This is one reason that palpation of the chest is necessary during the secondary assessment. As the intercostal muscles fatigue, the flail segment becomes more apparent on inspection.

As for other chest injuries, emergency management is aimed at establishing and maintaining an airway, effective ventilation, oxygenation, and circulation. Remember, the patient may be intentionally hypoventilating because of the pain and not as a result of some other respiratory pathology. If the respiratory rate or

tidal volume is ineffective, begin positive pressure ventilation with a bag-valve device. Maximize oxygenation by nonrebreather mask at 15 liters per minute (lpm) in the adequately breathing patient or attached to the bag-valve device through a reservoir if providing assisted ventilation.

Stabilization of the flail segment with sandbags or other devices is no longer recommended. The patient may be able to self-splint using a pillow and his own arm. Rapidly transport the patient to a medical facility capable of managing the chest injury.

Pain management is an important element of treating any chest wall injury including rib fractures. Frequently, pain impedes the patient's ability to move air. In many cases, patients will hypoventilate in response to the guarded respirations they are taking. Using a narcotic analgesic such as fentanyl can allow the patient to breathe more easily and adequately. When systems allow, paramedics should be aggressive with pain management and provide optimal relief to improve ventilations.

Hemothorax

A hemothorax is very similar to a pneumothorax; however, blood instead of air fills the pleural space and collapses the lung. The source of bleeding varies but is associated with laceration or rupture of the lung tissue itself or a vascular structure within the thoracic cavity as a result of blunt or penetrating trauma, causing the blood to collect in the pleural cavity.

As in a pneumothorax, as the blood continues to collect it places inward pressure on the lung tissue, collapsing the

lung (▶ Figure 43-5). Because of gravity, the blood is pulled downward and has a tendency to collect in the lower bases of the lung in the seated patient or posteriorly in the supine patient. This is important to consider when assessing the patient's breath sounds.

Stabilization of a flail segment with sandbags or other devices is no longer recommended.

In a pneumothorax, the air moves upward and collects in the superior portion of the lungs in the seated patient and the anterior portion in the supine patient. Thus, the breath sounds would be decreased or absent in the upper lobes in the seated patient or anteriorly in the supine patient, whereas in a hemothorax the breath sounds would be decreased or absent in the lower lobes in the seated patient or posterior in the supine patient. Because blood, and not air, is the source of lung collapse, not only is the patient prone to respiratory compromise, but he can also experience hypovolemia.

The patient with a hemothorax presents with signs and symptoms very similar to those of a patient with a pneumothorax; however, because of the blood loss, signs and symptoms of hypovolemia usually predominate. (It is common for a pneumothorax and hemothorax to occur together. This condition is referred to as a *hemopneumothorax*.)

The following are the signs and symptoms of a hemothorax:

- Dyspnea
- Tachypnea
- Decreased or absent breath sounds to the affected hemithorax
- Tachycardia

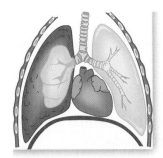

Figure 43-5 In a hemothorax, blood leaks into the chest cavity from lacerated vessels or the lung itself, and the lung compresses.

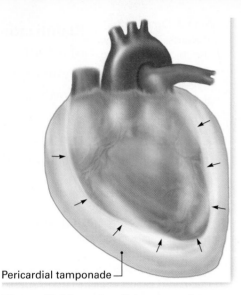

Pericardial tamponade

Figure 43-6 In pericardial tamponade, accumulating blood compresses the heart inward.

- Pale, cool, and clammy skin
- Decreasing systolic blood pressure
- Narrow pulse pressure
- Decreasing SpO₂ reading
- Evidence of blunt or penetrating trauma to the thorax

Emergency care focuses on management of the airway, ventilation, oxygenation, and circulation. The paramedic is limited in managing the hemothorax in the field and should focus on reversing life threats found in the primary assessment and on expeditious transport. Needle decompression will not relieve a true hemothorax, but providers should keep in mind that hemothorax and pneumothorax are frequently paired. If indications indicate, needle decompression may still be attempted in undifferentiated cases.

Administration of fluids to expand the existing blood volume should be restricted, even in a hemothorax. Fluids will dilute the blood, making it less viscous, and will increase the blood pressure, allowing the wound to bleed faster and potentially dislodge a clot. Follow your local protocol when infusing fluids in the trauma patient.

Acute Pericardial Tamponade

Acute pericardial tamponade is seen in approximately 2 percent of patients with penetrating trauma to the chest and upper abdomen. It is rarely seen in patients with blunt thoracic trauma and is most often associated with stab wounds to the chest. This is a critical chest injury that can cause the patient's condition to deteriorate in minutes. Rapid recognition and subsequent expeditious transport are imperative to patient survival.

Pericardial tamponade occurs when an injury to the heart causes blood to collect in the pericardial sac, a tough fibrous sac surrounding the heart. As the volume of blood in the pericardial sac increases, it compresses the atria and ventricles and does not allow them to fill adequately (▶ Figure 43-6). This reduces the stroke volume—the amount of blood being ejected with each ventricular contraction.

A decrease in stroke volume causes a decrease in cardiac output. A decrease in cardiac output decreases the blood pressure. This, in turn, affects perfusion of the vital organs. As the blood pressure decreases, the body attempts to compensate by increasing the heart rate and total peripheral vascular resistance (PVR) through vasoconstriction. Thus, tachycardia and pale, cool, clammy skin are signs of pericardial tamponade. Because the blood is not moving forward effectively through the heart, aorta, and arteries, the blood backs up in the venous system, causing the veins—especially the large veins close to the heart, such as the jugular veins—to become distended.

Signs and symptoms of acute pericardial tamponade are very similar to those of a tension pneumothorax, with the exception of significant dyspnea because there is no associated lung injury in pericardial tamponade. Therefore, the breath sounds will remain equal bilaterally, and there will be no tracheal deviation. Signs and symptoms include the following:

- Tachycardia
- Anxiety or anxiousness
- Hypotension
- Cyanosis
- Pulsus paradoxus (decrease in systolic blood pressure by >10 mmHg during inhalation)
- A reduction in peripheral pulse amplitude during inspiration
- JVD

Emergency care focuses on management of the airway, ventilation, oxygenation, and circulation. The paramedic is limited in managing a pericardial tamponade in the field; however, early recognition of the condition and expeditious transport could be lifesaving. The emergency care should focus on reversing life threats found in the primary assessment.

Differentiating among these chest injuries could be difficult (see Table 43-1). Some of the injuries may present with more subtle signs and symptoms initially. Having a high index of suspicion is imperative to making a good clinical decision and differential field diagnosis.

CHEST TUBES

Any seasoned paramedic has probably encountered patients in need of a chest tube—whether they are medical patients with a spontaneous pneumothorax or trauma patients with an acute simple or tension pneumothorax. The main reason any patient requires a chest tube is physiologically very simple—to return the inherent negativity of the thoracic cage, allowing adequate lung expansion. In addition, chest tubes can be used for a variety of other reasons, including to drain blood, pus, or other fluids from the chest cavity; to instill medications such as talc or chemotherapeutic agents for some medical conditions; or to reexpand a partially collapsed lung (pneumothorax).

Chest tubes are placed through surgical stab wounds or via a trocar—a sharp, pointed metal stylet on which the chest tube is mounted, much like an IV catheter. The inserting clinician must ensure that the chest tube completely enters the pleural space, so that all drainage eyelets on the tube end up inside the thorax in order to form an air-tight seal. Sutures are then used to secure the tube, and an occlusive dressing is placed around the tube at the insertion site to further enhance the integrity of the system. The goal should be that atmospheric air cannot enter the chest cavity during inspiration, which would create an open pneumothorax.

The paramedic must assess stability before transporting patients, and patients receiving emergent chest tubes are unstable by their very nature. The paramedic must consider whether the treatment (i.e., the chest tube) has sufficiently stabilized the patient to allow safe transport. Patients receive emergent chest tubes for any number of conditions, including significant simple pneumothorax, tension

TABLE 43-1 — Differential Field Diagnosis of Chest Injury

Sign or Symptom	Tension Pneumothorax	Open Pneumothorax	Flail Chest	Hemothorax	Pericardial Tamponade
Breath sounds	Severely decreased or absent unilaterally and possibly decreased on the uninjured side	Decreased on the injured side	Decreased on the injured side	Decreased on the injured side	Present, clear, and equal bilaterally
Blood pressure	Decreased with a narrow pulse pressure	Normal if not associated with other trauma	Normal if not associated with other trauma	Decreased with a narrow pulse pressure	Decreased with a narrow pulse pressure
Pulse	Weak and rapid peripheral pulses	Tachycardia possibly present owing to hypoxia, but peripheral pulses normal unless with other associated trauma	Tachycardia possibly present owing to hypoxia, but peripheral pulses normal unless with associated trauma	Weak and rapid peripheral pulses	Weak and rapid peripheral pulses
Jugular veins	Distended (late finding) if patient not hypovolemic	Normal	Normal	Flat	Distended (late finding) if patient not hypovolemic
Respiratory distress	Severe	Present	Present	Present	Possible
Pulsus paradoxus	Present	Absent	Absent	Absent	Present
Asymmetrical chest	Present	Absent	Absent	Absent	Absent
Paradoxical chest movement	Absent	Absent	Present	Absent	Absent
Decreased SpO_2	Severe	Present to severe	Present to severe	Present	Present

pneumothorax, or hemopneumothorax. While the chest tube is inserted, the paramedic must be sure to keep monitoring the patient for changes in condition as well as the specifics of chest tube monitoring, which are outlined below.

Assisting with Chest Tubes

When assisting with chest tube insertion, the paramedic should be cognizant of the sterile nature of the procedure. The paramedic assistant does not need to be "sterile" but must be sure not to contaminate the clinician's sterile field or objects. After the chest tube is inserted, the assistant may pass the nonsterile end of the drainage tubing to the clinician, who attaches it to the chest tube. Additional measures to secure the tubing to the patient's chest will be needed, including spiral-taping all chest tube-drain tube connections and placing reinforcing tape over the dressing site.

At insertion, the paramedic and clinician should note whether any subcutaneous emphysema is present at the insertion site. An increase in subcutaneous emphy-sema during transport should alert the paramedic that the chest tube may have become partially dislodged and prompt a complete reassessment of the patient, the chest drainage unit, and especially the insertion site.

Chest Tube Monitoring

Chest tube monitoring can be divided into four sections: insertion site care, chest drainage output, water/mechanical seal, and suction. In assessing the insertion site, the paramedic should look for increased drainage from the site on the dressing, palpate for subcutaneous emphysema, and inspect the tape connections for integrity. The chest tube should be secured in at least two spots to the patient's thorax—at the insertion site and also along the lower abdomen to prevent accidental dislodgement. This will allow dependent loops to form below the patient's chest so passive drainage may occur with gravity.

Chest drainage should be inspected for color, clarity, consistency, and total amount. A recently placed emergent chest tube should be inspected at least every 30 to 60 minutes, looking for total amount of output. The presence of bloody drainage of greater than 1500 mL on insertion or greater than 100 mL per hour for four consecutive hours is considered by many to be signs of the need for operative intervention (thoracotomy). Drainage amounts can be marked directly on the face of the chest drainage unit for easy reference. The paramedic should always remember that to ensure that a negative pressure is maintained in the chest drainage unit, the unit must be kept upright and below the level of the patient's chest (i.e., the insertion site).

The next step for the paramedic in assessing the chest tube and drainage unit is to check that the water seal or mechanical valve is at the ordered level. In a wet system, a column of water forms the seal and prevents air from reentering the patient's chest. Typically, a negative 20 cmH_2O is ordered by the clinician, although other amounts may be encountered in the settings of pediatric patients or chest surgeries. In a dry system, a one-way mechanical valve prevents air from entering the system and functions instead of a water column. The water column of the valve prevents atmospheric air from being drawn into the chest during inspiration.

The final item to assess in dealing with chest tubes is the presence or absence of wall suction. The use of suction with a chest tube is not mandatory unless the clinician orders it—suction simply helps the lung reexpand more quickly. Remember that it is the one-way valve in a dry system or water column in the wet system that provides the negativity to the system and prevents air entrainment back into the patient's chest through the chest tube. Suction just enhances the process and does not itself provide inherent negative pressure directly to the thoracic cage.

In addition, most commercial chest drainage units have a device called an *air leak indicator*. This is part of the water seal; bubbling in this section of the chest drainage unit alerts the paramedic that an air leak is present in either the patient's chest (more likely) or in the chest drainage unit/tubing/connections. Absence of bubbling or intermittent bubbling with a cough may suggest that the lung is fully expanded.

TRANSITIONING

REVIEW ITEMS

1. A patient with a stab wound to the anterior chest presents with a decrease in mental status; circumoral cyanosis; very weak and rapid radial pulses; pale, cool, and clammy skin; blood pressure 72/56 mmHg; heart rate 132 beats per minute (bpm); and respirations 28/minute with adequate chest rise. You note jugular venous engorgement on inspiration. The patient has equal and clear breath sounds bilaterally. You should suspect _____.

   a. tension pneumothorax
   b. hemothorax
   c. open pneumothorax
   d. pericardial tamponade

2. A patient with a penetrating chest injury has jugular venous engorgement and a decrease in pulse amplitude on inspiration. You should suspect _____.

   a. an increase in intrathoracic pressure
   b. excessive blood loss into the pleural space
   c. a decrease in peripheral vascular resistance
   d. fluid collection in the alveolar–capillary interface

3. A patient was kicked in the anterior chest during a fight. He complains of severe pain to the chest on inhalation and difficulty breathing. His radial pulse is 128/minute, respiratory rate is 38/minute and shallow, and blood pressure is 148/92 mmHg. His breath sounds are clear and equal but decreased bilaterally. You should suspect _____.

   a. a hemothorax
   b. a tension pneumothorax
   c. a chest wall contusion
   d. a pericardial tamponade

4. A patient with an open chest injury is anxious and agitated. You should suspect that this response is most likely caused by_____.

   a. pain associated with the injury
   b. a normal reaction to trauma
   c. a narrowing pulse pressure
   d. a decrease in oxygenation

5. Which of the following would most likely differentiate a tension pneumothorax from a pericardial tamponade?

   a. unilateral decreased or absent breath sounds
   b. jugular vein distention and a narrow pulse pressure
   c. severe tachycardia and hypotension
   d. peripheral and core cyanosis

6. You are providing emergency care to a patient with a gunshot wound to the chest. He is responding to verbal stimuli with moaning. His SpO_2 is 86 percent; radial pulse is absent; skin is pale, cool, and clammy; his carotid pulse reveals a heart rate of 123 bpm; his respirations are 22/minute with adequate chest rise; and his blood pressure is 66/48 mmHg. You should _____ .

   a. initiate two-large bore IVs and run both at a wide-open rate until the blood pressure reaches a normal range
   b. initiate one large-bore IV and run at a rate to achieve a systolic blood pressure of 80 to 90 mmHg or until radial pulses are regained
   c. initiate one large bore IV line and keep it at a to-keep-open rate
   d. not initiate an IV line in the chest-injured patient

APPLIED PATHOPHYSIOLOGY

1. Explain the difference in the presentation between a patient suspected of having a simple pneumothorax and a patient with a tension pneumothorax.

2. Explain the difference in the presentation between a patient suspected of having a hemothorax and a patient in hypovolemic shock with no chest injury.

3. Explain the difference in the presentation between a patient suspected of having a tension pneumothorax and a patient in hypovolemic shock with no chest injury.

4. Explain the pathophysiology of hypotension and hypoperfusion in a pericardial tamponade.

5. Explain the pathophysiology of hypotension and hypoperfusion in a tension pneumothorax.

6. Explain why a patient with a flail segment can become severely hypoxic.

CLINICAL DECISION MAKING

You are called to treat a 19-year-old male patient who was involved in an altercation. He is sitting upright against the wall outside a club. He is very anxious and agitated and is complaining that he cannot breathe. You note a large bloodstain on the front of his shirt.

1. Based on the scene size-up and characteristics of the scene, list the possible conditions you should suspect.

The primary assessment reveals that the patient is alert, anxious, agitated, and confused; complains of severe shortness of breath; and has circumoral cyanosis. His respirations are 38/minute; radial pulse is barely palpable at 148 beats per minute; skin is pale, cool, and clammy; and SpO_2 is 72 percent. You expose the patient and find what appears to be a stab wound to the right chest.

2. What are the immediate life threats?

3. What immediate emergency care should you provide based on the life threats found in the primary assessment?

4. Explain the related pathophysiology of the anxiousness and agitation.

5. Explain the related pathophysiology of the confusion.

6. What conditions have you ruled out from the scene size-up? What conditions seem more plausible based on the primary assessment?

During the secondary assessment, you note that the patient is becoming less agitated; however, his mental status continues to decrease. His jugular veins appear to be engorged, and you note subcutaneous emphysema when palpating the neck. The breath sounds are absent on the right and decreased on the left. A small stab wound is noted to the right anterior chest at approximately the fourth intercostal space at the midclavicular line. No evidence of trauma is noted to the abdomen, pelvis, or extremities. The abdomen is soft and nontender, and the pelvis is stable. The peripheral pulses are absent, and the skin is extremely pale, cool, and clammy. You note cyanosis to the distal extremities, face, and neck. The blood pressure is 72/60 mmHg, heart rate is 148 beats per minute, respirations are 42/minute and labored, and SpO_2 is 68 percent.

7. What condition should you suspect?

8. Explain the differential indicators as to why you suspect that condition.

9. What further emergency care should you provide?

10. Why is the patient's blood pressure only 72/60 mmHg? Explain the reason for the narrow pulse pressure.

11. Explain why the patient became less agitated. Why is this a critical finding in this patient?

TOPIC

44

Standard Trauma

Competency Integrates assessment findings with principles of epidemiology and pathophysiology to formulate a field impression to implement a comprehensive treatment/disposition plan for an acutely injured patient.

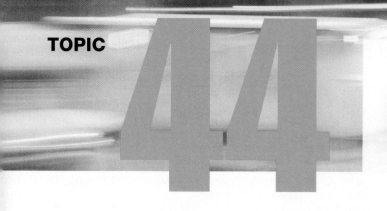

ABDOMINAL TRAUMA

TRANSITION highlights

- Overview of the three types of organs in the abdominal cavity (hollow, vascular, solid).
- Mechanisms that cause blunt and penetrating trauma.
- Assessment findings with abdominal trauma and current recommendations for the management of these injuries.

INTRODUCTION

Children sometimes play a game called mystery box, in which they take turns guessing about an unknown object contained within a closed box. In many ways, this game is similar to the assessment and treatment of a patient with an abdominal injury. You cannot see what is inside the abdomen, and, indeed, it is full of surprises.

As a paramedic, you have some clues, however. You have a working knowledge of anatomy, and you have an assessment that will allow you to gather information and help you form reasonable conclusions. In some cases, your assessment of the abdomen will point you to likely problems. In other cases, you may never know for sure what is wrong.

That said, it is important to remember that in our game of mystery box, the goal is not necessarily to pinpoint the exact problem but, rather, to identify when that problem is causing a critical life threat. With abdominal trauma, the focus must always be on the big picture.

EPIDEMIOLOGY

Trauma is the leading cause of death of patients between the ages of 1 and 44. The specific frequency of death associated with isolated abdominal trauma is difficult to pinpoint. However, when you consider internal bleeding and multisystem trauma

cases, blunt abdominal trauma is consistently among the leading causes of trauma-related death.

PATHOPHYSIOLOGY

The abdomen itself is a container. Housed within this container are a series of vital structures that can be generally classified among three categories: hollow organs, solid organs, and blood vessels. Although these structures are generally well protected, they are subject to damage associated with trauma.

Damage can come in the form of direct force, such as a blow to the abdomen; compression forces, such as organs being squeezed between a seatbelt and the spinal column; and shearing/deceleration injury, such as an organ being torn out of place as the body decelerates. How these organs will respond to these offending forces will depend largely on their specific makeup.

HOLLOW ORGANS   Hollow organs in the abdomen include (among others) the stomach, intestines, urinary bladder, and gallbladder. Hollow organs generally respond well to trauma, as they tend to be flexible and possess the capability of stretching. However, when excessive force is exerted on these organs, the internal pressure changes will often cause the hollow structure to rupture.

Rupture of the structure and associated bleeding can be problematic in itself, but often the larger problem is the release of air and fluid contents into the abdominal vault. Depending on the organ, spilled contents can cause inflammation and life-threatening infection.

SOLID ORGANS   Solid organs in the abdomen include the liver, spleen, pancreas, and kidneys. Solid organs are dense and are often very rich in blood supply. Because of their solid makeup, they do not respond well to trauma. External forces often cause direct damage to the organ, which can result in excessive bleeding.

BLOOD VESSELS   Several large blood vessels make their way through the abdominal cavity. The abdominal aorta and the inferior vena cava are among the largest. Trauma to these vessels can lead to massive blood loss that is not visible; this is the leading cause of death in abdominal injuries.

Trauma to the Abdomen

Abdominal structures can be damaged by a variety of forces. When considering abdominal injuries, it is important to understand the nature of the energy exerted on them.

DIRECT FORCE INJURY Direct force results from energy being applied specifically onto a point in the abdomen. This can come in the form of penetrating trauma, such as a gunshot wound, or in the form of blunt trauma, such as a poorly placed lap belt striking the lower abdominal quadrants. In direct force injuries, the energy of the offending object is transferred directly to whatever organ or structure happens to be in its path.

COMPRESSION INJURY With a mechanism similar to that of direct force, compression injuries exert forces directly onto organs and other structures. In this case, an organ is squeezed, or compressed, between other structures. For example, when an unbelted driver in a car crash is thrown forward into the steering wheel, the wheel will be driven into his abdomen. As it drives backward into the area of his liver, that organ will be compressed between the wheel and the spinal column, potentially resulting in organ damage.

SHEARING/DECELERATION INJURY Isaac Newton found that objects in motion tend to stay in motion. When a body is stopped abruptly, as in a motor vehicle crash, its organs continue moving forward until they are stopped. If the force is great enough, these organs may be torn from their tethering structures. Often this rapid deceleration can damage the organ. In some cases, the tethering ligaments may actually slice through the solid organs they normally hold in place. This shears the organ into pieces and results in massive hemorrhage. Shearing injuries are common in both the liver and aorta.

Abdominal trauma can penetrate the muscular walls and skin and cause an open injury. Occasionally, internal organs can protrude through holes (this is called an *evisceration*). More commonly, however, injuries are caused by blunt forces that do not penetrate the abdominal walls. This type of injury is referred to as a *closed abdominal injury.*

ASSESSMENT FINDINGS

Abdominal injuries frequently result in severe internal bleeding. Therefore, the real focus of the assessment of abdominal trauma is the rapid identification of life threats. We will discuss techniques that may assist you in identifying a likely abdominal problem; however, you should never become so focused on the differential diagnosis that you neglect the larger priorities.

A thorough primary assessment is critical in a patient with abdominal trauma. Remember that although the abdominal wound may be dramatic, airway and breathing issues may still be the higher priority. It is assuredly true that the best way to keep a trauma patient alive is to manage the airway and ventilation. This is true regardless of the nature of the patient's injuries.

Your primary assessment may also reveal signs of shock that would indicate internal bleeding long before you examine the abdomen. Keep in mind that if you identify shock, treatment must begin immediately regardless of what part of the abdomen is causing the problem.

Once you have completed the primary assessment (and treated any necessary deficits), you can use your knowledge of abdominal anatomy to help you identify other potential problems that may be associated with trauma. Here, you will consider both the mechanism and location of injury to better understand the potential for damage.

Recall that the abdomen is divided into four quadrants (▶ Figure 44-1). The umbilicus is the center and divides both upper and lower and left and right. Knowing the general location of key organs (Table 44-1) will help you predict the potential for damage.

When assessing the abdomen, consider the mechanism of injury. What forces impacted the abdomen? How much energy was transferred? High energy can be expected to cause more damage than low energy. Consider, for instance, the difference between being struck by a rock and being struck by a bullet. Consider also the path that the energy took.

Certain areas of the abdomen are more vulnerable to damage caused by trauma. Recall the location of the solid organs. For example, when trauma impacts the right upper quadrant, the liver is vulnerable. Because the liver is a vascular, solid organ, damage to this area often results in severe

> **Although the abdominal wound may be dramatic, airway and breathing issues may still be the higher priority.**

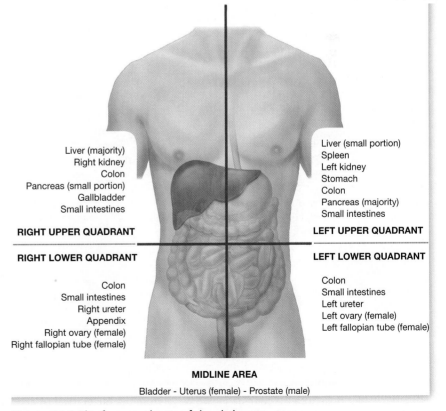

Liver (majority)
Right kidney
Colon
Pancreas (small portion)
Gallbladder
Small intestines

RIGHT UPPER QUADRANT

RIGHT LOWER QUADRANT

Colon
Small intestines
Right ureter
Appendix
Right ovary (female)
Right fallopian tube (female)

Liver (small portion)
Spleen
Left kidney
Stomach
Colon
Pancreas (majority)
Small intestines

LEFT UPPER QUADRANT

LEFT LOWER QUADRANT

Colon
Small intestines
Left ureter
Left ovary (female)
Left fallopian tube (female)

MIDLINE AREA

Bladder - Uterus (female) - Prostate (male)

Figure 44-1 The four quadrants of the abdomen.

TABLE 44-1 Contents of the Abdominal Quadrants

Right Upper Quadrant	Left Upper Quadrant
• Liver	• Liver
• Gallbladder	• Spleen
• Right kidney	• Stomach
• Colon/small intestine	• Left kidney
• Pancreas (head)	• Colon/small intestine
	• Pancreas (tail)

Right Lower Quadrant	Left Lower Quadrant
• Appendix	• Colon/small intestine
• Colon/small intestine	• Ovary/fallopian tube (women)
• Ovary/fallopian tube (women)	• Bladder
• Bladder	

bleeding. Use your knowledge of anatomy to predict which structures are most likely to be involved in the injury.

Penetrating Versus Blunt Trauma

PENETRATING TRAUMA Penetrating trauma disrupts the integrity of the abdominal wall. Some object, such as a knife, a bullet, or a handlebar, has physically been inserted into the abdominal cavity and displaced and destroyed the tissue and structures that happened to be in the way. In some cases, the path of damage is easy to predict. In a truly open wound, the path may actually be visible. However, you should always remember that penetrating trauma is not always easy to assess.

Small external holes can result in huge internal injuries. Consider a small bullet hole (▶ Figure 44-2). Although the offending object is small, the energy behind it is great. This impact can cause massive organ damage beneath the skin, despite leaving only a small entrance wound.

Occasionally, with penetrating trauma, an exit wound may be visible as well. This may help predict the path of destruction, but the process is inherently unreliable because of bullet fragmentation and ricochet.

Consider also a cone of damage with penetrating weapons such as a knife. By looking at the object we may be able to predict depth, but remember that the object may have been moved inside the body and therefore may have caused damage to a larger area than the immediate pathway.

When assessing penetrating trauma, be sure to fully expose patients. Small puncture wounds are often difficult to find. Be sure also to examine all four sides of the abdomen: anterior, posterior, and the two flanks or sides.

BLUNT TRAUMA Blunt trauma results from force spread out over a larger area such that the abdominal wall is not disrupted (a closed abdominal injury). Make no mistake, however; the energy behind the offending force can be immense. The difficulty in assessing a closed injury is that there is no clear pathway. In some cases, you can identify the likely point of impact, but even in these cases the damage beneath the skin is often unpredictable.

In blunt trauma, you will need to assume the worst and use other findings, such as vital signs, to indicate shock and other life threats. When assessing closed abdominal injuries, consider the patient's position at the time of impact. Is the patient guarding his abdomen (▶ Figure 44-3)?

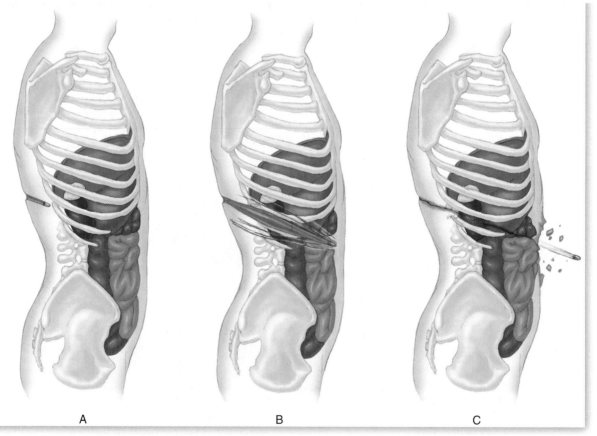

A	B	C

Figure 44-2 Bullets cause damage in two ways: from the bullet itself (A and C) and from cavitation, which is the temporary cavity caused by the pressure wave (B).

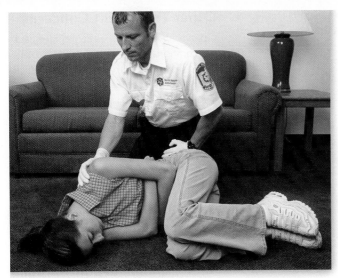

Figure 44-3 A typical "guarded" position for a patient with acute abdominal pain.

Look for pain, rigidity, and discoloration that may indicate an underlying injury (▶ Figure 44-4). Use palpation of all four quadrants to assess for tenderness, rigidity, and guarding. Remember also that abdominal injury is often missed when treating a patient with multisystem trauma. Often blunt trauma (a closed injury) is difficult to identify when the patient is unconscious or distracted by other injuries. When possible, complete a secondary survey that includes palpation of the abdomen to help better identify abdominal problems.

Abdominal Pain

Abdominal pain is a useful indicator of injury. Localizing abdominal pain can be helpful in identifying likely injured structures. Discuss pain with the patient. Palpate the abdomen to identify point tenderness.

Remember that abdominal pain can also be referred to other areas (called *referred pain*), such as a spleen injury causing shoulder pain. At the same time, keep in mind that damaged organs may be bleeding rapidly without causing significant pain. Other injuries, such as extremity trauma or spinal cord injury, can often distract the patient from abdominal pain. A lack of pain should never rule out a potential abdominal injury, especially in the presence of other physical findings.

Abdomen or Lung

Injuries to the abdomen quite frequently involve lung tissue. Remember that on inspiration, the diaphragm can drop as low as the umbilicus and therefore expose lung tissue to what would otherwise be an abdominal injury. Always suspect a lung injury with abdominal trauma and carefully assess breathing to identify possible lung and/or chest complications.

DECISION MAKING: SHOCK AND ABDOMINAL TRAUMA

Mechanism of Injury + Shock = Critical Patient

You should always keep this formula in mind when assessing a patient with abdominal trauma. In the presence of any abdominal injury (even a minor one), keep a keen eye out for the signs and symptoms of shock, including altered mental status, tachycardia, increased respiratory rate, and delayed capillary refill. Any of these signs can indicate an underlying critical injury.

Pediatric Considerations

The organs in a pediatric abdomen are more exposed, as they are covered less by the rib cage than those in an adult. The abdomen also makes up a larger portion of the overall torso and therefore is more exposed to trauma. Always consider abdominal injuries in blunt force trauma in children. Your index of suspicion should be especially high in car-versus-pedestrian injuries, as often the abdomen is directly in the line of the majority of the energy being transferred by the car.

EMERGENCY MEDICAL CARE

The most important elements of care for a patient with abdominal trauma are directed by findings in the primary assessment. Treat airway, breathing, and circulation with the highest priority.

Airway and Breathing

Regardless of how dramatic the abdominal injury, airway and breathing will always take precedence. Providing oxygenation and ventilation to the trauma patient is a crucial element in improving outcomes.

Open abdominal injuries may disrupt not only the abdominal cavity, but also the chest cavity. If the penetration is high enough to involve lung tissue, the hole in the abdomen may be interfering with respiratory mechanics. Consider using a nonporous dressing with any question of lung involvement. These dressings seal abdominal wounds to prevent air entry and potentially preserve the integrity of the chest cavity as well.

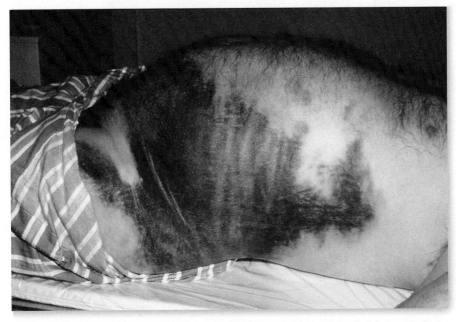

Figure 44-4 Abdominal bruising is a sign of blunt trauma and probable internal bleeding.

Circulation

Recognize and treat shock. Apply high-concentration oxygen to maintain normal oxygen saturations, maintain normal temperature, and initiate rapid transport to an appropriate facility. Manage external hemorrhage when possible, and always have a high index of suspicion for internal bleeding in abdominal trauma. Transport patients with suspected shock rapidly.

Initiate a large-bore IV with normal saline, and administer as necessitated by the patient's clinical picture and per local protocol.

Other Treatment Concerns

Open abdominal injuries sometimes cause eviscerations. Be sure to cover exposed internal organs with a moistened saline dressing and then seal the wound with a nonporous dressing (▶ Figure 44-5). Never replace protruding internal organs.

First take Standard Precautions.

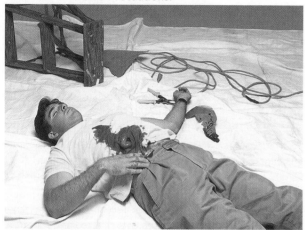

Open abdominal wound with evisceration.

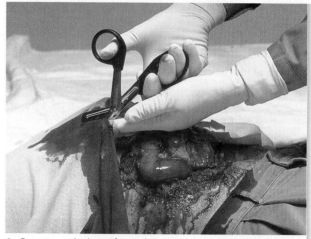

1. Cut away clothing from the wound.

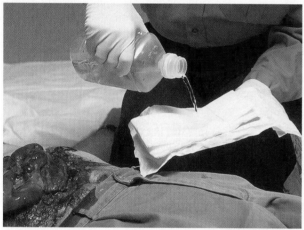

2. Soak a dressing with sterile saline.

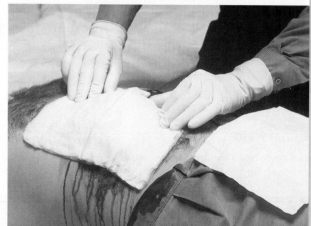

3. Place the moist dressing over the wound.

Cover the dressed wound to maintain warmth. Secure the covering with tape or cravats tied above and below the position of the exposed organ.

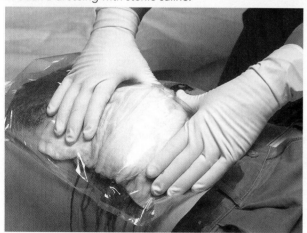

4. Apply an occlusive dressing over the moist dressing if local protocols recommend that you do so.

Figure 44-5 Steps in dressing an open abdominal wound.

When treating an impaled object, stabilize it in place. Never remove the object.

Constantly reassess patients with abdominal injuries, as their status can change rapidly. Internal bleeding can quickly lead to a decompensated patient, and it is your obligation to recognize such deterioration.

When appropriate, transport the patient with abdominal injuries in a position of comfort. Often a knee-flexed position will be preferred. Ensure that your destination choice has the capability to care for the injuries that may be present.

In the past, analgesics were discouraged in abdominal trauma. However with today's relatively short-acting pain medications, such as fentanyl, pain management can be used safely in the case of abdominal trauma. Follow local protocols, but consider pain management in any trauma patient.

Always remember that identification of the specific abdominal injury is less important than treating immediate life threats. Refer back to the primary assessment and treat life threats first.

TRANSITIONING

REVIEW ITEMS

1. Which of the following would be considered a hollow organ?
   - a. gallbladder
   - b. liver
   - c. spleen
   - d. kidney

2. You are treating a patient who was struck in the abdomen by a hockey stick. He complains of left shoulder pain despite the fact he sustained no trauma to the shoulder. You should suspect _____.
   - a. a spleen injury
   - b. a prior shoulder injury that has been exacerbated
   - c. a shoulder injury that is referring pain to the abdomen
   - d. a gallbladder injury

3. You are treating a patient with a puncture wound to the upper right quadrant. The organ you should be most concerned about is the _____.
   - a. liver
   - b. spleen
   - c. stomach
   - d. appendix

4. You are assessing a patient who has been stabbed in the upper left quadrant. He complains of difficulty breathing and is coughing up blood. These findings are most likely caused by _____.
   - a. lung tissue damage from the abdominal injury
   - b. referred pain from the abdomen
   - c. a chest injury you missed on your assessment
   - d. a stomach injury

5. You are treating a patient with an abdominal evisceration. Your primary assessment reveals vomit in his airway, 6 respirations per minute, and a carotid pulse of 130. You should first _____.
   - a. suction the airway
   - b. ventilate with a bag-valve mask
   - c. apply moist sterile dressings
   - d. apply an occlusive dressing

APPLIED PATHOPHYSIOLOGY

1. For each of the following organs, indicate in which quadrant it is found and whether it is a hollow or solid organ.

4. Describe how a deceleration/shearing force would injure an abdominal organ.

Organ	Location	Hollow or Solid
Spleen		
Liver		
Stomach		
Gallbladder		

2. List three signs of a closed abdominal injury.

3. Describe why a solid organ might be more vulnerable to trauma compared with a hollow organ.

5. Discuss why penetrating trauma to the abdomen is often difficult to assess. Why is it unpredictable?

CLINICAL DECISION MAKING

You are called to respond to a 17-year-old male patient who has been struck by a car. On arrival, bystanders note that he was hit by the grille of a car traveling approximately 35 miles per hour and was thrown 10 feet onto the street. The scene is safe, and you approach. Your general impression finds the patient on the ground with an angulated femur fracture. He is moaning in pain. You note that he is pale and diaphoretic.

Your primary assessment reveals a patent airway, rapid breathing with bilateral lung sounds, and no radial pulse. He does, however, have a carotid pulse at a rate of 124.

1. Is this patient critical? Why or why not?

2. What immediate actions must you take?

The patient states, "My leg hurts!" He denies any further complaint. Your rapid trauma assessment finds tenderness and guarding in the upper left quadrant of his abdomen, and the obviously fractured femur.

3. Is this patient in shock? If yes, what is the most likely cause of the shock?

4. Given the tenderness in the upper left quadrant, what organ(s) might you be concerned is/are affected?

5. Explain the pathophysiologic cause for the following:

   a. Absent radial pulse

   b. Pale skin

   c. No complaint of pain even though his belly is tender to palpation

6. You begin a large-bore IV on the patient and run normal saline. What is the goal for your fluid resuscitation?

Standard Trauma

Competency Integrates assessment findings with principles of epidemiology and pathophysiology to formulate a field impression to implement a comprehensive treatment/disposition plan for an acutely injured patient.

TOPIC

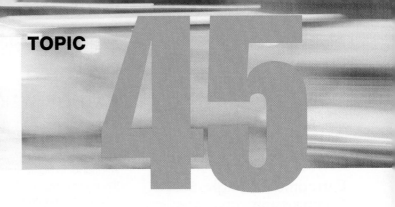

SOFT TISSUE INJURIES: CRUSH INJURY AND COMPARTMENT SYNDROME

INTRODUCTION

Crush injuries and compartment syndrome damage tissues in a very specific way. Crush injury is a form of blunt trauma, whereas compartment syndrome is a complication of blunt trauma. These particular types of injury present the paramedic with very specific challenges to patient assessment and care. Compartment syndrome requires a paramedic to think long term and prevent ongoing injury, whereas crush injuries force the provider to consider some very different treatment modalities. In this topic, we discuss both of these specific circumstances as they pertain to blunt trauma.

Even with these specific circumstances in mind, remember the basic principles of assessing and treating blunt force trauma. In particular, recall that when dealing with soft tissue injuries you must consider not just the outside of the skin, but also the potential for injury beneath the skin.

Blunt trauma damages by applying force and stretching tissues beyond their normal tolerances. A *crush injury*—a particular type of blunt trauma—damages tissues by compressive force

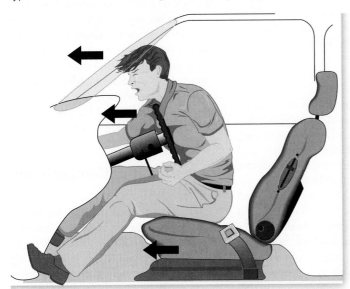

Figure 45-1 Direct force can cause crush injuries, some resulting in open wounds.

(▶ Figure 45-1). This force is generally applied over larger areas and damages more tissue, either through direct compression (direct, crushing force) or by compressing tissues and limiting blood flow (perfusion) to the cells in that area. Crush injuries can occur over a relatively small area, such as striking the thumb with a hammer, or over a large area, such as traumatic asphyxia of the chest. The mechanism of injury remains similar.

This type of injury can occur from either external or internal forces. An example of external direct compression might be a beam that has fallen and trapped a patient's leg. A different mechanism that might have a similar net effect would be *compartment syndrome*. In compartment syndrome, internal swelling causes high pressure to build up within the relatively closed muscular compartment of an extremity. This pressure can damage nerve, muscle, and vascular tissue and limit perfusion to that area. As compartment syndrome emerges, tissue is destroyed just as it would be by direct force.

EPIDEMIOLOGY

The broad definition of soft tissue injury (nonbony, nonorgan injury) accounts for the vast majority of traumatic injuries. Crush injuries are only a small portion of this category, but they result from a wide range of mechanisms.

Direct Force

Direct force crush injuries are the most common types of crush injuries. In this case, an object (or objects) applies force and destroys tissue by direct compression. Examples of this include injuries caused by falling objects and blunt trauma distributed over larger areas.

Entrapment/Weight-Based Compression

In this situation, compression of tissue is caused by the patient's position. This damage typically manifests over hours—and sometimes days. The inability of a patient to shift position causes compression and restricts blood flow. Cells are deprived of oxygen and waste products build up. Dramatic examples of this include victims trapped and pinned by earthquakes and bomb blasts, but more common examples occur in patients who fall and are unable to get up; their weight causes the crushing force on dependent structures.

> **Crush injuries can restrict and even stop blood flow to the areas that are being compressed.**

Consider a stroke patient who collapses and pins her own leg beneath her body weight (▶ **Figure 45-2**). Her stroke renders her unable to get up or even change her position. Her own body weight compresses her leg and causes a crush-type injury.

Internal Compression

Internal swelling causes compartment syndrome and damages tissue by direct, internal compression and by limiting perfusion.

PATHOPHYSIOLOGY

Direct compression destroys cells in a similar manner as any other direct force trauma does. Energy is transferred from an offending object into the tissues. When tissues are stretched beyond their normal tolerances, damage occurs. With crush injuries, that damage can be spread over wide areas and extend deep into tissues below the skin.

Blood flow is essential to the cells for the delivery of oxygen and nutrients and for the removal of waste products. Crush injuries can restrict and even stop blood flow to the areas that are being compressed. These types of injuries are common when, for example, a patient's lower extremities are pinned under rubble after a building collapse. As the legs are compressed, cells are destroyed, not just by the direct force but also by the lack of perfusion. If compression continues over an extended time (typically longer than four hours), the muscle tissue will actually begin to break down.

Poor perfusion and direct cellular damage result in destruction of skeletal cell membranes and the release of myoglobin (a protein found in skeletal muscle), uric acid, and potassium. This process is referred to as *rhabdomyolysis*. If severe enough, these byproducts can be leached into capillary circulation and distributed systemically. The distribution of potassium and myoglobin can have devastating systemic effects. Serum potassium levels spike and can cause life-threatening cardiac dysrhythmias, and excess myoglobin can cause damage to the kidneys leading to renal failure. Other acids that are also released and are now circulating can cause a rapid drop in body pH, leading to severe metabolic acidosis and subsequent systemic vasodilation.

In cases of extended compression, as in a victim pinned by a heavy object or even an immobile patient unable to move, the release of compression can also lead to a sudden and abrupt distribution of waste products into systemic circulation. This immediate release of toxic byproducts is extremely dangerous and can lead to sudden death.

Compartment Syndrome

Compartment syndrome is compression from the opposite direction. *Fascia* is a fibrous membrane that serves to separate areas of muscle. Because fascia does not stretch, these muscular compartments form relatively closed containers. When bleeding or swelling occurs inside these compartments, pressure can build up. If this pressure continues to rise, it can reduce perfusion and destroy cells; this buildup of pressure is compartment syndrome.

ASSESSMENT FINDINGS

Remember that all assessment begins with a thorough primary assessment. Although your attention may be immediately grabbed by pinned extremities, the airway and breathing still take precedence. Treat life-threatening emergencies first.

Crush injuries often cause massive internal hemorrhage. Be vigilant for the signs and symptoms of shock. Again, dramatic injuries may mask more serious underlying issues.

The actual crush injury will generally appear similar to any other blunt trauma wound. Typically, the chief complaint will be pain in the affected area. Discoloration—such as bruising, tenderness, and even deformity—can indicate such an injury. In prolonged or massive compression injuries, blood vessels and nervous tissue may be destroyed. As such, it is common to see diminished circulatory, sensory, and motor function in distal areas (▶ **Figure 45-3**).

Assessment may be extremely difficult if the patient is trapped under an object. Understand the limitations of your assessment at this point, and be prepared for further injuries and unexpected complications once the patient is disentangled.

Assessment of Compartment Syndrome

Compartment syndrome typically occurs in the extremities; however, it can also occur in the buttocks and even the abdomen. Compartment syndrome is generally not an acute problem and typically takes hours and even days to develop. As such,

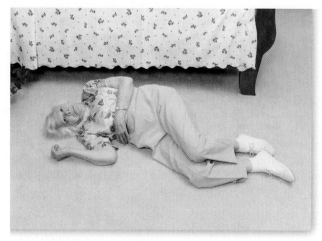

Figure 45-2 A stroke patient who has fallen and trapped her right leg beneath her body weight.

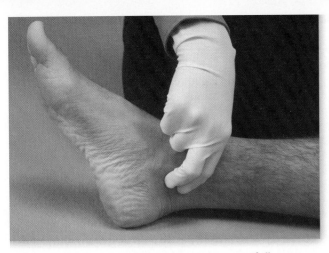

Figure 45-3 Assess circulation in an extremity following a crush injury.

much of your assessment will be geared to preventing compartment syndrome rather than identifying it.

Signs and symptoms of compartment syndrome include the following:

- Pain, discomfort, and/or burning sensation in the affected extremity, especially pain that continues or increases after immobilization
- Tenderness (pain on palpation) in the affected extremity
- Unusual firmness or rigidity in the affected area
- Altered motor function, circulation, or sensation in the distal areas of the extremity (Note: Loss of a distal pulse is an unusual finding in compartment syndrome. Typically a pulse is present, even though circulation may be impaired. This pulse may feel weaker than the same pulse in the unaffected extremity. Delayed capillary refill time may be a more important finding.)
- Weakness or paralysis of the muscles

Remember that assessment of soft tissue injuries will often be a lower priority than treating the ABCs. Always ensure that the primary assessment has been completed prior to evaluating such wounds.

EMERGENCY MEDICAL CARE

Scene safety will be an important element in treating crush injuries. Before initiating any patient contact, ensure that the mechanism of injury that injured the patient will not injure you. Treating patients in a collapse zone requires specialized training and rescue resources. Be sure to know what resources are available in your area and how to access those resources when necessary.

The most important care in crush injuries will be to treat immediate life threats first. Always address airway and breathing complications and life-threatening hemorrhage immediately. Only after treating these, more important priorities should you be concerned with addressing soft tissue injuries. Beware of being distracted by a dramatic soft tissue injury while more subtle complications rapidly kill your patient.

Crush injuries can encompass virtually any area of the body. As a result, you will have to tailor your treatment to best treat the affected area. For example, crush injuries to the chest, such as traumatic asphyxia, might require immediate ventilatory support. Massive crush injuries will also require immediate and rapid transport to an appropriate trauma facility.

Often, soft tissue injuries will mask more serious internal injuries, such as internal bleeding. Always think of the structures that lie beneath the outer injury and consider how damaging those structures might affect your patient's overall status.

In compression-related injuries (whether they are caused by an external force or by the patient's position), relieving the pressure is important. Restoring blood flow to the affected area will limit tissue damage.

Keep in mind that patients who have been trapped for prolonged periods may have systemic complications as a result of their compression-related injuries. When compression is released, waste products and toxins from the affected area may be released into the patient's system. These toxins can cause cardiac dysrhythmias, hypotension, and other systemic complications. With patients who have been trapped longer than four hours, consider starting a large-bore IV line and hydrating with normal saline. This additional fluid helps maintain kidney function and dilute toxin concentration. Run IV fluids at a rate guided by medical direction or local protocol.

Remember also that large, entrapping objects may be limiting hemorrhage in the affected area and, when released, may allow massive bleeding to occur. Always be prepared for rapid patient deterioration after removal from entrapment.

Prior to removing entrapping objects, consider the risk of cardiac dysrhythmia. Prepare for sudden cardiac arrest and have a defibrillator ready. If protocol allows, consider the administration of sodium bicarbonate. This medication treats acidosis and also helps preserve kidney function in the face of severe metabolic acidosis.

In general, treat crush injuries as you would any other blunt force trauma. Immobilize potential fractures, elevate the involved extremity, and use ice to reduce swelling. Consider spinal immobilization when appropriate. Pain control is another important consideration. Crush injuries can be severely painful, so always consider analgesia as local protocol allows.

Preventing and Treating Compartment Syndrome

As stated, compartment syndrome generally develops over long periods of time. As a result, it is typically not a major concern for the short contact times of most EMS systems. However, in many situations EMS may be in prolonged contact with patients, and in such circumstances preventive measures will help avoid compartment syndrome.

The following actions are necessary to prevent compartment syndrome:

- **Elevate extremities.** Although some experts disagree, it is generally accepted that keeping an extremity elevated above the level of the heart will help minimize swelling and maximize the work of the lymphatic system to remove accumulated fluid from the area.
- **Beware of constricting immobilization.** Although splinting material may be just right at the time of initial immobilization, remember that swelling can cause these same bands to become

> **Beware of being distracted by a dramatic soft tissue injury while more subtle complications rapidly kill your patient.**

constricting. Monitor equipment frequently to ensure appropriate tightness. Remove any constrictive jewelry.
- **Apply cold.** Appropriately applied cold packs and ice can help limit edema and mitigate pain.

- **Monitor distal circulatory, sensory, and motor function.** Changes in these findings can indicate rising pressure and could identify a reason to modify response and/or transport modalities.

Crush injuries and compartment syndrome are infrequent circumstances that require critical decision making. Use good patient assessment to identify life threats and treat specific injuries appropriately.

TRANSITIONING

REVIEW ITEMS

1. Which of the following would be considered a mechanism of injury leading to a crush injury?
   a. an angulated tibia/fibula fracture
   b. a stab wound to the left thigh
   c. a syncope patient who falls and strikes his head against the dresser
   d. a stroke patient who falls and traps his leg under his body weight for eight hours

2. Which of the following signs would potentially indicate compartment syndrome in an injured extremity?
   a. firmness or rigidity
   b. swelling at the site of the fracture
   c. red discoloration
   d. decreased capillary refill time in the distal areas

3. Which of the following is a step you might take to prevent compartment syndrome?
   a. Use compression bandages to wrap the extremity.
   b. Elevate the extremity.
   c. Place the extremity in a position below the heart.
   d. Apply heat packs.

4. Which of the following patients would have the potential for systemic effects of a crush injury?
   a. a patient recently freed after having his extremities pinned for four hours
   b. a patient recently freed after having his extremities pinned for four minutes
   c. a patient who has crushed his thumb with a hammer
   d. a patient who has broken his leg while inline skating

5. Which of the following would cause damage as the result of compartment syndrome?
   a. internal compression
   b. direct compression
   c. entrapment/weight-based compression
   d. organic/inorganic compression

APPLIED PATHOPHYSIOLOGY

1. List three signs of compartment syndrome.

2. Describe how the mechanism of entrapment/weight-based compression damages soft tissue.

3. Describe the relationship between fascia and compartment syndrome.

CLINICAL DECISION MAKING

You respond to a roof collapse with people trapped. On arrival, you stage and wait for rescue personnel to secure the scene. About four hours later, you are directed in. Rescue workers bring you to a patient whose legs are trapped beneath a collapsed beam. The workers state they are almost ready to lift the beam off the patient.

1. What types of injuries would you expect from this mechanism?

2. What immediate assessment steps should you take?

Your partner completes the assessment as you prepare the stretcher. Your partner tells you the patient is breathing only four times per minute. At that moment, the captain of the rescue team tells you to step back, as rescue workers are now ready to move the beam.

3. What should your next action be?

4. Is ventilating the patient worth delaying extrication?

The beam is moved, and you move the patient to the backboard for transport. Your partner tells you, "I don't think he has a pulse."

5. Explain why the patient may have gone into cardiac arrest now (there may be more than one reason).

6. Why might having advanced life support on scene prior to removal of the beam be important?

Standard Trauma

Competency Integrates assessment findings with principles of epidemiology and pathophysiology to formulate a field impression to implement a comprehensive treatment/disposition plan for an acutely injured patient.

TOPIC

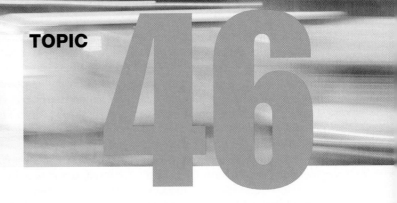

46

ORTHOPEDIC TRAUMA

INTRODUCTION

"No one ever died from a broken bone" is an inaccurate myth sometimes heard among circles of less-informed health care providers. It is true that orthopedic trauma is often classified as a lower priority than airway and breathing, and it is true that a broad spectrum of potential musculoskeletal injuries ranges from severe to minor; however, universally considering orthopedic trauma to be insignificant or benign in nature is a very serious mistake.

Broken bones *have* killed. Furthermore, the immediate treatment of orthopedic injuries can play a major role not just in life or death, but also in the overall impact of the injury on the patient. The assessment and proper prehospital treatment you provide play a direct role in the outcome of the injury.

EPIDEMIOLOGY

According to the U.S. Centers for Disease Control and Prevention, traumatic injuries are the leading cause of death for people under the age of 44; each year, roughly 1 in 10 people will visit an emergency department to seek treatment for a traumatic injury. The tragic loss of life, loss of productivity, and the enormous cost of rehabilitation place a tremendous burden on the health care system.

On a personal level, orthopedic injuries are a major life-changing event for many of our patients. Aside from being potentially life-threatening injuries, musculoskeletal trauma may also threaten patients' well-being, psychological health, and general independence.

Often, care of orthopedic trauma is mistakenly delegated to a lower priority. Although there certainly may be higher priorities of care in a trauma patient, appropriate treatment of a musculoskeletal injury may significantly affect the severity of the injury and, in general, improve the overall outcome of the patient.

PATHOPHYSIOLOGY

The adult body contains 206 bones. These bones are connected to each other by ligaments and articulated with muscles and tendons. Together these bones and connective tissues form the

TRANSITION *highlights*

- *Brief description of the frequency of traumatic injuries and deaths, and the personal ramifications of these types of injuries.*

- *Pathophysiology of injury to the skeletal bones, and how some can be either life threatening or limb threatening.*

- *Assessment steps and clinical findings consistent with orthopedic trauma.*

- *Current treatment parameters and key elements of splinting specific types of injuries:*
  - *Pelvis fracture.*
  - *Femur fracture.*

- *Effect of orthopedic trauma as it pertains to pediatric and geriatric patients.*

musculoskeletal system. Before we consider what can go wrong, we should first consider the basic functions of the musculoskeletal system. Bone, muscle, and connective tissue work together to provide the body with five basic functions:

- Giving the body shape
- Protection of important structures
- Movement
- Creation of red blood cells
- Storage of key minerals the body uses for metabolism

When we consider orthopedic injuries, we need to think about how injuries affect these basic functions. In addition, when considering injuries, we should examine how the musculoskeletal system works in concert with other body systems. For example, most long bones are anatomically located next to very large blood vessels (arteries and veins) and nerves. Therefore, an injury to such a bone may, in fact, have an impact on the circulation of blood as well. With those factors in mind, let us now consider damage to the musculoskeletal system.

The most obvious injury to the musculoskeletal system is the fracture. In this case, bone is actually broken. A fracture can physically displace bones, as in an angulated fracture, or simply crack the bone, as in a greenstick fracture. Major concerns regarding fractures fall back to the musculoskeletal system function. Examples of this include loss of mobility (Did the fracture hinder movement associated with a particular bone, as it usually does?), loss of protection (Did the force that broke the bone also damage underlying organs?), and impact on associated systems (Did the fracture damage proximal blood vessels and or nerve tissue?).

In addition to fractures, connective tissue can be damaged in the form of strains and sprains. Generally, these injuries occur when movement of a joint exceeds the normal range of motion.

> **Assessment of the injury must consider function.**

Excessive motion can stretch and tear tendons and ligaments. Again, assessment of the injury must consider function. Sprains and strains are typically limited to disruption of movement and structure but can also have an impact on other systems, such as circulation and nervous function.

A joint can be dislocated when the junction of two or more bones is disrupted. These types of injuries can have a serious impact on structure and movement and can seriously impair blood flow and nervous function.

Life-Threatening Orthopedic Injuries

Most orthopedic injuries are not life threatening. However, certain injuries present an immediate lethal potential. For the most part, these injuries are the ones that directly affect the circulatory system. Fractures of the pelvis—a basin-shaped structure composed of large irregular bones that require tremendous force to fracture—are among the most dangerous orthopedic injuries. Because large blood vessels, such as the iliac arteries, pass through the pelvis, fractures (and the force required to fracture) can result in massive hemorrhage and blood loss.

In addition to adjacent blood vessels, large bones also have their own network

of internal circulation that is vulnerable when the bone is fractured (▶ Figure 46-1).

Along with the pelvis, the femurs are very susceptible to severe bleeding associated with a fracture. A loss of up to 1.5 liters of blood can be associated with a single fractured femur. This blood loss can be serious in itself, but it would be even more dangerous when it contributes to blood loss from other injuries. If a force is great enough to break a large bone such as the femur, we must always be concerned with potential injuries to other parts of the body.

Always remember that the total blood loss may be made up of a variety of different sources of bleeding. We must consider (and treat) all the causes of blood loss. A fractured femur alone is serious; a fractured femur plus a lacerated liver is deadly.

Limb-Threatening Injuries

Some injuries may not be immediately life threatening, yet they may still be considered critical. Although an orthopedic injury may not threaten the life of the patient, it might threaten the viability of a limb.

When fractures displace bones and when dislocations interrupt the joint space, circulation is frequently compromised. If a bone is displaced and impinges a major blood vessel, circulation in the distal parts of the limb may be compromised. In this case, tissues downstream from the site of the fracture will go without perfusion, critical nutrients and oxygen will not be delivered, and waste products will build up. Thus, tissue will rapidly become hypoxic and, without correction, will die.

Part of your assessment must include ensuring distal circulation. Injuries that threaten circulation must be rapidly resolved or the entire limb may be threatened.

Orthopedic Injury: A Life-Changing Event

Even simple, non-life-threatening orthopedic injuries may significantly alter the life of your patient. Consider a simple sprain. This joint injury is likely not to kill the patient, but if he lives alone on the second floor and needs to climb stairs

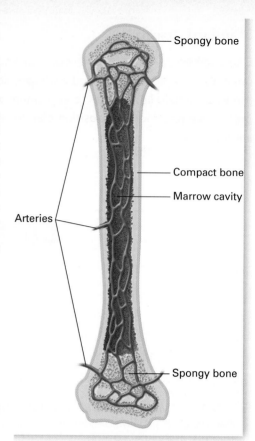

Figure 46-1 Bones have both arteries and veins, although only arteries are shown here. Because they are so richly supplied with blood vessels, bones can bleed profusely when fractured.

— Spongy bone
— Compact bone
— Marrow cavity
Arteries
— Spongy bone

each day to go to work, his lifestyle will be changed significantly. How will he buy groceries? How will he fill his prescriptions? Even this minor injury can have a major impact. Remember that your appropriate immediate treatments may help minimize the patient's recovery time.

Furthermore, you should consider the emotional impact of such an injury. Although it may be a minor injury to you, this may be a life-changing disaster to the patient. Your empathy might be as important an element of treatment as any splint you carry.

ASSESSMENT FINDINGS

Mechanism of Injury

Mechanism of injury will play a critical role in assessing an orthopedic injury. Many orthopedic injuries will be hidden behind intact skin. As a result, you will need to assess the forces at play in order to predict potential underlying injuries and their

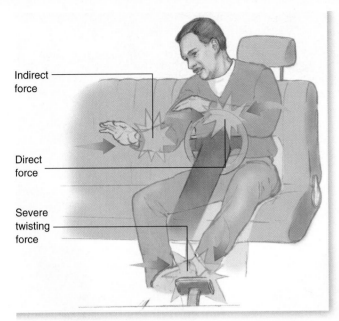

Indirect force

Direct force

Severe twisting force

Figure 46-2 Three basic mechanisms of orthopedic injury.

severity. Orthopedic injuries are typically the result of direct force, indirect force, or twisting force (▶ **Figure 46-2**).

DIRECT FORCE In direct force injuries, force is transferred by a direct blow to the site of injury. An example of a direct force injury would be a fracture as a result of being hit by a baseball bat. Force is transferred directly from the bat onto the bone and tissue that it strikes.

INDIRECT FORCE In indirect force injuries, force strikes one area and is transferred to an area away from the point of impact. For example, when a person falls from a height and lands on his feet, the force of impact may be transferred up his legs and result in pelvic fractures. The force never directly strikes the pelvis, but the transferred energy still results in a fracture.

TWISTING FORCE In twisting force, one end of a bone is held in place while the opposite end is turned. An example of this would be a runner stepping into a hole. His foot stays in place, while his leg is thrust forward. The mechanism can result in fractures to the bones of the leg.

Assess these forces when performing the scene size-up. Look not just at the nature of the forces, but also at how severely they were applied. Consider factors such as the speed of a crash, height of a fall, and surface of impact.

Assessing Orthopedic Injuries

The primary assessment should always take priority. Although an orthopedic injury may be dramatic to look at, the more severe and life-threatening injury may be subtle. Always assess and treat airway, breathing, and circulation before committing to the care of orthopedic injuries.

Fractures may be easy or difficult to identify. In general, you should always err on the side of caution and treat a suspected fracture in the same manner as you would treat an obvious fracture. Fractures may be rapidly identified by deformity, such as displaced bones and unusual angulation.

You may also see bones protruding from the skin, as in an open fracture. Closed fractures (fractures where the overlying skin remains intact) may be more difficult to assess. In these cases, it may be useful to consider the "Six Ps of Assessment":

1. **Pain.** Does the patient have pain in the injured area? Is the area sensitive to palpation (pain on palpation), or is the pain increased with movement?
2. **Pallor.** Is the injured area, or the area distal to the injury, pale, which would indicate compromised circulation?
3. **Paresthesia.** Does the patient complain of numbness/tingling or pins and needles in the affected extremity? These findings can indicate neurologic compromise.
4. **Pulses.** Are distal pulses present or lost?
5. **Paralysis.** Can the patient move the affected extremity?
6. **Pressure.** Does the patient complain of the sensation of pressure?

Another symptom of a potential fracture is guarding of the injury. In this case, the patient will position himself in such a way that the injured area is protected and immobilized. Consider also edema and crepitus as indicative signs of fracture.

The presence of any of these signs and symptoms would indicate the potential of a fracture. Without X-ray, it is very difficult to differentiate fractures from other soft tissue injuries, such as sprains and strains. Again, it is important to treat all injuries with signs and symptoms of a fracture as if they were, in fact, fractures.

Distal circulation, sensory, and motor (C/S/M) function must always be assessed. Deficits can indicate serious neurovascular compromise and may indicate a limb-threatening injury. Deficits in C/S/M function should be considered a true emergency.

A thorough assessment of an orthopedic injury must also consider the impact on other systems and/or organs. Remember that the force that broke the rib may also have injured the underlying lung. Beware the potential for spinal injury in forces great enough to fracture bones such as the pelvis and femur.

> **Distal circulation, sensory, and motor (C/S/M) function must always be assessed.**

EMERGENCY MEDICAL CARE

With most orthopedic injuries, other life-threatening problems need to be treated first. Use a thorough primary assessment to identify critical priorities before moving on to the treatment of orthopedic injuries. As stated previously, some orthopedic injuries in and of themselves may be life threatening. However, shock associated with blood loss from pelvic or femur fractures should be identified when assessing circulation in the primary survey and not based solely on a secondary assessment of an extremity.

After addressing immediate life threats, the basic principles of treating an orthopedic injury include immobilization, application of cold, and elevation. Remember that even in potentially critical orthopedic injuries, the basic application of these principles will generally provide the necessary immediate care that will help maximize outcomes.

Pain associated with an orthopedic injury may be severe. Analgesia is an important element of care for these types of injuries. Pain control medications, such as fentanyl, should be administered to ease pain and allow for easier immobilization. Always follow local protocol.

Immobilization

A key principle of treating (and transporting) a patient with an orthopedic injury is immobilization. Immobilization prevents jagged bone ends from damaging adjacent soft tissue, nerves, and blood vessels. It helps maintain normal circulation and prevents occlusion of vessels through movement. Immobilization can help slow and stop bleeding associated with a fracture and, finally, immobilization decreases pain. All these elements help improve both short-term and long-term outcomes of orthopedic injury and, as a result, should be important priorities of prehospital care.

In some cases, immediate treatment of airway and breathing may be your first priority. Remember that even in these cases, minimal immobilization may contribute to improved outcomes. Simply preventing movement is important. In short-term settings, this may mean using manual stabilization or fixation to a long board or another extremity. These simple steps should be considered even when larger priorities redirect your attention.

> **Immobilization can help slow and stop bleeding associated with a fracture.**

For example, with a patient with multisystem trauma, you might have an untrained person simply hold an obviously fractured femur in place while you complete your primary assessment. Although this would not be considered proper splinting, that quick manual immobilization might prevent jagged bone ends from damaging soft tissue as the leg moves. It might also help slow bleeding from the fractured area.

In a larger sense, *immobilization* refers to splinting or the application of a device to limit movement. Splinting can be accomplished with commercial or improvised devices. It is important to be creative when accomplishing the objectives of splinting. Immobilization of fractures and dislocations often requires nontraditional methods.

Key elements of splinting include the following:

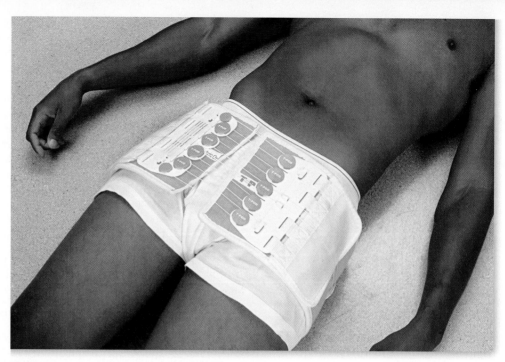

Figure 46-3 A commercially available pelvic splint may be used to immobilize a pelvic fracture.

- Assess C/S/M functions in the distal extremity prior to application of the splint. This assessment not only provides a baseline but will also help you identify changes that might occur as a result of the splinting process.

- Remove jewelry and cut away clothing before application of a splint. Edema associated with the injury can rapidly turn these items into constricting bands that limit circulation.

- Apply a dressing to open wounds prior to splinting. Often the direct pressure of splinting can aid in bleeding control. Clean dressings will also minimize the threat of infection.

The goal of splinting is to immobilize the joint above and the joint below the injury site. In a joint injury, you should immobilize the bone above and the bone below the injured joint. These goals can be accomplished in a variety of ways. Padded board splints, traction splints, vacuum splints, and air splints can all be used to accomplish the objectives of splinting. Remember to be creative.

Special Splinting Circumstances

PELVIS FRACTURES Always consider other internal injuries in association with a pelvic fracture. Typically, massive

forces have been applied to cause such an injury. Spinal injuries are common in pelvic fractures; therefore, you should consider using a backboard to immobilize the patient. Various commercially available pelvic binders are available to splint these types of fractures (▶ **Figure 46-3**). Such devices are used to limit lateral movement of an unstable pelvis. You may also consider (when local protocol allows) using a pneumatic anti-shock garment (PASG) to immobilize the pelvis.

FEMUR FRACTURES Recall that femur fractures alone can result in serious bleeding. Splinting not only treats the orthopedic injury but also potentially addresses a circulation problem. As a result, splinting such an injury might be a slightly higher priority than treating other isolated musculoskeletal trauma. When protocol allows, consider using a traction splint (▶ **Figure 46-4**) to immobilize the femur. Applying traction pulls displaced bone ends in line and also helps prevent muscle contraction that can lead to increased bleeding.

Splinting should always be assessed immediately after completion. Check distal C/S/M function. Improper splinting can often result in impaired C/S/M function. Remember also that improper splinting can lead to excessive movement

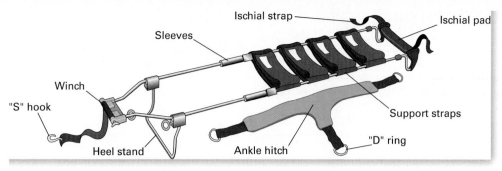

Figure 46-4 A bipolar traction splint.

and pressure-related injuries from inadequate padding.

Elevation and Cold

After the injury has been splinted properly, consider elevating it above the level of the heart. In theory, elevation helps decrease edema and minimizes pain. Elevate only if proper immobilization has been achieved first. Elevation without immobilization can actually aggravate an injury by causing excessive movement of displaced bone ends.

Application of cold packs and ice to an orthopedic injury is also thought to limit edema by causing peripheral vasoconstriction. As with elevation, the reduction in edema can help minimize pain. Never apply cold directly to bare skin, as this can cause cold-related injuries such as frostbite. Always wrap the ice or cold pack in a towel or similar cloth prior to application.

Orthopedic Injuries in Special Populations

Anatomic differences in pediatric and geriatric patients require special consideration. Pediatric patients often have less-calcified bones. As a result, their bones are more pliable and flexible. Because of this anatomic difference, true fractures are less common in younger patients than they are in adults. Although children certainly break bones, often more force is required. Furthermore, because children's bones are flexible, often more internal damage can occur even though the protective bones remain intact. Beware of underlying injuries in children.

In geriatric patients, diseases such as osteoporosis may require an alternative approach to the assessment of mechanism of injury. Decreased bone density, a condition common in elderly patients, can often lead to fractures with minimal force applied. A mechanism of injury that would be unlikely to break the bone of a younger person may indeed result in fractures in a person with a disease such as osteoporosis. Have a higher index of suspicion when evaluating orthopedic injuries in geriatric patients.

TRANSITIONING · · · · · · ·

REVIEW ITEMS

1. Which of the following would be a function of the musculoskeletal system impaired by a fracture?
   a. insulation
   b. heat retention
   c. fluid balance
   d. structure

2. Which of the following complications of a dislocation would indicate a critical patient?
   a. no distal pulse
   b. pain at the dislocation site
   c. deformity at the dislocation site
   d. swelling in distal extremity

3. A pelvic fracture is most often considered life threatening because of _____.
   a. pain
   b. hemorrhage
   c. sepsis
   d. vomiting

4. An unbelted driver fractures his femur as he is thrown forward into the steering wheel during a motor vehicle crash. This mechanism of injury would best be described as _____.
   a. direct force
   b. indirect force
   c. twisting force
   d. dislocating force

5. Which of the following assessment findings would indicate that splinting has been done improperly?
   a. flushed skin in an extremity following splinting
   b. continued pain in the extremity following splinting
   c. numbness in a hand following splinting
   d. inability to move the splinted extremity

APPLIED PATHOPHYSIOLOGY

1. List the "Six Ps of Assessment" that might indicate a fracture.

2. Why is a fractured femur considered a potentially life-threatening injury? How is this fracture potentially different from a tibia or fibula fracture?

3. How might your scene size-up and assessment of a potential fracture for an 85-year-old patient differ from that for a 35-year-old patient?

CLINICAL DECISION MAKING

You respond to an 11-year-old girl struck by a car. Bystanders note that the child was struck and thrown 10 feet onto the road.

1. What types of injuries would you expect from this mechanism?

2. What immediate assessment steps should you take?

On arrival you find the patient alert and oriented, breathing rapidly, with good distal pulses. The patient is crying and complains of pain in her pelvis and left upper arm. On inspection, you note that her pelvis is unstable and her arm is angulated and obviously fractured.

3. Given the nature of her injuries, what other systems might be affected?

4. Assuming her airway, breathing, and circulation are adequate, how would you deal with the unstable pelvis?

5. Should you take the time to splint her arm prior to leaving the scene?

6. After the arm has been splinted, what additional steps can you take to improve care of this injury?

Standard Trauma

Competency Integrates assessment findings with principles of epidemiology and pathophysiology to formulate a field impression to implement a comprehensive treatment/disposition plan for an acutely injured patient.

TOPIC

47

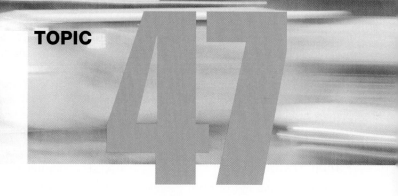

HEAD AND NECK TRAUMA

INTRODUCTION

Injuries to the head and neck pose a threat to the most vital systems of the body. Any force exerted in the head immediately threatens the brain, but in addition, head and neck trauma can also involve other especially vital structures, including the airway and major blood vessels. Moreover, significant trauma to these areas can also disrupt, alter, and obstruct normal anatomy that is essential to life-giving functions. For example, injuries to the mouth and jaw can displace the normal structures of the upper airway and disrupt the flow of air. These injuries are often immediately life threatening and are also difficult to correct rapidly. A variety of factors, from displaced anatomy to the time-sensitive nature of the pathophysiology, makes head and neck trauma patients among the most challenging calls to which a paramedic may respond.

These calls are not common. Statistically speaking, most paramedics will go their entire career without experiencing the most critical of head and neck trauma patients. That is fortunate for our patients, but it makes for little practice of skills necessary to deal with this type of patient. Interventions such as surgical airways are high risk in nature, and their infrequent use requires repetitive training by paramedics to maintain a competent skill level.

Traumatic brain injury is certainly a high risk in head and neck trauma. The next topic is devoted entirely to that subject. This topic specifically discusses the other life-threatening challenges of head and neck trauma, with special consideration given to airway maintenance.

EPIDEMIOLOGY

The Centers for Disease Control and Prevention estimates that roughly 1.7 million Americans suffer head and neck injuries annually. Of those, 275,000 are hospitalized and roughly 50,000 of them die. It is difficult to quantify exactly how many of those patients suffer from isolated brain injuries, but it suffices to say that many of those patients sustain life-altering head and neck trauma that involves systems other than just their brain. Frequently, these injuries involve additional airway and circulatory compromise.

TRANSITION highlights

- *Pathophysiology of head and neck injuries.*
- *Assessment steps and considerations for victims of head and neck trauma, including airway, breathing, and circulation considerations.*
- *Review of key treatment steps, including the airway decision-making process.*
- *Overview of surgical airway procedures.*

Trauma to the head and neck is sustained from a variety of sources. Injuries can result from both penetrating and blunt forces. Common etiologies include violence, motor vehicle crashes, falls, and sports-related injuries.

> **Injuries can result from both penetrating and blunt forces.**

PATHOPHYSIOLOGY

The pathophysiology of brain injuries will be discussed in great detail in the next topic. However, in this topic we describe additional pathophysiologies associated with head and neck trauma.

The pathophysiology of head and neck trauma is directly related to the external force causing the trauma. Structures are damaged by both blunt and penetrating trauma; the pathway of the offending force can be traced to identify the proximal damage. However, in head and neck injuries, we must also consider secondary pathologies associated with injuries. Secondary swelling is frequently a threat to surrounding structures and can be a major risk associated with airway maintenance. Bleeding, secretions, and dislodged teeth are also a major airway risk.

As the head sits atop the cervical spine, major facial, head, and neck trauma typically pose a high risk for cervical spinal fracture. In fact, 2 percent to 12 percent of major trauma victims have a cervical spine injury and 7 percent to 14 percent of these injuries are unstable. The following sections describe some specific pathophysiologies associated with head and neck trauma.

Facial Trauma

In addition to the risk of brain trauma, external forces applied to the face pose a risk for soft tissue damage, fractures, ocular injuries, and displacement of anatomy that threatens the airway.

The bones of the face are relatively unprotected and, with significant force, can be broken. These fractures can range from simple loss of integrity of the bones to gross instability of the facial structure. Most dangerously, facial fractures, particularly maxilla and mandible fractures, can displace anatomy and threaten the airway.

LEFORT FRACTURES   In the early 1900s, René LeFort categorized a series of fractures associated with the facial bones and the maxilla. He found that fractures to the anterior skull and jawbone followed predictable patterns and outlined three basic characterizations of facial/maxilla fractures:

- A LeFort I fracture consists of a break in the facial bones along a horizontal axis. The fracture typically travels from the nasal septum to the edges of the maxilla (the lateral pyriform rims) (▶ **Figure 47-1**). This fracture typically results from direct, blunt trauma to the lower portions of the face.

- A LeFort II fracture also usually results from direct, blunt trauma to the face, but in this case the fracture extends over the bridge of the nasal bones. It is sometimes called a *pyramidal fracture*, as the line of damage resembles a pyramid as it crosses the maxilla and

then travels superiorly to the nose (Figure 47-1). Common findings associated with LeFort II fractures include cerebrospinal fluid (CSF) discharge from the nose and diplopia (double vision).

- A LeFort III fracture not only involves the maxilla but also fractures the zygomatic bones and extends to the orbits (Figure 47-1). LeFort III fractures also produce CSF discharge from the nose and commonly cause facial deformity, including a "lengthening" of the face due to instability of fractured segments.

Although LeFort fractures are common patterns for fractured facial bones, not all fractures fit within these patterns. It is common to see both isolated fractures that do not involve all the structures described here and more extensive and devastating fractures that involve more structures than listed previously.

Mandibular fractures are also common in cases of blunt and penetrating trauma

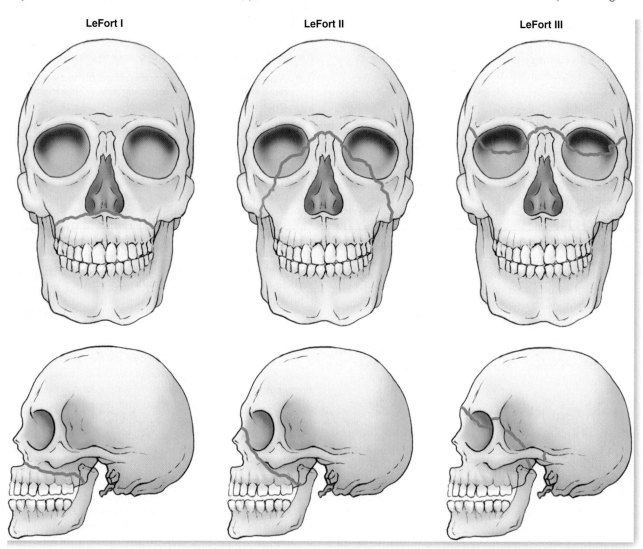

Figure 47-1 LeFort fracture classifications.

to the face. These fractures are sometimes evident through facial deformity, but can also be recognized through poor alignment of teeth (as a new finding), difficulty speaking, and difficulty opening and closing the mouth.

The greatest risk associated with facial fractures is, of course, traumatic brain injury, but facial fractures can also be a significant threat to the airway. As structures that form the mouth, jaw, and hard palate are destroyed and displaced, the pathway for air can be interrupted. Furthermore, these fractures are typically associated with bleeding and soft tissue injury; both these elements can further exacerbate an already serious injury.

Soft tissue injuries of the face can be significant even without secondary fractures. The face and mouth are rich with blood vessels, and bleeding can be severe. Arteries in the temporal scalp are especially vulnerable to trauma and can pose a serious risk if damaged. Bleeding in the mouth itself is not typically massive, but even minor bleeding can pose a risk of airway compromise.

Trauma to the Neck

Like facial trauma, trauma to the neck poses a series of different risks. Direct trauma can damage a wide array of vital structures, including the larynx and trachea, the esophagus, the spinal column, and the large vessels that supply blood to the brain.

AIRWAY INJURIES Airway issues are the prime concern with trauma to the neck. Although the trachea and larynx are relatively well protected, high energy forces can destroy, displace, and fracture the cartilaginous structures that form the upper airway. Anatomic displacement represents a critical injury in that air cannot reach the lower airway.

A secondary threat in any injury to the structures of the airway is edema. Swelling can cause airway occlusion in both an immediate and a delayed fashion. Frequently edema will develop over time, thereby transforming an otherwise patent airway into a severely threatened or even occluded airway. Recognizing the mechanism of injury and constant vigilance in assessment are the keys to identifying this subtle threat.

SPINAL INJURIES In addition to airway concerns, neck injuries also must elicit concerns regarding the spinal column and spinal injuries. Topic 49 discusses spinal injuries in much greater detail, but it is important to recognize the threat of spinal injury with any head or neck trauma, and it is equally important to recognize the risk of secondary spinal injury associated with the treatment of some facial and neck injuries.

VASCULAR INJURIES Large blood vessels, including the internal and external jugular veins and the carotid arteries, lie relatively exposed in the soft tissue of the neck. These vessels are vulnerable to both blunt and penetrating trauma. The most obvious risk of injury is hemorrhage. Violation of these large vessels can lead to rapid and exsanguinating bleeding. In addition, there is a relatively negative venous pressure in the jugular veins, creating the risk of embolism when their integrity is disrupted.

OTHER INJURIES TO THE NECK Finally, other injuries can occur secondary to neck trauma. The esophagus can be perforated, lacerated, or otherwise disrupted. This can lead not only to dysfunction of the GI system, but also to severe bleeding and infection.

Blunt and penetrating trauma can also cause air to accumulate outside the path of the airway, in a condition called *pneumomediastinum*. This free air is usually a symptom of larger airway problem, but can represent a loss of integrity along the tracheal and bronchial tree.

PATIENT ASSESSMENT

The scene assessment plays an important role in the management of head and neck injuries. Reviewing the mechanism of injury will help predict underlying damage. Review the forces in play. Consider how the energy affected the patient and what structures were in the path of the trauma.

Look for exsanguinating hemorrhage. Neck injuries can result in severe bleeding that could, under the right circumstances, require immediate action. Remember to assess for life-threatening bleeding even before moving on to other critical elements.

The primary assessment in head and neck injuries is desperately important. Head and neck injuries directly affect the airway, breathing, and circulation; a well-performed primary assessment will rapidly identify these critical life threats.

Airway Assessment

An assessment of the airway is always the immediate priority (except in the case of life-threatening bleeding). Patients with head and neck trauma have very real threats to the movement of air. Ensure that the patient has a patent airway; if necessary, open and secure it. Bleeding is an ever-present risk in head and neck trauma and suction may be an immediate necessity.

Besides assessing for the presence of an airway, you must assess for long-term patency. Will the airway stay open? Multiple threats to long-term airway security exist in the context of head and neck trauma; Table 47-1 details these threats to the airway.

As always, if an airway problem is identified in the primary assessment, take immediate steps to correct it. Airway treatment will be discussed in greater detail in later sections.

Breathing Assessment

Threats to breathing also abound in head and neck trauma. Anatomic displacement, bleeding, and free air in the mediastinum can all affect the ability to breathe effectively. Consider also the effects of changing mental status.

Assess for both the presence and adequacy of breathing. Expose and look at the chest. Often injuries involving the neck will also involve the chest, as lung tissue can be found as high as the subclavicle regions. Listen to lung sounds to identify the presence of a pneumothorax. Consider sealing open neck wounds with an occlusive dressing. This will help both to prevent the development of a tension pneumothorax if lung tissue is involved and to help prevent air from entering venous circulation. Feel the chest for deformity, equal rise, and the presence of subcutaneous air.

> Reviewing the mechanism of injury will help predict underlying damage.

Ensure that breathing is adequately meeting the needs of oxygenation and ventilation; if it is not, take steps to provide support.

Circulation

Head and neck injuries can lead to massive hemorrhage. Always assess circulatory

TABLE 47-1	Long-Term Airway Threats in Head and Neck Trauma	

Long-Term Threat	Assessment Findings
Mental status: Decreasing mental status leads to diminished control of the airway. Loss of muscle control and gag reflex can lead to airway failure.	Decreasing level of consciousness, snoring, gasping.
Hemorrhage and secretions: Ongoing bleeding and inability to maintain a gag reflex can lead to aspiration and airway obstruction.	Secretions in the airway, gurgling sounds, continued hemorrhage.
Foreign objects: Often foreign objects can threaten the airway. Always check the airway for loose or broken teeth, chewing tobacco, and other foreign objects that could become an obstruction.	Mechanism of injury, presence of foreign objects, stridor.
Edema: Swelling of soft tissue in the airway can lead to impairment and obstruction of airflow.	Stridor. Voice changes are a very important finding that can demonstrate increasing edema in the airway. Look for hoarseness and difficulty speaking. Trends toward worsening speech quality are ominous findings.

status and take corrective action when necessary. Control hemorrhage using direct pressure and monitor for ongoing bleeding. Beware that direct pressure can affect air movement and weigh priorities accordingly. Hemostatic agents can be helpful in neck injuries, but obviously tourniquets should never be placed around the neck.

Mental Status

A rapid mental status examination is an important element of any primary assessment for a head or neck trauma patient. Determining a baseline mental status is essential so as to identify downward trends that could impact airway control and breathing adequacy. Mental status is also valuable in recognizing early signs of hypoxia, shock, and traumatic brain injury.

Secondary Assessment and Reassessment

Head and neck trauma patients require constant vigilance and frequent reassessment. Subtle signs can indicate major problems to come. Use a detailed physical examination to find more subtle indicators of life-threatening problems. Look for the typical signs of trauma (DCAP-BTLS), as well as signs common to head and neck injuries (▶ Figure 47-2). Check the ears and nose for the presence of CSF. Examine the patient's eyes and

vision. Assess the patient's mouth and the alignment of his teeth and jaw. Is there malocclusion (misalignment of the jaw when the mouth closes)? Listen to speech patterns by the patient. Are there

changes? Look for soft tissue injuries to the neck. Remember that inferior injuries can affect the lungs.

The patient with head and neck trauma is in a rapidly evolving situation. New problems can emerge and existing problems can worsen. Constantly reassess the patient to identify potential issues.

EMERGENCY MEDICAL CARE

Head and neck injuries are frequently life threatening, and treatment is often necessary as early as the primary assessment. Paramedics should be prepared to intervene swiftly to correct life threats.

Spinal Immobilization

A patient who sustained supraclavicular trauma is considered to have a C-spine injury until proven otherwise. The mechanism of injury alone should indicate at least an evaluation for spinal injury, if not full spinal immobilization. That said, often the risk of spinal injury adds complexity to other highly important treatments. For example, holding manual cervical spinal immobilization makes endotracheal intubation (ETI) significantly more difficult.

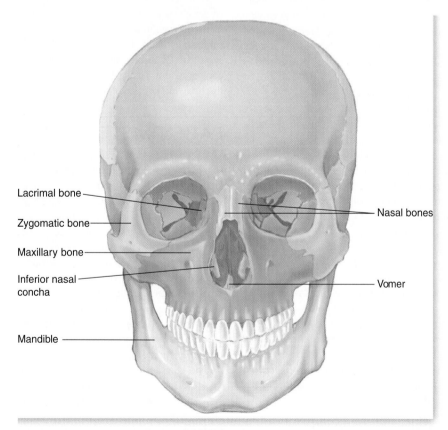

Figure 47-2 Detailed assessment of the face.

Lacrimal bone
Zygomatic bone
Maxillary bone
Inferior nasal concha
Mandible
Nasal bones
Vomer

Although there are methods to improve success, a cost–benefit analysis should be considered before attempting ETI, especially if basic life support (BLS) methods are effective.

Just as some interventions are made more difficult with spinal immobilization, you should also consider how other interventions can affect spinal injuries. For example, ETI has been shown to cause movement of cervical vertebrae. Even simple basic maneuvers such as a jaw thrust can cause movement in the cervical spine. Might it be better to simply insert an oral airway? These costs must be considered as you order your priority lists.

Airway

Airway management is a complex subject with regard to head and neck injuries. A wide range of both life-threatening and time-sensitive challenges face paramedics as they assess and treat these patients. Simply speaking, many of these patients do not have an airway and require immediate intervention. Resolution can be simple. Basic maneuvers, such as suction and positioning, may be effective. However, with trauma to the head and neck, often more complicated interventions may be necessary.

BLIND INSERTION AIRWAY DEVICES
In some cases, unprotected airways can be assisted using a blind insertion airway device such as a King airway or a laryngeal mask airway. By sealing off the esophagus and, at least in theory, isolating the glottis opening, airway security can be improved. Aspiration risk can be lowered and ventilations can be made more effective by improving the channel of air. Unfortunately, in many cases, blind insertion airway devices do not provide the security necessary to fully protect an airway. Because, in most cases, these devices are periglottic and not transglottic in nature, they do not protect against glottis edema. Also, because they are inserted blindly, it is difficult to determine whether anatomy has been displaced secondary to trauma. Although they may protect against bleeding, they are of little use if the anatomic pathway for air has been disrupted.

ENDOTRACHEAL INTUBATION
Definitive airway management in the head and neck trauma patient typically comes in the form of ETI. Although it is certainly not necessary in every patient, inflating the distal balloon in the trachea seals off the pathway of air and prevents occlusion by edema. It also stops the threat of aspiration. That said, the choice to move to ETI must come only after a careful cost–benefit analysis. The paramedic must weigh the goal of airway security, oxygenation, and ventilation against the risks of the procedure—ETI, especially in trauma care, is fraught with risks.

At a minimum, ETI is simply more difficult in the trauma patient. Spinal immobilization prevents optimizing the patient's position (the sniffing position) and limits neck motility and cervical extension. Head and neck trauma can also compound the difficulty by adding bleeding, soft tissue trauma, and even displaced anatomy to the mix. Under the best circumstances, this intubation may be the most challenging of your career. Edema also can complicate matters. Although the threat of airway occlusion forces consideration of ETI, the very findings that indicate this threat also indicate that the intubation will be more difficult. Typically these patients are awake; if they are exhibiting voice changes, it is implied that the lumen of their glottis opening is narrowing with inflammation.

The choice to move to intubation must be made with careful consideration of many factors. This choice must include the efficacy of BLS efforts, the immediacy of the threats, and the capabilities and resources of the responding crew. Could the attempt be made at the hospital where conditions are more optimal? Sometimes the answer is yes, but sometimes it is no.

Consider also the impact of intubation on your patient. Of course, airway security is a high priority, but intubation comes with its own set of costs. Intubation has been shown to raise intracranial pressure, manipulate cervical vertebrae, and cause hypoxia during the apneic procedure. There is also the hugely important risk of esophageal intubation. The cost–benefit analysis must carefully weigh the benefits of the procedure against the underlying risks.

Consider also that ETI may not be effective in securing an airway in trauma. If anatomy has been displaced or the airway is fully obstructed, more aggressive procedures may be necessary.

SURGICAL AND PSEUDOSURGICAL AIRWAYS
Some cases of head and neck trauma will require immediate surgical intervention. When anatomy is displaced or when the path of air is fully occluded, the oropharynx must be bypassed.

Surgical airways are a controversial topic in EMS. Many systems have removed the skill from the scope of practice of paramedics, citing infrequent use, inability to maintain skill proficiency, and dismal patient outcomes even with successful application of the skill. That notwithstanding, for those who have retained the skill, surgical airways may be a rapidly required intervention for the head and neck trauma patient.

Surgical airways are generally divided into three categories: needle cricothyroidotomy, open surgical airways, and pseudosurgical airways. A needle cricothyroidotomy uses a needle and a transtracheal jet insufflation set to oxygenate patients through the cricothyroid membrane. An open surgical airway exposes the cricothyroid membrane; after cutting a hole through it, the paramedic inserts a tube through which the patient can be ventilated. A pseudosurgical airway uses a combination of a needle cricothyroidotomy and an open surgical procedure to create a ventilation tube (usually a wide-lumen needle is used to puncture the cricothyroid membrane, and then a tube is inserted). Each of these procedures has its benefits, but each also has costs. Before discussing specific procedures, however, we should first review the techniques common to all three types.

Each of these procedures should be used when no other method of moving air is possible. Specifically speaking, surgical airways should be used when trauma or obstruction prevent oxygenation and ventilation by other means. Studies have shown that surgical airways used for other indications have universally poor outcomes.

Most EMS surgical airways access the trachea via the cricothyroid membrane. This membrane spans the anterior gap between the thyroid cartilage and the cricoid ring (▶ Figure 47-3). Roughly speaking, the membrane itself is about the size of the patient's thumbnail, so space is at a premium. To further complicate matters, the membrane is rimmed on its lower border by the supercricothyroid vessels and on its lateral aspect by the middle thyroid vein and anterior jugular vein. Penetration of the membrane ideally should avoid these vessels, but frequently lacerates them simply because of the small size of the membrane.

Externally, this landmark is usually identified by locating the thyroid cartilage (the Adam's apple) and then palpating for the inferior cricoid ring. The indentation

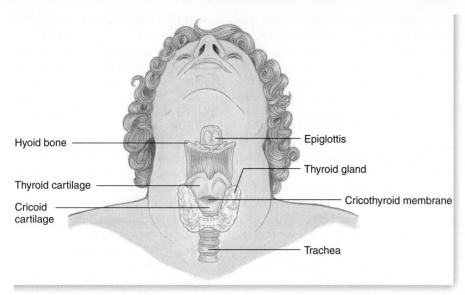

Figure 47-3 The cricothyroid membrane and surrounding structures.

Labels: Hyoid bone, Thyroid cartilage, Cricoid cartilage, Epiglottis, Thyroid gland, Cricothyroid membrane, Trachea

between the structures would therefore represent the cricoid membrane. Identification of this landmark becomes more difficult with very small patients and with obese patients. It can also be a challenge in patients with anterior neck trauma. In fact, the only absolute contraindication to surgical airway is the inability to identify landmarks.

A needle cricothyroidotomy is typically performed on pediatric patients (although it can be used in adults as well). The challenge of a needle cricothyroidotomy is the small lumen through which air is moved. In most cases, transtracheal jet ventilation is administered through a 14-gauge needle. Although, with pressure, oxygen can be delivered, there is little opportunity for ventilation and the removal of carbon dioxide. Ventilation can be improved by using a 4:1 ratio of inspiration/exhalation, but little evidence exists that proper ventilation will occur. In most cases, use of a needle cricothyroidotomy is essentially a race against the clock. It assumes that the patient can tolerate hypercapnia in exchange for minimal oxygenation.

In a needle cricothyroidotomy, a large-bore needle (typically 14-gauge), attached to a syringe, is inserted through the cricothyroid membrane at roughly a 45-degree angle until it reaches the inner lumen of the trachea. At that point, the catheter is advanced into the trachea and the stylet is removed. A jet insufflation kit is then attached to the hub of the catheter and the patient is ventilated via a 50-psi bypass on the oxygen regulator.

An open surgical airway is the generally preferred method to bypass the upper air-

way. It is preferred in that it enables a larger tube to be placed through the cricothyroid membrane. Typically either a commercially available tracheostomy tube or a modified 5.0–6.0 endotracheal tube is used. The larger-lumen tube allows for better oxygenation and ventilation and is generally achievable in the adult population. Unfortunately, this skill is not simple either. Even in an adult, the cricothyroid membrane is small and because of the proximity of relatively large blood vessels, bleeding is often a complication that obscures visibility. Most experts now recommend using a vertical incision to expose the underlying membrane and then using a retractor or specially designed tracheotomy hook to initially penetrate the membrane and secure the landmark. If bleeding does occur, having the hook in place will allow for continued identification of the membrane, even in poor visibility. Some systems go as far as to advocate the use of a pediatric gum-elastic bougie (tube changer). This device can be placed through the membrane prior to passing the tube and can be used as a guide to introduce the tube into correct placement. Always follow local protocol.

Safety is a prime concern during this procedure. There have been many cases of health care professionals cutting themselves with a scalpel blade as they make secondary incisions while palpating landmarks. The use of specially made hooks and/or retractors can help mitigate this concern.

Pseudosurgical airways combine the previous two procedures. Many specially designed devices are available that use

the simplicity of the needle cricothyroidotomy procedure to introduce a much larger tube. These devices can be thought of as extra-large cricothyroidotomy needles. Membrane puncture is completed with the device, and then the larger-lumen catheter is advanced as in the previous techniques.

As with any airway procedure, the decision to move to a surgical airway must be made after a careful cost–benefit analysis. These techniques should never be used if less-invasive techniques are available.

Breathing

Breathing can be a specific challenge to patients with head and neck trauma. We have previously discussed airway issues that can significantly interfere with oxygenation and ventilation, but remember that all deficits in breathing may not be simply the result of airway problems. Consider the impact of brain injuries and spinal injuries on the mechanism of breathing. Each of these types of injuries can interfere with the stimulus and message transmission necessary to maintain adequate respirations. Damage to the medulla can disrupt breathing control, and damage to the spinal cord can halt movement of the diaphragm, the intercostal muscles, or both. Consider also the effect of decreasing mental status on breathing effort. Simple changes in the level of consciousness may cause inadequate respirations.

If inadequate ventilations are identified, positive pressure ventilations must be initiated. This, in and of itself, can be challenging. Patients with severe facial trauma may be very difficult to ventilate with a bag-mask device. Obtaining a seal on displaced anatomy may be impossible. Creative positioning may create a seal, but in many cases, more advanced techniques such as blind insertion airways or ETI may be necessary.

As stated previously, many neck injuries also involve the lungs. Carefully assess for pneumothorax in any neck injury and use occlusive dressings to care for penetrating trauma.

Other treatments of head and neck injuries include spinal immobilization, bleeding control (including the dressing and bandaging of soft tissue injuries), and analgesia when appropriate. More in-depth discussions concerning the treatment of traumatic brain injuries and spinal injuries will be forthcoming in later topics.

REVIEW ITEMS

1. Which of the following facial fractures typically involves the orbital bones?
   a. LeFort I
   b. LeFort II
   c. LeFort III
   d. LeFort IV

2. Which of the following findings would commonly indicate a mandibular fracture?
   a. diplopia
   b. epistaxis
   c. CSF leaking from the nose
   d. difficulty speaking

3. Which of the following findings would most likely indicate an airway edema problem?
   a. diplopia
   b. difficulty speaking
   c. wheezing
   d. hemoptysis

4. Which of the following would be a negative side effect of intubation in a trauma patient?
   a. decreased intracranial pressure
   b. tachycardia
   c. hyperoxia
   d. movement of cervical vertebrae

5. The landmark used for placement of a surgical airway is known as the _____.
   a. cricothyroid membrane
   b. thyroid ring
   c. angle of Louis
   d. tympanic membrane

APPLIED PATHOPHYSIOLOGY

1. Describe how breathing can be affected by head and neck trauma.

2. Discuss why it is important to seal neck wounds with an occlusive dressing.

3. Describe why an open surgical airway might be preferable to a needle cricothyroidotomy.

CLINICAL DECISION MAKING

A 16-year-old male patient was struck in the neck by a tree branch while riding an ATV at moderate speed. He was thrown from the vehicle and is now seated on the ground complaining of pain in the anterior aspect of his neck.

1. What immediate concerns does this mechanism of injury point to?

2. Please describe specifically the steps of your primary assessment. Specifically, what would you examine?

The patient has a patent airway and is breathing with clear lung sounds. He is coughing up a bit of blood, and you note a reddening of the skin on the anterior aspect of his neck. This area is also very tender to touch. You also note that the patient is speaking with a very hoarse voice.

3. Do you need to manage this patient's airway—and, if so, why?

4. Does the quality of the patient's voice indicate anything—and, if so, what?

5. What, if any, role does spinal immobilization play in this patient?

6. What would be the most appropriate method of airway management for this patient?

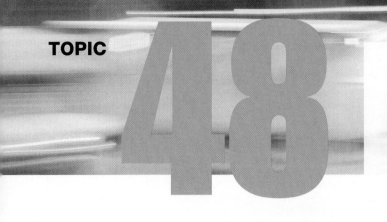

Standard Trauma

Competency Integrates assessment findings with principles of epidemiology and pathophysiology to formulate a field impression to implement a comprehensive treatment/disposition plan for an acutely injured patient.

TRAUMATIC BRAIN INJURY

TRANSITION *highlights*

- *Incidence and death rates for traumatic brain injury along with age and gender predispositions for these injuries.*

- *Pathophysiology of brain injuries to include types of injuries, effects on cerebral tissue, and effects on normal brain functioning:*
  - Intracerebral hemorrhage.
  - Diffuse axonal injury.
  - Concussion.
  - Epidural hematoma.
  - Subdural hematoma.
  - Subarachnoid hemorrhage.

- *Assessment steps and considerations for victims of brain injury, with special emphasis on four topics:*
  - Brain herniation.
  - Importance of mental status.
  - Decorticate and decerebrate posturing.
  - Glasgow Coma Scale.

- *Current treatment parameters for patients with both herniating and nonherniating brain injuries.*

INTRODUCTION

As a paramedic, on a regular basis you will be faced with caring for patients suffering from head injuries. In the United States, 1.5 million people per year incur a head injury. These injuries require a high level of suspicion, as signs and symptoms can manifest days and even weeks after the original injury, especially in the very young and elderly. Assessment of these patients can be complicated because altered mentation is a common presentation in head injuries. In addition, drugs or alcohol may compound the situation, making assessment even

more difficult. You must overcome these challenges in order to promptly evaluate the condition and prevent further neurologic damage to your patient.

Understanding the anatomy of the skull and its contents is imperative for determining the specific type of head or traumatic brain injury (TBI) your patient is displaying. The skull is the part of the skeletal system that protects the brain and a portion of the spinal cord. It is formed by the fusion of several flat bones held together by cranial sutures. The brain occupies 80 percent to 90 percent of the space within the skull. Therefore, the space in which the brain can swell or bleed is grossly limited. The other 10 percent to 20 percent of the space is filled with cerebrospinal fluid (CSF), which cushions the brain within the skull.

Inside the skull, the meninges protect the surface of the brain. The three *meninges*, or layers of tissue, are the dura mater, the arachnoid layer, and the pia mater. The *dura mater*, literally meaning "hard mother," is composed of a double layer of thick, fibrous tissue and is the outermost protective layer. Directly beneath the dura mater is the *arachnoid layer*. The *pia mater* is the layer that is in direct contact with the brain.

The gap between the arachnoid and pia mater is called the *subarachnoid space*. It is composed of fibrous, spongy tissue and CSF. The brain itself is divided into three parts: the cerebrum, cerebellum, and brainstem.

EPIDEMIOLOGY

Head injuries are the leading cause of death among accident victims younger than 45 years of age. Each year 50,000 people die from traumatic brain injuries. About 50 percent of head injury patients requiring surgical intervention arrive to the emergency department with a Glasgow Coma Scale (GCS) score ranging from 9 to 15. These patients have improved results if surgical intervention takes place prior to their neurologic demise—which emphasizes the importance of transport to a trauma center.

Epidemiologies specific to intracerebral hemorrhage, diffuse axonal injury (DAI), epidural hematoma, subdural hematoma, and subarachnoid hematoma are discussed in the following section.

PATHOPHYSIOLOGY

Intracerebral Hemorrhage

Intracranial hemorrhage is classified as extraaxial or intraaxial. *Extraaxial hemorrhage* takes place outside the brain and includes epidural, subdural, and subarachnoid hematomas. *Intraaxial hemorrhage* occurs within the brain tissue itself and is called *intracerebral hemorrhage*. Intracerebral hemorrhage is further divided into intraparenchymal and intraventricular hemorrhages. Intracerebral hemorrhage is a serious medical emergency because of the increase in intracranial pressure (ICP). If left untreated, intracerebral hemorrhage leads to coma and death.

Traumatic *intraparenchymal hemorrhage* is likely caused by penetrating trauma. However, this kind of hemorrhage can also be caused by depressed skull fractures and acceleration–deceleration trauma. The mortality rate for intraparenchymal hemorrhage is over 40 percent. The risk for death is especially high when the injury occurs within the brainstem. Bleeding in the medulla oblongata is even more lethal because breathing and circulatory mechanisms are controlled in this portion of the brain.

Intraventricular hemorrhage is characterized by bleeding into the brain's ventricular system, where CSF is produced. This type of hemorrhage is found in 35 percent of adults with moderate to severe head injury. An extensive amount of force is necessary to create this injury; therefore, other associated injuries are common. The prognosis for intraventricular hemorrhage is fairly dismal because of increased ICP and the likelihood for the brain to herniate through the opening at the base of the skull.

Intracerebral hemorrhage is frequently associated with altered mentation. Altered levels of consciousness, as well as nausea and vomiting, are seen in nearly 50 percent of cases. Forty percent of patients also complain of a headache with intracerebral hemorrhage. Other signs and symptoms commonly seen in this injury include systolic hypertension, unequal pupils, neurologic deficits, and seizures.

Diffuse Axonal Injury

Diffuse axonal injury (DAI) is one of the most devastating types of TBI. The damage from this type of head injury occurs over a more widespread area of the brain rather than in a focal area.

DAI typically stems from traumatic acceleration–deceleration injuries. It is a pathologic process in which axons are stretched and twisted by rotational shearing forces that occur during rapidly changing movement. The damaged axons begin to swell and separate from each other, causing interference between the communication and transmission of nerve impulses throughout the brain. This injury is one of the major causes of unconsciousness and persistent vegetative state after head trauma.

DAI occurs in 50 percent of all cases of severe head trauma. It is commonly seen in victims of motor vehicle crashes, falls, and assault. Frequently, the outcome of this injury is coma. More than 90 percent of patients with DAI never regain consciousness. The few patients who do eventually wake up remain significantly impaired neurologically.

CONCUSSION *Concussion* is a milder form of DAI. It is a synonym for mild TBI, which is a head injury associated with a GCS score of 13 to 15. Concussion is defined as a trauma-induced alteration in mental status or other neurologic function that may or may not involve loss of consciousness. This injury is caused by an impulsive force transmitted to the head. The result is a rapid, short-lived impairment of neurologic function that resolves spontaneously. Concussive injuries produce structural injuries to the brain; however, they exhibit only temporary functional disturbances.

An average of 80 percent of the 1.5 million reported traumatic brain injuries in the United States are mild. Mild head injury may result in cortical contusions from coup and contrecoup injuries. Milder degrees of axonal damage play a role in this TBI. It causes the hallmark signs and symptoms of confusion, retrograde and anterograde amnesia, and typically no preceding loss of consciousness. If loss of consciousness occurs, it is brief and does not recur.

Other signs and symptoms of concussion include headache, dizziness, lack of awareness, inability to concentrate, slurred speech, ataxia, nausea, and vomiting. Remember that these signs and symptoms are immediate after impact and subside gradually. Signs and symptoms that present several minutes after the original impact or worsen with time are indicative of a more serious head injury and not concussion.

Epidural Hematoma

Epidural hematoma is an accumulation of blood between the potential space of the dura and the bone of the skull (▶ Figure 48-1). This is considered to be the most serious complication of head injury and must be repaired quickly. Prognosis is excellent with aggressive treatment, including immediate surgical intervention. Therefore, the time required to diagnose this injury and transport the patient to an appropriate medical facility greatly affects the outcome.

Epidural hematoma complicates 2 percent of head injury cases, or approximately 40,000 cases per year. Alcohol and other intoxicating agents have been associated with increasing the incidence of these injuries. Morbidity and mortality are associated with level of mentation and location of the hematoma. The mortality rate for patients who are awake prior to surgery is nearly zero, for obtunded patients it is 9 percent, and for comatose patients it is 20 percent.

When looking at the location of the injury, patients with bilateral epidural hematomas have a 20 percent mortality rate. Those with epidural hematomas occurring in the posterior fossa of the brain have an even higher mortality rate: 26 percent. Few epidural hematomas are located in the frontal or occipital portions of the brain. Men are more likely to incur this injury than women with a 4:1 ratio; however, there is no delineation between races.

> **If left untreated, intracerebral hemorrhage leads to coma and death.**

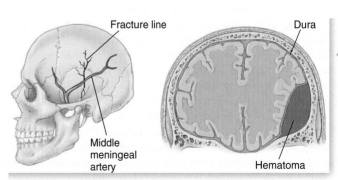

Figure 48-1 Epidural hematoma.

Epidural hematoma originates from deceleration injuries or low-velocity impact to the head. Skull fractures are common with these injuries, occurring in 90 percent of adult patients. Epidural hematoma is frequently seen in the temporoparietal region, where the skull fracture crosses the path of the middle meningeal artery.

The bleeding takes place between the protective covering of the brain (dura) and the skull. The bleeding is profuse and rapidly expands within the space, causing a sudden increase in ICP. This rise in ICP causes the cascade of signs and symptoms, including decreased mental status, severe headache, fixed and dilated pupils, vomiting, altered or absent breathing, posturing, and systolic hypertension with associated bradycardia (Cushing reflex, a late finding). Among patients with an epidural hematoma, 20 percent have a lucid interval. The patient will suffer from a loss of consciousness and then a period of responsiveness. Shortly thereafter, his level of consciousness will deteriorate rapidly.

Subdural Hematoma

Subdural hematoma is a collection of blood over the surface of the brain, between the dura mater and arachnoid meninges (▶ **Figure 48-2**). Subdural bleeding is typically the result of deceleration injuries and low-pressure venous bleeding. The bleeding occurs as a result of shearing action along the subdural space and traumatic stretching of small bridging veins. This hematoma is frequently associated with trauma but can also occur spontaneously in patients who receive anticoagulant therapy such as warfarin (Coumadin) or have a coagulopathy condition (prolonged bleeding time).

Subdural hematoma is classified based on the time elapsed from the inciting event and diagnosis. The three phases are acute, subacute, and chronic. Signs and symptoms begin immediately in the acute phase. If left untreated, the subacute phase begins three to seven days after the injury, and the chronic phase begins two to three weeks later.

Subdural hematoma is the most common intracranial lesion, occurring in one-third of patients with severe head injury and a GCS score of less than 9. Chronic subdural hematoma is reported in an average of 3 in 100,000 persons. It is more common among patients over 60 years of age owing to the predisposition for cerebral atrophy and decreased resiliency of bridging veins.

The highest incidence, 7.35 in 100,000 patients, is among patients 70 to 79 years of age. These patients with chronic subdural hematoma often present with headache, personality changes, and ataxia, progressing over weeks. Subdural hematoma is also seen in child abuse cases and incidents involving shaken baby syndrome. The typical mortality rate for this type of hematoma is around 60 percent.

Manifestations of subdural hematoma can vary greatly, ranging from clinically silent to expansion large enough to cause brain herniation. Signs and symptoms of acute subdural hematoma include declining level of consciousness, abnormal or absent respirations, dilation of one pupil, weakness or paralysis to one side of the body, vomiting, seizures, increasing systolic blood pressure, and decreasing heart rate.

Subarachnoid Hemorrhage

Subarachnoid hemorrhage refers to an accumulation of blood in the subarachnoid space. Subarachnoid hemorrhage can be both traumatic and nontraumatic in nature. The most common cause is a spontaneous rupture of an aneurysm.

When looking at the traumatic causes of subarachnoid hemorrhage; it is seen that the elderly often incur this injury from a fall. Younger patients usually sustain this injury as a result of a motor vehicle crash. It is the most common intracranial hemorrhage as a result of blunt force trauma and is often associated with some other bleeding within the skull. Approximately 373,000 people are hospitalized with a subarachnoid hemorrhage each year. Of these patients,

56,000 succumb to their injuries, whereas 99,000 survive with permanent disabilities.

The immediate danger in subarachnoid hemorrhage is ischemia, in which portions of the brain that do not receive adequate blood and oxygen supply suffer irreparable injury. This can lead to permanent neurologic damage or death. The three most common complications that promote ischemia to the brain are vasospasm, hydrocephalus, and intracranial hypertension.

In vasospasm, blood vessels constrict in response to chemicals released when blood breaks down in the subarachnoid space. *Hydrocephalus* is an accumulation of fluid in the ventricles of the brain. This occurs in 15 percent of subarachnoid hemorrhage because CSF cannot drain properly. Thus, pressure builds up on the brain, promoting further ischemic complications. Intracranial hypertension can lead to further bleeding and damage to the blood vessels. This complication is associated with a 70 percent mortality rate.

The classic symptom of nontraumatic subarachnoid hemorrhage is a thunderclap headache. It is described as the worst pain ever felt. The majority of studies have shown that patients progress from being pain free to experiencing severe excruciating pain in a matter of seconds. Loss of consciousness typically follows but can take several hours. Other signs and symptoms of subarachnoid hemorrhage include restlessness, confusion, motor and sensory dysfunction, vomiting, and seizures. Severe neurologic deficits develop and become irreversible within minutes.

ASSESSMENT FINDINGS

Assessment of head injury begins with your dispatch information and general impression. Information provided by the

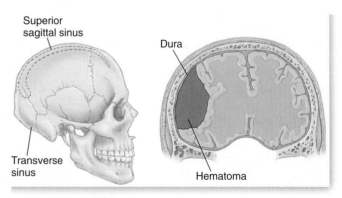

Figure 48-2 Subdural hematoma.

dispatcher can paint a picture of whether the patient is suffering from a traumatic incident or medical event. On arrival at the scene, evaluation of the mechanism of injury can help you ascertain whether a head injury is suspected. Obvious signs of a possible head injury include facial lacerations, scalp hematomas, a starred windshield, a cracked helmet, or evidence of a fall.

Primary assessment of a patient suffering from a head injury begins with manual stabilization of the spine. The forces applied to the head that cause these head injuries have the potential of causing injury to the spine as well. Therefore, the airway should be opened using a jaw-thrust maneuver while maintaining manual stabilization of the spine. If necessary, clear the airway of any potential obstruction and keep suction available at all times.

Maintaining the airway and providing oxygenation to the brain are vital to preventing further neurologic demise. Provide oxygen via a nonrebreather mask with 15 liters per minute (lpm) supplemental oxygen. Should the breathing be inadequate, administer positive pressure ventilation with supplemental oxygen via a bag-valve mask. Control any major bleeding as needed, as scalp lacerations have a tendency to bleed heavily.

If the patient displays definite signs of brain herniation, where you suspect the brain is being pushed through the opening at the base of the skull, you should consider hyperventilating the patient with supplemental oxygen. (This remains somewhat controversial and may not be included in your specific protocol.) Signs of brain herniation include unequal pupils, fixed pupils, posturing, hemiplegia or hemiparesis, Cushing reflex, or a deteriorating GCS score of two or more points. Begin positive pressure ventilation with a bag-valve mask and supplemental oxygen at a rate of 20 ventilations per minute. Do so with caution because ventilating at a rate greater than 20 can inversely cause a reduction of cerebral blood flow and worsen the head injury.

It is critical to maintain the systolic blood pressure above 90 mmHg in the traumatic brain-injured patient. A decrease in blood pressure will lead to a reduction in cerebral perfusion pressure and cerebral blood flow. Hypotension (systolic blood pressure <90 mmHg) in the TBI patient is a devastating complication that leads to worsened outcomes.

Therefore, you will initiate an intravenous line with a large-bore catheter and administer normal saline or lactated Ringer's to maintain a systolic blood pressure above 90 mmHg. Never use a fluid containing glucose, such as 5% dextrose in water (D_5W). A brain injury is a special situation in a trauma patient, when you must maintain the systolic blood pressure above 90 mmHg; avoid intentionally restricting fluid administration as in other trauma patients, when you want to raise the systolic blood pressure no higher than 80 to 90 mmHg.

A patient suffering from an injury to the head must have his mental status assessed and reassessed frequently. The AVPU mnemonic (**A**lert, **V**oice, **P**ain, **U**nresponsive) is used to assess mentation. Keep in mind that the patient may be alert originally but then may decline according to the location and type of injury to the head.

During evaluation of the patient's response to pain, he may react in one of two ways: purposeful or nonpurposeful. The patient may attempt to remove the source of the pain or try to move away. These responses are considered purposeful and show a higher level of functioning in the brain. However, the patient may respond by inappropriately moving the extremities or parts of the body but with no effort to stop the pain. This is considered to be nonpurposeful movement and indicates a deeper level of unresponsiveness.

Nonpurposeful movement can be exhibited in one of two ways: decorticate or decerebrate posturing (▶ **Figure 48-3**). Decorticate posturing is evidenced by flexion of the arms across the chest and extension of the legs. Decorticate posturing is associated with an injury in the upper portion of the brainstem. On the other hand, decerebrate posturing is indicative of an injury in the lower portion of the brainstem. In decerebrate posturing, the patient extends both arms down at the side of the body with extension of

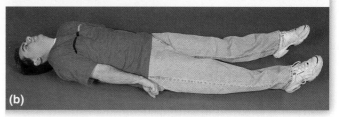

Figure 48-3 Nonpurposeful responses to painful stimuli include (a) flexion (decorticate) posturing and (b) extension (decerebrate) posturing.

the legs and arching of the back.

The patient is considered unresponsive when there is no response to verbal or painful stimuli. This is an ominous sign of head injury.

Be sure to document the patient's level of mentation accurately and often. A baseline level of mentation and continuous reassessment of mentation is crucial for determining if the patient is deteriorating. Further evaluation of mental status can be done by using the GCS. This assessment applies a numerical value to the patient's eye opening as well as best motor and verbal responses. To ensure accuracy, be certain that you are observing the patient's eye opening as you approach. Review the adult GCS as listed in **Table 48-1** and the pediatric GCS found in Topic 50.

During the secondary assessment, a physical exam paying particular attention to the brain and neurologic status is necessary. When evaluating the head, inspect thoroughly through the hair for abrasions, lacerations, and impaled objects (▶ **Figure 48-4**). Assess for deformities, depressions, and hematomas around the head and face. Use caution when palpating, though, as you do not want to cause further harm to any depressed areas of the skull.

Check the patient's pupils with a bright light for size, equality, and reactivity. If

> **A patient suffering from an injury to the head must have his mental status assessed and reassessed frequently.**

TABLE 48-1	Glasgow Coma Scale	
Eye Opening		
Spontaneous		4
To verbal command		3
To pain		2
No response		1
Verbal Response		
Oriented and converses		5
Disoriented and converses		4
Inappropriate words		3
Incomprehensible sounds		2
No response		1
Motor Response		
Obeys verbal commands		6
Localizes pain		5
Withdraws from pain (flexion)		4
Abnormal flexion in response to pain (decorticate rigidity)		3
Extension in response to pain (decerebrate rigidity)		2
No response		1

one or both pupils are fixed and dilated, increased ICP is likely. When you are evaluating the eyes, does the patient track and focus, as indicated by his looking and following you with his eyes? Is there a purplish discoloration around the soft tissue of the eye? This "raccoon" sign may be indicative of an intracranial injury and is also a delayed sign of skull fracture.

Finally, leakage of blood or CSF from the ears or nose can indicate a skull fracture or intracranial injury.

If the patient is awake and alert, you will want to assess his motor and sensory function. Begin by having the patient move his fingers and toes. Assess hand grasps for strength and equality. Have the patient push down on your hands with his feet and then pull up against your hands. When assessing dorsiflexion and plantar flexion, you are evaluating the strength and equality of this motor movement. You can assess sensory function by pinching the arm or touching a toe and having the patient identify which extremity is being touched.

Vital signs may be able to help you delineate between a head injury and some other disease process. Vital signs in head injury patients should be checked and recorded every 5 minutes. Variations in blood pressure, respiratory rate, and heart rate can also lead you to suspect impending deterioration of your patient (see Table 48-2).

History taking from bystanders at the scene can provide vital information about the mechanism of injury. As patients with head injury frequently have an altered mental status or loss of consciousness, bystanders can offer information that the patient is unable to provide.

The most crucial question is in regard to loss of consciousness. Determine how long the patient was unresponsive, when the loss of consciousness occurred in relation to the time of the injury, whether the loss of consciousness was sudden or

gradual, and whether there was more than one episode of unconsciousness.

Ascertain where and how the incident took place and whether the patient was moved after the injury. Obtain complaints the patient may have had specifically relating to dizziness, numbness, weakness, tingling, and paralysis. Also, in addition to past medical history, ask whether the patient has a prior history of head injury and, if so, when it occurred.

EMERGENCY MEDICAL CARE

Unfortunately, head injuries can be severe and life threatening. Prompt recognition and treatment of these injuries is paramount for patient survival and limiting permanent disability. Head injuries require a standard systematic approach for treatment and include the following:

- **Establish manual inline stabilization of the spine.**
  - Inline stabilization involves keeping the head, neck, and spinal column in alignment until the patient is fully immobilized to a backboard. This includes maintaining cervical stabilization even after a cervical collar is applied. Once immobilization including the head is complete, you may then release manual stabilization.
- **Maintain a patent airway.**
  - Use a manual jaw-thrust maneuver to open the airway.

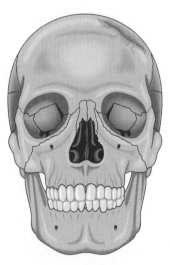

Soft area or depression.

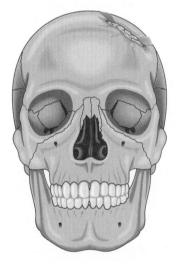

Open wound with bleeding and/or exposed brain tissue.

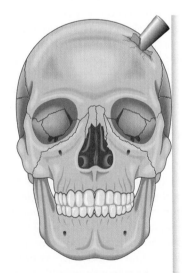

Impaled object in skull.

Figure 48-4 Examine the head for deformities, depressions, lacerations, or impaled objects.

TABLE 48-2

Implications of Changes in Vital Signs with Head Injuries

Vital Sign	Decreased	Increased
Blood pressure	Suspect hemorrhagic shock or head injury that has injured or compressed the brainstem	Suspect increased intracranial pressure
Respiratory rate	Respirations can be slow, shallow, or irregular with compression of the brainstem	Respirations can be fast, shallow, or irregular with compression of the brainstem
Heart rate	Suspect increased intracranial pressure or severe hypoxia	Suspect hemorrhage somewhere else in the body or early onset of hypoxia

– Remove any foreign bodies in the mouth and suction any secretions that may compromise the airway.

– The patient might vomit; therefore, protect him from aspiration. Keep suction available at all times, and be prepared to log-roll the patient.

– Consider advanced airway options when indicated.

• **Assess the adequacy of respirations and provide oxygen therapy.**

– If the respiratory status is adequate, administer oxygen at 15 lpm via a nonrebreather mask to maintain oxygen saturations at 95 percent.

– If the respiratory status is inadequate, provide positive pressure ventilation via a bag-valve mask with supplemental oxygen at a rate of 10 to 12 breaths per minute.

– Consider hyperventilation in patients with severe head injury and suspected brain herniation. (Note that the concept of hyperventilation in head injury is controversial. It may produce some short-term improvement but has no role in long-term management of herniation or elevated ICP. Always follow your local protocol.)

• **Control bleeding, as head injuries are likely to bleed heavily.**

– Dress and bandage open head wounds with sterile gauze.

– Do not apply pressure to open or depressed areas of the skull.

– Never remove a penetrating object from the head or face.

– Do not stop the flow of any CSF emitting from the ears or nose.

• **Transport the patient immediately to an appropriate medical facility.**

– Initiate an intravenous line of normal saline or lactated Ringer's using a large-bore catheter.

– Infuse the fluid at a rate to maintain a systolic blood pressure above 90 mmHg.

– Be careful not to be overly aggressive in fluid administration or make the patient hypertensive. Fluids can contribute to a worsened cerebral edema and increased ICP; however, maintaining an adequate mean arterial pressure is imperative in achieving adequate cerebral perfusion pressures and cerebral blood flow.

• **Be prepared for emergency care of seizures.**

• **Monitor the airway, breathing, circulation, and mental status continuously for any signs of deterioration and treat appropriately.**

TRANSITIONING

REVIEW ITEMS

1. You believe your head injury patient is displaying a Cushing reflex. This is evidenced by _____.
   a. hypotension and bradycardia
   b. hypertension and bradycardia
   c. hypotension and tachycardia
   d. hypertension and tachycardia

2. Which head injury is commonly associated with a skull fracture in the temporal region of the skull near the meningeal arteries?
   a. intracerebral hemorrhage
   b. epidural hematoma
   c. subdural hematoma
   d. subarachnoid hematoma

3. What type of head injury interferes with the communication and transmission of nerve impulses throughout the brain?
   a. diffuse axonal injury
   b. epidural hematoma
   c. skull fracture
   d. intraventricular hemorrhage

4. A 15-year-old baseball player is hit in the head with a fly ball. He immediately drops to the ground and is unconscious. As you approach his side, he immediately wakes up and is temporarily confused and amnestic to the event. As you continue to spend time with him, his mentation improves, and he begins to complain of a headache. Which type of head injury do you believe your patient has sustained?
   a. epidural hematoma
   b. subdural hematoma
   c. concussion
   d. intracerebral hemorrhage

5. Your 37-year-old male patient was sitting on the couch when he started complaining of a headache. He states that it is the worst headache he has ever felt in his life, and it is rapidly getting worse. This symptom is associated with which type of hemorrhage?

a. epidural hematoma

b. subdural hematoma

c. subarachnoid hemorrhage

d. intracerebral hematoma

6. A 42-year-old woman is on a skiing trip when she suddenly loses control and strikes a tree head-on. After a temporary loss of consciousness, the patient is awake and alert and complaining of a headache. She continues to act normally for a short time until suddenly she becomes lethargic and inappropriate. This lucid interval can be associated with which type of hematoma?

a. epidural hematoma

b. subdural hematoma

c. subarachnoid hematoma

d. intracerebral hematoma

APPLIED PATHOPHYSIOLOGY

Discuss fluid administration in the brain injured patient and how it differs from fluid administration in other non–brain-injured trauma patients.

CLINICAL DECISION MAKING

You are dispatched for a 42-year-old lumberman who reportedly fell 30 feet from a tree. When you arrive on scene, you find the patient supine on the ground. He does not open his eyes, nor does he speak or groan. When you rub his sternum, he flexes his arms to his chest and extends his legs.

1. What is this patient's Glasgow Coma Scale score?

2. How would you open the patient's airway?

You open the patient's airway to find blood and vomitus in the mouth. The patient is breathing regularly at 6 times per minute. His SpO$_2$ reading is 74 percent.

3. How would you manage this patient's airway and breathing?

You observe a large pool of blood behind the head. On closer exam, you notice a depression in the occiput of the skull. His blood pressure is 76/40 mmHg, and his heart rate is 108 mmHg.

4. How would you control the bleeding from the head?

5. Does this patient require expeditious transport? Why or why not?

6. What treatment would you provide en route to the hospital?

7. Would you administer fluids? If so, what type and at what rate?

Standard Trauma

Competency Integrates assessment findings with principles of epidemiology and pathophysiology to formulate a field impression to implement a comprehensive treatment/disposition plan for an acutely injured patient.

TOPIC

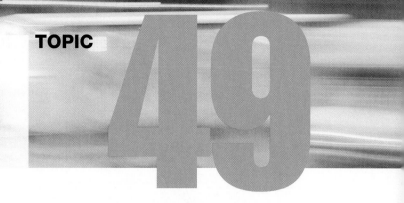

COMPLETE AND INCOMPLETE SPINE AND SPINAL CORD INJURIES

INTRODUCTION

Spinal cord injuries can be among the most traumatic injuries seen by the paramedic. They may arise from a wide variety of causes—motor vehicle crashes, diving accidents, falls, and sports injuries, to name just a few. The paramedic must be able to identify injuries that could damage the spinal cord or spinal column and to provide appropriate emergency care. Improper movement and handling of patients with spinal cord or spinal column injuries can lead to permanent disability or even death.

EPIDEMIOLOGY

An injury to the spinal cord could result in a catastrophic permanent disability to the patient. Approximately 11,000 new cases of spinal cord injury (SCI) occur each year in the United States. Most cases of SCI occur in men (80 percent), with an average age of 38 years. According to the National Spinal Cord Injury Database, the etiology of the majority of cases is associated with motor vehicle crashes, which account for close to half the cases, followed by falls, especially in the elderly; penetrating trauma; and sports and recreational activities.

Elderly patients are more prone to suffering from SCI from minor trauma resulting from degenerative vertebral disorders. In addition, elderly patients have become more active over the years; thus, the incidence of SCI in the elderly is on the rise.

SPINAL CORD ANATOMY

Understanding the basic anatomy of the spinal cord is important to adequately comprehend clinical assessment findings related to incomplete spinal cord injuries. The spinal cord is housed within the vertebral column and has 31 pairs of spinal nerves attached to it that exit at different levels. The spinal cord originates at the cervicomedullary junction inferior to the foramen magnum and terminates at the lower margin of the first lumbar vertebra (L1).

The most inferior portion of the spinal cord, known as the *conus medullaris*, narrows to a point and lies inferior to the lumbosacral enlargement. A series of nerve roots, referred to as the

TRANSITION *highlights*

- *Incidence with which spinal cord injury occurs, along with the predisposing factors of age, gender, and mechanism.*

- *Normal spinal cord anatomy, including important sensory and motor nerve tracts.*

- *Pathophysiology of spinal cord injury with basic mechanisms of injury, depending on amount of spinal cord involved:*
  - Complete spinal cord injury.
  - Incomplete spinal cord injury.
  - Spinal shock.

- *Motor and sensory findings consistent with various types of incomplete spinal cord injuries:*
  - Central cord syndrome.
  - Brown-Séquard syndrome.
  - Anterior cord syndrome.

- *Specific assessment tests that ascertain level of spinal cord involvement.*

- *General treatment strategies for the patient with a spinal cord injury.*

cauda equina, continues to extend inferiorly and exit through the lumbar and sacral vertebrae (▶ Figure 49-1). An injury below the level of the second lumbar vertebra (L2) is not necessarily considered an SCI because it involves segmental spinal nerves or the cauda equina. The dura mater, arachnoid, and pia mater meningeal layers extend from the brain to approximately the second sacral vertebra and provide protection to the spinal cord.

The spinal cord, like the brain, is composed of central nervous system tissue and requires a constant supply of oxygen and glucose. Blood supply to the spinal cord is provided by one anterior

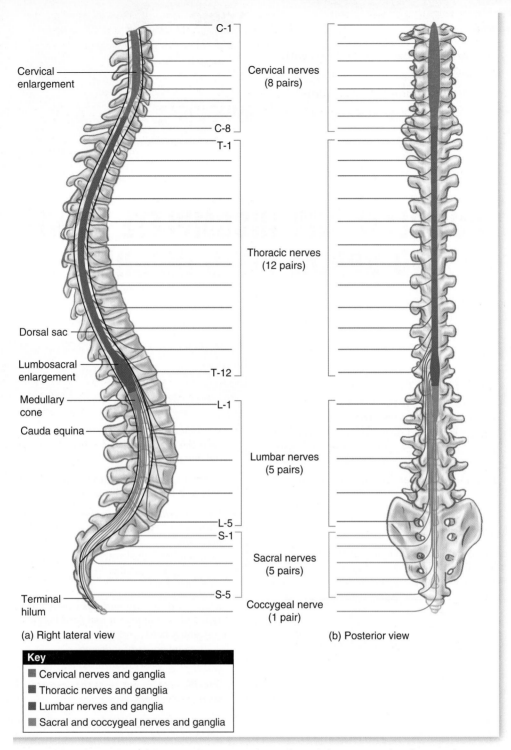

Cervical enlargement

Dorsal sac

Lumbosacral enlargement

Medullary cone

Cauda equina

Terminal hilum

(a) Right lateral view

C-1

C-8

T-1

T-12

L-1

L-5

S-1

S-5

Cervical nerves
(8 pairs)

Thoracic nerves
(12 pairs)

Lumbar nerves
(5 pairs)

Sacral nerves
(5 pairs)

Coccygeal nerve
(1 pair)

(b) Posterior view

Key
- Cervical nerves and ganglia
- Thoracic nerves and ganglia
- Lumbar nerves and ganglia
- Sacral and coccygeal nerves and ganglia

Figure 49-1 Illustration of the spinal nerves (a) laterally and (b) posteriorly. The ganglia are detailed as well.

spinal artery and two paired posterior spinal arteries. The anterior spinal artery supplies the anterior two-thirds of the spinal cord and extends the full length of the spinal cord. The posterior arteries supply the remaining posterior one-third of the spinal cord. An injury to the anterior spinal artery from laceration or compression by the vertebrae or a bony vertebral frag-

ment may result in anterior spinal cord damage and ischemia with neurologic dysfunction.

A cross section reveals that the cord is separated into a right and a left half by the anterior medial fissure and the posterior medial sulcus. The central portion of the cord contains gray matter that consists primarily of cell bodies of neurons and

forms an "H" pattern. Surrounding the gray matter is white matter that contains three major motor and sensory nerve tracts: (1) the dorsal or posterior column, which contains the gracile fasciculus and cuneate fasciculus; (2) the lateral pyramidal tract, which carries the corticospinal tracts; and (3) the anterior spinothalamic tract. Both the dorsal (posterior) column

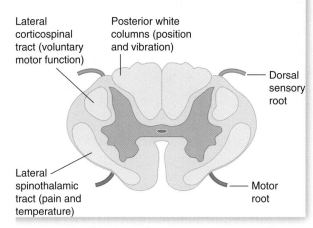

CROSS SECTION OF CERVICAL SPINAL CORD

Lateral corticospinal tract (voluntary motor function)

Posterior white columns (position and vibration)

Dorsal sensory root

Motor root

Lateral spinothalamic tract (pain and temperature)

Figure 49-2 Cross section of spinal cord showing corticospinal, spinothalamic, and posterior columns.

(gracile fasciculus and cuneate fasciculus) and anterior (spinothalamic) column contain sensory nerve tracts that carry information from sensory receptors up to the brain (▶ Figure 49-2).

The posterior (dorsal) column nerve tracts carry sensations of position (proprioception), vibration, and light touch from the skin, muscles, tendons, and joints to the brain. These posterior column nerve tracts cross over (decussate) at the cervicomedullary junction; therefore, the sensory impulse is carried by the ipsilateral (same side) portion of the spinal cord where the stimulus was received.

Thus, if light touch is applied to the right side of the body, the impulse is carried via the posterior column nerve tracts on the right side of the spinal cord. If an injury to the posterior column on the right side would occur, the patient would potentially lose the ability to feel light touch, vibration, and proprioception on the right side of the body below the site of the cord injury.

The spinothalamic nerve tracts carry pain, temperature, pressure, and crude touch sensations to the brain. Unlike the posterior column, these nerve fibers cross shortly after entering the cord and are carried on the contralateral (opposite side) of the spinal cord.

If an injury to the spinothalamic tract were to occur on the right side of the spinal cord, the patient would lose the ability to feel pain on the left side of the body; however, pain sensation would be preserved on the right. This may lead to some confusion in interpretation of the assessment findings for the emergency medical practitioner who is not familiar with the ascending nerve tracts. This, in turn, may

be perceived as an indication that an injury to the spinal cord has not occurred, as the pain response is preserved even though light touch and motor findings may be absent on one side of the body and pain response absent on the opposite side.

The lateral pyramidal (corticospinal) tract is a motor nerve (descending) tract that carries impulses from the cortex of the brain down the spinal column to muscles that cause fine and voluntary muscle movement. Like the posterior column, these nerve tracts cross over in the medulla. Thus, an injury to the spinal cord on the right side would produce loss of motor function on the right or ipsilateral (same) side.

An easy mnemonic that one can use to remember the spinal tracts and the associated sensory and motor response is LMNOP. This refers to **L**ight touch, **M**otor, and **NO P**ain. This means that light touch sensation and motor impulses are carried by nerve tracts on the same side of the spinal cord, but the pain sensation is carried by pain tracts on the opposite side of the spinal cord.

PATHOPHYSIOLOGY

The spinal cord can be injured by a variety of mechanisms, including flexion, rotation, compression, hyperextension, lateral bending, distraction, and penetrating wounds. An actual complete anatomic transaction of the spinal cord is rare, whereas a physiologic or functional transaction is more common, leading to a loss of function below the level of injury. Primary injury is associated with direct injury of the cord as a result of compression, tearing, stretching, or laceration.

The primary injury to the spinal cord initiates a complex cascade of events that leads to secondary SCI that results from ischemic gray and white matter. Hypoxia, hypoglycemia, hypotension, hyperthermia, and improper immobilization can lead to more significant secondary injury to the patient. The complete or maximum neurologic deficit is most often not exhibited by the patient immediately following the injury. Typically, as the secondary

injury progresses, the neurologic deficits continue to worsen.

Complete Spinal Cord Injury

Most EMS providers have been taught about complete spinal cord injury, which is defined as a total loss of motor or sensory function distal to the site of the cord injury. This condition is fairly easy to detect during the assessment, owing to the complete bilateral loss of neurologic function. It is rare that neurologic function will be regained. However, a complete SCI could be mimicked by spinal shock, in which the patient presents with complete neurologic dysfunction following the injury but recovers motor and sensory function within 24 hours after the injury.

For the paramedic, management of the patient will be the same, regardless of whether spinal shock (discussed later in this topic) or complete SCI is suspected, and it will include complete spinal immobilization.

Incomplete Spinal Cord Injury

Incomplete spinal cord injury, which implies that only a portion of the spinal cord is injured, is more common than a complete SCI. Because of the undamaged spinal nerve tracts, the patient will not present with complete loss of motor or sensory function below the level of injury. Instead, the patient may present with partial neurologic function, which contributes to confusing assessment findings if incomplete spinal cord injuries are not well understood by the paramedic.

For example, if the anterior portion of the spinal cord is injured, where spinal tracts carry the sensation of pain, the patient will lose the ability to feel pain while maintaining the ability to move his extremities and feel the sensation of light touch. Likewise, if the lateral portions of the spinal cord are injured, where the motor tracts are located, the patient may retain the ability to feel pain and light touch; however, he would lose the ability to move his extremities below the level of injury.

> **An injury to the spinal cord on the right side would produce loss of motor function on the right or ipsilateral (same) side.**

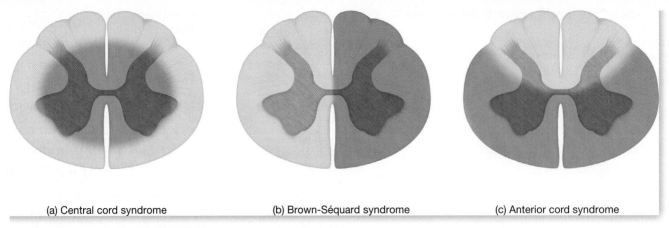

(a) Central cord syndrome   (b) Brown-Séquard syndrome   (c) Anterior cord syndrome

Figure 49-3 Cross sections of the spinal cord, showing the H-shaped gray matter surrounded by white matter. Illustrated here are the three most common types of incomplete spinal cord injury (the areas of the injury are highlighted in red): (a) Central cord syndrome results from injury to the central cord. (b) Brown-Séquard syndrome results from injury to the right or left half of the cord. (c) Anterior cord syndrome results from injury to the anterior cord.

These presentations conflict directly with the findings of complete SCI and may cause the paramedic to fail to provide complete spinal immobilization, especially if he was taught that all spinal injuries cause complete loss of motor and sensory function below the level of the SCI.

Specific presentations of incomplete spinal injury are central cord syndrome, Brown-Séquard syndrome, or an anterior cord syndrome in 90 percent of the incomplete injuries (▶ Figure 49-3). The most common is the central cord syndrome that is often associated with older patients with degenerative arthritis. Each syndrome results in different, distinct patient presentations (see Table 49-1).

CENTRAL CORD SYNDROME In central cord syndrome, the ligamentum flavum (▶ Figure 49-4) impinges on the central portion of the spinal cord, causing a concussion or contusion to the gray and inner portions of the spinal nerve tracts within the white matter. The sensory and motor tracts that innervate the lower extremities are located in the peripheral (outer) portions of the nerve tracts, whereas the upper extremities are controlled by the inner or central portions of the nerve tracts.

Thus, with central cord syndrome, the patient experiences weakness, paralysis, and sensory dysfunction in the upper extremities; however, the lower extremities have no or little neurologic dysfunction. This may appear confusing to many emergency care personnel because it is often thought that the sensory and motor dysfunction always occurs below the level of injury.

BROWN-SÉQUARD SYNDROME Brown-Séquard syndrome results from injury to only one side (hemisection) of the spinal cord, usually as a result of penetrating trauma. Because only one side of the cord is involved in the injury, the patient will exhibit loss of motor function and loss of light touch on the same side as the SCI; however, the pain response will be preserved to that side of the body. On the opposite side of the body, the patient will have motor function and light touch sensation but will have a loss of pain sensation.

ANTERIOR CORD SYNDROME Anterior cord syndrome results from injury to the anterior portion of the spinal cord from contusion of the cord, injury from bony fragments, and laceration or occlusion of the anterior spinal artery. Because the anterior portion of the cord is involved, the spinothalamic and corticospinal tract damage results in a loss of motor function and a loss of pain and temperature sensation below the level of injury. Because the posterior columns are not involved, the patient retains the ability to feel light touch.

Spinal Shock

Spinal shock is a temporary loss of neurologic function and autonomic tone distal to the injury to the spinal cord. The patient typically presents with the loss of motor and sensory function and urinary bladder incontinence. In addition, the patient may exhibit bradycardia, hypotension, and hypothermia.

TABLE 49-1	Incomplete Spinal Cord Injury Syndrome Assessment Findings	
Incomplete Spinal Cord Injury Syndrome	Motor Findings	Sensory Findings
Central cord syndrome	Paralysis or severe weakness of the upper extremities, less severe or no motor dysfunction in the lower extremities	Loss of pain sensation in upper extremities, less pain dysfunction in the lower extremities
Brown-Séquard syndrome	Loss of motor function to one side of the body below the level of injury	Loss of light touch to the same side of the body as motor dysfunction, loss of pain sensation opposite the light touch, and motor dysfunction
Anterior cord syndrome	Loss of motor function to both sides of the body below the level of injury	Loss of pain sensation to both sides of the body below the level of injury; patient is able to continue to feel light touch

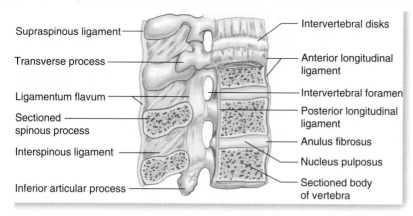

Supraspinous ligament

Transverse process

Ligamentum flavum

Sectioned spinous process

Interspinous ligament

Inferior articular process

Intervertebral disks

Anterior longitudinal ligament

Intervertebral foramen

Posterior longitudinal ligament

Anulus fibrosus

Nucleus pulposus

Sectioned body of vertebra

Figure 49-4 Ligaments and intervertebral disks of the spine. Lateral view of the spinal column (anterior to the right). The lower vertebrae have been cut sagittally to reveal the spinal canal and some of the ligaments.

TABLE 49-2	Differential Assessment Findings: Hypovolemic Shock Versus Neurogenic Shock	
Vital Sign Finding	Hypovolemic Shock	Neurogenic Shock
Blood pressure	Decreased	Decreased
Heart rate	Tachycardia	Bradycardia
Skin	Pale, cool, and clammy	Warm, dry, and flushed

Neurogenic hypotension may result from spinal shock. The loss of vasomotor control allows the vessels below the level of SCI to dilate, creating a distributive type of shock. Because the autonomic nervous system control to the body below the injury is blocked, loss of tone and vessel dilation remain unopposed. Blood begins to pool in the dilated vessels, causing a drop in the blood pressure. Administration of intravenous fluids may be the initial therapeutic measure to maintain adequate perfusion if the systolic blood pressure is below 90 mmHg. Vasoconstrictive agents may be added later in the patient's course of treatment.

Typically, the heart rate would increase as a reflex response to the decrease in blood pressure, as seen in hypovolemic shock; however, interruption of the sympathetic trunk that fails to elicit an appropriate sympathetic response, including epinephrine release, does not allow an increase in the heart rate. Thus, the patient presents with hypotension and bradycardia. The hypotension tends to be mild, with systolic blood pressure maintained above 90 mmHg.

Because of the peripheral vasodilation and pooling of blood, the skin is initially flushed. The skin is also dry owing to the lack of sympathetic stimulation of sweat glands. Most of these findings are totally opposite those associated with hypovolemic shock. If the patient presents with hypotension, tachycardia, and pale, cool, and clammy skin, always suspect blood loss and treat for hypovolemic shock (see Table 49-2).

ASSESSMENT FINDINGS

In assessment of the patient with an SCI, it is imperative to assess the various spinal tracts by testing for pain, light touch sensation, and motor function.

Testing for grip strength by having the patient squeeze one's fingers does not test the different nerve tracts and various levels of the spinal cord, and thus it is an incomplete and ineffective test.

A quick and effective method to test the corticospinal tract at various levels of the cord is to have the conscious patient perform the following motor function tests (see Table 49-3):

- Have the patient flex his elbows (tests C6).
- Have the patient extend his elbows (tests C7).
- Have the patient extend his arms with the hands out, palm down, fingers spread apart; have the patient resist as you squeeze the second and fourth fingers (tests T1).
- Support the patient's wrist and push on the extended hand while the patient resists (tests C7).
- Place your hands against the bottom of the feet and have the patient "push down" to test foot plantar flexion (tests S1 and S2).

TABLE 49-3	Spinal Cord Motor Assessment and Level of Loss of Function	
Level of Spinal Cord	Motor Function	Assessment
C6	Flexion at elbow	Have the patient flex his arms at the elbows.
C7	Extension at elbow	Have the patient extend his arms at elbows.
C7	Resistance to downward motion with hand extension	Have patient hold his arms out with hand extended and palm down. Provide support under the wrist while you push downward on the hand.
T1	Flexion of fingers	Have the patient flex his fingers.
T1	Resistance to abducted fingers	With the arm and hand extended with the palm facing downward, have the patient abduct (spread apart) the fingers. Squeeze the second and fourth fingers, attempting to push them together.
T1–T12	Intercostal and abdominal muscles	Observe the patient for inadequate ventilation effort.
L5	Dorsiflexion of the foot	Place your hands on the top of the patient's feet; have the patient pull up against them.
S1–S2	Plantar flexion of the foot	Place your hands on the bottom of the patient's feet; have the patient push down against them.

- Place your hands on top of the feet and have the patient pull up against your hands to test dorsiflexion (tests L5).

To test the posterior column (light touch), lightly touch each hand and foot while having the patient distinguish which hand or foot is being touched. To test the spinothalamic tracts (pain), pinch each hand and foot and have the patient distinguish which hand or foot is being pinched. One recommended method is to use a cotton swab with a wooden stick. Break the stick, and use the cotton swab end to test for light touch and the broken wooden end of the stick to poke the patient to elicit a pain response.

Be sure the patient's eyes are closed during the light touch and pain testing. Redundancy is built into the assessment to identify any neurologic dysfunction that may indicate the potential for an incomplete spinal injury (see Table 49-4).

EMERGENCY MEDICAL CARE

Because spinal cord tissue is basically the same as brain tissue, it is essential to establish and maintain an adequate airway, ventilation, and oxygenation. If the SpO$_2$ reading is less than 95 percent,

administer supplemental oxygen. If the tidal volume or respiratory rate is inadequate, provide positive pressure ventilation.

In all the following instances, the patient must be immobilized regardless of the neurologic assessment findings:

- A significant mechanism of injury is evident.
- The patient has an altered mental status.
- The patient complains of pain or tenderness to the vertebral column.
- The patient is unreliable because of intoxication, head injury, stress reaction, or other distracting injury (fractures, abdominal injury).
- Any sensory or motor dysfunction is found during the neurologic assessment.

En route to the medical facility, initiate an intravenous line of normal saline or lactated Ringer's. A large-bore catheter is recommended in case fluid must be administered to maintain the blood pressure. Run the fluid at a rate to maintain the

TABLE 49-4	Level of Spinal Cord Injury Correlated to Loss of Sensory Function
Level of Spinal Cord	Level of Loss of Sensation
C4	Suprasternal notch
C5	Below the clavicle
C6	Thumb
C7	Index finger
T4	Nipple line
T10	Umbilicus
L1	Femoral pulse
L4	Knee
S1	Lateral aspect of foot
S2–S4	Perianal region

systolic blood pressure at 90 mmHg or above.

If there is any suspicion that the patient is hypoglycemic, check the blood glucose level (BGL) using a glucose meter (glucometer). If the BGL is less than 60 mg/dL, administer 25 grams of 50% dextrose in water (D$_{50}$W).

Vasoactive agents may be necessary to maintain blood pressure in severe cases of spinal shock. Always follow local protocols.

TRANSITIONING

REVIEW ITEMS

1. A patient presents with bilateral loss of motor and sensory function below the nipple line. You should suspect _____.
   a. central cord syndrome
   b. unresolved spinal shock
   c. anterior cord syndrome
   d. neurogenic spinal shock

2. A patient loses the ability to feel pain to the left side of his body. You should suspect an injury to the _____.
   a. right corticospinal tract
   b. left posterior column
   c. right spinothalamic tract
   d. left cauda equina

3. A patient who has an isolated spinal cord injury to the right posterior column would present with _____.
   a. an inability to move the right side of his body
   b. a loss of pain sensation to the left side of the body

   c. a loss vibration sensation to the left side of the body
   d. an inability to feel light touch to the right side of the body

4. A suspected spinal cord injured patient exhibits sonorous sounds on inhalation and exhalation. This may result in _____.
   a. a worsened secondary spinal cord injury
   b. a decrease in circulating carbon dioxide
   c. the need for immediate advanced airway management
   d. application of continuous positive airway pressure (CPAP)

5. An elderly patient who was involved in a minor motor vehicle crash is walking around the scene when you arrive. Following your assessment, you note that the patient has noticeable weakness to both upper extremities; however, the lower extremities have normal motor function. The patient is able to feel light touch and pain in all four extremities. You should _____.

a. immobilize both upper extremities with splints to prevent further movement

b. place the patient in a position of comfort, apply a nonrebreather mask, and transport

c. place the patient in a lateral recumbent position to prevent aspiration of blood

d. manually stabilize the spine until you can perform full spinal immobilization

APPLIED PATHOPHYSIOLOGY

1. List the major motor and sensory tracts in the spinal cord and the general location of each.

2. Describe how to assess each of the three major sets of tracts.

3. Explain why it would be necessary to test for pain in a patient who has the ability to feel light touch.

4. Why would the patient with spinal shock possibly develop hypotension?

5. Explain the difference in the pathophysiology between hypovolemic shock and spinal shock.

6. Describe fluid administration in the spinal cord-injured patient.

CLINICAL DECISION MAKING

You arrive on the scene at a construction accident and find a 43-year-old male patient who fell approximately 30 feet off scaffolding. The patient landed on his side and is still in that position as you approach him. The patient appears to be alert and talking.

1. What are your initial considerations when entering the scene and approaching the patient?

2. What injuries should you suspect based on the mechanism of injury?

Following the primary assessment, you determine that the patient is alert and oriented to person, place, and time. His airway is patent. His respiratory rate is 22/minute with adequate chest rise. His radial pulse is 92/minute. His skin is warm and dry. His SpO2 reading is 98 percent on room air. His blood pressure is 84/56 mmHg.

3. Can you identify any life threats? If so, what are they?

4. What immediate emergency care should you provide based on the primary assessment?

5. What do the vital signs indicate?

During the secondary assessment, you note abrasions to the right temporal region and a contusion to the right lateral thorax. The pupils are equal and reactive, the nose and mouth are clear, and no evidence of trauma is noted to the neck. The trachea is midline, and the jugular veins are not distended or flat. The chest is rising and falling symmetrically, and no instability is noted on palpation. The breath sounds are

equal and clear bilaterally. The abdomen is soft and nontender. The pelvis is stable. The right upper and lower extremities have abrasions and contusions. The peripheral pulses are present in all four extremities.

During the neurologic exam, you note that the patient is unable to move on the right side of the body below the nipple line; however, he is able to move his hands and feet on the left side of the body. He cannot feel light touch when applied to the right side of the body; however, he is able to feel the light touch to the entire left side of the body. The patient is able to feel a pinch to the right hand and foot. Although he is able to feel light touch to the left side of the body, he is unable to feel a pinch when applied to the left hand and foot. The patient has no pertinent past medical history, takes no medications, and has no known allergies. His last oral intake was approximately two hours earlier at lunch when he ate a sandwich and drank a Coke. He explains that his fall was a result of tripping and losing his balance.

6. What condition(s) have you ruled out in your differential field impression?

7. Do you suspect a spinal cord injury? If so, what specific type? Why?

8. Explain the reason for the conflicting neurologic findings.

9. Based on your differential field diagnosis, what emergency care should you provide?

10. Would you administer fluids in this patient? If so, what fluid, at what rate, and for what reason?

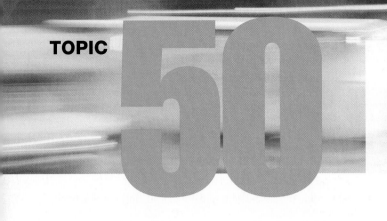

Standard Trauma

Competency Integrates assessment findings with principles of epidemiology and pathophysiology to formulate a field impression to implement a comprehensive treatment/disposition plan for an acutely injured patient.

TRAUMA IN SPECIAL POPULATIONS: PEDIATRICS

TRANSITION *highlights*

- *Incidence of pediatric trauma and death.*
- *Normal physiologic differences between pediatric and adult patients that contribute to heightened morbidity and mortality in pediatric patients.*
- *Disease patterns and assessment findings common in pediatric patients.*
- *Maintaining the vital functions of airway, breathing, and circulation while managing pediatric trauma patients.*
- *Importance for the paramedic to provide "organ-specific care" to the patient as well as care aimed at supporting lost function:*
  - *Cerebral blood flow.*
  - *Head, neck, and spine considerations.*
  - *Thoracic chest wall considerations.*
  - *Multiorgan system trauma.*
  - *Abdomen and pelvic considerations.*
- *General treatment strategies for the pediatric patient suffering from trauma.*

INTRODUCTION

Trauma is the leading cause of death and disability in children. It is a difficult concept to grasp, but trauma is a *disease* with recognizable and predictable contributing factors, seasonality, high-risk populations and behaviors, and proven but not widely adopted prevention strategies. Injuries are responsible for more deaths of our children than all other causes combined, but are only the tip of an iceberg that has huge financial and emotional effects on society from long-term disabilities. Most of the pediatric calls that EMS professionals respond to are because of trauma; thus, it is critical to under-stand the anatomic and physiologic differences between children and adults.

Children have unique anatomic and physiologic characteristics that predispose them to an exaggerated and poorly adapted response to acute injuries. Children are less able than adults to cope with life-threatening stress, and their coping mechanisms are quickly exhausted.

Because of their smaller body mass and inability to withstand intense forces, children are more likely to suffer multiorgan system involvement and have multiple injuries, often including injuries to the central nervous system. In children, as in adults, the presence of shock and hypotension is the strongest predictor for increased mortality—the difference is that these two cardinal features have a quicker onset time in children and are more difficult to recognize than in adults, leading to costly treatment delays and worse outcomes.

Blunt abdominal or thoracic trauma, closed head injury, long bone fractures, or spinal cord injury can all result in severe hypotension and shock that, if unrecognized and inadequately treated, will lead to poorer outcomes, more quickly, and with higher morbidity (associated injuries and long-term disabilities) and mortality (death) compared with adults with similar injuries.

Paramedics must learn to recognize both the anatomic differences and the subtle assessment findings that indicate critical injuries in children. We must adapt our assessment procedures and adjust our treatments according to physical size and physiologic norms. Moreover, we must also recognize that there is a vast difference in capabilities in handling pediatric trauma and develop transport guidelines to deliver patients to the most appropriate level of care.

EPIDEMIOLOGY

The burden of nonfatal injuries is enormous, with almost 10 million injuries in 2004 to the under-20-years-old population (www.cdc.gov/injury/wisqars/index.html). More than 300,000 children are hospitalized each year with trauma-related injuries. The cost of the associated morbidity to U.S. society is incalculable, as there are significant long-term rehabilitation issues, as well as neurologic impairments and secondary social and psychological aftereffects. Ripple effects from acute and chronic conditions are significant and affect whole families, leading to higher divorce rates, financial burdens, and persistent behavioral concerns.

Prevention is the most important strategy for controlling this epidemic of injury. Significant strides have been made with the adoption of mandatory seatbelt and helmet laws, increased fire safety, gun control, and education programs. Nonetheless, injury remains a significant killer of children.

Despite advances in prevention, detection, and resuscitation, the population of pediatric trauma patients continues to have the worst outcome. It is estimated that only 10 percent to 15 percent of traumatically injured children have life-threatening injuries. Despite that low figure, however, trauma is the leading cause of death for children, in no small part because medical care providers are not trained and equipped to provide a rapid and coordinated response focusing on the immediate threats to life and do not recognize the unique and sometimes subtle anatomic and physiologic differences between children and adults.

The pattern of pediatric injuries varies with the mechanism. Because trauma encompasses everything from nonaccidental, inflicted injury to submersions and burns, the age-related differences in the incidence and outcomes vary considerably. Motor vehicle trauma accounts for the majority of injuries in the United States. Pediatrics is no exception, with more than 40 percent of injuries reported to the National Trauma Data Bank (www.facs.org/trauma/ntdb/index.html) stemming from motor vehicle crashes, 20 percent from falls, and another 10 percent from nonaccidental, inflicted injuries.

When considering motor vehicle-related trauma, pediatric patients can be either passengers or pedestrians. The term *restrained passenger* in reference to a pediatric patient is one that should be questioned closely, as it is estimated that only 15 percent of children in child safety seats are properly harnessed in correctly installed seats (www.cdc.gov/ncipc/factsheets/childpas.htm).

Trauma Scoring Systems and Outcome

The introduction and spread of statewide trauma systems, the adoption of the American College of Surgeons' trauma center verification for hospitals, and the development of trauma registries and databases have allowed for categorization of trauma patients and increased attention to the necessary resources required for managing trauma, especially pediatric trauma.

Triage systems that pay attention to both physiologic criteria and mechanism of injury are important in the early management and referral of pediatric patients. Because trauma is a time-sensitive disease, early goal-directed therapy and prompt referral and transport of injured children to a higher level of care are critical to their survival and overall functional outcomes. In highly evolved trauma systems, triage and transport begin with prehospital EMS providers. Physicians and the public alike should insist on a high level of pediatric education and credentialing for EMS professionals, thereby creating an essential foundation that ensures optimal age-appropriate and competent resuscitation.

Trauma scoring systems are generally used for two purposes: as a tool for triage/treatment decision support or as a tool for predicting severity of illness or mortality. The triage tool should be simple and easy to calculate, but it must be accurate enough to include all patients who require a higher level of trauma services. The latter scoring system is usually more complex, using many variables, and is not considered relevant in the early resuscitation stages but is important for decision support later, for benchmarking, and for outcomes research. The most widely applied scoring system is the Glasgow Coma Scale (GCS). Modification of the GCS for pediatric patients has been an important advancement in the assessment of age-appropriate behavior in both verbal and preverbal children (see **Table 50-1**). As a gold standard in the rapid and early assessment of a trauma patient, it has outcome prediction value as well.

Reliability is experience dependent and can be difficult to obtain in an intubated patient; it is impossible to obtain in a sedated and/or paralyzed patient. Some studies have observed definite differences in outcome of patients with a low GCS score (3–4) compared with higher (7–8) scores, whereas the middle–severe range (5–6) is less prognostic of outcome.

Multiple studies have shown that the admission GCS is more predictive of injury severity than field GCS, and the motor component has been found to be the best predictor of outcome. That said, one study observed a significant improvement in GCS in almost one-third of pediatric trauma patients who had initial GCS scores between 6 and 8 following resuscitation, reminding us that (1) serial exams are more important than a single exam and (2) continual reassessment is important.

Because of their smaller body mass and inability to withstand intense forces, children are more likely to suffer multi-organ system involvement and have multiple injuries.

ASSESSING AND TREATING ANATOMIC AND PHYSIOLOGIC DIFFERENCES IN CHILDREN

"Airway, breathing, circulation" are the ABCs of resuscitation medicine and must be followed, in that order, every time. This is because children are more likely to have respiratory problems or airway complications from trauma that will respond to this approach. Failure to follow the ABCs, or "the basics," is a common error in medicine, especially in emergency and critical care, when a crisis situation may unexpectedly arise and the untrained are caught unprepared.

In the Pediatric Assessment Triangle, these ABCs have been modified to "appearance, [work of] breathing, and circulation" to incorporate the overall picture of the child as critical to one's early assessment and also to acknowledge the airway as a vital factor in the assessment of "breathing."

Understanding how blood loss can affect organ perfusion and cause shock, altered mental status, and cool and

Triage systems that pay attention to both physiologic criteria and mechanism of injury are important in the early management and referral of pediatric patients.

TABLE 50-1 Pediatric Glasgow Coma Scale

		>1 Year	<1 Year	
Eye opening	4	Spontaneous	Spontaneous	
	3	To verbal command	To shout	
	2	To pain	To pain	
	1	No response	No response	

		>1 Year	<1 Year	
Best motor response	6	Obeys		
	5	Localizes pain	Localizes pain	
	4	Flexion—withdrawal	Flexion—withdrawal	
	3	Flexion—abnormal (decorticate rigidity)	Flexion—abnormal (decorticate rigidity)	
	2	Extension (decerebrate rigidity)	Extension (decerebrate rigidity)	
	1	No response	No response	

		>5 Years	2–5 Years	0–23 Months
Best verbal response	5	Oriented and converses	Appropriate words and phrases	Smiles, coos, cries appropriately
	4	Disoriented and converses	Inappropriate words	Cries to pain
	3	Inappropriate words	Cries and/or screams	Inappropriate crying and/or screaming
	2	Incomprehensible sounds	Grunts	Grunts
	1	No response	No response	No response

"clamped down" extremities in a pediatric patient is essential to providing responsive and lifesaving care to these patients, most of whom have injuries that are *not* life threatening initially but can rapidly become so if too much time is wasted between injury and presentation to health care providers.

Airway, Oxygenation, and Ventilation

Anatomic differences in the pediatric airway must be considered when assessing and controlling the oxygenation and ventilation of injured infants and children. The prominent forehead and occiput and relatively small midface (the area between the eyes and jaw) of the infant and child, the smaller jaw and relatively large tongue, narrow nares and lower airways that are prone to edema and secretions during injury, the high position of the vocal cords (glottis) at C2–C3 (as opposed to C5 in the adult) with anteroinferior slanting vocal cords, floppy epiglottis, and short neck all create a potentially very difficult airway to control, especially in the settings of gastric reflux, relative obesity, and aspiration.

Add to these anatomic concerns the high likelihood of traumatic brain injury and one can easily envision how respiratory insufficiency can quickly progress to respiratory and then cardiorespiratory arrest. Thorough knowledge and appreciation of these anatomic differences in infants and children are essential for anyone managing a pediatric airway.

Breathing

Whether to control the pediatric airway with an endotracheal tube, a laryngeal mask airway, or another blind insertion airway versus continuing with bag-mask ventilations is a hot topic in prehospital pediatric care. It cannot be overstressed that the paramedic has all the skills necessary to provide lifesaving care, and the data support the fact that good bag-mask skills are not just essential but possibly better than advanced airway skills in certain circumstances.

Because hypoxia and both hypo- and hypercarbia are major factors contributing to morbidity and mortality, patients with an altered GCS or rapidly deteriorating mental status should have their airway and breathing continually assessed and their ventilation assisted. When in doubt that a pediatric patient is breathing adequately, understand that a GCS of less than 12 is not normal and that the patient may need assistance.

Decreasing mental status and subsequent inability to maintain airway security are indications for endotracheal intubation by ALS providers (when allowed by protocol). Keeping your patient from deteriorating to that point will have more effect on the overall outcome than anything else you can do in the prehospital environment.

Recent literature on severely head-injured patients has shown a direct correlation between the adequacy of ventilation and survival with poorer outcomes seen on arrival to the emergency department in patients who were hyper- or hypoventilated to partial pressure of end-tidal CO_2 ($PETCO_2$) <30 or >50 mmHg by EMS providers.

The dangers of hyperventilation are increasingly evident in the resuscitation literature. "Above all, do no harm" is our motto in medicine; it is important to consider this here. If you are assisting ventilations in your pediatric patient, be sure to keep an age-appropriate rate (infants, 0–1 year old: 20–30 breaths/minute; 1–6 years old: 25 breaths/minute; 6–12 years old: 20 breaths/minute; over 12 years old: 10–12 breaths/minute).

With assisted ventilation comes the transition from a spontaneously breathing patient to one who is now positive pressure (either mechanical or manual) ventilated. This commonly results in an alteration in the patient's cardiopulmonary status. In the hypovolemic condition commonly encountered in the traumatically injured patient, the application of positive pressure can result in a hemodynamic vise effect on the right atrium, leading to diminished atrial filling and decreased ventricular cardiac output. This vise effect, combined with overly aggressive airway pressures, can lead to pulseless electrical activity (PEA), in which venous return, and thus cardiac output, is impeded from the tamponade effect of the high afterload on an underfilled right ventricle owing to high intrathoracic pressures.

The lack of pulmonary blood flow results in no left-sided filling or systemic cardiac output. The only treatment is to ensure that assisted breaths are giving just enough pressure to move the chest and to provide adequate oxygenation and ventilation while avoiding overdistention and the vise effect. In the hypotensive or potentially hemodynamically unstable trauma patient, this is essential to avoiding the "second hit" of hypotension and hypoxemia, which are major contributors to mortality and morbidity.

Circulation

The blood volume of children varies by age, with infants having up to 100 mL/kg; this figure decreases inversely with age until adolescence, when the adult 50–60 mL/kg blood volume is the rule. For a newborn, this volume is the equivalent of a 12-ounce can of soda; for a one-year-old child, a liter bottle of soda; for a six-year-old, a two-liter bottle.

It does not take much blood loss to put a young child in shock; early recognition of and response to shock saves more lives than anything else you can provide in the field. Once the pediatric patient is packaged safely, rapid transport to the hospital is the most important therapy we can offer in the prehospital setting.

Pediatric patients respond to blood loss predictably. When faced with reduced preload and/or stroke volume, cardiac output is maintained by increasing the heart rate. Additionally, the body must increase the vascular resistance to keep the pressure up. Consider the following equation: Blood Pressure (BP) = HR × Stroke Volume/Systemic Vascular Resistance.

Tachycardia (that is, heart rate above the age-related norms) indicates shock in children. Shock can also be recognized by assessing signs of poor perfusion, such as cool, pale extremities, weak pulses, and altered mental status. Any child with an altered mental status—poor response to the environment, low tone, abnormal activity, weak or uncoordinated, unconscious—either has a closed head injury or, absent that possibility, is in shock.

Obtain IV access and administer up to 3 fluid boluses at 20 mL/kg or as directed in your protocols in response to the pediatric patient's presentation. Consider boluses of 10 mL/kg in neonates. Use caution in fluid administration so as not to overload the patient with fluid—something that is much easier done in pediatric patients than in adults. IV access should be obtained en route. Prompt transport to surgical intervention remains the definitive treatment in pediatric trauma for any level of EMS provider.

ORGAN-SPECIFIC CARE

Beyond their general anatomic differences, children require organ-specific care to maximize outcomes following trauma. After ensuring proper care of airway, breathing, and circulation, attention may be focused on the primary system affected by the trauma.

Cerebral Blood Flow

The acutely injured brain is highly susceptible to any disruption of perfusion and/or oxygenation. The same can be said for any organ; however, given the lack of regenerative properties of the central nervous system, this is the organ to target with our therapies.

Closed head injuries definitely disrupt regional (and potentially global) cerebral autoregulation. The unique ability of the cerebral vasculature to intrinsically constrict or dilate based on systemic arterial blood pressure is interfered with; this disruption potentially harms the ability to maintain a constant blood flow based on metabolic demands. The pressure-dependent autoregulation is usually the first to go in the setting of injury; with that loss, the cerebral arterial vascular bed will either passively dilate as the blood pressure rises or constrict as the blood pressure falls. As a last resort, the chemical regulatory properties usually remain intact except in areas of profound ischemia or necrosis; therefore, the treatment goals of maintaining normal oxygen and carbon dioxide levels are vitally important.

Head, Neck, and Spine

Pediatric pedestrians who are motor-vehicle trauma victims may suffer a pattern of injuries known as the *Waddell triad*, consisting of a femoral shaft fracture, intraabdominal and/or intrathoracic injuries, and a closed head injury that logically result from the three collisions that occur in succession: bumper versus leg, body versus hood, and head versus ground after being thrown. Although the incidence of all three injuries may be rare, a high index of suspicion should be maintained.

Given the disproportionately large head in children, the adage "Children lead with their heads" is an important one to remember when assessing the traumatically injured child. Head injuries are extremely common in children and may be difficult to assess. However, given that more than 80 percent of deaths from pediatric trauma are associated with severe traumatic brain injury, this needs to be at the top of any differential diagnosis of a child who is "not acting right."

An isolated closed head injury, combined with the limited developmental repertoire in children, makes these patients particularly difficult to assess. Therefore, thorough knowledge of age-appropriate developmental milestones coupled with a caretaker's report of the child's baseline functional status are the keys to accurate assessment. Use of the Pediatric Assessment Triangle, which focuses on appearance, breathing, and circulatory status, combined with the pediatric-modified GCS allows for an objective early and rapid assessment on which to base the need for intervention, consultation, and further testing.

Thermoregulation is an important factor in pediatric resuscitation; the head is a major source of this heat loss, contributing to stress and potentially affecting cardiovascular and coagulation properties. An increasing body of literature is now available regarding the use of controlled hypothermia in the setting of traumatic brain injury, but at this time no recommendations have been made for prehospital cooling in this population.

When the mechanism of injury is unknown or compatible with spinal cord injury, it is important to remember that the child's neck, being shorter and supporting a proportionately larger mass with less developed musculature, is particularly prone to spinal cord injury. For this reason, the paramedic should rapidly assess the child and the mechanism of injury, then proceed immediately with immobilization.

Spinal cord injury is more frequent in the upper cervical spine (C1–C3) in children under eight years of age (as opposed to adults, in whom injury is more common in C5–C7). Because of the relatively horizontal, nonstabilizing facet joints, active growth centers, and lax ligaments, lateral and rotational distraction injuries can occur without radiographic evidence (a condition called spinal cord injury without radiologic abnormality [SCIWORA]), making cervical and other spine injuries very difficult to diagnose.

Of the children presenting with spinal cord injury, half of them will have normal spine films. Thus, normal X-rays, though reassuring, cannot rule out spinal cord injury in the child. Complicating this is that when treating an unconscious or flaccid infant or child, the child must be assumed to have a high spinal cord injury until ruled out with physical exam and additional scans (MRI, helical CT). Because of the infant's and young child's prominent occiput, every effort must be made to maintain neutral

> **Normal X-rays cannot rule out spinal cord injury in the child.**

cervical alignment, avoiding hyperextension of the cervical spine during intubation or avoiding flexion when supine on a spine board.

Chest

An important characteristic of pediatric trauma is the fact that children can have significant solid and hollow organ damage with no external evidence or overlying fractures. The delayed ossification of the pediatric rib cage allows for blunt forces to be transmitted through the ribs onto the underlying organ, resulting in significant lung, cardiac, hepatic, splenic, or renal contusion with no radiographic findings of fractures and delayed plain radiographic findings of pulmonary contusion. For this reason, the mechanism of injury and a healthy amount of suspicion become important factors in the assessment, monitoring, and treatment of pediatric injuries.

It is well described that infants and children are 50 percent less likely to have rib fractures compared with adults, yet they are twice as likely to have intrathoracic (pulmonary or cardiac) injury with no bony abnormality, leading to twice the adult rate of lung contusion, pneumothorax, and hemothorax. This predisposes the pediatric patient to have early respiratory distress, hypoxia, and respiratory failure given the child's anatomic differences, smaller lung volumes, and increased metabolic (energy) requirements. Early recognition and management with oxygen and rapid transfer are keys to survival and improved outcomes.

Multiorgan System Trauma

Injuries to the chest have been reported in 8 percent to 62 percent of children with multiorgan system injuries and usually result in immediate physiologic compromise, carrying a 25 percent mortality rate when associated with traumatic brain injury or abdominal trauma. Traumatic cardiac arrest holds the worst survival of all out-of-hospital arrests; there is no difference between adults and pediatric patients in this regard.

In a large sample of pediatric patients with traumatic arrests who received cardiopulmonary resuscitation (CPR), 24 percent survived and one-third of those survivors had a good neurologic outcome, as opposed to another study of out-of-hospital pediatric cardiac arrest in

which only 8 percent survived, with only one-third of them having good neurologic outcomes. In the first study, pediatric patients who arrived with an undetectable pulse had poor outcome (4 surviving out of 269). Survival for those patients with a detectable pulse and respirations on arrival to the emergency department (39 percent survival) was significantly better than survival of patients arriving apneic with a detectable pulse (19 percent).

In patients who survive long enough to arrive at the hospital alive, the injuries most highly associated with death are cardiac tamponade (70 percent), massive hemothorax (50 percent), direct cardiac injury (48 percent), injuries to the aorta and great vessels (42 percent), flail chest (40 percent), and tension pneumothorax (39 percent). Although these are often complicated by and confused with aspiration, the treatment is the same: supporting the ABCs with supplemental oxygen, assisting ventilation as needed, and close monitoring and observation.

Cardiac contusion and resulting myocardial irritability can give rise to EKG abnormalities and myocardial dysfunction that, if unrecognized, can progress rapidly to cardiovascular collapse. Hypotension that is unresponsive to fluid resuscitation may be the result of myocardial dysfunction or, owing to the lax fixation of the mediastinum and propensity for more visceral shift, caused by compromise of preload or afterload. Commotio cordis is an entity that is increasingly reported as a cause of sudden traumatic cardiac arrest in children, caused by blunt sternal trauma and carrying a high mortality rate.

In the highly compliant chest wall of the child, the work of breathing can be amplified significantly, leading to subcostal, sternal, and supraclavicular retractions. The diaphragm is the major muscle of respiration in infants because of the lack of axillary and intercostal muscle development, but its muscle fibers are fatigue prone in the early stages of life and its horizontal insertion is mechanically disadvantaged. Combine this with gastric distention, supine positioning, and narrow airways, and the infant is at significant risk for respiratory failure owing to the increased work of breathing.

Because of the high chest wall compliance, infants and children are unable to maintain end-expiratory lung volumes, leading to lung collapse (atelectasis).

Infants and children are much more prone to atelectasis than adults and, with the high potential for aspiration and/or lung contusion following trauma, their condition can change rapidly.

It is well described that after these lung units have collapsed from underinflation (atelectasis), they require more pressure to open up once closed than they do to keep open once opened. An infant or child in distress, who is breathing rapidly and shallowly without any assisted positive pressure, is at high risk of atelectasis, especially when the condition is compounded by an altered mental status, lung contusion, and aspiration. The resulting atelectasis leads to worsening gas exchange with decreased oxygenation and ventilation (CO_2 removal).

The compensatory response to keep these lung units from collapsing is grunting, or laryngeal braking, and is an extremely costly sign of respiratory distress and an immediate precursor to respiratory failure. This anatomic mechanical disadvantage, coupled with the higher oxygen consumption per body mass, puts children under eight years of age at high risk for rapid progression to hypoxemia.

Abdomen and Pelvis

Internal abdominal injuries in the child can kill very quickly. Hepatic and splenic contusions from blunt trauma can be responsible for the child literally bleeding out into the peritoneum. Renal contusions involving the aorta and renal arteries can be quite severe as well, but most renal injuries are not as life threatening as intraperitoneal abdominal injuries.

In both peritoneal and retroperitoneal injuries, there may be no external sign of trauma (bruising, lacerations) but the patient's abdomen will be extremely tender and there may be some abdominal distention. This can be a subtle sign, but it is a very important one that is not to be overlooked, as it means that a significant amount of fluid (blood, urine, intestinal contents) has collected already.

Abdominal distention is poorly tolerated by children because their diaphragms are so easily compromised, making the work of breathing even more difficult. Similarly, when assessing a child with suspected abdominal trauma, the child may be splinting and not taking adequate-size breaths, making it appear as if the child is in mild or moderate respiratory distress, which again is not a clue to be overlooked but instead is one to be acted on: Transport the child as soon as it is safe to do so.

Eviscerating and penetrating trauma is fairly rare in pediatric patients but is treated as it would be in adults, with rapid assessment, stabilization, and transfer. Any vomiting of blood or bile should be a clue for significant abdominal trauma; the paramedic should suspect lower thoracic or lumbar spine injuries in children as well. Pelvic fractures can be quite severe and, because of the high risk for large vessel injuries (iliac and femoral arteries and veins), should be suspected in an immobile patient who has a high degree of pain with movement.

Because young children may be preverbal and unable to tell you where it hurts, it is critical that the paramedic be able to read their signs and interpret their actions and inactions, as those may be the only clues to what is bothering them. Diagnosing abdominal injury is one of the greatest challenges in pediatric medicine.

Skeletal Injuries

Skeletal injuries are the most common traumatic injuries to young and school-age children; they require medical attention even though they are rarely life threatening. The ability of a child to generate forces sufficient to cause a long-bone fracture is directly related to size and ability to get around. Toddlers are the youngest patients in whom accidental fractures are seen, as toddlers are ambulatory and can climb. Trauma in infants is very likely to be inflicted by others; therefore, the scene should be treated as a crime scene until proven otherwise. Keeping to fact-based, unbiased, and thorough documentation by the paramedic is of vital importance.

TRANSITIONING ● ● ● ● ● ● ●

REVIEW ITEMS

1. The leading cause of death of children is from trauma associated with _____.
    a. nonaccidental (inflicted) injuries
    b. falls
    c. motor vehicle crashes
    d. bicycle crashes

2. Factors associated with worse outcomes in pediatric trauma are _____.
    a. long bone fractures (e.g., femur)
    b. abdominal injuries
    c. hypotension and hypoxia
    d. pelvic fractures

3. Children's lungs are more prone to collapse (atelectasis) because of children's _____.
    a. highly compliant chest wall
    b. retained secretions
    c. weak cough
    d. small airways

4. Abdominal trauma in children is poorly recognized primarily because _____.
    a. children cannot communicate their injuries to caretakers
    b. children can mask the signs and symptoms well
    c. children tolerate shock well
    d. medical providers are poorly trained to read the signs and symptoms

APPLIED PATHOPHYSIOLOGY

1. Describe the signs of shock in a child.

2. Describe the Pediatric Assessment Triangle.

3. Explain the signs of altered mental status.

CLINICAL DECISION MAKING

You are called for a 7-year-old male patient who is complaining of abdominal pain after hitting a tree while riding his bicycle. You suspect that his handlebars turned as he crashed. He has no head injury, no neck pain, and no loss of consciousness but is having trouble catching his breath, is tearful, and reports that his pain is the "worst ever felt." His heart rate is 170/minute, and his radial pulse feels thready. His respiratory rate is 35/minute. His arms are cool and skin looks mottled. He will not lie flat because of the pain in his "stomach."

1. Is this child in shock?

2. What do you suspect his injury is?

3. What is your priority in management of this condition?

The child's mother arrives on scene and offers more medical history: He had hernia surgery as an infant, has multiple environmental allergies, and recently has not been feeling well. During this time, your patient moves from a sitting position to lying down and seems to fall asleep. He becomes difficult to arouse, and you notice he is very clammy and pale. His abdomen is distended.

4. What is your priority now?

Standard Trauma

Competency Integrates assessment findings with principles of epidemiology and pathophysiology to formulate a field impression to implement a comprehensive treatment/disposition plan for an acutely injured patient.

TOPIC

51

TRAUMA IN SPECIAL POPULATIONS: GERIATRICS

INTRODUCTION

Generally, when EMS providers receive a trauma call, almost automatically the first question in their mind is "What is the mechanism of injury?," as if the answer "penetrating trauma" or "blunt trauma" is the best descriptor of what to think or do. Although many times in EMS education we classify trauma this way, a more important criterion is "How old is the patient?" If the answer is older than 65 years of age, then that becomes a much more important determinant of how and what is done for the patient than the type of trauma (or mechanism of injury) into which they best fit.

Age alone, however, may not be the best descriptor of a geriatric patient. Take, for example, a 60-year-old man with a history of chronic obstructive pulmonary disease (COPD): This patient will have a different response to thoracic trauma than a 60-year-old man without COPD. Therefore, beyond the patient's age, also consider the patient's ability to withstand trauma from a hemodynamic event and what ability the body has to repair itself.

Generally, if a patient has a chronic medical condition typically associated with the elderly (cardiovascular disease [CVD], hypertension, myocardial infarction [MI], COPD, congestive heart failure [CHF], osteoporosis, diabetes, and the like), or if a patient simply looks older than 65 because of difficult life experiences prior to this event, the paramedic may also want to treat that patient as a geriatric trauma patient. A single preexisting medical condition raises the mortality from any specific injury by 30 percent, and two or more preexisting conditions increase the expected mortality by 60 percent. Failure to make this distinction and failure to consider the special challenges of the geriatric population may lead EMS to cause more harm than good. Often, assessment and treatment steps are based on research done on younger adult patients, who anatomically and physiologically are not the same as geriatric patients.

Simply put, the paramedic must reconsider the assessment approach and management techniques when faced with a geriatric trauma patient.

TRANSITION highlights

- **Shifting population demographics of older Americans to an increasing size of the overall population.**
- **Incidence rates for geriatric trauma and death, as well as utilization of health care and EMS.**
- **Pathophysiologic changes that accompany injuries in the geriatric patient:**
  - Brain trauma.
  - Neck trauma.
  - Spinal trauma.
  - Thoracic trauma.
  - Abdominal trauma.
  - Musculoskeletal trauma.
  - Burn trauma.
- **Early and late assessment findings with various specific types of injury patterns in the geriatric population.**
- **Current treatment strategies for the geriatric patient suffering from trauma.**

EPIDEMIOLOGY

Geriatric patients (those 65 years of age or older) numbered almost 40 million in 2008. This represented 12.8 percent of the U.S. population, or about one in every eight Americans. By 2030, this number will almost double, to more than 71 million elderly people. People over 65 years of age represented 12.4 percent of the population in 2000 and are expected to grow to 20 percent of the population by 2030. Although the U.S. numbers are not universal, most other developed countries are seeing a similar trend. People over age 65 disproportionately use ambulance services and health care facilities. Even though the elderly are only roughly 12 percent of the population, they account for more

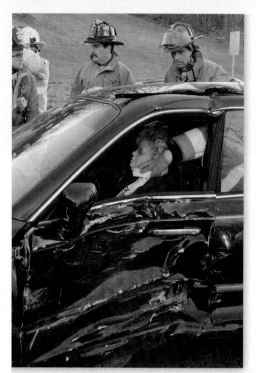

Figure 51-1 Motor vehicle collisions are the second leading cause of accidental death, after falls, in the geriatric population. (© Mark C. Ide)

> **Falls account for the majority of injuries in the geriatric population.**

than 36 percent of all ambulance transports and 25 percent of hospitalizations.

Falls account for the majority of injuries in the geriatric population. The most common resulting injuries from falls are hip fractures, femur fractures, wrist fractures, and head injuries. Although falls do not produce serious injuries most of the time, geriatric falls account for 75 percent of all fall-related deaths.

Complicating the hospitalization, rehabilitation, and recovery from falls is *postfall syndrome*. This is a sequence of events in which a geriatric patient falls and gets admitted to the hospital for treatment and rehabilitation. On returning home, the patient loses confidence about moving around the home and assumes a more sedentary lifestyle. With this inactivity, muscles atrophy, bones weaken, joints become stiffer, and so on. This then leaves the patient at greater risk of a more serious fall in the future. In fact, the largest predictor of falls in the geriatric population is a history of a previous fall. The causes of falls are fairly evenly divided between intrinsic causes, such as dizziness or syncope, and extrinsic causes, such as tripping on a rug or slipping on ice.

Motor vehicle collisions (MVCs) are the second leading cause of accidental death, after falls, in the geriatric population (▶ Figure 51-1). Even though the elderly drive fewer miles than those in the younger age bracket and tend to drive closer to home, they have a death rate that is three times that of patients aged 25 years per 100,000 population. Following MVC deaths, the next most common cause of accidental death in the geriatric population is auto-versus-pedestrian accidents, which carry the highest fatality rate of any specific mechanism. Accidental burns (both contact and inhalation) account for about 8 percent of geriatric deaths, followed by penetration injuries (usually from attempted suicide).

PATHOPHYSIOLOGY

Topic 58, "Geriatrics," contains an important discussion of the changes in anatomy and physiology of the body due to aging. In tandem with this are the effects of pathologic conditions that further alter body physiology and the response of the body to trauma. All these variables must be taken into consideration when dealing with traumatized geriatric patients.

Head and Brain Trauma

Head trauma is of particular concern in the geriatric population. Beyond the briskness of hemorrhage from scalp lacerations that can bleed significantly because of poor vasoconstriction from vascular disease is the increased incidence of concurrent brain trauma. During the aging process, the brain will atrophy, causing a void between the brain and skull within the cranium. This space will initially be filled with extra cerebrospinal fluid (CSF). Along with the shrinking brain tissue will be a stretching of the bridging vessels between the brain and skull.

When the geriatric patient sustains head trauma, the brain can actually shift within the cranial vault. This, in turn, tears blood vessels, resulting in epidural and, particularly, subdural hematomas. Unlike the younger patient with a cerebral bleed that will demonstrate symptoms more readily, in the geriatric patient the blood will continue to collect in the space left by the atrophied brain for a longer time before the patient becomes symptomatic from the head injury. In fact, enough time may pass between the initial injury and the symptoms of altered mental status or significant headache that the patient (and the family or care providers) may not recall the history of a fall or some other mechanism of injury.

In addition, assessment of the pupils may not yield reliable findings of brain herniation, as a large percentage of geriatric patients have a concurrent ophthalmic condition, such as cataracts, asymmetric pupils, or changes in light reflex from either ophthalmologic medications or other preexisting conditions. Complicating this in the geriatric patient as well may be organic brain syndromes, which will make gathering a reliable history of the patient's mental status more challenging.

Neck Trauma

Neck injuries are also common in patients with a history of either head or chest wall trauma (▶ Figure 51-2). In geriatric patients, sensory perception is diminished; they may not complain of neck pain despite the presence of an actual injury to the vertebrae. The absence of neck pain

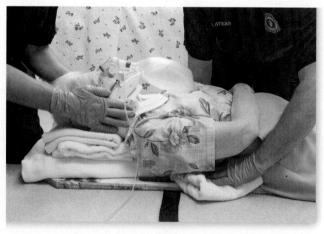

Figure 51-2 Neck injuries are common in patients with a history of either head or chest wall trauma.

in a geriatric patient, with or without tenderness on palpation, is not a sufficient criterion for ruling out cervical trauma. It has been noted in the elderly population that high cervical fractures (i.e., C1 and C2) are possible if not probable with even a "minimal" mechanism of injury, such as a fall from a standing position. This fact should be recalled for any geriatric victim who is found in a lying position on the floor (or in a bed) when there is not a clear history of no traumatic incident.

Spinal Trauma

Degenerative changes in the spinal column from osteoporosis or spondylosis can alter the strength and structure of the vertebrae. Arthritic "spurs" can narrow the spinal canal and the exiting points for the spinal nerves, ultimately increasing the pressure on the nerves and the spinal cord itself. Further damage to the spinal column from trauma can easily shatter vertebrae, causing increased likelihood of cord trauma (compression or laceration) and spinal nerve root damage. The presence of kyphosis or scoliosis in the spine also increases the likelihood of spinal and cord trauma and poses an additional complication when trying to immobilize the patient properly. Anterior cord syndrome is seen almost exclusively in the elderly population.

As mentioned, because the geriatric patient commonly has diminished sensory capability, there may be either no complaint of pain despite an injury being present or a minimal amount of pain that is out of proportion with the significance of the injury.

Thoracic Trauma

The aging process is particularly hard on the thoracic cage and pulmonary system. The ribs become much more brittle and easier to break in the geriatric patient because of osteoporosis and the calcification of the costosternal and costovertebral joints. Furthermore, age-related changes to the underlying normal lung physiology result in diminished vital capacity, weaker respiratory musculature, and diminished efficiency at exchanging oxygen and carbon dioxide across the alveoli to the perialveolar capillary membranes. With what may seem to be a minimal mechanism of injury to the chest, the resultant rib fractures and pulmonary contusions can severely hamper the effectiveness of the respiratory system. The mortality for a geriatric patient with even a single rib injury can be as high as 12 percent.

Added to this are the detrimental effects of chronic lung conditions—emphysema, asthma, chronic bronchitis, cancer, and others—that are more common in the elderly. The resultant efficiency of the respiratory system may not have the compensatory mechanisms needed to overcome this pulmonary insult, and the patient's respiratory status can fail rapidly. The provision of positive pressure ventilation (PPV) in the geriatric patient may also become problematic because of the lower airway pressures needed to cause barotrauma.

Abdominal Trauma

Because of the effects of aging and concurrent disease states, abdominal trauma is yet another condition that will likely present differently in the geriatric patient than it would in a younger patient. Owing to the brittle nature of the ribs and the atrophy of abdominal musculature, the liver and spleen are more likely to be injured from blunt trauma because of a lack of protection. The resulting hemorrhage from these organs may go unnoticed because of the general lack of pain perceived by the geriatric patient and the inability of the cardiovascular system to mount a tachycardic response, which is common in younger patients suffering from internal bleeding.

Blood pressure, another measure that is used to gauge the efficiency of the cardiovascular system, may be misleading for internal bleeding because the systolic pressure may still be within a "normal" range, but in the geriatric patient this could actually represent hypotension because the patient's preinjury blood pressure may typically be higher owing to a history of hypertension. Medications (mainly beta blockers) may also diminish the heart rate response seen with blood loss. If the paramedic should wait for either tachycardia or hypotension in the geriatric patient with abdominal trauma and internal bleeding, it could result in catastrophic consequences.

Musculoskeletal Trauma

In the geriatric patient, a drop in the amount of fat (adipose) tissue is relative to body weight, which leaves bones more susceptible to injury. Compounding this is the cartilaginous support of the skeletal system: With aging, it loses its adaptive

capabilities and cannot flex as efficiently, and, thus, is more likely to break when stressed. The presence of fat pads that are normally found around bony prominences diminishes and contributes not only to bedsores (pressure ulcers) in the bedridden patient but also to a higher likelihood of skeletal trauma with falls and other traumatic mechanisms.

As mentioned previously, falls account for a large percentage of the musculoskeletal trauma seen in the geriatric population. Osteoporosis, as a risk factor, is the most common concurrent disease state contributing to bone weakness and fractures. Hip fractures are the most common serious injury secondary to a fall, followed in significance and frequency by fractures of the femur, pelvis, tibia, and upper extremities. Even an isolated fracture can become life threatening to the geriatric patient, as the loss of tissue turgor and the negative effects of atherosclerotic changes to the vasculature can result in significant blood loss into the muscle compartment.

Burn Trauma

To provide a complete discussion of geriatric trauma, burn trauma must also be mentioned. As stated previously, burn trauma is the fourth leading cause of death in the geriatric population. The effect of aging on the integumentary system plays a significant role in contributing to the seriousness of a burn. The geriatric patient has thinner epidermal and dermal layers of the skin, and with a diminution of the subcutaneous layer as well, with geriatric exposure to a heat load (be it thermal, chemical, electrical, or radiation), exponentially more damage occurs to the skin and underlying structures. There is a linear increase in mortality for burn injuries based on age only.

Burn shock, which results from the loss of intravascular proteins and fluid shifting, typically does not occur in the younger patient unless 20 percent to 25 percent of total body surface area is affected by either partial-thickness burns or full-thickness burns. In geriatric patients, however, the changes in physiology, compounded by the presence of underlying disease states, result in the development of burn shock with much lower body surface involvement.

The geriatric patient is also at greater risk of airway closure and respiratory failure from inhalation injuries. The elderly patient will develop significant edema around the glottic opening from inhalation of superheated air, causing airway closure, and will sustain tracheal, bronchial, and alveolar damage, which results in the inability to ventilate the alveoli and diminishes the exchange of gases at the alveolar level. The end result is early and rapid failure of the airway and pulmonary system. Naturally, the presence of chronic lung or CVD states will only hasten and worsen the injury patterns seen.

ASSESSMENT FINDINGS

Assessment findings of trauma for geriatric patients exhibit some similarities, as well as some dissimilarities, with those for the younger adult. In remaining consistent with the aforementioned body location approach to geriatric trauma, Table 51-1 identifies common manifestations of trauma, with some delineation and differentiation on early versus late findings. In all the considerations listed in this table, the consistent feature assumed is that the paramedic has collected a detailed patient history and completed a thorough physical assessment to uncover these findings. Please remember that certain clinical conditions are very insidious in the geriatric patient, and the paramedic must remain vigilant during the assessment phase. Also remember that the older the patient and the more concurrent chronic conditions the patient has, the faster the progression from early clinical findings to late clinical findings and ultimate death.

Although Table 51-1 is not meant to be all-inclusive for all findings that may be present for each injury state, it is designed to provide a functional knowledge base to enable the paramedic to ascertain the significance of the traumatic event. It is of utmost importance that the paramedic keeps in mind that because of the effects of aging, pathologic findings, and concurrent medications, the presentation of trauma is different in the geriatric patient than in the younger adult. In addition, the relative absence of robust compensatory mechanisms in the elderly will allow the

TABLE 51-1	Common Manifestations of Trauma in Geriatric Patients	
Trauma Location	Earlier Clinical Findings	Later Clinical Findings
Head/brain trauma	• Scalp trauma • Facial contusions • Hematomas • Hemorrhage	• Headache • Altered mental status • Vital sign changes • Seizures
Neck trauma	• Limited motion • Discomfort • Vertebral deformity • Soft tissue trauma • Sensory–motor deficits • Hoarseness	• Vital sign changes • Expanding hematoma • Progressive paralysis • Dyspnea • Muscle spasms
Spinal trauma	• Vertebral deformity • Discomfort • Soft tissue trauma • Limited motion • Sensory–motor deficits	• Paralysis • Vital sign changes • Dyspnea • Altered mentation
Thoracic trauma	• Soft tissue trauma • Flail segments • Tachypnea • Dyspnea • Unequal breath sounds • Decreased breath sounds	• Dyspnea/apnea • Decreased oximetry • Tachypnea/bradypnea • Unequal breath sounds • Absent breath sounds • Vital sign changes
Abdominal trauma	• Soft tissue trauma • Abdominal guarding • Expanding hematomas • Pain/discomfort • Dyspnea	• Abdominal rigidity • Abdominal guarding • Vital sign changes • Severe dyspnea • Distended abdomen
Musculoskeletal trauma	• Obvious deformity • Soft tissue trauma • Limited motion • Discomfort/pain	• Absent distal pulses • Absent sensory • Vital sign changes • Altered mental status
Burn trauma	• Superficial burns • Partial thickness burns • Full thickness burns • Discomfort/pain • Dyspnea (airway burn) • Dyspnea (chest burn)	• Loss of motion • Vital sign changes • Altered mental status • Stridor (airway burn) • Dyspnea or apnea • Vital sign changes • Pulmonary edema (acute respiratory distress syndrome [ARDS])

clinical progression from stable to unstable to occur extremely rapidly.

Although not an assessment step per se, part of recognizing and managing trauma in the geriatric population includes notification of the receiving facility as early as possible. Have a lower threshold for transporting a geriatric trauma patient to a trauma center. If transporting the patient to a facility with an in-house trauma team, consider activating the team. Aggressive management of the geriatric trauma patient is associated with minimized complications and overall improved outcomes. Consider the

patient's mechanism of injury, the patient's age and concurrent medical conditions, the current clinical status of the patient, transport times, local protocols, and medical direction when determining the receiving facility.

EMERGENCY MEDICAL CARE

The assessment and management of a geriatric trauma patient must be appropriate for the situation, specific for the injury, efficient in its rendering, and thorough in its completeness to realize the best possible scenario for the patient's survival. Geriatric trauma is often debilitating and too often fatal. The skills performed by the on-scene paramedic will have just as great an impact on survivability as any treatment that will be rendered in the hospital setting:

1. **Ensure inline immobilization.** Recall that kyphosis, scoliosis, and other skeletal anomalies may make the fitting of a cervical collar impossible. Be creative by using rolled towels and tape for a makeshift collar if necessary.

2. **Maintain patency of the airway.** Geriatric patients may have previous dental work that can complicate airway maintenance. Constantly assess and reassess the patency of the airway and provide suctioning as needed for secretions, vomitus, or hemorrhage. If sonorous airway sounds cannot be relieved by positioning or manual airway maneuvers, consider the insertion of an oropharyngeal airway or a nasopharyngeal airway to help keep the tongue off the posterior pharynx. Consider an advanced airway when appropriate.

3. **Ensure adequacy of breathing.** Secondary to head, cervical, thoracic, or multisystem trauma, the breathing mechanics and strength of the respiratory muscles can easily fatigue and fail. Note the patient's speech patterns and quality of alveolar breath sounds if he is conscious to help guide the need for PPV. If the patient is unconscious, assess the chest wall excursion and quality of alveolar breath sounds to determine whether PPV is needed. Seal any open chest wounds with an occlusive dressing, and stabilize any flailed segment with a bulky dressing. If breathing is adequate, apply oxygen via a nonrebreather mask or nasal cannula, depending on the status of the patient. If breathing is inadequate, provide high-flow oxygen in conjunction with PPV (always ventilate gently to lower the chances for barotraumas). Provide supplemental oxygen to all geriatric trauma victims.

4. **Support cardiovascular function.** Any external hemorrhage should be treated immediately with direct pressure. Assess the quality of peripheral perfusion by the quality of the skin findings and peripheral pulses. The heart rate in a geriatric patient may not become tachycardic in response to hypoxia or hypovolemia because of cardiac disease and concurrent medications. Remember also that what may be a normal blood pressure in a younger adult may actually be hypotension in a geriatric patient with underlying hypertension. Management of hypoperfusion includes the administration of high-flow oxygen, proper patient positioning, and maintaining normothermia.

IV fluids should be administered according to protocol and patient presentation, keeping in mind that geriatric patients may have preexisting conditions (e.g., CHF) that can be worsened by excess fluid administration. Administer fluids cautiously, and monitor lung sounds and respiratory status frequently during transport.

Management of other issues, such as soft tissue injuries, musculoskeletal trauma, and the like, should follow the same treatment principles as with other trauma victims. It is important to note again that full spinal immobilization of the patient may need to be modified because of the presence of skeletal deformity from kyphosis, scoliosis, osteoarthritis, and other skeletal diseases.

Constantly reassess the patient's airway, breathing, and circulatory components en route to the hospital, and ensure the quality of the ongoing interventions.

In conclusion, thousands of geriatric patients are victims of accidental trauma and traumatic injuries. The paramedic, always first on the scene, has the opportunity and responsibility to ensure that a rapid and thorough interview and assessment are performed so treatment decisions will have a positive impact on the patient and ensure an optimal patient outcome. To do this, the paramedic must remain abreast of changes in geriatric curricula, injury presentation, emergency management, and destination protocols to the appropriate facility.

TRANSITIONING

REVIEW ITEMS

1. Which of the following factors is most contributory to hip fractures in a geriatric fall victim?
   a. osteoporosis
   b. failing eyesight
   c. joint stiffening
   d. weight gain

2. A 78-year-old female patient has wrecked her car, has injured her sternum, and is complaining of respiratory distress. Of the following factors, which one would be most contributory should she go into respiratory failure?
   a. weakening of the abdominal musculature
   b. diminution of the number of functional alveoli
   c. drop in carbon dioxide levels from hyperventilation
   d. loss of strength and coordination of respiratory muscles

3. When providing mechanical ventilation to an elderly trauma victim in severe respiratory distress, why should the paramedic ventilate slowly with low airway pressures?
   a. Failure to do so will result in inadequate oxygenation.
   b. Geriatric patients are more susceptible to barotrauma.
   c. It avoids the likelihood of wiping out the breathing reflex.
   d. It prevents accidental overventilation.

4. An elderly female patient has been assaulted and beaten during a robbery. You find her unresponsive on the floor. Her vital signs are blood pressure 108/78, heart rate 94 beats per minute, and respiratory rate 26. She has two stab wounds to

the abdomen, which is distended and rigid, and she has an open fracture of the radius and ulna, which is not actively bleeding. Pupils are unresponsive to light. The pulse oximeter reads 90 percent on room air. Of the following, which would be most contributory to acute deterioration?

    a. possible head injury

    b. the long bone fracture

    c. occult bleeding in the abdomen

    d. respiratory failure

5. Why would a geriatric patient be more likely than a younger adult to suffer a brain injury secondary to head trauma?

    a. because of atrophy of the brain and accumulation of blood in the subdural cavity

    b. because the geriatric patient is clumsier than the younger adult

    c. because medications that the geriatric patient is taking tend to make the brain bleed more easily

    d. because the geriatric patient is typically hypertensive, which makes the blood vessels rupture

6. A 78-year-old male patient has fallen in his bathroom while getting out of the shower, landing on his side on a tile floor. Given this mechanism, what is the most likely significant injury he may sustain?

    a. fractured clavicle from falling on outstretched hand

    b. abdominal trauma with hidden internal bleeding

    c. pulmonary contusion with resultant dyspnea

    d. hip fracture or dislocation

7. Normal or expected early findings of hypoperfusion are typically absent in geriatric patients because _____.

    a. they typically cannot sustain tachycardia due to cardiac disease or medications

    b. owing to the effects of aging, geriatric patients are often hypotensive anyway

    c. it is too difficult to obtain accurate vital signs in the geriatric population

    d. the systolic pressure in geriatric patients tends not to decrease until significant blood loss has occurred

8. In a geriatric patient with a history of head trauma, the paramedic identifies unequal pupils. Why may this not be an accurate indication of a brain injury?

    a. because the geriatric pupil needs more intense light to respond

    b. because geriatric pupils normally do not constrict to light

    c. because of the possible presence of cataracts

    d. because of deterioration of the optic region of the brain

APPLIED PATHOPHYSIOLOGY

Family members have noticed that their elderly grandfather is not acting "normal." They summon EMS; on your arrival, you determine that the patient's mental status is diminished. Vital signs are normal, and the pulse oximeter is 97 percent on room air. The family stated that about a week ago they got home and found him lying on the floor, where he had fallen, in the kitchen. Because he was fine then, they didn't call for an ambulance.

1. What is the most likely cause for this patient's deterioration a week or so after the incident?

2. Discuss the problems with trying to obtain a good baseline mental status on geriatric patients.

3. Discuss why vital signs in a geriatric patient may not be truly representative of the underlying physiologic status.

4. For the following injuries, identify how the aging process changes the presentation of common injuries as seen in the geriatric patient:

    a. Head/brain trauma

    b. Thoracic trauma

    c. Neck and spinal trauma

    d. Musculoskeletal trauma

5. Why may pupil inequality found in a geriatric head trauma patient not be representative of the degree of actual brain injury present?

CLINICAL DECISION MAKING

You are called to an extended-care facility where a geriatric patient with Alzheimer disease was able to walk out an unlocked door and escape into the wooded area behind the facility. After about four hours, the patient was located by the local fire department at the foot of a ridge from which he apparently had fallen. The fire department personnel extricated the patient to your location using a Stokes basket. The patient is not currently immobilized, he appears unresponsive, his clothes look wet and cold, and dried blood is visible on the side of his head.

1. Based on this brief history, what would be at least three etiologies for this patient's unresponsiveness?

The primary assessment reveals the patient to be responsive to noxious stimuli with nonpurposeful motion. The airway is patent, but breathing is slow at 8 per minute, with minimal chest wall excursion and no alveolar breath sounds. The soft tissue trauma to the head is not actively bleeding anymore, and the pulse is found to be diminished peripherally with a rate of 89 beats per minute. The skin is cold to the touch, capillary refill is delayed, and you have noted that the patient's right leg is angulated awkwardly at the mid-femur location. The pulse oximeter reads 78 percent.

2. Would this patient be considered a high or low priority?

3. What action should you take to initially care for this patient?

After managing the situation described, you continue with your secondary assessment. You find the pupils to be unequal in size, but cataracts are present. A depressed right temporal skull fracture has an overlying laceration. The airway remains clear, breathing is now adequate, and peripheral perfusion has not changed. Your assessment of the injured leg reveals a suspected midshaft closed fracture of the femur.

4. How else could you confirm that the patient has a brain injury from the fall, as he also has cataracts?

5. Explain why the vital signs may be misleading regarding the degree of instability this patient may be experiencing.

6. Identify the appropriate treatment for this patient given his age, injuries, and present clinical status.

7. What would be key indicators of patient improvement with treatment?

8. What would be key indicators of deterioration with treatment?

TOPIC

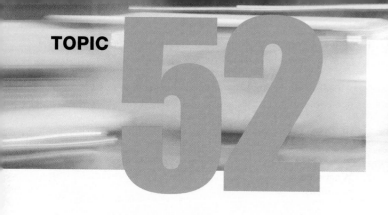

Standard Trauma

Competency Integrates assessment findings with principles of epidemiology and pathophysiology to formulate a field impression to implement a comprehensive treatment/disposition plan for an acutely injured patient.

TRAUMA IN SPECIAL POPULATIONS: PREGNANCY

TRANSITION *highlights*

- Incident rates at which pregnant females are traumatized, and the most common mechanisms of injury causing the trauma.

- Normal anatomic and physiologic variations in the pregnant woman.

- Complications that can occur from trauma in the pregnant woman:
  – Uterine contractions.
  – Preterm labor.
  – Spontaneous abortion.
  – Abruptio placentae.
  – Uterine rupture.
  – Penetrating trauma.
  – Pelvic fractures.
  – Hemorrhage and shock.
  – Cardiopulmonary arrest.

- Assessment findings with various specific types of injury patterns in the traumatized pregnant patient.

- Current treatment strategies for the pregnant patient.

INTRODUCTION

The study of trauma care teaches that insults to the body result in predictable and recognizable findings. In EMS, we use these findings to identify pathologies such as shock and aggressively treat our patients. Pregnant patients who are involved in trauma pose a special challenge to providers in that their physiologic makeup changes greatly as a baby grows within the uterus. Not only are there specific risks of trauma to pregnancy, but the responses of the woman's body systems may also be vastly differ-

> **Trauma is the leading cause of death for pregnant women.**

ent from those of a nonpregnant person. Furthermore, in many cases the effects of trauma impact not just the mother, but the unborn fetus as well. To handle a pregnant trauma victim properly, paramedics must understand the physiology of pregnancy, recognize the effects of trauma, and adjust treatment to give maximum benefit to those in this special population.

EPIDEMIOLOGY

Trauma occurs in approximately 6 percent to 7 percent of all pregnancies and is the leading cause of death for pregnant women. The morbidity and mortality of the patient depend in part on the mechanism of injury, gestational age of the fetus, and severity of the trauma. It is estimated that 1 percent to 3 percent of minor traumas involving pregnant women result in fetal loss and that 41 percent of fetuses die when the mother suffers a life-threatening injury. In addition, keep in mind that approximately 8 percent of pregnant female trauma patients do not know they are pregnant.

Motor vehicle collisions account for more than 50 percent of all the injuries sustained by pregnant trauma patients. Maternal death is the primary cause of fetal death in this type of mechanism of injury. Pregnant women, especially those after their 20th week, are also prone to falling because of physiologic changes such as weight gain and cardiovascular alterations (▶ Figure 52-1). About 2 percent of pregnant women sustain repeated blows to the abdomen because they have fallen more than once.

Violence is also a significant risk. Approximately 4 percent to 17 percent of women will experience physical abuse while pregnant. Penetrating trauma to the abdomen alone accounts for approximately 36 percent of overall maternal mortality. Gunshot wounds and stab wounds are the most frequent causes of penetrating trauma to this population; penetrating trauma directly to the uterus has a 67 percent fetal death rate.

ANATOMY AND PHYSIOLOGY

Various anatomic and physiologic changes occur during pregnancy (▶ Figure 52-2). These changes can influence how the patient presents in the prehospital environment.

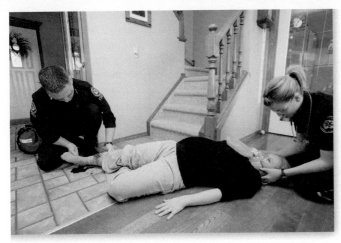

Figure 52-1 Pregnant women may sustain all types of trauma and are especially susceptible to falls and physical abuse.

4 mmHg in the systolic pressure and a decline of 5 to 15 mmHg in the patient's diastolic pressure. The woman's blood pressure will return to almost a normal prepregnancy level by the third trimester.

An increase in estrogen levels results in a 10- to 15-beat-per-minute increase in the patient's heart rate, as well as a 30 percent to 50 percent increase in cardiac output. Blood flow to the pregnant patient's uterus increases from 60 mL/min prepregnancy to 600 mL/min by the third trimester. These cardiovascular changes can mask the signs of shock in the trauma patient.

Other anatomic and physiologic changes occur in the pregnant woman's other body systems. The diaphragm gradually elevates 4 cm upward into the thoracic cavity, which results in decreased functional residual capacity in the lungs and contributes to an increase in oxygen consumption. The abdominal viscera are pushed upward and stretched, making injury to the bowel more likely. This change may also desensitize the patient's perception of pain despite the severity of an abdominal injury. A decrease in gastrointestinal motility and an increase in acid production make the patient prone to aspirating and vomiting.

The uterus grows throughout the pregnancy and rises out of the pelvis into the abdominal area. Besides containing the vulnerable fetus, the uterus is also a highly vascular organ that can bleed heavily if exposed to trauma. As the fetus grows, the uterus stretches and becomes more and more vulnerable to external forces.

Cardiovascular changes are important to keep in mind when considering trauma. The total blood volume in a pregnant female is increased by about 25 percent. There is a decrease in the patient's total peripheral resistance during the first two months of pregnancy. This change precipitates a gradual decline of about 2 to

A variety of other changes occur in the pregnant patient's body. The bladder is displaced into the abdominal cavity. Renal blood flow is increased. Pelvic joints are loosened, and the woman's center of gravity changes. All these issues can make trauma more serious in the pregnant woman.

The patient's presentation may be influenced by the gestational age and size of the fetus. The growing uterus and fetus can compress the patient's vena cava, which may result in supine hypotensive syndrome. When the compression of the vena cava occurs, the patient's cardiac output can be decreased by 28 percent, which causes a reduction in the patient's systolic blood pressure of about 30 mmHg. This reduction in venous blood flow can lead to signs and symptoms of shock if left untreated.

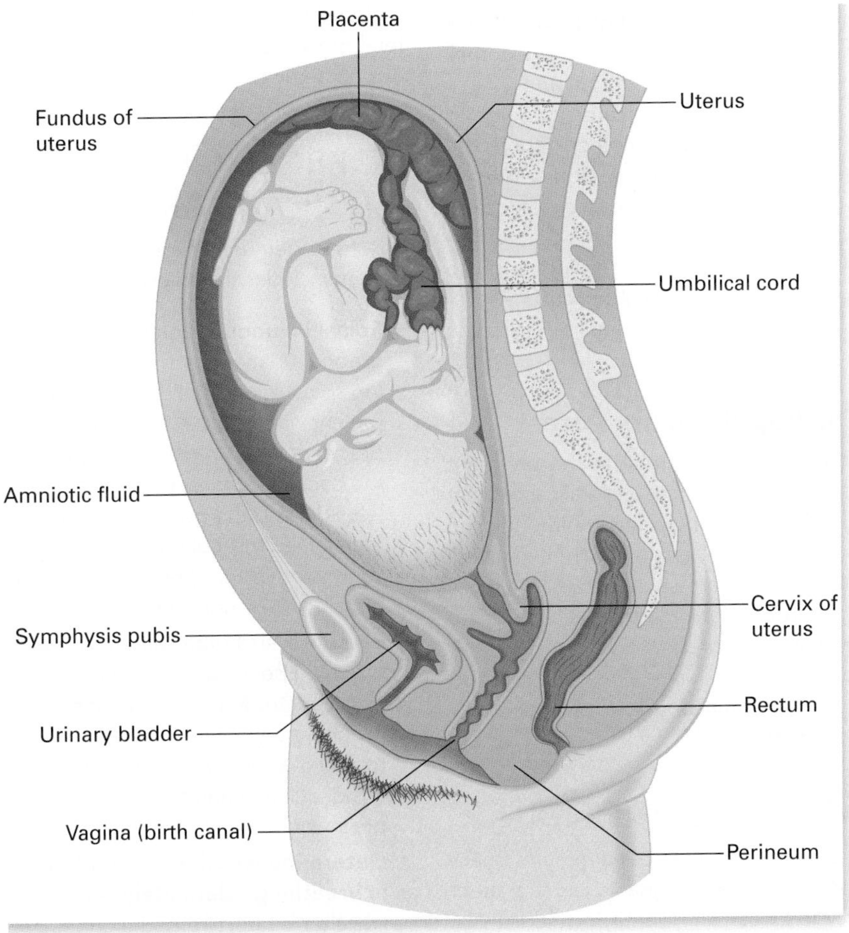

PATHOPHYSIOLOGY— COMPLICATIONS OF TRAUMA

Some of the most frequent complications resulting from traumatic injury to the pregnant patient are described here.

Uterine Contractions and Preterm Labor

The most common complication resulting from traumatic injury in the pregnant patient is uterine contractions. In cases of direct trauma, the uterus can respond

Placenta

Fundus of uterus

Uterus

Umbilical cord

Amniotic fluid

Cervix of uterus

Symphysis pubis

Rectum

Urinary bladder

Vagina (birth canal)

Perineum

Figure 52-2 The anatomy of pregnancy.

with contractions. Depending on the nature and severity of the trauma, these contractions may be self-limited or they may progress into preterm labor. In cases of severe trauma, it is a common response for a pregnant woman's body to attempt to sacrifice the pregnancy in a struggle to stay alive. Therefore, preterm labor (and associated contractions) is common.

Preterm labor is defined as labor occurring before the 38th week of gestation. For a fetus to be viable, it must be at least at 24 weeks of gestation. The longer the fetus remains in the mother, the better are its chances of survival. A major concern with any potentially pregnant trauma victim is not only the injuries she has sustained, but also the potential for preterm delivery and the threat to the pregnancy itself.

Spontaneous Abortion

Blunt or penetrating traumatic injuries can result in spontaneous abortions if the injury occurs before the 20th week of gestation. The most common signs and symptoms include abdominal pain or cramping, as well as vaginal bleeding.

Abruptio Placentae

Abruptio placentae, resulting mostly from blunt trauma experienced during pregnancy, accounts for 50 percent to 70 percent of fetal losses. Abruptio placentae commonly occur in the second and third trimesters of pregnancy. As the uterus grows, it becomes more and more vulnerable to trauma. In abruptio placentae, trauma causes a separation of the placenta from the uterine wall. This separation can be either partial or complete in nature. It results in impaired gas exchange between the mother and fetus and potentially massive intrauterine hemorrhage. This bleeding can occur with—or, more commonly, without—external signs of hemorrhage. Signs and symptoms associated with this condition are maternal abdominal pain, uterine tenderness, vaginal bleeding, and hypovolemia.

Uterine Rupture

Uterine rupture occurs in fewer than 1 percent of pregnant trauma victims. The most common cause is severe blunt force trauma to the abdomen. Uterine rupture often presents with maternal shock and palpable fetal parts inside the abdomen. It is one of the most fatal complications for the mother and fetus.

Penetrating Trauma

Penetrating trauma also can result in fetal injury or death. The size of the uterus may help shield the mother against some abdominal injuries, but it puts the fetus at greater risk for injury. The location of the penetrating trauma has a direct impact on the patient's outcome. Bowel and abdominal injuries occur more frequently in the upper abdomen and can cause injury to the mother, whereas direct trauma to the lower abdomen can result in more injuries or death to the fetus.

Pelvic Fractures

Pelvic fractures in pregnant patients result most frequently from blunt trauma to the abdomen. The patient may experience significant hemorrhage and may sustain bladder, urethral, or intestinal injuries. Pelvic fractures are associated with a 25 percent fetal mortality rate.

Hemorrhage and Shock

Hemorrhage is a common finding associated with trauma during pregnancy and can result in shock. It can result from any of the conditions previously described in this section or as a result of another injury. Hemorrhage, both internal and external, should be suspected after trauma.

Shock is a frequent cause of death to both the fetus and the mother. It should be anticipated and managed aggressively. It is possible for a pregnant patient to lose 30 percent of her blood volume before normal signs and symptoms of shock begin to appear. If the traditional signs of hypovolemic shock appear, the fetal mortality can be as high as 85 percent.

Cardiopulmonary Arrest

Cardiopulmonary arrest in the pregnant trauma patient poses a significant threat to the viability of the fetus. Although the chance of the fetus surviving maternal cardiopulmonary arrest because of trauma is poor, resuscitative attempts should be provided for pregnant patients in their third trimester, unless instructed otherwise. Rapid transport to a medical facility is imperative.

ASSESSMENT FINDINGS

The prehospital assessment and management of the pregnant trauma patient are focused on identifying, ensuring, maintaining, and supporting the vital functions of the patient's airway, breathing, and circulation. Unlike other traumatic emergencies, two patients must be considered by the paramedic. The best way to help both the mother and fetus involved in trauma is to take a proactive approach and to treat the mother aggressively. All pregnant women who have suffered an injury, regardless of the severity of the injury, should be evaluated by a physician in the emergency room.

The assessment of the pregnant trauma patient should be conducted in basically the same fashion as other trauma assessments. However, you should pay particular attention to the abdomen and uterus. The uterus will be palpable above the iliac crest after the 12th week of pregnancy. It will continue to grow and progress upward throughout the pregnancy. The normal uterus will be firm and round. When contractions occur, the uterus will usually harden. If the uterus is asymmetrical or irregular in shape, it may suggest a uterine rupture.

In addition to the usual trauma assessment, it is important to obtain information related directly to the pregnancy, if possible. Questions may include asking about the pregnancy, due date, gestational age, fetal movement, contractions, and previous obstetric history.

EMERGENCY MEDICAL CARE

The management of a pregnant trauma patient includes the following:

- **Spinal immobilization** is required for pregnant patients suspected of having spinal injury. Once the pregnant patient who is more than 20 weeks pregnant is secured appropriately, the backboard must be tilted to the left side, and this position must be maintained throughout the duration of your care. This will help prevent supine hypotensive syndrome.

- **Establish and maintain an open airway.** Use advanced airways as appropriate. Anticipate vomiting with pregnant patients and have suction readily available. Airway compromise is more likely when the patient is pregnant.

- **Determine whether the patient is breathing adequately** and whether bilateral breath sounds are present. If the patient's breathing is inadequate, provide positive pressure ventilation with supplemental high-flow oxygen. If breathing is adequate, provide oxygen via non-rebreather or nasal cannula so you maintain the patient's oxygen saturation at 100 percent. Remember that the fetus is very vulnerable to any reduction in oxygen and will require as much oxygen as possible to prevent hypoxia, even if signs of maternal hypoxia are not present.

- **Assess the patient's circulation, and check for major bleeding.** If vaginal bleeding is present, absorb the blood flow with a pad but do not pack the vagina. Anticipate, prevent, and treat shock.
- **Treat hypotension aggressively.** Volume replacement should be considered in all shock patients. Use isotonic crystalloids to maintain a systolic blood pressure of 80 to 90 mmHg.

In the event of traumatic brain injury, consider slightly higher levels (typically, 90 mmHg). Remember that preventing hypotensive shock in the mother preserves perfusion in the fetus. Be aggressive, but always follow local protocol.

- **Perform a visual exam at the vaginal opening** to assess for crowning or bleeding. If labor occurs as a result of the trauma, additional resources will be needed to help care for both patients.
- **Consider the pregnancy when administering analgesics.** Viable pain control options are available, but some narcotics can be detrimental to the fetus. Consult medical direction advice and follow local protocols.
- **Treat and manage any other injuries.**
- **Transport the patient to a medical facility that preferably has obstetric**

capabilities. Consider air medical transport for major traumas. Inform the trauma center as soon as possible that the patient is pregnant.

- Some systems allow for the option of delaying the effects of labor using medications such as magnesium sulfate. The use of such medication prehospitally is controversial. Always follow local protocols and consult online control when in doubt.

The best method of caring for the fetus is by anticipating injuries and shock and aggressively managing the mother.

> **The best method of caring for the fetus is by anticipating injuries and shock and aggressively managing the mother.**

TRANSITIONING

REVIEW ITEMS

1. A pregnant trauma patient who is in her third trimester presents with a palpable fetus in her upper abdomen. Based on that finding, you should suspect _____.
   a. eclampsia
   b. uterine rupture
   c. abruptio placentae
   d. pelvic fracture

2. A 26-week-pregnant trauma patient is suffering from supine hypotensive syndrome. After properly securing the patient to a backboard, the board must be _____.
   a. tilted downward
   b. tilted upward
   c. tilted to the right
   d. tilted to the left

3. What is the most common complication resulting from traumatic injury in the pregnant patient?

   a. uterine rupture
   b. uterine contractions
   c. pelvic fractures
   d. abruptio placentae

4. Which of the following mechanisms of injury account for more than half of all injuries sustained by pregnant patients?
   a. falls
   b. gunshot wounds
   c. stab wounds
   d. motor vehicle collisions

5. What percentage of fetal loss is accounted for by abruptio placentae due to mostly blunt trauma?
   a. 10–25 percent
   b. 25–45 percent
   c. 50–70 percent
   d. 1–10 percent

APPLIED PATHOPHYSIOLOGY

1. Explain how the physiologic changes experienced during pregnancy may mask the signs and symptoms of shock resulting from trauma.

2. Why is maximum oxygenation important in the management of a pregnant trauma patient?

3. Why can fetal growth influence the patient's perception of abdominal pain?

4. Explain how the gas exchange between the mother and fetus is inhibited if the patient has abruptio placentae.

CLINICAL DECISION MAKING

You are dispatched to a residence for a patient who fell. When you arrive, a teenager emerges from the residence and states that his aunt has fallen while in the shower. You determine that the scene is safe, and you approach the 26-year-old female patient, who is lying in the bathtub.

1. Based on the scene size-up characteristics, list the possible conditions you suspect the patient may be experiencing.

The primary assessment reveals that the patient is anxious, alert, and oriented. She states she slipped on some shampoo left inside the tub. She is complaining of severe abdominal pain. Her respiratory rate is 22/minute with adequate chest rise and fall. Her radial pulse is strong and regular at a rate of 112 beats per minute. You note no external bleeding. Her skin is warm and still very wet from the shower. The SpO$_2$ reading is 97 percent.

2. What are the life threats to this patient?

3. What immediate emergency care should you provide based on the primary assessment?

4. What conditions have you ruled out from your initial considerations in the scene size-up?

5. What conditions are you still considering as the possible cause? Would you add any conditions as a possible cause?

During the secondary assessment, the patient continues to complain of severe abdominal pain and cramping. She states that she is 24 weeks pregnant. In addition, she has a headache and her lower back hurts. Her abdomen is tender, her pelvis is stable, and no deformities or trauma to the extremities are evident. You note no crowning or external bleeding. The peripheral pulses are all present. The patient is allergic to aspirin, has a history of depression, and takes no prescription medication aside from her prenatal vitamins. She had lemonade and a turkey sandwich about 30 minutes prior to your arrival. Her blood pressure is 112/66 mmHg, her heart rate is now 112 beats per minute, and her respirations are 18 per minute.

6. What conditions have you ruled out in your differential field diagnosis? Why?

7. What should your emergency care include?

8. Why is it important to anticipate shock in this patient?

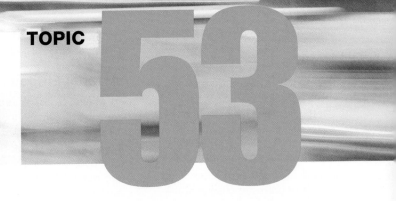

Standard Trauma

Competency Integrates assessment findings with principles of epidemiology and pathophysiology to formulate a field impression to implement a comprehensive treatment/disposition plan for an acutely injured patient.

DIVING EMERGENCIES: DECOMPRESSION SICKNESS AND ARTERIAL EMBOLISM

INTRODUCTION

According to the Divers Alert Network (DAN), between 1.5 and 3 million people scuba dive commercially or recreationally each year. The popularity of this sport means that many of our friends, neighbors, colleagues, and, potentially, patients will have participated in compressed air diving. Many of these people will dive in deep water. Although the vast majority of these participants will dive safely, a small portion of diving excursions will result in decompression-related injuries and air emboli. As a paramedic, you must be prepared to recognize and treat these injuries properly.

EPIDEMIOLOGY

Until recently, the incidence of diving-related injuries has been difficult to track. Between 1998 and 2002, DAN reviewed more than 50,000 dives and found that recompression treatment was required 28 times. Although these are perhaps the best data we have, there may be many more unreported incidents. Again, according to DAN, as many as 500,000 divers will take their first dive each year. That means that at any moment, up to nearly a quarter of the scuba diving population is relatively novice.

Given that most decompression-related injuries occur because of incorrect diving procedures or mistakes, it is reasonable to expect a potentially higher rate of injuries. On the other hand, we do know that severe injuries and death resulting from decompression injury and air emboli are rare. A U.S. military study estimated death rates among compressed air dives to be quite rare, with a ratio of roughly 1.3 deaths per 100,000 dives.

PATHOPHYSIOLOGY

There are several different pathophysiologies of diving emergencies. These issues can be traced back to the distinct physiologic dysfunction and to the improper diving procedure that led to the problem.

Dysbarism

Dysbarism, or decompression sickness, results from expanding pressures between diving depths and the surface. Divers who fail

TRANSITION *highlights*

- **Overview of the popularity of diving (including recreational), and documented occurrence of dive-related emergencies.**
- **Causes of dysbarism, and the laws of physics that contribute to it:**
  – Boyle law.
  – Dalton law.
  – Henry law.
  – Charles law.
- **Common assessment findings when caring for a patient with a dive-related emergency.**
- **Types of decompression sickness (type I and type II).**
- **Current treatment strategies for diving emergencies.**

to employ safe ascending techniques expose themselves to the risks of nitrogen bubbles and rapid gas expansion. Dysbarism is best described by relating it to the physics of diving.

DIVING AND PHYSICS   Four laws of physics play an important role in decompression-related injuries:

- **Boyle law.**   *At a constant temperature, the volume of a gas varies inversely with the pressure.* For example, at the pressures of 50 feet of depth, the volume of air in the lungs is roughly half of what it would be on the surface. If a diver were to ascend rapidly without the necessary safety precautions, gases in gas-filled organs such as the lungs would quickly expand and potentially rupture. Pressure

> Most decompression-related injuries occur because of incorrect diving procedures or mistakes.

changes can also damage air-filled structures such as the eardrum and sinus cavities.

- **Dalton law.** *The total pressure of a mixture of gases equals the sum of the partial pressures of the individual gases that make up the mixture.* Simply put, the total pressure of the air we breathe is made up of a series of individual pressures of gases. These individual pressures change as the external pressure changes. For example, nitrogen comprises about 78 percent of total pressure of the air we breathe. If you were to descend to a depth of 50 feet, the ambient pressure would significantly increase and therefore increase the pressure of nitrogen. At high pressures (greater depths), the increased pressure of nitrogen can cause higher levels of nitrogen to dissolve into the bloodstream. This can cause a central nervous system disturbance called *nitrogen narcosis.* It has been said that the effect of every 50 feet of depth is similar to the intoxicating effects of one alcoholic beverage.

- **Henry law.** *At a constant temperature, the amount of gas dissolved in a liquid is proportional to the surrounding pressure.* For example, at high pressures (great depth), gases, especially nitrogen, dissolve into the blood and tissues of the body. If a diver were to ascend too rapidly, pressure would quickly increase and nitrogen would be returned to a gaseous state while still in the blood and tissues. This gaseous nitrogen forms bubbles in fats and other body tissues and can cause tissue damage and severe pain. Compression from these bubbles harms tissue and can cause nerve and blood vessel disruption. The immune system often responds to the presence of nitrogen bubbles and can cause allergy-related symptoms. In addition, nitrogen bubbles can cause clotting-related problems in the form of obstructions called *emboli.*

- **Charles law.** *The volume of a gas is proportional to the temperature.* Cold temperatures cause the volumes of gases to decrease. As temperatures increase rapidly, as in a rapid ascent from the cold depths, the volume of gas will increase rap-

idly. This increased volume can cause trauma to gas-filled organs.

Arterial Emboli

In severe cases of decompression sickness, barotrauma in the lungs can lead to air entering the pulmonary vein. Air bubbles, also called *air emboli,* are then returned to the left side of the heart and are potentially distributed to the arterial side of the cardiovascular system. When the bubbles reach small arterioles, they can result in an obstruction to flow and impair perfusion to tissues beyond the obstruction. Emboli commonly cause major problems when they occlude blood flow in the lungs (pulmonary embolism) or when they occlude blood flow in the arteries of the brain (embolotic stroke).

ASSESSMENT FINDINGS

Mechanism of injury will be the most important finding when assessing a diving injury. Although many of these injuries will be acute onset and therefore obviously diving injuries, some will not. If your patient is wearing a wetsuit, you would suspect a diving injury, but remember that symptoms of diving injuries can be delayed.

Also remember that decompression injuries are exacerbated by air travel. Even though your current location might not include diving venues, be sure to investigate recent history when symptoms point you in the direction of decompression sickness. Remember also that dysbarism occurs in divers of all skill levels, not just in first-time novices.

Important considerations with decompression sickness include the following:

- History of diving
- Use of compressed air (scuba)
- What types of compressed air mixtures were used
- Depth of diving
- Recent air travel after diving
- Any complications during the dive (entrapment, injuries, etc.)

Complicated Diving Injuries

When assessing a diving injury, remember that these injuries often involve more than one significant problem. Although we have been discussing dysbarism exclusively, the overwhelming number of fatalities associated with diving result from drowning.

Keep in mind that decompression sickness often results from the rapid ascent used to escape another injury or problem. For example, the diver might have had to ascend rapidly because of an injury, entanglement, or equipment failure.

Always be sure to consider the entire picture, not just the decompression sickness. Complete a thorough primary assessment, consider spinal immobilization (when indicated), and look for other associated injuries.

Assessing Decompression Sickness

The signs and symptoms of dysbarism/decompression sickness are typically divided into two categories.

- *Type I decompression sickness* is most commonly typified by pain. Often referred to as *the bends,* this pain is typically dull, achy, and worst in major joints, such as the shoulder. This pain is most commonly caused by nitrogen bubbles in the blood and tissues and can come on rapidly or more chronically. Occasionally pain will worsen with time (especially if the diver flies too soon after deep-water diving). Skin rash and irritation are also common complaints.

- *Type II decompression sickness* is the more severe variant and can affect a number of body systems:
  - **Respiratory system.** Pulmonary air emboli are rare but potentially life threatening. Symptoms include respiratory distress, bloody sputum, and acute-onset chest pain. Decompression sickness in the lungs, also called *the chokes,* can also be life threatening. These symptoms can be immediate or delayed 12 to 48 hours and include burning sensation on inhalation and a nonproductive cough. Nonspecific symptoms also include pallor, cyanosis, low oxygen saturations, and accessory muscle use.
  - **Circulatory system.** Decompression sickness can cause fluid to shift out of the blood vessels and can thereby cause hypovolemia. This disorder is characterized by the signs and symptoms of shock, including tachycardia and low blood pressure. Coagulation disorders can also lead to clot formation and perfusion-related problems.
  - **Nervous system.** The brain and spinal cord can be affected by

> **Decompression injuries are exacerbated by air travel.**

nitrogen bubbles and small emboli. Nitrogen narcosis, compression damage, and perfusion problems can cause neurologic symptoms such as altered mental status, vision disturbance, weakness, numbness and tingling, and even loss of bowel and bladder control. Air emboli can cause strokelike problems and include similar symptoms, including seizures, motor and sensory deficits, and pupil changes.

Arterial emboli are related to decompression sickness but may exist independently. Recall that barotrauma in the lungs can cause air to enter the arterial bloodstream. Emboli then obstruct the flow of blood and cause perfusion deficits to tissue. In the extreme, this can cause a pulmonary embolism, but it can also cause more local signs and symptoms. Always assess for signs of barotrauma, including the following:

- Shortness of breath
- Use of respiratory accessory muscles
- Pallor, cyanosis, and low oxygen saturation
- Subcutaneous emphysema (air trapped beneath the skin, especially in the neck area)
- Bleeding from the ears
- Vertigo

Signs of pulmonary air embolism include the preceding signs and symptoms plus chest pain, blood-tinged sputum, and cardiac arrest. Signs of localized emboli include increasing pain, especially in the joints.

When assessing a person with a potential dive injury, also consider that certain conditions make decompression sickness more likely. Predisposing risk factors include the following:

- Flying too soon after diving (typically sooner than 12 to 24 hours)
- Not following standard safety procedures while diving
- Diving at extreme depths (or prolonged exposure to extreme depths)
- Manual exertion (work) while diving
- Cold water
- Obesity
- Age
- Dehydration
- Prior heart/cardiovascular conditions

EMERGENCY MEDICAL CARE

As stated, decompression sickness may be only one of a variety of concerns when responding to a diving accident. Consider spinal precautions when indicated and treat life threats based on the findings of your primary assessment.

When treating decompression sickness, consider the position of the patient. When spinal injury is not a consideration, place the patient in a lateral recumbent position. Do not place the patient in a Trendelenburg or head-down position.

As always, treat airway and breathing problems aggressively. High-flow oxygen is exceptionally important because it diminishes the effects of nitrogen. Advanced airway management, such as endotracheal intubation, may be important both to secure the airway of patients with altered mental status and to improve oxygenation

and ventilation. As always, assess the situation and use the correct airway management tool for the desired outcome.

Obtain venous access as a precautionary measure en route to the hospital. Administer fluids per protocol.

Pain management may be a very important element of care. Many diving emergencies, particularly the bends, can result in severe, debilitating pain. Use appropriate analgesics according to local protocol to ease the pain of these situations.

> **Many diving emergencies, particularly the bends, can result in severe, debilitating pain.**

Appropriate Transport

Aside from oxygen, few prehospital treatments are therapeutic in decompression sickness. As a result, rapid transport may be the most important therapy. When you identify a patient with type II decompression sickness and/or signs of arterial embolism, rapid transport to an appropriate facility is the highest priority.

When making a transport decision, consider that the treatment of severe decompression sickness often requires the use of a decompression chamber. It may be advisable to facilitate transport to a facility with this type of capability. That may mean alternative transport methods, such as air medical transport. You should advise the crew that diving-related accidents are being considered so that the crew will fly at the lowest possible altitude (and/or the cabin will be appropriately pressurized). Always follow local protocol.

TRANSITIONING

REVIEW ITEMS

1. Which of the following would be a diving injury associated with the Boyle law?
   a. ruptured alveoli from increased air volumes
   b. nitrogen bubbles in the fatty tissue
   c. nitrogen narcosis
   d. nitrogen emboli

2. Which of the following would be a diving injury associated with the Dalton law?
   a. nitrogen bubbles in the fatty tissue

   b. ruptured alveoli from increased air volumes
   c. air emboli in arteries
   d. ruptured eardrum

3. A diver working in cold water ascends quickly and now complains of ear pain and bleeding from his ears. This would best be an example of a problem associated with the _____.
   a. Charles law
   b. Henry law
   c. Dalton law
   d. Boyle law

4. A deep-water diver ascends but is now acting confused and has difficulty answering questions. He has no other complaints. Which of the following conditions might best explain his altered mental status?

    a. nitrogen narcosis   b. barotrauma

    c. pulmonary emboli   d. the chokes

5. A deep-water diver had an equipment failure and had to ascend at an unsafe rate. He now complains of shortness of breath, coughing up blood, and chest pain. The most likely cause would be _____.

    a. pulmonary embolism   b. nitrogen narcosis

    c. hyperventilation   d. pneumonia

APPLIED PATHOPHYSIOLOGY

1. Describe the effects of type II decompression sickness on the following systems:

    a. Respiratory system

    b. Circulatory system

    c. Nervous system

2. Describe how barotrauma might result in an arterial gas embolism.

3. Describe why high-flow oxygen is important in treating type II decompression sickness.

CLINICAL DECISION MAKING

You are called to the local airport. Dispatch tells you that a man has just been taken off an arriving plane. Prearrival questioning indicates that the patient is complaining of severe pain in his back, arms, and knees. He also is complaining of shortness of breath. No other passengers have had similar complaints. Dispatch notes that airline staff will meet you in the terminal.

On arrival you find a 35-year-old man seated in a wheelchair. He is restless and in obvious distress from pain. You notice that he is also tachypneic and has a cough. Airport staff tell you he was fine when he got on the plane but now is "very sick."

1. As you begin to consider a differential diagnosis, what are some potential causes for this patient's pain and shortness of breath?

2. What immediate assessment steps should you take?

Your primary assessment notes a patent airway and somewhat labored breathing. His respiratory rate is 36/minute, and he has crackles in the bases of his lungs. His pulse is also fast at 128. His skin is slightly pale and moist. He is alert but agitated. He tells you he is in severe pain. His knees, shoulders, and back "are killing him."

3. What other questions might you ask to make a better differential diagnosis?

The patient tells you he was just returning from a scuba weekend. He has been diving all weekend but now needs to get home for work on Monday. He tells you it was a great "party weekend," but he "may have overdone it."

4. What elements of the history of the present illness might indicate decompression sickness?

5. Does this patient have predisposing factors that might make decompression sickness likely?

6. What are the most important elements of treatment for this patient?

Standard Trauma

Competency Integrates assessment findings with principles of epidemiology and pathophysiology to formulate a field impression to implement a comprehensive treatment/disposition plan for an acutely injured patient.

TOPIC

54

LIGHTNING STRIKE INJURIES

INTRODUCTION

Lightning is a very dramatic natural phenomenon that captures the attention of many people. A lightning strike can produce a catastrophic or mortal outcome for the victim, or it can leave very little to no residual physical or physiologic effects. It is very important to recognize that a lightning strike is both a medical and a traumatic event.

EPIDEMIOLOGY

Lightning strikes the earth approximately 8 million times a day. Most of these strikes are benign and cause little damage to property or physical structures and even less injury to humans. Because humans are rarely struck by lightning, this fascinating electrical phenomenon is often disregarded as a potential immediate danger. It is the second leading cause of storm-related deaths in the United States and consistently one of the top three leading causes of death from a natural or environmental phenomenon. Although a standardized reporting system is lacking, it is estimated that 90 percent of lightning strike victims survive but experience some type of acute or permanent disability.

The highest incidence of lightning strikes occurs between May and September, with the largest numbers reported in June, July, and August. This is associated with an increase in recreational, work-related, or other outdoor activity. Approximately one-third of the strike injuries are work related, one-third are associated with recreational or sports activity, and the remaining one-third occur in other situations, such as being struck while on the telephone. The most common days to be struck are Saturdays and Sundays, with the most common time being between noon and 6:00 PM.

Children under age 16 and adults between 26 and 35 years of age experience the highest incidence of lightning strikes. Compared with females, males have a five times greater likelihood of being struck, primarily because of the types of activities in which they engage.

Being indoors provides the greatest protection during lightning events because of the large amount of electrical wiring and

TRANSITION highlights

- Incident rates of lightning strikes, including morbidity and mortality rates and predispositions as to the time of year, locations, and age distributions.
- The physics of lightning strikes.
- How a lightning strike alters normal body physiology to cause presenting signs and symptoms.
- Format for triaging when confronted with multiple patients struck by lightning (such as at large outdoor events).
- Current treatment strategies when managing a patient struck by lightning.

plumbing, which disperse the current throughout the structure. Owing to this unique conduit of current, however, a lightning strike can occur indoors if the victim is in contact with sinks, showers, toilets, indoor pools, and other plumbing, or if the victim is near or using electrical appliances or devices that are hard wired to the structure, such as a computer, telephone, or electronic game. Interestingly, the incidence of lightning strikes involving 911 and other emergency service call takers increased when the personnel began using headsets that were wired to the communications console.

Hundreds of people are struck each year while talking on the telephone. For this to occur, they must be using a landline phone that is hard wired to both the receiver and the jack. The lightning energy is transmitted through the phone line up to the receiver and to the person's ear and head. If a portable phone is being

> Ninety percent of lightning strike victims survive but experience some type of disability.

> **The contact temperature of lightning is 15,000 to 60,000 degrees Fahrenheit; however, its duration is only 0.01 to 0.001 second.**

used, a complete electrical circuit is not present; thus, no direct current can be transmitted to the person. However, it has been reported that a loud crack from static electricity has produced acoustic injury in lightning strikes when a portable phone was in use.

Cars, buses, and other enclosed vehicles also provide good protection from lightning strikes. This is a result not of the rubber tires but, rather, of the ability of the metal structure to dissipate the electrical current along the outside of the vehicle, leaving the occupants inside relatively safe and unharmed, provided that they are not in contact with the metal frame, the radio, or any other electrical device.

PHYSICS OF LIGHTNING

Lightning occurs from a transfer of an electrical charge. An electrical potential is created when warm low-pressure air rises through high-pressure air. The inferior portion of the cloud becomes negatively charged, but the ground remains positive. Static electricity generates lightning channels that are dissipated within the cloud or extend downward toward the ground. Objects on the ground send positively charged strokes upward. If both the downward and upward strokes make contact, a lightning strike is observed. It is important to realize that not all upward strokes result in a visible lightning strike; however, these strokes contain enough energy to cause potential electrical injury to a person.

It is important to recognize that lightning can occur 10 miles ahead of a thunderstorm. The sky may appear clear and blue with no rain in sight when a lightning bolt takes shape. This type of lightning, which is a side cloud discharge that is carried by wind current, is often referred to as *anvil lightning*, or a

> **The initial presenting rhythm immediately following the event is often asystole.**

"bolt from the blue." Most important, as an EMS provider you must recognize that even though the sky is clear, the patient may have been struck by lightning if a thunderstorm is in the area.

Lightning current is not considered to be alternating current (AC) or direct current (DC) but is often referred to as "cosmic direct current." It is a massive electrical discharge that can create a current with 100 million to 2 billion volts, with amperage as high as 200,000 amps. The contact temperature of lightning is 15,000 to 60,000 degrees Fahrenheit; however, its duration is only 0.01 to 0.001 second.

A common misconception about a lightning strike is that it produces massive and critical full-thickness burns; however, the short duration time of the strike allows for only minimal internal and external burns to occur. The energy flashes over the body, typically producing only superficial burns. If the victim has metal on his person, such as coins in his pocket, however, the metal may retain the heat for a longer period of time after the strike and produce deeper partial-thickness or full-thickness burns to that isolated area of the body. No source (entry) and ground (exit) wounds are associated with a lightning strike.

PATHOPHYSIOLOGY

A lightning strike is both a serious medical and a traumatic event that can lead to significant injury, permanent disability, and sudden death. The central, autonomic, and peripheral nervous systems are extremely sensitive to electrical energy that can lead to acute and chronic neurologic disruptions and damage.

Confusion, altered mental status, coma, headache, seizures, personality changes, and a decrease in cognitive ability are some of the manifestations of central nervous system involvement. The sympathetic nervous system may respond with massive vasoconstriction, producing hypertension and mottling of the extremities. The electrical energy may cause the autonomic nervous system to shut down the vital respiratory and cardiac centers in the medulla, resulting in cardiopulmonary arrest.

Cardiopulmonary arrest is typically the cause of death of a lightning strike victim. The immense electrical energy enters the body and acts as a massive defibrillation. As with a standard defibrillation, the electrical energy depolarizes the myocardium and produces a period of asystole. How-

ever, as a result of the dysfunction of the autonomic nervous system and lack of a functioning medullary cardiac center to provide stimulation to the myocardium, the heart remains in asystole. Thus, the initial presenting rhythm immediately following the event is often asystole; however, the patient could also present in ventricular fibrillation. Eventually, the inherent automaticity property of the cardiac conduction system produces electrical impulses and the heart begins to contract. However, the respiratory center in the medulla remains shut off as the result of the lightning strike.

Because of the lack of adequate ventilation, the heart begins to become severely hypoxic and acidotic, resulting in a secondary cardiac arrest from ventricular fibrillation. Contrary to the normal thinking in initial rhythms in cardiac arrest, the lightning strike victim may be more viable in the initial asystolic cardiac rhythm. The ventricular fibrillation rhythm may reflect a severely acidic and hypoxic state associated with a secondary cardiac arrest that may be more difficult to resuscitate.

The sudden and immense electrical stimulation may produce a severe muscular contraction that may cause the victim to be thrown several yards. Likewise, the air around the strike is rapidly and massively heated and then cooled, causing a sudden explosive and implosive displacement of air, propelling the victim and potentially causing blunt trauma to the head, spine, chest, abdomen, pelvis, and extremities; soft-tissue trauma; internal organ damage; and barotrauma to air-containing structures. Because of this mechanism, maintain a high index of suspicion of traumatic injury and consider spinal immobilization of lightning strike victims.

ASSESSMENT FINDINGS

As previously mentioned, superficial burns are normally present in lightning strike injuries. Severe burns are usually associated with a thermal source from the ignition of clothing or metal objects retaining heat and causing more extensive burns. Linear burns may occur and appear as lines on the body. These result from sweat or rainwater running down the body at the time of the strike, being substantially heated, and then vaporizing.

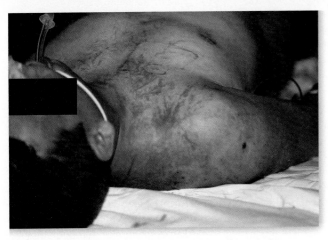

Figure 54-1 A feathering pattern on the skin resulting from a lightning strike. (© *David Effron, M.D.*)

Punctuate burns may occur and appear similar to cigarette burns. A feathering or pathognomonic fernlike pattern (also called a Lichtenberg figure) is not actually a burn but a discoloration to the skin in a fernlike pattern due to an electron shower (▶ **Figure 54-1**). Other assessment findings are listed in **Table 54-1**.

Triage of Multiple Lightning Strike Victims

Approximately 90 percent of lightning strikes involve only one victim, with the remaining 10 percent involving two or more. The most common cause of death is from immediate cardiac arrest following the strike. If a patient is not apneic or pulseless following a lightning strike, it is highly unlikely that he will deteriorate to cardiac arrest or not survive the event. Thus, when performing triage at a lightning strike scene with more than one patient, it is done in a manner reverse of what is typical, even if several patients are involved. The patient in respiratory or cardiac arrest is the priority and the first person to receive emergency care.

EMERGENCY MEDICAL CARE

Lightning strike patients may require a wide variety of interventions, based on their specific pathophysiology; these might range from very minimal emergency medical care, such as oxygen therapy, to complete respiratory and cardiac resuscitation. Emergency care should include the following:

- **Ensure your own safety at the scene.** Move the patient indoors or into the ambulance as quickly as possible to eliminate your risk of being struck. It is a myth that lightning strikes the same place only once. The Empire State Building is struck thousands of times each year!
- **Consider complete spinal immobilization**, as a lightning strike also has a blunt traumatic mechanism.
- **If the clothing is on fire or smoldering, douse the area with water.** Remove hot or smoldering jewelry or

TABLE 54-1	Assessment Findings in Lightning Strike Injuries
Assessment Finding	**Associated Pathophysiology**
Cardiac dysrhythmias (atrial fibrillation, premature ventricular contractions, supraventricular tachycardia, and persistent tachycardia)	Electrical disturbance in the conduction system
Apnea	Disruption to the respiratory center in the medulla
Cyanosis	Hypoxia from respiratory insufficiency owing to disruption to the respiratory center in the medulla or cardiac arrest
Low SpO$_2$ reading	Hypoxia from respiratory insufficiency owing to disruption to the respiratory center in the medulla or cardiac arrest or severe vasoconstriction in the extremities from excessive sympathetic stimulation from the electrical energy
Retrograde amnesia	Disruption of the central nervous system from the electrical energy
Hemiplegia or temporary paralysis to an extremity	Disruption of the central nervous system or peripheral nervous system from the electrical energy
Aphasia	Disruption of the central nervous system from the electrical energy
Vertigo or dizziness	Disruption of the central nervous system from the electrical energy
Mottling to an extremity	Severe vasoconstriction from arterial spasm in the extremities from excessive sympathetic stimulation from the electrical energy
Pain, numbness, burning or tingling sensation	Disruption of the central nervous system or peripheral nervous system from the electrical energy
Fixed and dilated pupils	Disruption of the central nervous system from the electrical energy
Transient hypertension	Severe vasoconstriction from excessive sympathetic stimulation from the electrical energy
Sight disturbance or corneal burn	Intense heat and light associated with the strike, retinal detachment, or retinal hemorrhage
Hearing loss and ruptured tympanic membrane	Disruption of the central nervous system from the electrical energy or barotrauma owing to explosive force, or a basilar skull fracture
Fracture or dislocation	Severe muscular contraction or propulsion of the victim

any other objects that may retain heat and continue to burn the patient.

- **Establish, and maintain a patent airway.**
- **If the tidal volume or respiratory rate is inadequate, begin positive pressure ventilation.**
- **Maintain adequate oxygenation.** Assess the patient for evidence of hypoxia. Apply a pulse oximeter and determine the SpO_2 reading. If either clinical evidence of hypoxia exists, the patient complains of dyspnea or exhibits signs or respiratory distress, or the SpO_2 reading is less than 95 percent on room air, administer oxygen via a nasal cannula at 2 to 4 liters per minute (lpm). Titrate the oxygen

by increasing the liter flow and possibly changing the delivery device to maintain a SpO_2 of greater than 95 percent, and abolish the signs of respiratory distress or complaint of dyspnea.

- **Assess circulation.** Be cautious when assessing peripheral perfusion and pulses because the sympathetic dysfunction may have produced arterial spasm with mottled extremities and absent or weak peripheral pulses. Establish an intravenous line of normal saline. Titrate the fluids to the patient's blood pressure and perfusion status. Keep in mind that a lightning strike injury is a medical and traumatic event; therefore, fluid administration may be necessary

if blood loss is associated with an injury that occurred during the strike.

- **Apply sterile dressings to any soft tissue injuries.**
- **Immobilize any suspected fractures or dislocations.**
- **If the patient is in or was to deteriorate into cardiac arrest, perform cardiopulmonary resuscitation.**
- **Assess for a shockable rhythm** and provide early defibrillation.
- **Perform 12-lead ECG and cardiac monitoring** to identify any ongoing cardiac dysrhythmias. Although they are unlikely, treat dysrhythmias according to Advanced Cardiac Life Support guidelines.

TRANSITIONING

REVIEW ITEMS

1. On arrival at the scene, you find four patients who have been struck by lightning. Which of the following patient presentations would be the first patient to receive priority emergency care?
   a. partial thickness burns involving 40 percent of the body
   b. a patient presenting with strokelike signs and symptoms
   c. a pulseless and apneic patient
   d. a patient with mottled extremities

2. A lightning strike patient has a left shoulder dislocation. The injury is most likely caused by _____.
   a. deep muscle injury from vasospasm
   b. severe muscular contraction
   c. a seizure following the lighting strike
   d. an injury prior to the lighting strike

3. Secondary cardiac arrest following a lighting strike is typically caused by _____.
   a. failure of the sinoatrial node to generate an electrical impulse

   b. severe myocardial tissue damage from the extreme electrical energy
   c. myocardial ischemia and acidosis from persistent respiratory arrest
   d. dysrhythmias resulting from blunt myocardial trauma and a cardiac contusion

4. Which assessment finding would heighten your suspicion that the patient has been struck by lightning?
   a. blood pressure of 198/132 mmHg
   b. linear burns to the body
   c. a mottled extremity
   d. unequal pupils

5. Pupillary assessment findings that would indicate a possible lightning strike are _____.
   a. pinpoint pupils that are nonreactive to light
   b. unequal pupils that remain reactive to light
   c. midsize pupils that are reactive to light
   d. dilated pupils that are nonreactive to light

APPLIED PATHOPHYSIOLOGY

1. Explain the reason that burns associated with a lightning strike are typically only superficial.

2. Explain why a lightning strike injury is considered a traumatic event.

3. Explain why a lightning strike injury is considered a medical event.

4. Why is a lightning strike patient prone to cardiopulmonary arrest? Explain the difference in the pathophysiology associated with the lightning strike cardiac arrest as compared with a typical cardiac arrest.

5. Why does a secondary cardiac arrest occur in the lightning strike patient?

6. Explain the triage performed for multiple victims of lightning strike and how and why it differs from the normal triage.

CLINICAL DECISION MAKING

You arrive on the scene of a residence and find a 56-year-old male patient lying on the garage floor. The garage door is open and rain appears to have wet the garage floor. A passerby saw the man lying there and called 911. As you approach, the patient is not alert, and you note that his lower extremities are cyanotic and mottled.

1. Based on the scene size-up, list the possible conditions you suspect.

During the primary assessment you find that the patient responds to verbal stimuli; however, he is confused and disoriented and has slurred speech. His respirations are 14 per minute with adequate chest rise, radial pulse is 138 beats per minute and irregular, and his skin is pale, cool, and clammy. His SpO$_2$ is unobtainable in the upper extremities.

2. What are the life threats?

3. What immediate emergency care would you provide based on the primary assessment?

4. Explain the possible causes for the pale, cool, and clammy skin.

During the secondary assessment, you note no trauma to the head, fixed and dilated pupils, and burns around the ears. There is no tracheal deviation or subcutaneous emphysema, and the jugular veins are normal in engorgement. The chest is symmetrical, and breath sounds are equal and clear bilaterally. The abdomen is soft and nontender. The pelvis is stable. The lower extremities are cool and mottled, and the distal pedal pulses are absent in both feet. The upper extremities have cigarette-like burn lesions and are cool, pale, and clammy. His blood pressure is 214/164 mmHg, heart rate is 138 beats per minute and irregular, and respirations are 14 per minute with an adequate chest rise. The blood glucose reading is 102 mg/dL.

5. What condition do you suspect? Explain the reason(s) why.

6. Explain the pathophysiology of the following assessment findings:

   a. Fixed and dilated pupils

   b. Cool and mottled lower extremities

   c. Cigarette-like burn lesions to the upper extremities

   d. Blood pressure of 214/164 mmHg

   e. Irregular heart rate of 138 beats per minute

7. What further emergency care should you provide?

TOPIC

Standard Special Patient Populations

Competency Integrates assessment findings with principles of pathophysiology and knowledge of psychosocial needs to formulate a field impression and implement a comprehensive treatment/disposition plan for patients with special needs.

OBSTETRICS (ANTEPARTUM COMPLICATIONS)

TRANSITION *highlights*

- *Rates of complications seen during pregnancy, including morbidity and mortality numbers.*

- *Expanded explanation of specific pathology as it relates to obstetric emergencies:*
  - – Placenta previa.
  - – Abruptio placentae.
  - – Ectopic pregnancy.
  - – Preeclampsia and eclampsia.
  - – Abortion.

- *Assessment parameters for the patient suffering from antepartum complications.*

- *Specific questions to ask while obtaining a history.*

- *Current treatment standards for a patient with antepartum emergencies.*

INTRODUCTION

*A*ntepartum refers to the period of pregnancy before the onset of labor. Therefore, antepartum emergencies entail obstetric complications that can occur any time between conception and delivery of the fetus. These emergencies carry a variety of clinical manifestations that can be as subtle as abdominal cramping and as life threatening as massive hemorrhage. Antepartum emergencies can pose a significant risk not only to the pregnant patient, but also to the fetus. These complications require the paramedic to maintain a keen level of awareness to protect the lives of the mother and her unborn child.

EPIDEMIOLOGY

Pregnancy is a natural process that can result in complications over the course of nine months. Four percent of pregnancies develop complications during the third trimester alone. Of that

4 percent, placenta previa occurs 22 percent of the time and abruptio placentae 31 percent of the time. In other cases, a cause for these complications cannot be identified. Further epidemiology of placenta previa, abruptio placentae, ectopic pregnancy, preeclampsia, eclampsia, and abortion is discussed in the next section.

PATHOPHYSIOLOGY

Placenta Previa

Normal implantation of the placenta should occur in the posterior portion of the fundus, or top portion of the uterus. In *placenta previa*, the placenta implants over the internal cervical os (or opening) (▶ Figure 55-1). The three variants of this condition are complete, partial, and marginal. *Complete* placenta previa covers the entire cervical os, *partial* covers the os to some extent, and *marginal* approaches the border of the os.

In placenta previa, placental implantation is initiated by the embryo adhering to the lower end of the uterus. As the placenta grows, it may cover a portion of the cervix. Then when the cervix thins for impending labor, the placental attachment is disrupted, which leads to bleeding at the implantation site.

The uterus is unable to contract properly to stop the flow of blood from the open blood vessels. Thrombin releases from the bleeding sites, causing further uterine contractions and thus a vicious cycle of bleeding, contractions, and worsening separation of the placenta. Generally, the abdomen is not tender between contractions. Placenta previa can occur in the first trimester of pregnancy; however, it is more typical to present in the second and third trimesters.

Placenta previa complicates 5 out of every 1,000 pregnancies and is responsible for 0.03 percent of maternal deaths. The incidence for placenta previa increases by 10 percent after a woman has had four or more Caesarean births. The risk of neonatal mortality is higher for placenta previa babies than for those not exposed. A great majority of maternal deaths are related to uterine bleeding and complications from disseminated intravascular coagulopathy.

Several risk factors are associated with placenta previa. Women younger than 20 years of age and those over 35 years of

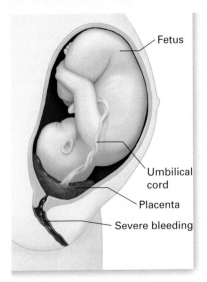

Figure 55-1 Placenta previa.

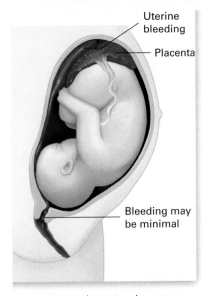

Figure 55-2 Abruptio placentae.

age are at the greatest risk. Other factors include multiparity (more than two deliveries), multiple gestation (more than one fetus), rapid succession of pregnancies, recurrent abortions, infertility treatments, residence at a higher altitude, and cocaine and cigarette use.

Vaginal bleeding occurs 80 percent of the time in placenta previa. The classic presentation of placenta previa is painless, bright red vaginal bleeding; however, the color of the blood should not preclude the consideration of placenta previa. Bleeding starts slowly and may increase in flow as the separation continues. On abdominal examination, the uterus will appear soft, nontender, and relaxed. The absence of abdominal pain and uterine contractions is used primarily to distinguish between placenta previa and abruptio placentae.

However, up to 10 percent of women may experience painful uterine contractions. In addition, bright red blood is not always present and the blood may be dark or an intermediate color. Any vaginal bleeding occurring after 24 weeks gestation should be a consideration for placenta previa, as it is a major cause of third-trimester hemorrhage.

Abruptio Placentae

Abruptio placentae, or placental abruption, is an obstetric catastrophe in which the placental lining separates from the uterus prematurely. It is referred to as a separation that occurs after 20 weeks gestation and before birth. Incidence of abruptio placentae peaks at 24 to 26 weeks gestation. It is a common cause of

late-term pregnancy bleeding in women, occurring in 1 percent of pregnancies worldwide. In the United States, placental abruption complicates 1 in 100 births and results in stillbirth in 1.2 of every 1,000 deliveries. Abruptio placentae carries a fetal fatality rate of 20 percent to 40 percent and is also a significant contributor to maternal mortality.

Abruptio placentae begins with avulsion of the anchoring placental villi from the expanding lower uterine segment (▶ Figure 55-2). This leads to bleeding into the tissue between the uterine wall and the placenta, which, in turn, pushes the placenta away from the uterus, causing further bleeding. In addition to severe maternal blood loss, abruptio placentae initiates a cascade of events that results in reduced maternal–fetal oxygen and nutrient exchange, membrane rupture, uterine contractility, and clotting abnormalities. Clinical manifestations include abdominal pain, vaginal bleeding (80 percent), premature contractions, and fetal distress or death.

Abruptio placentae can present in one of two types: complete or partial. In *complete* abruption, the placenta separates completely from the uterine wall. This type carries a 100 percent fetal mortality rate. *Partial* placental abruption is an incomplete or partial separation from the uterine wall. Because the placenta is partially attached and functioning, it is associated with a lower fetal mortality rate, rather than 100 percent.

There are several risk factors for placental abruption. Maternal hypertension is responsible for 44 percent of all abrup-

tions. Other risk factors include maternal trauma, short umbilical cord, prolonged or premature rupture of membranes, previous abruption, infection, and toxins such as cocaine intoxication and cigarette smoking. Another major risk factor for placental abruption is maternal age. Pregnant women younger than 20 years of age and older than 35 are at an even greater risk.

Patients with placental abruption display specific signs and symptoms. Painful, dark vaginal bleeding is ominous in abruptio placentae. However, vaginal bleeding does not always take place, nor is the blood always dark in color. Bleeding can transpire internally, causing the uterus to appear disproportionately enlarged. Be watchful for hypovolemic shock, as evidenced by tachycardia, hypotension, and signs of poor perfusion. Contractions are commonly painful and palpable on exam. They may be so frequent as to seem continuous. Tenderness in the abdomen and pain in the uterus are also frequent findings in abruptio placentae.

Abruptio placentae with greater than 50 percent separation is considered to be severe. The presence of severe abruption causes both maternal and fetal compromise. Unfortunately, the amount of vaginal bleeding does not correlate with the degree of placental separation and is a poor indicator to the extent of impending compromise.

In summary, there are no clinical findings that definitively suggest placenta previa or placental abruption; however, bleeding in the second or third trimester requires expert evaluation.

Ectopic Pregnancy

Ectopic pregnancy is a complication of pregnancy in which the ovum implants outside the uterine cavity (▶ Figure 55-3). Ninety-eight percent of ectopic pregnancies occur in the fallopian tube; therefore, they are called *tubal pregnancies*. Implantation, although unlikely, can occur in other places, such as the cervix, ovaries, or abdomen. Almost 100 percent of ectopic pregnancies end in fetal death. Furthermore, ectopic pregnancy can be very dangerous for the mother because of the risk of internal bleeding. Hemorrhage from ectopic pregnancy is still a leading cause of pregnancy-related maternal death in the first trimester.

In a typical ectopic pregnancy, the embryo does not reach the uterus and instead adheres to the lining of the

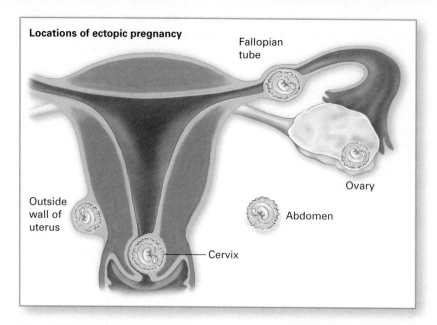

Figure 55-3 Ectopic pregnancy.

fallopian tube. The implanted embryo burrows into the tubal lining and invades the blood vessels of the tube, which causes bleeding. The pain from an ectopic pregnancy is caused by the release of prostaglandins at the implantation site and free blood in the peritoneal cavity. Fifty percent of ectopic pregnancies that are left untreated will resolve without treatment.

Overall, the incidence of ectopic pregnancy increased during the mid-20th century. It plateaued at 20 per 1000 pregnancies and an average of 7 percent of all pregnancy-related deaths. At present, ectopic pregnancy occurs in 1 out of every 44 pregnancies in the United States. For unclear reasons, there is a seasonal incidence for ectopic pregnancy, with increasing frequency between June and December.

There are many risk factors for ectopic pregnancy, including pelvic inflammatory disease, infertility, the use of an intrauterine device, previous ectopic pregnancy or tubal ligation, adhesions from surgery, and smoking. However, nearly half of all ectopic pregnancies are found to have no risk factor identified.

Early signs and symptoms of ectopic pregnancy are extremely subtle, or even absent. Early findings include pain in the lower abdomen, pain while urinating or during a bowel movement, and mild vaginal bleeding. Patients with a late ectopic pregnancy or rupture of the fallopian tube typically experience pain and hemorrhage. Hemorrhage will be both vaginal (external) and internal. The vaginal bleeding is caused by the falling progesterone levels, and the internal bleeding comes directly from the affected fallopian tube. Severe internal bleeding may be evidenced by low back pain, abdominal pain, and referred shoulder pain from free blood irritating the diaphragm.

Preeclampsia and Eclampsia

Preeclampsia is a medical condition that may develop after 20 weeks gestation, in which hypertension, edema, and protein in the urine develop during the pregnancy. Diagnostic criteria for hypertension include blood pressure greater than 140/90 mmHg in two consecutive measurements four hours apart. If the patient has preexisting hypertension, then a systolic pressure more than 30 mmHg over the patient's baseline and diastolic pressure more than 15 mmHg over the baseline are considered diagnostic.

In addition to hypertension and proteinuria, other diagnostic clinical manifestations include visual disturbances, headaches, edema, and scant urine output. Patients having hypertension as described with no other associated signs and symptoms are diagnosed with pregnancy-induced hypertension. Once the patient develops these signs and symptoms, preeclampsia is diagnosed. *Eclampsia* refers to the development of generalized tonic–clonic seizures in women with pregnancy-induced hypertension or preeclampsia, when the seizures cannot be attributed to another cause.

In preeclampsia, abnormal formation of placental arteries causes susceptibility to vasoconstriction. The vasoconstriction causes hypoperfusion to the placenta. This, in turn, promotes ischemia and even infarction of the placenta. Once this occurs, a release of vasoactive substances causes a cascade of events, including inflammatory response, vasoconstriction, clotting disorders, and increased capillary permeability. All these responses present the clinical manifestations of preeclampsia and eclampsia.

Preeclampsia occurs in approximately 5 percent to 8 percent of all pregnancies in the United States. Ten percent of preeclampsia cases occur at less than 34 weeks gestation. It is the third leading cause of pregnancy-related death, with hemorrhage being the first cause and embolism the second. Preeclampsia is estimated to cause 790 maternal deaths out of 100,000 live births.

Preeclampsia is more common among women under 20 years of age and over 35 years of age. The frequency varies across race and ethnicity, however; African American women have a higher mortality rate than other groups. A history of preeclampsia is also a strong risk factor for recurrence. Other risk factors include a history of diabetes, heart disease, kidney problems, preexisting hypertension, first pregnancy, or multiple gestations.

Several signs and symptoms are specific to preeclampsia. Mild cases can present very subtly and sometimes even go unnoticed. Common signs and symptoms of preeclampsia include hypertension, sudden increase in edema, angioedema (facial swelling), proteinuria, complaint of sudden weight gain, headache, nausea and vomiting, and visual disturbances. In severe cases and development of eclampsia, the patient will present with generalized tonic–clonic seizures.

Hypertension, as described, should be greater than 140/90 mmHg or, with preexisting hypertension, more than 30/15 mmHg over the patient's typical blood pressure. Edema in pregnancy is not

> **Preeclampsia is the third leading cause of pregnancy-related death, with hemorrhage being the first cause and embolism the second.**

uncommon. However, a sudden increase in edema or angioedema is consistent with preeclampsia and should not be considered normal.

Proteinuria is a very specific sign of preeclampsia; however, at present there is no means of testing for it in the prehospital environment. Weight gain is also expected in pregnancy. If a pregnant patient expresses a gain of more than 2 pounds in a week or 6 pounds in a month, you should suspect preeclampsia. In the first trimester of pregnancy, nausea and vomiting are extremely common; however, a sudden onset of nausea and vomiting in the second or third trimester is another indicator of preeclampsia when accompanied with other associated signs and symptoms.

Spontaneous Abortion

Also known as miscarriage, *spontaneous abortion* is a loss of pregnancy before the age of viability. A pregnancy is considered viable at 20 weeks gestation. Abortions can be spontaneous or induced. Spontaneous abortions are unintentional, involuntary, and occur because of a wide variety of natural causes. Induced abortions are intentionally performed for medical reasons (therapeutic) or personal reasons (elective).

Spontaneous abortion is extremely common in early pregnancy. Fortunately, the frequency for miscarriage decreases with increasing gestational age. As many as 20 percent of clinically recognized pregnancies under 20 weeks gestation will have vaginal bleeding, and 10 percent will have a spontaneous abortion. Abdominal cramping or pain and vaginal bleeding are common in miscarriage. The further along the gestation, the heavier the bleeding. Refer to Table 55-1 for the various types of abortion and patient presentation.

Maternal causes for spontaneous abortion include structural problems, incompetent cervix, infection, poor nutrition, substance abuse, smoking, and trauma. Maternal age is also a significant maternal risk factor. Women over 40 years of age have a 40 percent risk of miscarriage, and women over 50 years of age have an 80 percent risk of miscarriage. Abnormal placental implantation and placental separation are abnormalities involving the placenta that are capable of inducing abortion. Also, abnormal genetics and fetal implantation complications can both result in spontaneous abortion.

ASSESSMENT

Antepartum emergencies can be extremely stressful not only for the patient, but also for the paramedic. Anxiety and stress can inhibit the accuracy of information communicated among everyone involved. Use your dispatch informa-tion as well as scene size-up to help you determine the extent of the emergency at hand.

Once you ensure proper Standard Precautions and scene safety, perform a primary assessment. Your primary assessment should thoroughly evaluate the patient's airway, breathing, and circulation, as well as mental status. Use the same assessment and treatment techniques for a pregnant patient as you would for a patient who is not pregnant.

Use the history and secondary assessment to determine specific information about the patient and her pregnancy. Keep in mind that not all patients are aware that they are pregnant at the time of your interview and that those who are may not be accurate in the gestational age. In some cases, the patient's current emergency may be her first sign of pregnancy. Include the following questions as appropriate:

- When was your last menstrual period?
  - Was your last period normal for you (color and amount)?
  - Have your periods been regular?
  - Have you missed a period?
  - Have you experienced breast tenderness, nausea, vomiting, or fatigue?
- Have you been pregnant before?
  - How many times have you been pregnant (gravida)?
  - How many live children did you deliver (para)?
  - How many births were vaginal? Caesarean?
  - What complications did you have with your pregnancy?
  - Have you had a spontaneous or therapeutic abortion?
- Are you experiencing any pain or discomfort?
  - What is the quality of your pain (sharp, dull, achy, or crampy)?
  - Is the pain constant or intermittent?
  - Did the pain come on suddenly or gradually?
  - Does anything make the pain better or worse?
  - Does the pain radiate anywhere?
  - Can you point to the pain with one finger?
  - Do have any other associated symptoms, such as nausea or vomiting?
- Are you experiencing any vaginal discharge?
  - What color is it?
  - How much was discharged (pad count)?

TABLE 55-1	Types of Abortion
Type	Description
Spontaneous (unintentional)	Involuntary termination of the pregnancy before viability, 20 weeks gestation
Threatened	Abdominal cramping and lower back pain with light spotting; cervix remains closed with no products of conception passed
Inevitable	Increased vaginal bleeding and abdominal cramping; cervix dilates
Incomplete	Vaginal bleeding, abdominal cramping; dilation of the cervix with partial passage of products of conception
Complete	Passage of all the products of conception; cervix closes, vaginal bleeding stops
Missed	Fetus dies in utero but is not expelled; uterine growth stops
Recurrent	Two or more consecutive spontaneous abortions
Induced (intentional)	Voluntary termination of the pregnancy before viability, 20 weeks gestation
Therapeutic	Intentional termination of the pregnancy to preserve the health of the mother
Elective	Intentional termination of the pregnancy for reasons other than preserving the health of the mother (e.g., fetal anomaly)

- Does it have an abnormal or foul odor?
- If the patient knows she is pregnant, ask the following:
  - Have you had any prenatal care?
  - When is your due date?
  - How many babies are you expecting?
  - Are you having a high-risk pregnancy?

Assessment of the abdomen during the secondary assessment may reveal very valuable findings related to an antepartum condition. Inspect for abnormal distention or signs of injury. Palpate the abdomen to determine where the patient's pain is located. Assess for guarding, tenderness, and abnormal masses. Obtain a baseline set of vital signs, and reassess frequently looking for a trend, especially one pointing to hemorrhage and shock.

Pregnancy is a natural process. Should the patient experience complications, however, she will typically present with one or more of the following signs and symptoms: abdominal pain, vaginal bleeding, passage of tissue or clots, weakness or dizziness, nausea and vomiting, edema, hypertension, and even seizures. Table 55-2 summarizes the signs and symptoms you may see on assessment of a patient with an antepartum emergency.

Remember, these are considered classic or hallmark signs and symptoms that are typically seen in these emergencies. They are not absolutes, and patients do not present in this manner 100 percent of the time. Use these hallmark signs and symptoms to accurately diagnose your patient and treat her according to her presentation.

EMERGENCY CARE

Prehospital emergency care for antepartum complications is primarily supportive. When providing emergency care to the pregnant patient you must always consider the status of the fetus. Although the pregnant patient may appear to be relatively well, especially in the early stages of shock and hemorrhage, the fetus may be severely compromised.

Emergency care of antepartum emergencies should include the following:

- **Establish and maintain a patent airway**.
  - Altered mental status, seizures, and coma are possible findings in these emergencies. It may be necessary to manually maintain the airway or use an airway adjunct, such as an oropharyngeal or nasopharyngeal airway. Advanced airway placement may be necessary in some cases.
- **Establish and maintain adequate oxygenation and ventilation**.
  - Determine the patient's SpO_2 reading and assess for evidence of hypoxia. The pregnant patient is one situation in which, regardless of the SpO_2 reading, a high concentration of oxygen should be administered via a nonrebreather mask at 15 liters per minute (lpm). Application of high-concentration oxygen maxi-

mizes oxygenation to the fetus, as hypoxia due to vasoconstriction is possible. If the patient's respiratory rate and tidal volume are inadequate, provide positive pressure ventilation with high concentrations of oxygen delivered via the ventilation device.

- **Place the patient in a left lateral recumbent position**.
  - Left lateral recumbent positioning prevents supine hypotensive syndrome during the later phases of pregnancy by displacing the gravid uterus off the maternal aorta. This will prevent any further reduction of placental perfusion and help increase fetal oxygenation.
- **Provide supportive care for seizures**.
  - Maintain airway management, adequate oxygenation and ventilation, and circulation in a patient having seizures. Maternal seizures cause hypoxia to the fetus. Ensure adequate oxygenation and ventilation to prevent the increasing hypoxic state of the fetus.

  Stopping convulsions in a pregnant woman is an important advanced therapy, as the seizure poses a dramatic risk to the fetus. Paramedics should be more aggressive with anticonvulsant therapies in this specific population. In cases of eclampsia, magnesium sulfate is traditionally used as the first-line anticonvulsant, as it is not as toxic to the fetus as traditional benzodiazepines are. However, because it has a relatively slow onset, many EMS systems continue to use lorazepam and midazolam with the idea that a prolonged seizure poses greater risk than the administration of benzodiazepines. Always follow local protocol.
- **Initiate expeditious transport**.
  - Antepartum complications can pose a serious risk to the mother. In some circumstances, definitive treatment is delivery of the fetus and placenta. Choose a medical facility that is capable of managing acute obstetric compromise.
- **En route, establish an intravenous line of normal saline**. If the patient is exhibiting signs and symptoms of shock, run the fluid at a rate to maintain perfusion. If no signs of hemorrhage or shock are present, run the fluid at a to-keep-open rate.

TABLE 55-2	Antepartum Complications and Associated Signs and Symptoms
Complication	**Signs and Symptoms**
Placenta previa	Painless, bright red vaginal bleeding; soft, relaxed uterus with minimal uterine contractions
Abruptio placentae	Painful, dark vaginal bleeding; firm, tense uterus with frequent uterine contractions
Ectopic pregnancy	Abdominal cramping or pain that can be associated with voiding; vaginal bleeding, usually early in the pregnancy
Preeclampsia	Hypertension and proteinuria; edema, weight gain, headaches, nausea and vomiting, usually later in pregnancy
Eclampsia	Hypertension and proteinuria with the onset of generalized tonic–clonic seizures not associated with another cause
Abortion	Abdominal cramping and vaginal bleeding; possible passage of tissue or blood clots

TRANSITIONING

REVIEW ITEMS

1. During your secondary assessment of a 32-year-old woman with abdominal pain, the patient explains that her physician terminated her pregnancy because the fetus had a genetic anomaly. What kind of abortion is this?
   a. spontaneous abortion
   b. inevitable abortion
   c. therapeutic abortion
   d. elective abortion

2. Who has the higher mortality rate in ectopic pregnancy?
   a. mother
   b. fetus

3. A blood pressure of 140/70 mmHg with associated signs and symptoms is indicative of preeclampsia.
   a. true
   b. false

4. Implantation of the placenta near the edge of the cervical os is what kind of placenta previa?
   a. complete
   b. partial
   c. marginal
   d. minimal

5. External vaginal bleeding is always present in abruptio placentae.
   a. true
   b. false

APPLIED PATHOPHYSIOLOGY

1. Describe the pathophysiology of placenta previa.

2. Describe the pathophysiology of abruptio placentae.

3. Describe how ectopic pregnancy can cause severe internal bleeding.

4. Describe how preeclampsia is different from eclampsia.

CRITICAL DECISION MAKING

You and your partner are dispatched for a 42-year-old pregnant patient with abdominal pain. She is 32 weeks pregnant with a history of seven pregnancies, two miscarriages, and one stillbirth.

1. What are the patient's gravida and para?
   a. Gravida _____
   b. Para _____

On exam, you observe a round, distended abdomen. The patient states that her abdomen appears larger than usual. There is no vaginal bleeding, but she is having contractions.

2. What is your diagnosis?

3. Why is the patient's abdomen expanding?

The patient's vital signs include blood pressure 90/50 mmHg, heart rate 124 beats/minute, respiratory rate 20/minute, and SpO$_2$ 94 percent.

4. Would you administer oxygen to this patient? If so, how much and why?

5. Why is the patient hypotensive and tachycardic?

6. What emergency care would you provide to this patient?

TOPIC

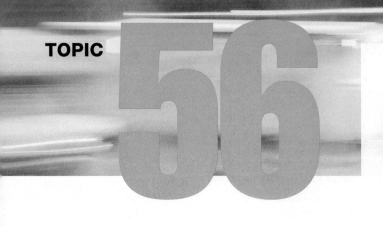

Standard Special Patient Populations

Competency Integrates assessment findings with principles of pathophysiology and knowledge of psychosocial needs to formulate a field impression and implement a comprehensive treatment/disposition plan for patients with special needs.

NEONATOLOGY

TRANSITION *highlights*

- *Incidence and morbidity/mortality of neonatal complications as well as rates that illustrate the commonality with which the neonate will need additional resuscitation following birth.*

- *Leading causes of death according to age brackets from <1 year of age to >65 years.*

- *Assessment format for a newborn child, including critical care interventions at each step.*

- *Mnemonic to assist the paramedic in remembering the steps and interventions when caring for a neonate.*

INTRODUCTION

From the time we are born, our lives are guided by the need to cope with the stressors nature throws at us. To be unable to cope with these stresses is to not survive—and life is survival.

In utero, the fetus can see, feel, hear, and breathe, although he is totally dependent on the mother for protection, warmth, oxygen, nutrition, waste removal, and immune function. After birth, the infant must begin to fend for himself by breathing air, depend on his own circulatory and respiratory systems for an adequate cardiac output and oxygen delivery, be capable of feeding effectively to allow for rapid growth, and develop an immune system that can protect him from the many bacterial, viral, and fungal pathogens that he will encounter from the moment of birth.

When one considers how complex our development is, from embryo to neonate, the true miracle in life is that anyone comes

> **About 10 percent of all newborns will require some medical interventions at birth.**

out able to survive at all. The spectrum of birth defects, either passed on through the genes or acquired from insults during pregnancy, fills textbooks and is growing every day as new ones are discovered from unlocking the human genetic code. Most women carrying fetuses with congenital anomalies spontaneously abort or miscarry in the first trimester (3 months) of pregnancy. Many fetuses with such anomalies, however, go on to be born prematurely or even at full term; it must be the assumption of every medical professional who approaches a neonate that the baby *may* have a congenital anomaly.

The most important advice to the EMS professional is that (1) you can never trust or assume that an ill infant does *not* have an anomaly and (2) the diagnosis, management, and ultimate treatment of that anomaly will require specialized practitioners found at children's hospitals.

EPIDEMIOLOGY

Not all infants are born equipped to cope with the stresses and huge changes, both anatomic and physiologic, that occur with the transition from an intrauterine to an extrauterine environment. Congenital anomalies—birth defects or anatomic maldevelopments affecting one or more organ systems—are the leading cause of death in the pre- and postnatal periods (▶ Figure 56-1).

It is estimated that about 20 percent to 30 percent of perinatal deaths are the result of congenital anomalies and that they are present in 2 percent to 5 percent of all live births. About half are due to genetic or inheritance causes, and the other half are either unknown or caused by teratogenic or uterine factors—injuries that occurred during the pregnancy itself from exposure to toxins (alcohol, drugs, and the like) or maldevelopment of the placenta.

About 10 percent of all newborns will require some medical interventions at birth, mostly to help them begin to breathe effectively. Of those, about 10 percent (or 1 percent of all newly born infants) will require resuscitation in order to survive the immediate neonatal period. Resuscitative measures include, but are not limited to, assisted bag-mask ventilations with oxygen,

10 Leading Causes of Death by Age Group—2001

Rank	<1	1–4	5–9	10–14	15–24	25–34	35–44	45–54	55–64	65+	Total
					Age Groups						
1	Congenital Anomalies 5,513	Unintentional Injury 1,714	Unintentional Injury 1,283	Unintentional Injury 1,553	Unintentional Injury 14,411	Unintentional Injury 11,839	Malignant Neoplasms 16,559	Malignant Neoplasms 49,562	Malignant Neoplasms 90,223	Heart Disease 582,730	Heart Disease 700,142
2	Short Gestation 4,410	Congenital Anomalies 557	Malignant Neoplasms 515	Malignant Neoplasms 493	Homicide 5,237	Homicide 5,204	Unintentional Injury 15,945	Heart Disease 38,399	Heart Disease 62,486	Malignant Neoplasms 390,214	Malignant Neoplasms 553,768
3	SIDS 2,234	Malignant Neoplasms 420	Congenital Anomalies 182	Suicide 272	Suicide 3,971	Suicide 5,070	Heart Disease 13,326	Unintentional Injury 13,344	Chronic Low Respiratory Disease 11,166	Cerebro-vascular 144,466	Cerebro-vascular 163,536
4	Maternal Pregnancy Comp. 1,499	Homicide 415	Homicide 137	Congenital Anomalies 194	Malignant Neoplasms 1,704	Malignant Neoplasms 3,394	Suicide 6,635	Liver Disease 7,259	Cerebro-vascular 9,608	Chronic Low Respiratory Disease 106,904	Chronic Low Respiratory Disease 123,013
5	Placenta Cord Membranes 1,018	Heart Disease 225	Heart Disease 98	Homicide 189	Heart Disease 999	Heart Disease 3,100	HIV 5,867	Suicide 5,942	Diabetes Mellitus 9,570	Influenza & Pneumonia 55,518	Unintentional Injury 101,537
6	Respiratory Distress 1,011	Influenza & Pneumonia 112	Benign Neoplasms 46	Heart Disease 174	Congenital Anomalies 505	HIV 2,101	Homicide 4,268	Cerebro-vascular 5,910	Unintentional Injury 7,658	Diabetes Mellitus 53,707	Diabetes Mellitus 71,372
7	Unintentional Injury 976	Septicemia 108	Influenza & Pneumonia 46	Chronic Low Respiratory Disease 62	HIV 225	Cerebro-vascular 601	Liver Disease 3,336	Diabetes Mellitus 5,343	Liver Disease 5,750	Alzheimer's Disease 53,246	Influenza & Pneumonia 62,034
8	Bacterial Sepsis 698	Perinatal Period 72	Chronic Low Respiratory Disease 42	Benign Neoplasms 53	Cerebro-vascular 196	Diabetes Mellitus 595	Cerebro-vascular 2,491	HIV 4,120	Suicide 3,317	Nephritis 33,121	Alzheimer's Disease 53,852
9	Circulatory System Disease 622	Benign Neoplasms 58	Cerebro-vascular 38	Influenza & Pneumonia 48	Influenza & Pneumonia 181	Congenital Anomalies 458	Diabetes Mellitus 1,958	Chronic Low Respiratory Disease 3,324	Nephritis 3,284	Unintentional Injury 32,694	Nephritis 39,480
10	Intrauterine Hypoxia 534	Cerebro-vascular 54	Septicemia 29	Cerebro-vascular 42	Chronic Low Respiratory Disease 171	Liver Disease 387	Influenza & Pneumonia 983	Homicide 2,467	Septicemia 3,111	Septicemia 25,418	Septicemia 32,236

Note: Homicide and suicide counts include terrorism deaths associated with the events of September 11, 2001, that occurred in New York City, Pennsylvania, and Virginia. A total of 2,926 U.S. residents lost their lives in these acts of terrorism in 2001, of which 2,922 were classified as (transportation-related) homicides and 4 were classified as suicides.
Source: National Center for Health Statistics, (NCHS) Vital Statistics Systems.
Produced by : Office of Statistics and Programming, National Center for Injury Prevention and Control, CDC.

Figure 56-1 Ten leading causes of death by age group. Courtesy of the Centers for Disease Control and Prevention.
Source: Morbidity and Mortality Weekly Report, Vol. 58, No. RR-1 (2009)

Because the infant is so fragile and dependent on his environment for survival, seemingly little things, such as ambient or room temperature, can make the difference between successful and failed resuscitation efforts. Because our assessments and interventions require physical examination of a naked infant and because infants are at such high risk for hypothermia, we must ensure normal body temperature when infants are well, but even more so when they are ill.

This is important to mention at the outset, as it is something the paramedic needs to think about and be prepared for ahead of time (e.g., while en route to the call, warm up the back of the ambulance). For this reason, forethought and preparation are keys to good treatment. In no other population is attention to detail more important than in the care of the neonate.

chest compressions, and even administration of medications.

Having the appropriate equipment and skill set to provide temperature control, airway suctioning, assisted ventilations, chest compressions, and glucose monitoring are among the most important aspects of neonatal resuscitation. This topic focuses on those lifesaving skills.

TERMINOLOGY RELATED TO NEWBORNS

Before discussing how to assess and treat a newborn, one must start with the terminology used by health care professionals to describe the stages of development.

The fetal or *in utero* period is the prenatal (literally, before birth) development of the human. The average duration of fetal development—called the *gestational period*, which begins with conception—is 9 months or around 40 weeks; this is referred to as the baby's *gestational age*, measured in weeks.

Babies born before 37 weeks gestational age are considered *premature*, those born within the 37-to-40-week period are called *term* infants, and those born after 40 weeks are considered *late term* gestations. For many reasons, premature infants are at especially high risk for complications; any EMS call to one should be considered a true emergency.

The term *perinatal* is used to define the immediate period around labor and delivery, which includes the late *prenatal* into the immediate *postnatal* times. The *neonatal period* refers to the first 30 days of life.

Infancy refers to the first year of life following the neonatal period (ages 1–12 months).

Having an understanding of this sometimes confusing terminology can help one both communicate with other health care professionals and understand why issues in one period of time can affect the infant in others.

Understanding the anatomic and physiologic transition from in utero to the extrauterine environment is crucial to appropriate assessment and management of the neonate or infant requiring medical attention. Those changes are the subject of introductory textbooks and will not be discussed in depth here, the assumption being that the paramedic should already have a working understanding of these changes.

ASSESSMENT AND EMERGENCY CARE

The most obvious and dramatic transition for neonates is going from an amniotic fluid-filled, "underwater" environment to an oxygen-rich, aerated (and colder) environment in which they are no longer able to receive oxygenated blood from their mothers via the placenta but are totally dependent on their lungs opening up to (1) the air they now need to breathe and (2) the pulmonary blood flow from the heart. The lungs need to literally open with air and redistribute the watery amniotic fluid, drying out in a way, and allowing the alveoli to begin gas exchange (CO_2 for O_2) for the first time.

If this amniotic fluid that was filling their lungs contained any of the meconium (or stool) that they have been producing in utero, their lungs may not function properly; they can quickly develop respiratory distress and then respiratory failure, characterized by cyanosis (blueing of the skin from deoxygenated blood), tachypnea, grunting, retractions, and even apnea. Cardiorespiratory failure and arrest are soon to follow if appropriate interventions are not taken.

If the newborn infant has a structural defect in the heart that does not permit adequate blood flow to the lungs or to the body, he will develop similar signs and symptoms. If the newborn develops an infection from delivery because his immune system is inadequately developed, he will present with the same signs and symptoms of respiratory distress, impending respiratory failure, and ultimately cardiorespiratory arrest. Respiratory failure can occur quickly—within minutes to hours—and requires immediate attention. Any deterioration must be acted on without delay.

> **Having the right equipment is the first rule of rescue for the neonatal and pediatric populations.**

Having the right equipment is the first rule of rescue for the neonatal and pediatric populations. There is no excuse for not having appropriately sized resuscitation equipment, from oral and nasal airways, to bag-valve masks (BVMs), to suctioning equipment.

One of the most important pieces of airway equipment (and the one most often overlooked) is something that gives you the ability to suction the airway. For the neonate and infant, a bulb suction may be all that is necessary to clear the airway and allow the infant to breathe.

Because infants are obligate nose breathers (meaning they are literally hard-wired by their nervous systems to breathe through their noses and do not yet know how to breathe through their mouths), infants with upper respiratory infections that cause swelling and mucus production of the already narrow nasal passages can present in respiratory distress. Simple suctioning with saline drops can open an airway very effectively.

ABCs: "In That Order, Every Time"

AIRWAY   The use of bag-mask ventilation in a neonate should never require force or much strength. Keeping a good facial-mask seal and avoiding pressure on the infant's eyes is easy if the appropriate mask size is available (▶ Figure 56-2). Use of an adult mask covering the infant's entire face may be required if an appropriately sized mask is not available—but this may require two rescuers for an adequate seal and to provide breaths.

Avoid pressure on the trachea, as it is not rigid and can easily collapse. Light downward pressure on the face with the mask, together with a corresponding light upward pressure from a one-fingered chin lift, is usually all that is required to maintain a good seal and open the airway. For infants with small jaws and possible craniofacial abnormalities (e.g., Pierre-Robin sequence), placing them prone may open their airways and allow for better air movement if they are breathing spontaneously.

Use of soft, rubber nasopharyngeal airways may be necessary to help keep the airway open if these infants are not breathing spontaneously. Use of an appropriately sized oral airway in the apneic infant can be very important in keeping the tongue forward enough to allow for adequate ventilation.

Remember that the infant's head, neck, and airway anatomy is significantly different from that of the older child: The head is proportionately much larger and heavier, with a prominent occiput and small midface (the part between the eyebrows and the chin) and a large tongue with limited mobility; the neck cannot support the head unassisted in the neonatal age range and must be supported by the caretaker; the airway structures of the neck—being collapsible, tracheal rings—are incompletely formed and flexible; and the entire airway, from nostrils to alveoli, is much smaller, easily blocked by

secretions and highly resistant to airflow when edematous.

The soft tissue and joint laxity of the neonate and infant allow for easy manipulation, and it should be obvious that overly vigorous resuscitative efforts (such as jaw lift or neck extension) could cause harm. Because of the large occiput of the infant, it is important to be familiar with how to position the infant supine and to use warm, dry towels to aid in positioning for the neck/shoulder roll.

Just as flexing the head (chin to chest) or even inadequate head extension (chin away from chest but not far enough) can close the airway because the tongue can cause occlusion, overextension of the head and jaw can actually compress the upper trachea and lead to more airway resistance, making ventilation more difficult. Find the middle ground between not enough extension and too much by listening with your stethoscope to the inspired (or delivered) breaths along the infant's neck.

BREATHING   When the airway patency has been established, assisted ventilation should be performed in any neonate with respiratory distress, apnea, or significant hypotonia (i.e., a floppy baby) and at a rate of 40 to 60 breaths per minute for a newborn, 30 to 40 per minute for an older neonate. High airway pressures during BVM ventilation can lead to trauma in the lungs and should be avoided.

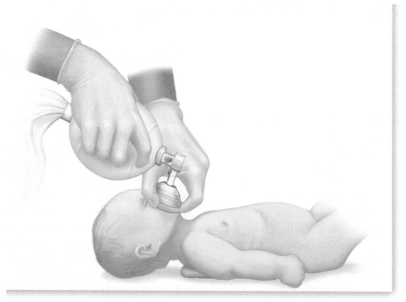

Figure 56-2 To provide positive pressure ventilation, use a bag-valve mask. Maintain a good mask seal. Ventilate with just enough force to raise the infant's chest. Ventilate at a rate of 40–60 per minute for 30 seconds, then reassess.

Having the appropriately sized manual resuscitator bag is also important. The paramedic should seek to use only size-appropriate tidal volumes (15–25 mL for a newborn, 25–50 mL for neonates up to 1 month of age) during assisted ventilation. The best rule is "just enough to move the chest" but no more than that because of the risk for causing a pneumothorax.

In the heat of the resuscitation, it is easy to forget these little things—once again reinforcing the need for attention to details as the key to successful resuscitation. Whenever possible, a manometer on the BVM apparatus should be used and peak inspiratory pressures kept below 30 cmH$_2$O. Aggressive use of positive end-expiratory pressure (PEEP) is usually not necessary because of the very compliant lungs and chest walls of the infant.

The efficacy of assisted ventilation will be obvious during a physical exam of the newborn or infant. One should see a rapid improvement in color and perfusion. If the infant was bradycardic when manual ventilations began, you should see an increase to normal or elevated heart rates if your ventilations are successful. An apneic infant will usually begin spontaneous respirations once adequately oxygenated and not overventilated.

Allowing the infant to continue breathing on his own is advised, but do not trust him to not become apneic again and require more assistance. According to the 2010 American Heart Association (AHA) Guidelines for Cardiopulmonary Resuscitation and Emergency Cardiovascular Care, a blended mix of oxygen and air should be titrated to achieve a targeted preductal SpO$_2$ after birth at 60 to 65 percent after 1 minute, 65 to 70 percent after 2 minutes, 70 to 75 percent after 3 minutes, 75 to 80 percent after 4 minutes, 80 to 85 percent after 5 minutes, and 85 to 95 percent after 10 minutes. If the heart rate is less than 60 beats per minute (bpm) after 90 seconds of resuscitation, the oxygen concentration should be increased to 100 percent until the heart rate increases to more than 100 bpm.

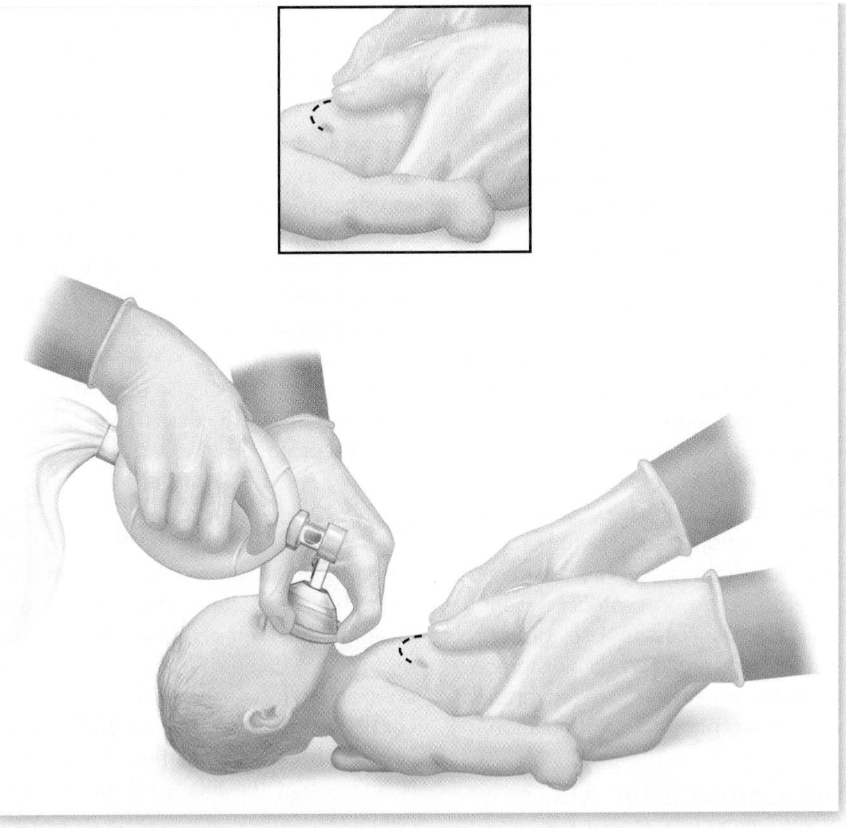

Endotracheal intubation is rarely necessary, but may be required to maintain long-term airway patency. If meconium is present in a hypotonic (distressed) baby, it is still recommended to aspirate meconium from the trachea prior to stimulation and ventilation. Prior to stimulating or ventilating the hypotonic baby, use a meconium aspirator attached to suction and aspirate meconium under direct laryngoscopy. Repeat this procedure taking care to monitor both preductal saturation and heart rate. Once aspiration is complete, you may consider intubation. It is very important to understand that meconium aspiration is limited to distressed babies—a baby with meconium staining that is active requires no tracheal suctioning.

CIRCULATION   In the infant with persistent bradycardia (heart rate less than 60 bpm and not increasing) and signs of poor perfusion (cool extremities, mottling, capillary refill time more than 3 seconds, cyanosis) after 1 minute of adequate assisted bag-mask ventilation, chest compressions should be delivered. Review of the technique is important to prevent injury.

With two hands encircling the chest, and using the thumbs to depress the inferior half of the sternum, this so-called thumb technique is very effective if the rescuer's hands are large enough, and it is not as fatiguing as the two-finger technique (▶ Figure 56-3). If the rescuer is unable to encircle the chest with his hands, the "two-finger" technique is recommended. Two fingers of one hand compress the chest while the other hand is used to support the infant's back. In both techniques, the depth of compression should be one-third of the anterior-to-posterior diameter of the infant's chest, the thumbs or fingers should not be lifted off the chest but full recoil allowed, and chest expansion should be allowed.

The compression:breath ratio is 3:1 with a total 2-second cycle time such that the rescuer providing compressions counts "one-and-two-and-three-and-BREATHE." In one minute, there should be 90 compressions and 30 breaths delivered. Practicing this is important to ensure good timing when and if the real need arises.

If the heart rate does not increase after proper ventilations and compressions, consider the administration of 1:10,000 epinephrine at 0.01mg/kg. Pharmacology is not typically necessary, but paramedics

Figure 56-3 To provide chest compressions, circle the torso with the fingers and place both thumbs on the lower third of the infant's sternum. If the infant is very small, you may need to overlap the thumbs. If the infant is very large, compress the sternum with the ring and middle fingers placed one finger's depth below the nipple line. In the newborn, compress the chest one-third the depth of the chest at the rate of 120 per minute and a ratio of 3:1 compressions to ventilations.

should be prepared to intervene in bradycardia if necessary.

For the infant who has a perfusing rhythm, circulation is a critical part of the exam, as shock in infants is poorly tolerated and blood pressure can be either difficult to obtain or normal in the setting of shock. Accounting for the environmental temperature, capillary refill time in the newborn or infant should always be brisk. In the setting of an adequate cardiac output, the extremities will be warm to at least the wrists and ankles, and the capillary refill time immediate. The presence of cool extremities and/or mottling of the skin with *any* delay of the capillary refill over 2 seconds is cause for concern and is a true emergency.

Because the infant's heart is relatively immature and stiff, any drop in cardiac output is compensated for by an increase in heart rate. Having a thorough knowledge of age-related normal (and abnormal) vital signs is crucial to appropriate triage and management of this population. In any suspected ill or injured infant, tachycardia (HR > 180 bpm) is never good until proven otherwise. Heart rates over 220 bpm usually signify a problem with the heart's conduction system and represent a true emergency requiring interventions.

> **Heart rates over 220 bpm usually signify a problem with the heart's conduction system and represent a true emergency requiring ALS interventions.**

Blood pressure is probably the trickiest vital sign to obtain on an infant. Often the monitors are not sensitive enough because the infant is moving (or the ambulance is) or rescuers do not have the appropriately sized cuffs. Because studies show that blood pressure is "the last to go" (unlike in adults, in whom shock is present when the systolic BP is less than 90 mmHg), a low-for-age BP is not necessary for the diagnosis of shock in infants and children. The presence of tachycardia and poor perfusion are all that is necessary. For this reason, it is crucial that the paramedic perform a thorough physical exam and pay attention to the other vital signs (heart rate, respiratory rate, capillary refill time, mental status/activity level, and muscle tone).

For newborns, a mean systolic blood pressure equal to or greater than the gestational age in weeks is considered acceptable but, again, this is in an otherwise healthy-looking infant. In the first month of life, a systolic BP less than 60 mmHg is considered hypotensive, in the infant (1 month–1 year) it is 70 mmHg, and up to 10 years of age the lower acceptable systolic limit is 70 + (2 × age in years).

Assessing the blood volume (i.e., hydration status) of a newborn or infant is probably one of the most challenging skills in all of medicine. Because the infant cannot communicate thirst or discomfort other than by crying, we must (again) rely on the details of the history, physical exam, and impressions of caretakers and rescuers together. A history of poor feeding, vomiting, copious diarrhea, a decreased number of wet diapers that day, any fever, sweating, or respiratory difficulties during feeding should all clue you in to the fact that the infant may be dry.

On exam, as mentioned, look for resting tachycardia, tenting of the skin, absence of tears, and, most important but latest to show, a lethargic infant with mottling and cool extremities, reflecting the increased systemic vascular resistance (SVR) required to maintain blood pressure in the setting of a decreased cardiac output from a low stroke volume owing to dehydration. Remember that:

$$BP = SVR \times Cardiac\ Output, and$$
$$Cardiac\ Output = Heart\ Rate \times Stroke\ Volume$$

Thus, the increase in heart rate is the first and most subtle sign of a diminished cardiac output and will precede frank shock by hours in many cases.

IV access in the neonate is challenging. If fluid or medications (e.g., $D_{10}W$) must be administered, attempt peripheral vascular access. Intraosseous access may be considered based on protocol if peripheral IVs are unsuccessful. Use a buretrol whenever fluids are to be administered to a neonate to prevent overhydration, which occurs rapidly in this population.

What Comes after ABC? DEFG—"Don't Ever Forget Glucose!"

Because the fuel stores of glycogen in infants are so quickly exhausted by their rapid metabolic rates, hypoglycemia is a very frequent finding in the ill or injured infant. Just as it is impossible to resuscitate a cold infant, so is it impossible to resuscitate a hypoglycemic one. All key metabolic pathways rely on rapid uptake and utilization of glucose, especially the brain, and it is crucial to remember that infants are at higher risk for this than any other age group. If the paramedic does not consider hypoglycemia in the differential diagnosis, he will never think to check for it. Because oral glucose can be absorbed rapidly, failure to check and treat for hypoglycemia is an unfortunately common mistake.

Feeding for newborns and infants is their exercise. It can be exhausting for a sick infant to feed, to coordinate the muscles of respiration and those of swallowing. This is especially true for premature or fragile infants with medical conditions. For this reason, questions about the infant's feeding (amount, duration, frequency, and whether there was any emesis, sweating, or frequent coughing) can be very important clues to the underlying problem. In a sense, the newborn infant's "day" can be reduced to four-hour cycles of sleeping, crying to communicate discomfort, feeding, and some period of alertness before sleeping again.

Understanding this routine, asking the caretaker about it, and paying particular attention to any deviations from it are crucial tips to getting a good history. Any lethargic infant with a history of poor feeding should be assumed to be hypoglycemic, and his blood sugar should be checked as soon as possible.

If glucose is to be administered to a neonate, $D_{10}W$ should be used at a dose of 5 to 10 mL/kg IV over 20 minutes. Follow local protocols.

H Is for Hypothermia

Once again, it cannot be overemphasized how important attention to the environmental temperature is to the care of an infant. Even the best resuscitation skills and efforts will fail if the infant is cold. A corollary to the old EMS adage "They're not dead until they're warm and dead" is that the infant will not survive until he is warm.

The inability of the neonate to generate enough heat is directly related to heat loss from the head's large surface area, the lack of insulating fat, and the high proportion of metabolically active brown fat—called "brown" because of the high density of energy-producing mitochondria that, when in a condition of inadequate fuel (oxygen and/or glucose) are unable to produce heat to keep the infant warm.

I Is for Infection

Infection is a major killer of neonates and can have a very rapid presentation. Sometimes the history is only of a fussy baby who was not feeding very well, whose breathing became more labored and then would stop occasionally (apnea) and have episodes of turning blue (cyanosis). This is the common introduction to the story of a potentially very sick and dying neonate and cannot be overlooked or discounted by health care professionals.

Any history of fever in an infant, *any* cyanosis, *any* apnea, and *any* history of rapid or shallow breathing requires immediate transport for evaluation. *Any* history of poor feeding, decreased urine output from the usual number of wet diapers per day, vomiting, or sweating, which all can lead to dehydration, requires that the infant be seen by a pediatric professional. *Any* history of blood in the stool, urine, or emesis and *any* rash beyond "baby acne"—especially a petechial rash, which is not raised and is nonblanching because it is, in fact, ruptured capillaries just under the skin and associated with severe infections (i.e., meningitis)—requires evaluation by a pediatric professional.

In short, any infant who is "not acting right" requires examination and is assumed to be ill until proven otherwise. Because the ways infants have to tell us that something is wrong are so few, we must be looking for the clues and pay attention to the little details—this can literally mean the difference between life and death.

No other patient age group encountered by EMS professionals will require such basic resuscitative care and yet have such a high potential for recovery and good outcome. That said, these calls are rare and highly stressful. Seeking out and receiving additional training such as that offered through the American Academy of Pediatrics' Neonatal Resuscitation Program is a good way to develop the confidence and skill set necessary to care for this most fragile population.

Safe Transport of the Infant

Every EMS provider should be familiar with how to safely transport a patient of any size and age. Entire chapters in EMS textbooks are devoted to lifting, packaging, and moving adult patients, but only a paragraph or two are given to safely packaging and transporting the most tenuous and fragile pediatric patient. Transporting an infant or child in the arms of a properly restrained caretaker is absolutely unacceptable. The force generated by a 10-pound patient on the arms of the parent involved in a 30-miles-per-hour crash

is beyond anyone's ability to resist.

Having a convertible child passenger restraint system (car seat) with two belt paths and a five-point harness system that can be adjusted to the size of the child is standard of care. Transporting the neonate in an isolette is ideal, as the chamber can be heated. In the absence of that, a car bed that lies across the stretcher and is strapped down using the stretcher's harnessing is next best. Few EMS systems have these, however, and most may not even have car seats (although that should change).

Unfortunately, most neonates (<5 kg) may not fit properly in these car seats. The restraining straps may not fit their shoulders and/or the seat may cause their heads to fall forward and obstruct their airways. For this reason, having a tested system that can be readily available for use during a neonatal emergency is crucial to our ultimate goal: safely transporting that patient to the hospital. Resources exist to help train EMS services in proper restraint of neonatal and pediatric patients, and they should afford themselves those opportunities.

> Any infant who is "not acting right" requires examination and is assumed to be ill until proven otherwise.

TRANSITIONING

REVIEW ITEMS

1. What percentage of newborns will require resuscitation with delivery?
   - a. 1 percent
   - b. 3 percent
   - c. 5 percent
   - d. 10 percent

2. You are transporting an infant who is having periods of apnea, but you don't have the appropriate-size mask to provide assisted ventilations. Before starting mouth-to-mouth/nose-assisted ventilations, what else could you try?
   - a. a nonrebreather mask on high-flow oxygen, using the reservoir bag to assist ventilations
   - b. an oral airway, blowing through it instead of using mouth-to-mouth/nose

   - c. an adult-size mask, creating a seal over the infant's entire face
   - d. nothing, just stimulating the baby to breathe

3. What is the normal range of heart rates for an awake newborn infant?
   - a. 60–80/minute
   - b. 80–100/minute
   - c. 100–120/minute
   - d. 120–140/minute

4. The recommended breath-to-compression ratio for infant cardiopulmonary resuscitation (CPR) is ____.
   - a. 3:1
   - b. 2:1
   - c. 1:2
   - d. 1:3

5. For the past two days, according to the mother's report, a three-week-old infant is more sleepy than usual, has been fussing continually when awake, cries when picked up but then falls quickly to sleep, has had some fever, and has not had the normal number of wet diapers per day. What is your assessment?

   a. This is normal for three-week-old infants—because of their rapid growth, they frequently need more fluid and are more tired.

   b. This is not normal but happens frequently, and the infant should be evaluated in the next couple of days.

   c. This is not normal, and the infant should be transported immediately to a facility capable of managing the infant.

APPLIED PATHOPHYSIOLOGY

1. Describe the proper positioning for performing chest compressions on a newborn.

2. Explain how to assess for an altered mental status in a neonate.

3. Describe the signs of respiratory distress in a newborn.

4. Explain transitional circulation in the newborn.

CLINICAL DECISION MAKING

You are called to the home of a two-week-old infant who turned blue for 20 seconds according to her 16-year-old mother. She has been feeding poorly for the past few days but has had no fever. You notice that the infant looks tired, has low muscle tone but is working to breathe, and is showing signs of respiratory distress (tachypnea, grunting, nasal flaring, subcostal and sternal retractions) with a respiratory rate of 80–90, heart rate 220 beats/minute, and unpalpable distal pulses.

1. What is your major concern about this patient?

2. Could this represent congenital heart disease? Infection? Dehydration?

3. What are normal vital signs (heart rate and respiratory rate) for a two-week-old?

The mother reports that the baby is looking better and that she does not want to go to the hospital, stating that she will call her baby's doctor or take her into the clinic.

4. Is this acceptable for her to do?

Standard Special Patient Populations

Competency Integrates assessment findings with principles of pathophysiology and knowledge of psychosocial needs to formulate a field impression and implement a comprehensive treatment/disposition plan for patients with special needs.

TOPIC

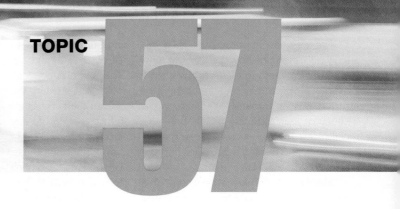

PEDIATRICS

INTRODUCTION

Before responding to any pediatric calls, one needs to look into three mirrors: one reflects yourself, your attitudes and beliefs; the second reflects your EMS service's unique abilities and weaknesses (whether from an educational, resource, or equipment standpoint) for handling pediatric patients during an emergency; and the third requires looking at your capabilities from a regional prehospital and hospital-based *systems* perspective: Does your region have the needed elements in place to fully care for critically ill and injured children? This topic will discuss these three views that need to be examined to provide best care for our most precious resource—our children.

INTO THE LOOKING GLASS: PERSONAL PERSPECTIVE

Few EMS calls provoke more anxiety than the pediatric cases. Most paramedics would prefer *any* sick adult to a screaming, ill, or injured child. The reasons cited for this are many ("I can't talk to them," "I'm afraid of hurting them," "They always fight me when I'm trying to help," "I can never remember what are normal vital signs," "The parents always try to tell us what to do," "We don't carry the right-size equipment"). If you fall into this majority of EMS professionals, doing some self-analysis to discover your reasons is very important—ideally before that call comes in.

If we do not examine and address those reasons, we will seek to avoid these calls, discount them when they do not go as well as they should, and blame others, and—fundamentally—we will not perform as well as we could for our patients, for our professional colleagues, and for ourselves.

When you can understand the reasons why caring for children provokes anxiety in you, you can begin to work with them to better suit the environment and the patient. Asking yourself "What would I want if it were my child?" will help guide you to become the best pediatric EMS professional you can be.

Pediatric calls present unique challenges, for a wide variety of reasons, and most EMS educational curricula do not adequately

TRANSITION *highlights*

- *Personal, EMS system, and health care system resources necessary to manage pediatric patients.*

- *How to approach the pediatric patient, and how to incorporate the primary caregiver's needs/wants/fears into the paramedic's assessment and treatment plans.*

- *The Pediatric Assessment Triangle (PAT) and its ability to help guide the paramedic into a thorough assessment.*

- *Common underlying pathology for disturbances in the pediatric airway, breathing, and circulatory functions.*

- *Current treatment standards when caring for a patient with a pediatric emergency.*

address our fears about caring in these situations for the most dependent and fragile members of our society.

APPROACHING THE CHILD: FIRST IMPRESSION

The first step in caring for children is to be able to get down to their level, both figuratively and quite literally. Standing above a child, as an adult stranger in a uniform with equipment and a squawking radio, is terrifying to any child. First impressions matter more to children because they cannot make the assumptions about you, based on your appearance, that adults can—from your gender, hairstyle, uniform, type of footwear, height, tone of voice, and demeanor—because children do not yet have the experience to make such judgments.

> Ask yourself, "What would I want if it were my child?"

The way you approach the child initially will determine how the next few minutes will go. Getting down to the child's eye level, which may mean crouching or sitting on the ground near him, while keeping your distance initially until the child "lets you in," is crucial to engaging that child and making a good first impression (▶ Figure 57-1).

Ideally, the primary assessment of a child is done as you approach him. Any child with "attitude" is one you need to take some time getting to know. The critically ill or injured child, for whom you need to intervene right away, will not care about your approach and interventions or will have little energy to spare to fight or disagree with you. For other children who are not so time-critical, a slow and respectful initial approach is critical to establishing that relationship.

For any conscious, alert child over six months of age, you are a potential threat until you prove that you aren't. Even though you may not be able to adequately treat his pain from an injury or relieve his respiratory distress right away, you can provide reassurance by reading his signs and respecting them.

Even an infant has signs or cues that, if you are looking for them, will alert you to when you are being too imposing, aggressive, or frightening; when it is okay to approach him; and when it is okay to touch him. This becomes even more important as the child grows and develops the autonomy to self-determine and control his environment. Illness and injury threaten that autonomy by stressing the child and his environment, including his parents or caretakers, and this puts an added dimension of stress back on the child.

Although you know you are there to help, the child does not and may need some convincing. Putting aside some of your need to hurry (i.e., your desire to minimize on-scene time) in order to spend an extra minute or two engaging the child is time well spent and may afford you an opportunity to learn something that could affect the course of that child's treatment.

Many children perceive looking them in the eyes, talking to them loudly, and reaching out to touch them all at once as threats. This approach can quickly overwhelm the scared child and cause him to retreat, cry inconsolably, and fight any further advances. Limiting your approach to just talking to him but not looking at him, or talking to the parent while visually assessing the child from a distance, can help the child adjust to your presence and give him time to assess you. The child will take many cues from the parent's response to the prehospital provider.

Working with the child by respecting his space, addressing him by name, and asking permission to examine him cannot be underestimated or overemphasized. Using toys or stuffed animals to approach the child is a good tactic, and they can also be used to help quiet and distract a crying child, allowing you to auscultate breath sounds or heart tones.

Be careful not to try to trick the child or lie to him—if you are caught, you will lose his trust. For example, do not tell the child that something will not hurt when it will, do not tell him medicine tastes good when it will not, and do not distract him with a toy and check a finger stick glucose without offering a warning.

PARENTS AND CARETAKERS

Certainly caretakers understand that you are there to help, but they will place their trust in you even more quickly if they see that you respect their child and value the child's cues. Respecting the child is respecting the parent and has an added benefit for working with the child: When the child sees that his caretaker trusts you, he will look at you differently, less as a stranger, and will be more likely to open up to you.

To further help this process, understanding the stress the caretakers are under will allow you to help them cope with what is likely one of the biggest crises in their life: having to call for emergency

> **Work with the child by respecting his space, addressing him by name, and asking permission to examine him.**

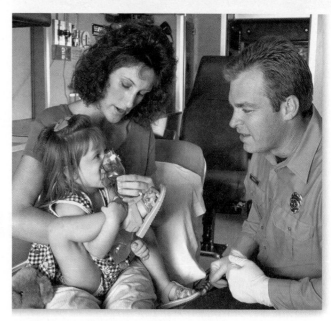

Figure 57-1 Approach a young child on the child's level, with the caregiver present.

help because of a sick or injured child. "Value passion wherever you find it" is a phrase that EMS personnel should always remember when dealing with parents and caretakers of sick and injured children. Valuing passion refers to the fact that they care most about their child and, during the stress from an illness or injury, nothing else matters as much to them—not you, not the doctors or nurses, not the police.

Furthermore, if you betray the caretakers' trust or do not align yourself with them in caring for and respecting their child, you have in essence betrayed them. When seen in this light, it becomes clear that allying yourself with parents or caretakers is much easier than not doing so and having them turn against you. Sometimes we must swallow our pride and be humble with stressed parents, but this is a sign not of weakness but of compassion.

Medical professionals have coined the term *difficult parents* to refer to parents who are stressed by a having a sick or injured child, who are having trouble coping, and who feel that the environment that is supposed to be caring for their child is instead uncaring, hostile, and unsafe. These parents can be bossy, very directive, and rigid and will sometimes order health care professionals around or be oppositional.

As professionals, it is our first responsibility to the patient and family members to make them feel safe and cared for, to always communicate with respect. Taking the time to listen to them and to address their fears and concerns honestly (saying "I don't know" when you do not is acceptable and preferable to making something up) is as important as performing a good history and physical exam.

ASSESSMENT OF THE PEDIATRIC PATIENT

For the reasons discussed in the preceding section, the physical assessment of a child is more art than science and requires a high degree of personal investment, professionalism, and expert communication skills. The knowledge base required is an understanding of the developmental and physical differences among infants and children of different ages.

Even within the first year of life (infancy), significant changes occur physically, neurologically, emotionally, and cognitively. Parents are well aware of these changes in their own children and are also aware of unique or subtle differences if their child has a chronic medical condition.

It is crucial to your assessment to use the parents' knowledge of these differences and, in so doing, build that bond of trust with the parent. Once you have an understanding of the growth and development of children through the first 12 to 15 years, age-related differences in vital signs and equipment become second nature, instinctual, and easy to remember.

Adult-oriented physical exam skills have limited applicability in assessing the ill or injured child. In terms of appearance, when one understands what should be the child's baseline normal activity, attitude, and appearance, one can quickly assess an altered mental status, a depressed level of functioning, or abnormalities in gait, posture, or coordination that make the difference in diagnosis and management.

Vital sign differences are sometimes misinterpreted and can lead to delays in management and outcome. Knowing, for example, that the response of an infant or a child to shock is to increase cardiac output through a dramatic increase in heart rate and systemic vascular resistance allows one to know to look for tachycardia and delayed capillary refill time, mottling, and low urine output (a decrease in the number of wet diapers when asked of the parent on history taking), which will prompt you to intervene quickly, without waiting for the low blood pressure of decompensated shock.

As delays in resuscitation of the child in shock are an independent variable that increases mortality rates by more than 20 percent, early intervention in pediatric shock has a proven benefit to the child's ultimate outcome.

Pediatric Assessment Triangle

No contribution to our assessment armamentarium is more important than the Pediatric Assessment Triangle (PAT; ▶ Figure 57-2), which modifies the traditional ABCs of airway–breathing–circulation to appearance–breathing–circulation, incorporating the adult-focused *airway* into pediatric *breathing* and elevating the importance of *disability*, which is sometimes forgotten, into *appearance*.

Outside of the Apgar scoring system for neonates, the PAT has allowed for a more objective and reproducible set of criteria for assessing the ill or injured child than any other system to date. It also follows the logical progression of the paramedic as he or she enters the scene: Looking at the child's appearance, level of activity, and "attitude" can be done from across the room; assessing breathing requires one to be a bit closer to the child to look and listen for signs of increased work of breathing (grunting, stridor, nasal flaring, retractions, and an increased respiratory rate); and the assessment of circulation requires a hand on the child's extremity to assess warmth and capillary refill time and to check the heart rate either by pulse or monitor.

Thinking of your assessment and triage as starting from the moment you enter the room or arrive on scene allows you to quickly determine the life support decisions you need to make: Do you have time to further assess the awake and screaming infant, or do you need to initiate immediate interventions for the unresponsive toddler lying in front of you? The paradigm

is intuitive to those experienced in pediatric assessment and should be the cornerstone of your assessment, triage, intervention, and reassessment strategy for pediatric care.

APPEARANCE Because of the high metabolic requirements of the infant and child (think in terms of the body's energy production and utilization, oxygen delivery and consumption, and carbon dioxide production), significant disturbances in the child's health from illness or injury will manifest themselves early and profoundly in the child's appearance. For this reason, appearance is the most important and first of the ABCs in pediatric assessment.

> Adult-oriented physical exam skills have limited applicability in assessing the ill or injured child.

Recognizing an abnormal appearance in a child requires a more detailed system than the traditional AVPU used in adult-oriented care. The **TICLS** mnemonic has proven itself over time and can help detect subtle but crucial deficits in the child's appearance and behavior:

- **T**one
- **I**nteractiveness
- **C**onsolability
- **L**ook/gaze
- **S**peech/cry

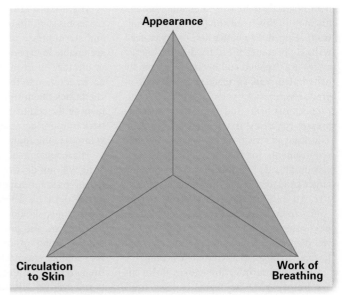

Figure 57-2 The Pediatric Assessment Triangle (PAT).

It is important to evaluate one's own contribution to the child's appearance, as a rapid and loud entry of the EMS team can, as previously mentioned, lead to an agitated and difficult-to-console child.

> **Respiratory distress and failure are the leading cause of hospitalization and second-leading cause of death and disability in children.**

Even though it should be somewhat reassuring that the child has this much attitude and is not likely to be critically ill, bear in mind that children do have effective, though somewhat limited, compensatory mechanisms.

A good rule of thumb is to not trust the child: His clinical condition can change very quickly as his limited ability to compensate is overwhelmed by the underlying illness or injury. This requires continued observation and reassessment, especially if transport times are long. On the other hand, a lethargic child who cannot muster the energy to cry is one to be very worried about: He needs immediate evaluation in a hospital equipped to resuscitate children and thus triggers a true "load and go" response.

Abnormal appearance is never good and can be caused by shock from inadequate perfusion, hypoglycemia, respiratory distress leading to respiratory failure and hypoxemia, hypercarbia and acidosis, neurologic compromise from a closed head injury, or poisoning.

BREATHING The process of *respiration* actually refers to our cellular engines (*mitochondria*) in which the consumption of oxygen and fuels (carbohydrates, fat) and production of energy and carbon dioxide (exhaust) allow us to cope with our environment and to grow and thrive. Cellular respiration requires homeostasis (balance and health), sufficient fuel intake, delivery (cardiac output and hemoglobin), and adequate mechanisms for getting oxygen in (oxygenation) and carbon dioxide out (ventilation) through the lungs (breathing).

The respiratory systems of the infant and child are poorly designed to handle an increased workload and thus are at a unique disadvantage when it comes to the mechanics of breathing when the lungs are sick. The paramedic should have a thorough knowledge and understanding of why that is, as this will allow for early recognition and management of pediatric respiratory distress and failure, which are the leading cause of hospitalization and the second-leading cause of death and disability in children. The significantly higher metabolic requirements of the infant and child make them unique from adults and more prone to fatigue and failure, with less ability to communicate their needs.

To elucidate the issues, consider the following case:

CASE STUDY

A three-month-old boy develops viral bronchiolitis during the winter, acquired from his two-year-old sister who attends day care; it starts with nasal congestion. With small nares with swollen mucosal lining and secretions, the increased resistance of breathing through his smaller nasal passages takes more energy. Because he is an obligatory nose breather and is literally not "wired" neurologically to be able to breathe through his mouth, this nasal congestion keeps him from being able to bottle-feed or breast-feed well. He becomes more tired as his energy stores are depleted and begins to get mildly dehydrated, which is made worse by his low-grade fever.

Both his heart and respiratory rates increase, requiring more energy from him. This leads to a vicious cycle, as his metabolic requirements for fuel, oxygen, water, and carbon dioxide removal all increase, placing larger and larger requirements on his already stressed cardiorespiratory system. He becomes more tired and begins to look lethargic, unable to cry or interact for very long. His wet diapers are much fewer in number, and he does not seem as interested in feeding.

As the viral infection moves down his respiratory tract, he begins to have trouble breathing because of the secretions and inflammation that are now affecting his bronchiolar tree. His coughing spells lead to more exhaustion, and his work of breathing increases even more to compensate. As his respiratory rate increases, so does his effort to inhale, as his lungs become heavier with mucus and fluid and his compliant chest wall does not give him any mechanical advantage the way a rigid, adult-like rib cage would.

His diaphragm-dependent breathing causes his sternum to retract because his ribs and sternum are mostly cartilaginous and are unable to expand in diameter with each inspiratory effort in the way adult rib cages do. In addition to the softer rib cage, infants' chests lack the normal bucket-handle movement of the adult rib cage, which also translates into an increase in thoracic and lung volumes in the adult.

His diaphragm has fatigue-prone muscles, as he will not develop a majority of type II, fatigue-resistant diaphragmatic muscles until he is as old as his sister. His accessory muscles (intercostals, shoulder girdle, and neck strap muscles) are also poorly developed, as he is not yet sitting up unassisted and only uses his shoulder and neck muscles with gravity from a supine position, not being old enough to roll over yet. His lung congestion worsens from the airway inflammation and mucus production, making him have to pull harder to get an adequate tidal volume.

His chest wall retracts with each breath, and he begins to laryngeal brake or "grunt" (it is impossible to do this quietly), closing off his glottis or vocal cords at the end of inhalation, bearing down with a Valsalva maneuver briefly before quickly exhaling and breathing in again. It is an extremely inefficient and only temporarily effective way of keeping his lung units from collapsing at the end of every breath.

This method of breathing—faster than normal, using what accessory muscles he has (mostly nasal flaring), sternally retracting and grunting—causes his normal oxygen requirements for breathing to go up by a factor of 5 to 10, leaving little oxygen reserve for anything else, such as attitude, interaction, crying, or physical activity.

The end result is an infant in severe respiratory distress and impending respiratory failure, with hypoxemia, hypercarbia, tachycardia, and tachypnea, resulting in respiratory and metabolic acidosis from dehydration. The infant will, from across the room, appear lethargic with decreased activity and tone, and without any attitude, and on exam will have all the preceding signs of increased work of breathing—until he cannot hold on anymore.

CIRCULATION Assessment of a child's circulatory system involves consideration of three essential elements that are in constant communication with each other: the pump (heart), the pipes (vasculature), and the fluid filling them (the blood volume). Dysfunction in any one of these will lead to the other two needing to compensate for it. The principles of circulation follow strict laws of nature. Most important is the Ohm law, in which Pressure = Flow × Resistance, which is the equation for blood pressure (BP = Cardiac Output × Systemic Vascular Resistance [SVR]), incorporating the three components (Cardiac Output = Heart Rate [HR] × Stroke Volume).

Volume Loss Take the most common form of shock, hypovolemic shock from bleeding or dehydration, as an example: Because the blood volume is low, the vasculature will clamp down to increase SVR, which will temporarily increase BP and the venous return to the heart (preload), which increases stroke volume and cardiac output. At the same time, the heart will pump faster to further increase cardiac output and maintain delivery of oxygen and life-sustaining nutrients to the tissues.

If these mechanisms are inadequate to compensate for the primary problem, the body will begin to shut down blood flow to nonvital organs, starting with the peripheral muscle beds of the arms and legs, by further increasing SVR until these extremities are cool to the touch, mottled in appearance, and pale. End-organ perfusion is affected with the findings of dry mucous membranes and low or no urine output. Because BP might be preserved, the rapid assessment of shock in a child involves tachycardia and these signs of compensatory increases in SVR.

A normal BP in a child with these findings is called *compensated shock*; this child requires emergent transport and advanced life support interventions. *Decompensated shock* refers to the late and preterminal phase when the BP starts to drop. Never wait for hypotension to begin rapid transport and intervention.

Pump Failure Primary pump dysfunction from a cardiomyopathy will lead to findings of increased heart rate and SVR, and poor end-organ perfusion. When the cardiac output is inadequate to keep up with the demands, these compensatory mechanisms ironically make matters worse. Increasing the metabolic needs of an already sick heart by increasing the rate and force with which it pumps while also increasing the load against which it has to pump (afterload) is a vicious cycle.

Cardiomyopathy can result from prolonged tachydysrhythmias such as supraventricular tachycardia (SVT), from viral infections of the myocardium, or from congenital heart disease. Because the myocardium is stiff and poorly contractile, increasing preload gently is important but aggressive fluid management is dangerous; decreasing heart rate and SVR is critical but requires specially trained pediatric practitioners.

Children with this form of shock require immediate care available in a children's hospital. As our ability to surgically treat congenital heart disease improves, more and more of these children are living to older ages and will be patients you will see.

Low Vascular Tone In this last example—distributive shock from sepsis, anaphylaxis, or a neurogenic etiology associated with a spinal cord injury—the problem is one of low vascular tone in which the body's catecholamines are unable to increase the SVR so vital to maintaining BP, perfusion, and preload to the heart. The heart rate will increase immediately (except in cases of spinal trauma), which is always the first sign and is never good, but the blood volume cannot increase by itself and will be distributed in a larger vascular bed, resulting in hypotension, a widened pulse pressure, and, paradoxically, skin that appears warm and well perfused.

In this situation, the child's appearance will be consistent with shock in that he will be lethargic, tachycardic, and tachypneic but not in respiratory distress, which is the child's attempt to remove carbon dioxide and compensate for the acid production from inadequate perfusion.

Rapid assessment of a child's circulation requires consideration of the three components of the circulatory system: the pump, the pipes, and the fluid in them. In all these categories, rapid transport and resuscitation are critical to outcome.

TREATMENT GUIDELINES AND PROTOCOLS

Thorough knowledge and understanding of pediatric emergency care will be reflected in an EMS service's patient care protocols. Although many protocols and guidelines are available on the Internet, going through the process of developing one's own set of protocols can be highly educational and empowering. Color-coded, length-based resuscitation tapes can form the foundation of color-coded guidelines for patients of different sizes and ages.

For advanced EMS providers, vascular access may be required on the pediatric patient. Access may be obtained through IV catheters or intraosseous (IO) insertion. Although IO is now widely used in the adult population, not long ago it was limited to the pediatric patient. The IO route is used in the critical patient when IV access cannot be obtained or would cause delay in care in the critically ill or injured pediatric patient. Fluid challenges are used in shock and are recommended at 20 mL/kg (10 mL/kg in infants). Follow local protocols for vascular access and fluid challenges.

Although ideally the EMS medical director should take the lead in the development and implementation of these guidelines, frequently this is not the case. EMTs and advanced providers should insist on some minimum treatment guidelines to handle the majority of pediatric calls: trauma (accidental and nonaccidental), respiratory distress, asthma, seizures, hypoglycemia, poisonings, cardiopulmonary arrest, environmental emergencies, and shock.

An essential component of any high-quality service is the use of quality improvement and case review strategies to analyze areas of weakness in education, equipment, systems of care, and other resources. It is important to ensure that the pediatric communities of interest, from the families to the hospital-based providers, are involved in the review process.

Pediatric Champion

It is recommended that an EMS service designate a "pediatric champion" who can serve as a resource for others in the department, keep an eye on the latest developments in prehospital pediatric management, serve as a liaison with the state Emergency Medical Services for Children (EMSC) program and the local community, develop and maintain treatment guidelines, and help facilitate continuing pediatric education.

REVIEW ITEMS

1. The Pediatric Assessment Triangle refers to what ABCs?
   a. attitude, behavior, consolability
   b. activity, breathing, cardiovascular
   c. appearance, breathing, circulation
   d. appearance, behavior, cuddliness

2. The equation for blood pressure is _____.
   a. BP = Stroke Volume × Heart Rate
   b. BP = Systemic Vascular Resistance × Heart Rate
   c. BP = Systemic Vascular Resistance × Stroke Volume
   d. BP = Systemic Vascular Resistance × Cardiac Output

3. The main reason that infants and children are poorly equipped to handle respiratory distress is because _____.
   a. their lungs are immature and airways are small
   b. after infancy, their immune systems are poorly developed
   c. their chest walls are so compliant that they cave in with the increased work of breathing

   d. they do not know how to cough effectively

4. Children with special health care needs are especially challenging primarily because _____.
   a. they frequently have conditions that require advanced life support (ALS) to manage
   b. their parents are often difficult to work with
   c. they are medically complex and frequently have baseline conditions that are very abnormal
   d. they cannot tell the paramedic what is wrong with them

5. The pediatric airway is different from the adult airway because _____.
   a. the child's tongue is proportionately smaller than the adult's
   b. the adult's head is bigger and neck is longer than the child's
   c. the child's airway structures are proportionately smaller
   d. the child produces more secretions

APPLIED PATHOPHYSIOLOGY

1. Differentiate between the Pediatric Assessment Triangle (PAT) and the adult primary assessment.

2. Explain why blood pressure is not the most critical finding in determining a shock state. Explain what vital signs are more important to assess in determining shock.

3. Explain the vicious cycle associated with respiratory distress that leads to failure in the pediatric patient.

4. Describe the signs and symptoms of respiratory distress.

5. Explain the difference between the presentations of respiratory distress and respiratory failure. What is the difference in emergency care?

6. Explain why children with special health care needs are most challenging to manage.

CLINICAL DECISION MAKING

You are called to the home of a three-year-old child with croup. She is sitting in her mother's lap and breathing quickly, with a respiratory rate of 50/minute, with audible inspiratory stridor. She is calm until you approach her, but when you get to within six feet of her, she begins to cry and her breathing becomes more audible and labored. She appears warm and well perfused, and her mother says she has had good liquid intake today but is not interested in solid foods. She has had some upper airway congestion but no fever. Her past medical history is unremarkable.

1. How would you describe her clinical condition? Stable? Urgent? Emergent?

2. Is her behavior normal for her age?

3. Is she in respiratory distress? Respiratory failure?

4. What are your treatment priorities?

Because her agitation makes her respiratory condition worse and her mother can calm her, you decide to let her mother hold her in her lap en route to the hospital. You secure her mother to your stretcher and have her hold her daughter in her arms.

5. Is this an appropriate arrangement in which to transport the child and mother?

Standard **Special Patient Populations**

Competency Integrates assessment findings with principles of pathophysiology and knowledge of psychosocial needs to formulate a field impression and implement a comprehensive treatment/disposition plan for patients with special needs.

TOPIC

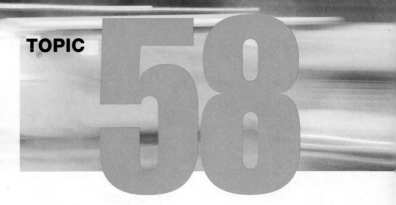

GERIATRICS

INTRODUCTION

A significant number of EMS calls you receive as an paramedic involve geriatric patients—understandably so, given that people over the age of 65 constitute the fastest-growing segment of population, and the largest users of health care, in the United States today. Therefore, it is important that you understand the characteristics of geriatric patients and how to tailor your assessment and treatment to their special needs.

Geriatric patients differ from their younger counterparts in many ways, largely owing to changes in physiology from lifestyle and aging. The geriatric patient often has very different signs and symptoms of an acute illness or traumatic injury as compared with younger patients. Compounding this is the fact that geriatric patients often have one or more coexisting long-term condition(s) that require multiple medications, which also affects how problems present.

The key to remember is that geriatric patients may not display common presentation patterns for emergency conditions that paramedics are called on to treat; as such, always maintain a high index of suspicion.

EPIDEMIOLOGY

Although it is not news that we are constantly aging, it is interesting to see *how* the population of the United States is aging. The elderly (those 65 years or older) numbered almost 40 million in 2008. This represented 12.8 percent of the U.S. population, or about one in every eight Americans. By 2030, this number will almost double, to more than 71 million elderly people. People over age 65 represented 12.4 percent of the population in 2000 but are expected to grow to 20 percent of the population by 2030.

Cardiovascular diseases, primarily heart attacks, are the leading cause of death in the elderly. Cancer is a close second, and strokes and chronic obstructive pulmonary disease (COPD) disorders comprise cause numbers three and four, respectively. The fifth-leading cause of death in the elderly is accidental injuries. The death rate per 100,000 population is three times higher for elderly victims of trauma than that for young adults, despite

TRANSITION highlights

- How the U.S. population is aging, and what percentage of the geriatric population uses health care services; incident rates for common chronic conditions as it pertains to the geriatric population.

- Pathophysiologic body changes that occur to geriatric patients:
  - Cardiovascular.
  - Respiratory.
  - Nervous.
  - Gastrointestinal.
  - Endocrine.
  - Musculoskeletal.
  - Renal.
  - Integumentary.

- Common assessment findings in geriatric patients and how to use a differential diagnosis process to determine the most likely field impression of the patient's emergency.

- Current treatment strategies for the geriatric patient with emphasis on supporting lost function.

the fact that trauma is thought of as a "young person's disease." Other chronic conditions present as well, but collectively they account for a minority of geriatric mortality. In addition, the elderly commonly have more than one chronic condition, and they use one-third of all prescription medications—an elderly patient takes, on average, 4.5 medications per day (▶ Figure 58-1).

The lesson to be learned is that elderly patients comprise a very significant percentage of calls seen by EMS providers. It behooves the paramedic to be familiar with the effects of aging on the body and how these effects manifest themselves during instances of injury or illness.

PATHOPHYSIOLOGY

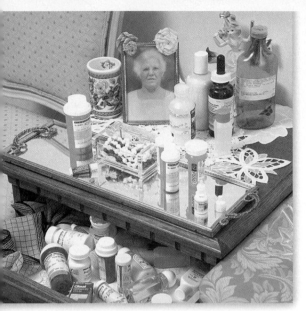

Figure 58-1 Elderly patients often take multiple medications.

The human body changes with age. As a person ages, cellular, organ, and system functioning changes. This change in physiology—which typically starts around age 30—is a normal part of aging. Although people may try to slow the aging process by diet, exercise, health care, and so on, it cannot be stopped entirely. To further compound the picture, most elderly patients will have not one but a combination of different disease processes in varying stages of development. Unfortunately, the aging body has fewer reserves with which to combat disease, and this ultimately contributes to the incidence of acute medical and traumatic emergencies.

It is important for the paramedic to understand and recognize changes in geriatric body systems so that appropriate care for elderly patients can be provided. Remember that the physiologic effects (summarized in **Table 58-1** and ▶ **Figure 58-2**) result from the normal aging process, not from disease progression per se. However, any disease or injury the patient experiences will only worsen—or be made worse by—these changes.

Cardiovascular System

With age, degenerative processes affect the ability of the heart to pump blood. Calcium is progressively deposited in areas of deterioration, especially around the valves of the heart. Damage to the valves of the heart caused by this degeneration can result in different problems. One problem is *stenosis* (narrowing of the

TABLE 58-1	Effects of Aging on Body Systems
Cardiovascular	The heart grows weaker even though it must pump against a higher resistance in the arteries, there may be abnormal heart rates or rhythms, the systolic blood pressure may start to rise because of increased arterial resistance to blood flow, and the blood vessels will not react as efficiently in response to brainstem stimulation that complicates blood pressure regulation during times of stress or emergency. Maximum cardiac output drops by 1 percent every year after age 35.
Pulmonary	The net effect of pulmonary changes in an elderly patient is that the body is less able to detect hypoxia or hypercapnia, less air enters and exits the lungs, less gas exchange occurs, the lung tissue loses its elasticity, and many of the muscles used in breathing lose their strength and coordination.
Nervous	As the nervous system fails, sensory functions diminish, reflexes become slower, proprioception diminishes, autoregulation of vegetative functions begins to fail, eyesight begins to fail, and pain perception diminishes, which can contribute to unrecognized injury or illness (such as heart attacks).
Gastrointestinal	Degeneration of the intestinal lining causes nutrients to be not as readily absorbed, which contributes to malnutrition. Fecal impaction and constipation are common because smooth muscle contractions of the large intestine diminish. Degeneration of the rectal sphincter muscle can also cause loss of bowel control. The liver does not function as effectively in metabolizing medications.
Endocrine	Changes to the endocrine system may cause fluid imbalance (resulting in either fluid retention or dehydration) and can alter the blood pressure (resulting in high or low blood pressure); changes in insulin secretion and effects may cause the blood sugar level to be elevated higher after a large meal and take longer to return to normal.
Musculoskeletal	The elderly are more prone to falls because of general weakness, worsening balance, and a loss in joint mobility; unfortunately, because of the changes in bone structure, these falls commonly result in skeletal fractures that take longer to heal than in younger people and may also contribute to medical emergencies.
Renal	Declining kidney function typically leads to a secondary disturbance in fluid balance and electrolyte distribution; because many drugs are filtered out by the kidneys, it is common for the elderly to suffer from drug toxicity if they take too much medication or take it too frequently. The geriatric renal system may be functional enough to meet the demands of the body on a day-to-day basis, but as a result of acute illness or injury the elderly patient's renal system may fail.
Integumentary	With injury, generation of new skin cells occurs less rapidly, so wounds heal slowly. Less perspiration is produced, and the sense of touch is dulled. As the skin ages, sores and tearing injuries tend to occur. This diminishes the effectiveness of the skin as a protective barrier in keeping microorganisms out of the body. Less subcutaneous fat leads to less protection against hypothermia.

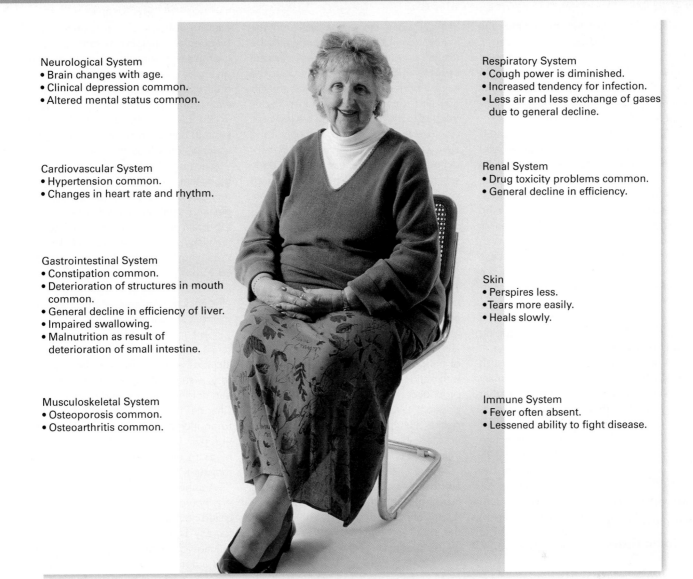

Neurological System
• Brain changes with age.
• Clinical depression common.
• Altered mental status common.

Cardiovascular System
• Hypertension common.
• Changes in heart rate and rhythm.

Gastrointestinal System
• Constipation common.
• Deterioration of structures in mouth common.
• General decline in efficiency of liver.
• Impaired swallowing.
• Malnutrition as result of deterioration of small intestine.

Musculoskeletal System
• Osteoporosis common.
• Osteoarthritis common.

Respiratory System
• Cough power is diminished.
• Increased tendency for infection.
• Less air and less exchange of gases due to general decline.

Renal System
• Drug toxicity problems common.
• General decline in efficiency.

Skin
• Perspires less.
• Tears more easily.
• Heals slowly.

Immune System
• Fever often absent.
• Lessened ability to fight disease.

Figure 58-2 Changes in the body systems of the elderly.

valve opening); another problem occurs when the valve fails to seal correctly, causing regurgitation (backward flow of blood).

With aging, fibrous tissue also begins to replace muscle tissue throughout the cardiovascular system. The walls of the heart generally become thickened without any increase in the size of the atrial or ventricular chambers. This thickening of the heart walls is known as *cardiac hypertrophy*. It causes a decrease in the stroke volume of the heart (because the heart is unable to hold as much blood), resulting in less blood being ejected from the heart with each contraction and a consequent decrease in cardiac output.

Another cardiovascular change that occurs as the body ages is that the arteries lose their elasticity (their ability to constrict and dilate easily), which creates greater resistance against which the heart must

pump. Widespread hardening of the arteries, or *arteriosclerosis*, tends to occur with age, which causes the arteries to become stiff and leads to further increases in the pressure the heart must pump against—and reducing cardiac output. This also leads to an increase in the systolic blood pressure with increasing age.

Compounding the stiffness of the arteries is a drop in baroreceptor sensitivity, which monitors the body's blood pressure. With a drop in baroreceptor sensitivity, it becomes harder for the geriatric patient to regulate blood pressure under normal circumstances as well as during emergencies.

Respiratory System

Changes in the aging respiratory system occur mainly as a result of alterations in the

respiratory muscles and in the elasticity and recoil of the thorax. Specifically, the size and strength of the muscles used for respiration decrease, and calcium deposits begin to form where the ribs join the sternum, causing the rib cage to become less pliable and increasing lung compliance. Diffusion of oxygen and carbon dioxide across the alveolar membrane decreases progressively as more and more alveolar surfaces degenerate.

Chemoreceptors located in the aortic arch, in the carotid bodies, and on the

> As the body ages, the arteries lose their elasticity, which creates greater resistance against which the heart must pump.

surface of the brainstem that monitor the levels of carbon dioxide and oxygen in the blood become less sensitive over time. This results in a relative inability to detect oxygen depletion (hypoxia) or increased carbon dioxide levels (hypercapnia) in the blood and tissues.

Airflow in and out of the lungs changes as well. In a younger person, the smaller airways (bronchioles) are supported by smooth muscle, which allows the bronchioles to keep their open shape so oxygen is easily inhaled with each incoming breath and carbon dioxide is easily exhaled with each exiting breath. With aging, both the number and size of these smooth muscle fibers that support the smaller airways decrease. The result is turbulent airflow, which diminishes air delivery to the terminal alveoli during inspiration and can result in air trapping during exhalation.

A number of pathologic diseases (such as COPD) aggravate this pulmonary decline. These factors become further exaggerated with the heightened respiratory activity needed during episodes of stress, shock, or pulmonary dysfunction from acute illness or injury (▶ Figure 58-3).

> **Sensory perception tends to diminish over time.**

The ability of the lungs to inhibit or resist disease and infection is also diminished with age. The cough reflex, which helps eliminate inhaled particles from the airway, may not trigger as readily, and the resulting cough may be less forceful because of the weakening muscles. The hairlike projections (cilia) that line the airway and help remove foreign particles trapped in the mucous lining are less able to move the material up and out of the airway. In addition, the nose and breathing passages secrete less of an antibody substance, which protects the body from viruses, into the mucus. Dehydration, common in the elderly, increases the tendency for respiratory infection as well.

Nervous System

The neurologic (nervous) system also becomes impaired by the normal effects of aging. Nerve cells (neurons) begin to degenerate and die as early as the mid-20s, and this ultimately impedes the ability of the body to adapt rapidly to changes within and outside the body. Reflexes slow, proprioception (sensing of one's body position) falters, sight diminishes (especially at night), and although hearing loss is not inevitable, the ability to discern higher-frequency sounds may slowly be lost.

The mass and weight of the brain actually decrease (atrophy), resulting in an increase in the amount of cerebrospinal fluid (CSF) to occupy the extra space in the skull. As brain neurons degenerate, waste products can collect in tissues, causing abnormal structures called *plaques* and *tangles* to form. As these changes from atrophy, plaques, and tangles take place, the overall ability of the brain to operate as it did when the person was younger becomes increasingly impossible (e.g., the ability of the elderly brain to control many of the body's processes becomes less efficient).

Because of changes that occur in the brainstem and other neurologic regulatory centers, the ability to perceive hunger and thirst are altered. The ability of the brain to monitor and regulate vital functions such as the rate and depth of breathing, heart rate, blood pressure, and core body temperature can become impaired and not operate with the same efficiency during stressful times as in the younger patient.

Sensory perception, as mentioned, tends to diminish as well over time; this includes everyday senses such as auditory, visual, olfactory, touch, pain, hot and cold sensations, and body position. Changes in both vision and balance lead to an increased incidence of falls in the elderly. Diminished tear production leads to eye irritation from inadequate moisture.

Another neurologic disorder is *peripheral neuropathy* (which is sometimes just called neuropathy); this is a generic term for any type of deranged or abnormal function of the peripheral motor, sensory, and autonomic nerve tracts. It could be *diffuse*, involving multiple neurons and nerve tracts that affect many parts of the body, or *focal*, involving neurons that affect a single, specific nerve and part of the body.

Gastrointestinal System

The sense of taste and smell is reduced in elderly patients, resulting in decreased food enjoyment (and possibly causing the person to stop eating regularly). Structures in the mouth deteriorate; periodontal disease can cause a loss of gum tissue and consequent tooth loss. Salivary flow lessens from degeneration of the salivary glands.

The smooth muscle contractions of the esophagus decrease, and the opening between the esophagus and the stomach loses tone, which can result in chronic heartburn as gastric acid enters the esophagus from the stomach.

The amount of hydrochloric acid secreted into the stomach also drops.

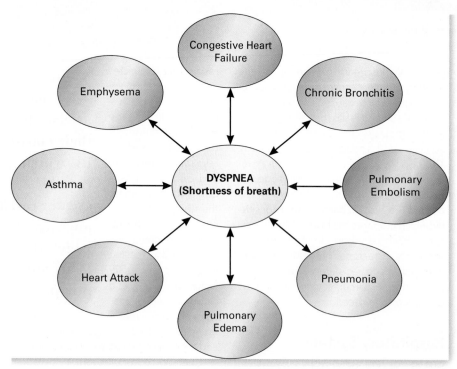

Figure 58-3 Common causes of dyspnea in the elderly.

This contributes to less efficient breaking down of ingested food before it enters the small intestine.

The liver decreases in size, weight, and function; this in turn decreases hepatic enzymes, causing a loss in the liver's ability to aid in digestion and metabolize certain drugs. This is further hampered by the drop in blood flow that occurs over time to the liver. Smooth muscle contractions (peristalsis) throughout the rest of the gastrointestinal tract diminish; therefore, it takes much longer for food to move through the system.

Because the lining of the small intestine degenerates, nutrients are not as readily absorbed, further contributing to malnutrition. Fecal impaction and constipation are common because smooth muscle contractions of the large intestine diminish. In some patients, degeneration of the rectal sphincter muscle can cause loss of bowel control.

Endocrine System

The progression of age-related changes of the endocrine system is unique. For most people, the changes in the endocrine system have no noticeable effect on overall health, but in some the changes may increase the risk of health problems (e.g., the changes in insulin effectiveness increase the risk of type 2 diabetes). Both hormone levels and target organ response are altered in the aging endocrine system.

Levels of certain hormones that elevate blood pressure (e.g., norepinephrine and vasopressin) can increase and contribute to hypertension, whereas other hormones that help regulate the body's fluid balance (such as renin and aldosterone) become deranged and contribute to fluid imbalance.

Furthermore, target organ response to beta adrenergic (sympathetic) stimulation in the heart and vascular smooth muscle decreases because of a loss of sensitivity of receptor cells. Aging produces mild carbohydrate intolerance and a minimal increase in fasting blood glucose levels from a drop in receptor cell responsiveness to insulin. Atrial natriuretic hormone (ANH) from atrial muscle tissue acts to help regulate water, sodium, potassium, and fat. The serum level of this hormone is also typically increased in the elderly and contributes to fluid imbalance. Aging also decreases the metabolism of thyroxine, a hormone that influences overall metabolic activity of the body.

Musculoskeletal System

The most significant musculoskeletal change resulting from aging is a loss of minerals in the bones, which is known as osteoporosis. This makes the bones more brittle and susceptible to fractures and slows the healing process. The disks located between the vertebrae of the spine start to narrow, which causes the characteristic curvature of the spine, seen in two out of every three elderly patients, known as kyphosis.

Joints begin to lose their flexibility with aging. The cartilage that covers the articular surfaces where joints meet begins to thin. The synovial fluid that surrounds these joints starts to thicken, causing joint stiffness. The ligaments that provide joints with stability start to weaken as well.

Renal System

The normal aging process also affects the renal system. The kidneys become smaller in size and weight because of a loss of the functional parts of the kidney, the nephrons. The effect is a decrease in the surface area of the kidney available to filter blood. The arterial system supplying the kidneys is also subject to the changes in the cardiovascular system, which results in a drop in renal blood flow. In combination, these changes result in a lesser amount of blood per minute passing through the kidneys for filtration, in addition to the decrease in available filtration surface area.

Because the kidneys play a vital role in fluid and electrolyte balance, kidney malfunction or injury typically leads to a secondary disturbance in fluid balance and electrolyte distribution. Because many drugs (including antibiotics) are filtered out by the kidneys, it is common for elderly patients to suffer from drug toxicity if they take too much medication or take it too frequently.

Integumentary System

Aging results in tremendous changes in the integumentary system (the skin). The skin becomes thinner from a deterioration of the subcutaneous layer, and less attachment tissue separates the dermis (inner layer) and epidermis (outer layer). An elderly person's skin is much more prone to injury than is the younger person's skin. Replacement cells are produced less rapidly, so wounds heal more slowly and skin is slow to replace itself.

Less perspiration is produced, and the sense of touch is dulled. In addition, the loss of subcutaneous fat results in less insulation against the cold and a higher incidence of hypothermia in the elderly. As the skin breaks down, sores and tearing injuries tend to occur. This diminishes the effectiveness of the skin as a protective barrier in keeping microorganisms out of the body.

ASSESSMENT FINDINGS AND DIFFERENTIAL CONSIDERATIONS

Because of the general decline in body systems, the elderly are prone to certain traumatic and medical emergencies that can cause rapid deterioration. As stated, aging may change the individual's response to illness and injury. For example, pain may be diminished or absent, and consequently the patient or paramedic may underestimate the severity of the patient's condition.

It is important that the paramedic be able to recognize these emergencies and provide appropriate emergency care. Having an understanding of what is occurring physiologically in these emergencies will help in recognizing and providing prompt, appropriate care. Table 58-2 is designed to assist you in interpreting several common complaints of the geriatric patient and differential field impressions that are consistent with them as you are completing your assessment. In addition, refer to the special considerations for scene size-up (Table 58-3) and for primary assessment (Table 58-4).

EMERGENCY MEDICAL CARE

Remember, a geriatric patient's condition can deteriorate rapidly. Therefore, it is critically important to anticipate problems and to continually reassess the patient. In the geriatric patient, the injury or failure of one body system can rapidly cause the failure of others. The following are key considerations and emergency care steps for the geriatric patient:

1. **Airway.** Geriatric patients often wear dentures; if these dentures become dislodged, they can create an airway obstruction. If necessary, suction and clear the airway immediately before assessing the breathing status. If the

TABLE 58-2 **Potential Differential Diagnoses Based on Clinical Findings in Geriatric Patients**

Clinical Finding	Changes Due to Altered Physiology	Common Assessment Findings	Potential Differential Diagnosis
Chest pain	• Altered pain perception, from neuropathies • Difficulty maintaining heart rate and regularity, from heart disease • Cardiac output lowered, from hypertrophy • Inability to maintain blood pressure regulation, from cardiovascular disease • Concurrent finding of dyspnea, from rapid onset of pulmonary edema • Acute decompensation, from failing body systems	• Severe, mild, or no chest pain • Respiratory distress • Weakness • Fatigue • Confusion • Dizziness • Nausea/vomiting • Aching shoulders • Abdominal pain	• Myocardial infarction (MI) vs. angina • Pleuritis • Pneumonia • Congestive heart failure (CHF) • Hypertensive disorder • Chronic obstructive pulmonary disease (COPD) • Pulmonary embolism • Gastrointestinal dysfunction • Possible recent thoracic injury or trauma
Dyspnea	• Failure to detect hypoxia or hypercapnia as readily because of failing chemoreceptors • Diminution in alveolar exchange cause by lowered tidal volume • Loss of alveoli decreases actual gas exchange • Weakening respiratory muscles contribute to rapid development of inadequate breathing	• Inability to speak in full sentences • Loss of alveolar breath sounds • Decreasing pulse oximetry • Vital sign changes • Crackles or wheezing • Possible fever • Altered mental status • Tachypnea, orthopnea • Tripod positioning • Sharp chest pain • Prolonged bed rest • Recent trauma • Gradual or rapid onset	• Asthma • Emphysema • Pneumonia • Pleurisy • Pulmonary emboli • Pulmonary edema • Chronic bronchitis • Spontaneous pneumothorax • Acute MI
Altered mental status	• Altered memory recall • Slowing of the reflexes • Global diminishing of the senses • Development of neurologic plaques and tangles that slow mental processing • Poor proprioception • Altered nutrition and thirst perception	• Mild to significant changes in mental status • Unresponsiveness • Headache • Changes in muscle coordination • Inequality of pupils • Changes in vital signs • Altered speech patterns • Seizures • Sensory loss • Changes in blood glucose level	• Cerebrovascular accident (CVA or stroke) or transient ischemic attack (TIA) • Syncope • Alzheimer disease • Drug overdose • Brain tumor • Hypertensive crisis • Seizure disorder • New/old brain injury • Electrolyte imbalance • Diabetic emergency • Dementia versus delirium • Thyroid disorder
Seizure	• Lowered seizure threshold with certain concurrent medical conditions • Increased risk of stroke or TIA • Changes in renal function cause electrolyte disturbance	• Tonic–clonic muscular activity • Tongue biting • Incontinence • Unresponsiveness • Changes in blood glucose level • Focal muscle spasms or hypertonicity	• Seizure disorder • CVA/TIA • Renal failure • Traumatic brain injury • Drug overdose • Infections • Electrolyte imbalance
Syncope	• Loss of normal autoregulation possibly leading to poor cerebral perfusion with sudden standing • Drop in cerebral perfusion caused by effects of drugs/meds	• Passing out after standing suddenly • History of strong emotional event • Possible loss of bowel/bladder control	• Seizure disorder • CVA/TIA • Drug overdose • Massive MI • Diabetic emergency • Cardiac arrhythmia

TABLE 58-2 (*Continued*)

Clinical Finding	Changes Due to Altered Physiology	Common Assessment Findings	Potential Differential Diagnosis
Drug toxicity (or overdose)	• Delayed gastric emptying • Forgetfulness regarding medication compliance • Renal and hepatic dysfunction lead to elevated blood levels	• Altered mental status • Seizures • Nausea • Vomiting • Vital sign changes • Diarrhea • Abdominal pain	• Diabetic emergency • CVA/TIA • Gastrointestinal emergency • Liver or kidney failure
Hypoperfusion	• Diminished cardiovascular performance • Failing pulmonary system • Hydration status usually diminished • Minor trauma can afflict multiple body systems negatively • Inability to aggressively counter acute illnesses or injuries from weak compensatory mechanisms • Side effects of medications	• Diminished orientation • Tachycardia • Normal to low blood pressure • Dyspnea • Poor peripheral perfusion • Diminished muscle tone • Tachypnea • Capillary refill >4 seconds • Skin cool and diaphoretic • Possible increased temperature (septic shock)	• Cardiogenic shock • Hypovolemic shock • Distributive shock

neck is stiff and not flexible enough to perform a head-tilt, chin-lift maneuver, perform a jaw thrust to establish a patent airway. Decreased range of motion in the neck may also make endotracheal intubation more difficult, as the sniffing position may be difficult to achieve. Take steps to properly pad and position geriatric patients prior to undertaking advanced airway procedures.

2. **Assess and be prepared to assist ventilations.** If the rate or depth is inadequate, initiate positive pressure ventilation immediately. Be careful not to ventilate the patient with excessive pressure or volumes, which could cause lung injury. Although loose dentures could cause an airway obstruction, if they are still firmly seated in the elderly patient in need of positive pressure ventilation, it

may be advisable to leave them in place. The dentures will help support the soft tissues around the mouth on which the mask of the ventilation device will be seated.

3. **Establish and maintain oxygen therapy.** Be sure to provide supplemental oxygen with positive pressure ventilation if the patient's breathing is inadequate. If the patient has adequate respirations, administer oxygen

TABLE 58-3   Clues to Illness Found in the Scene Size-Up

Clues	May Indicate
Bucket next to bed	The patient suffers from nausea and vomiting.
Hospital bed	The patient has no or limited mobility and a preexisting chronic illness.
Nebulizer setup	The patient has a chronic respiratory disease process.
Oxygen tank setup or oxygen concentrator	The patient has a chronic respiratory or cardiac disease.
Medications found at the scene	These may provide a clue as to the patient's preexisting condition(s).
Washcloth on the patient's forehead or near the patient	The patient has a severe headache or fever.
Patient in nightclothes in the middle of the afternoon	The patient has been sick all day.
Tripod position	The patient has significant respiratory distress.
Patient propped up on pillows	The patient has difficulty breathing when lying flat, commonly because of congestive heart failure.
A hot room temperature in the summer months	The patient has a possible heat emergency caused by dehydration or hyperthermia (elevated core body temperature).
A cold room temperature in the winter months	The patient has a possible cold emergency, hypothermia (decreased core body temperature).

TABLE 58-4	Special Considerations in the Primary Assessment of the Geriatric Patient
Chief complaint	The elderly patient may not complain of pain because of a preexisting central nervous system condition, such as stroke. However, any complaint of pain in the elderly must be taken seriously.
	Some elderly patients will not experience pain when suffering a serious condition, such as a heart attack, because of a disease process that affects the nerve endings. This is common in diabetic patients.
	Prickling and burning-type pain is usually caused by a condition affecting the superficial structures of the body, whereas an aching-type pain usually indicates that an organ is involved in the condition.
	Changes in the peripheral nerves in the skin can affect the elderly patient's ability to distinguish between hot and cold.
	A sudden loss of vision in one eye is not normal in the elderly and generally indicates a retinal artery occlusion or retinal detachment.
	Depression in the elderly is a serious complaint and must be managed properly. A depression state may cause the patient to not report or to minimize significant symptoms. The rate of suicide is high among the elderly.
	Alcohol abuse is more common in the elderly. Keep a higher index of suspicion and look for evidence of alcohol abuse in the scene size-up.
	Side effects of medications or interactions with other medications may cause the presenting signs and symptoms.
	Fainting may be a serious complaint associated with conditions affecting the brain, lungs, heart, or circulatory system, such as heart attack, pneumonia, blocked pulmonary artery (pulmonary embolism), shock, head injury or stroke, or congestive heart failure.
Mental status	Hypoxia causes agitation and aggression. High levels of carbon dioxide cause confusion and disorientation.
	A sudden onset of an altered mental status is not a normal part of aging and is not considered to be dementia. It is usually an indication of a serious illness or injury.
	Altered mental status may be caused by inadequate perfusion to the brain, hypoxia in the brain, dehydration, electrolyte disturbances, change in the blood glucose level, infection, cold emergency (hypothermia), stroke, head injury, tumors, drugs, or alcohol intoxication.
Airway	A reduction in the patient's reflexes may cause a high incidence of choking and aspiration of food or other substances.
	Cervical arthritis may make performing an effective head-tilt, chin-lift maneuver difficult because of the stiffness of the neck structures. A jaw-thrust maneuver may provide a better manual airway.
	Loose dentures may cause an airway obstruction. If the dentures are loose or poorly fitted, remove them. If the dentures are well fitted and snug in place, do not remove them. In a patient without dentures or teeth, it is much more difficult to get an effective mask seal if ventilation needs to be performed.
Breathing	Elderly patients have higher resting respiratory rates. A resting respiratory rate greater than 20 per minute may be completely normal.
	Elderly patients have lower tidal volumes. This can lead to early onset of hypoxia.
	Retractions are less likely to occur in the elderly because of the less elastic and compliant chest wall muscles.
Circulation	Elderly patients have higher resting heart rates, typically greater than 90 beats per minute, unless they are taking beta blockers.
	An irregularly irregular pulse (no regular rhythm or pattern) may be normal in an elderly patient.
Skin	The skin will normally appear to be dry and less elastic. Assessment of skin turgor in the elderly is not a reliable test of skin hydration. Inspect the inside of the mouth or under the lower eyelid to check for hydration status.
	Cold skin may indicate hypothermia, even when the elderly patient is found in the home. This is referred to as "urban hypothermia." A reduction in subcutaneous fat and skin vessel response may cause the body core temperature to decrease faster.
	Hot skin may indicate a heat emergency, such as heat stroke. Elderly patients are more prone to heat emergencies because of their inability to dilate the vessels to assist in cooling the body.
	Fever is less common in the elderly patient, even with serious infections.

if the SpO_2 is less than 95 percent or signs of hypoxia are present.

4. **Position the patient.** Exercise extreme caution when preparing the patient for transport, based on the type of emergency as outlined in the following guidelines:
   - If the emergency is medical in nature and the patient is alert and able to protect his own airway, place the patient in a position that is comfortable for him. This is typically a Fowler (sitting up) position.
   - If the patient has an altered mental status and is unable to protect his own airway, he should be placed in a left lateral recumbent position (recovery position) to prevent aspiration.
   - If spinal injury is suspected, the patient needs immediate stabilization of the spine during primary assessment, followed by immobilization to a long backboard. One limitation, however, is the geriatric patient with severe curvature of the spine caused by kyphosis. You may need to be creative and construct the cervical immobilization devices out of blankets to accommodate the curvature of the spine.
   - If the patient is unresponsive, assume a possible cervical spine injury and immobilize the patient fully as a precautionary measure.

5. **Intravenous access.** Obtaining access may be more challenging in the geriatric patient because of smaller, more fragile veins. Patients on warfarin may develop bleeding and hematomas at the IV start site. Finally, use caution when administering fluid boluses to patients with existing cardiac conditions, especially heart failure. IV access should be obtained en route in many cases.

6. **Medications.** Frequently, geriatric patients will have difficulty metabolizing administered medications because of decreased renal or liver function. If such history is present, beware of administering medications with a narrow therapeutic index, such as amiodarone and lidocaine. Normal doses of such medications can be rapidly toxic if the patient cannot process the medication normally. In some cases, half doses or longer administration times may be indicated. Follow local protocol.

7. **Transport.** Reassess the patient en route to the hospital, remembering that the geriatric patient's condition can rapidly deteriorate without warning.

To ensure appropriate care, reevaluate the geriatric patient frequently. The length of time spent with the patient or the condition of the patient will assist in establishing how to and how often to repeat the reassessment phase. Repeat and record the assessment at least every 15 minutes for a stable patient. If the patient is unstable, repeat and record at a minimum of every 5 minutes.

TRANSITIONING

REVIEW ITEMS

1. An elderly patient presents with a sudden onset of weakness, nausea and vomiting, dyspnea with inspiratory crackles, and an irregular heartbeat. This collection of findings may be representative of _____.
   a. a heart attack
   b. hypoglycemia
   c. seizures
   d. stroke

2. An elderly patient has fallen down three steps, which has resulted in a compound fracture of his left femur with heavy bleeding. On assessing the patient you find a blood pressure of 96/70, a heart rate of 88 beats per minute, respirations 22 per minute, and a pulse oximetry reading of 94 percent. Which of these described assessment findings *is not* consistent with hypovolemic shock but *is* consistent with geriatric trauma?
   a. blood pressure
   b. heart rate
   c. respiratory rate
   d. pulse oximetry reading

3. Failure of the chemoreceptors would lead to what disturbance in the geriatric patient?
   a. diminished perception of hypercapnia
   b. overproduction of insulin by the pancreas
   c. poor autoregulation of the systolic blood pressure
   d. increased intracranial pressure and diastolic hypertension

4. Which of the following is *not* an effect of aging that would contribute to the increased incident of falls in the elderly population?
   a. loss of proprioception
   b. kyphosis of the spine
   c. limited night vision
   d. atrophy of the brain

5. What medical emergency may present atypically in the elderly patient as a result of being diabetic with peripheral neuropathy?
   a. seizures
   b. syncope
   c. vertigo
   d. myocardial infarction

APPLIED PATHOPHYSIOLOGY

An elderly male patient was attempting to cross the street when he was stuck by a car traveling at a low rate of speed. The patient was thrown back about 4 feet and landed on his side.

1. Given the changes in the cardiovascular, pulmonary, nervous, and musculoskeletal systems, discuss how the patient may be at risk for significant trauma.

2. Discuss the differences in presentation that may occur in an 87-year-old patient suffering a heart attack compared with a 45-year-old suffering a heart attack.

CLINICAL DECISION MAKING

You are called for an "unknown unresponsive" elderly woman found by the driver for the meal-delivery service for the elderly. On your arrival, the police escort you into the house, where you find the patient lying unresponsive on the couch. It is midday, the ambient temperature is warm, and no sign of struggle is evident. The patient is alone, and no family members or friends from whom to gather information are present.

1. Based on the scene size-up characteristics, describe possible ways to learn about the patient's medical history.

2. For each body system (nervous, respiratory, cardiac, vascular, endocrine, etc.), list at least one differential diagnosis that could cause this unresponsiveness.

The primary assessment reveals the patient to be unresponsive to external stimuli. There is vomitus in the airway, breathing is slow and shallow, the heart rate is about 44 beats per minute and peripherally absent, and the skin is cool to the touch. The SpO_2 reading is 74 percent.

3. Of what life threats to the patient are you currently aware?

After managing and supporting the patient's lost function, further assessment reveals the pupils to be pinpoint, blood glucose level of 111 mg/dL, and the pulse oximeter increased to 94 percent with treatment. Breath sounds are bilaterally equal. No clinical findings of trauma are anywhere on the body. Your partner returns from the kitchen with a prescription bottle of Percocet (a narcotic pain medication) and a bottle of metoprolol (beta blocker), which was filled two days earlier. Both bottles are empty.

4. What conditions have you ruled out from your initial consideration in the scene size-up?

5. What conditions are you still considering as the possible cause? Would you add any conditions as a possible cause?

6. Explain the pathophysiologic cause for the following:
   a. Unresponsiveness
   b. Vomitus in the airway
   c. Poor peripheral perfusion but slow heart rate

During the secondary assessment, you learn from a family member who just arrived on scene that this patient had been upset the past week because of the recent death of her spouse. The pain pills, the person explains, were for a hip injury the patient suffered a few days earlier.

7. What conditions have you ruled out in your differential field diagnosis? Why?

8. What conditions are you considering as a probable cause? Why?

9. Based on your differential diagnosis, what are the next steps in emergency care? Why?

10. Explain how you came to a differential field diagnosis based on specific history and physical assessment findings.

Standard Special Patient Populations

Competency Integrates assessment findings with principles of pathophysiology and knowledge of psychosocial needs to formulate a field impression and implement a comprehensive treatment/disposition plan for patients with special needs.

TOPIC

59

PATIENTS WITH SPECIAL CHALLENGES

INTRODUCTION

Because of changes in medicine and lifestyle, the life span of Americans is increasing. Despite this, however, some people are still born with congenital defects, and some suffer significant trauma or endure critical illnesses that leave residual deficits.

In today's world, though, advances in medical care and medical technology allow people with certain deficits, who previously could only have been properly cared for within an extended care facility, to live at home (either independently or with family). Deficits that are compensated by medicine and technology could be as minimal as hearing impairment, or as advanced as mechanical ventilators for people who have lost the ability to breathe spontaneously.

There may be a mixing of lost function as well. For example, a patient who experienced severe brain trauma may be paralyzed on one side of the body and also may be unable to feed himself normally, so a feeding tube may be inserted into the abdominal wall.

Common causes of impairments include, for example, aging, birth defects, chronic illnesses, traumatic accidents, and abuse and/or neglect.

In your EMS career thus far, you have almost certainly encountered patients who have special medical challenges or whose lives are dependent on medical technologies. When their preexisting special challenges worsen, their medical devices fail, or they experience some other emergency independent of the chronic condition, EMS is the first one called to intervene.

The challenge to the paramedic is determining how to properly assess, intervene, and transport a patient with special challenges—especially in light of medical equipment or conditions that further complicate the situation—while still focusing on and treating the initial call for help.

EPIDEMIOLOGY

Trying to determine the number of people living in the United States with some type of special challenge is next to impossible, because there is neither a common registry for these individuals

TRANSITION *highlights*

- **Complexity of problems when people are living at home with medical technology or are victims of abuse.**

- **Pathophysiology of certain special challenges the patient may have, which necessitated the call to EMS:**
  - Abuse (children and the elderly).
  - Mental illnesses.
  - Disabilities:
    - ◆ Paralysis.
    - ◆ Obesity.
    - ◆ Traumatized patients.
  - Technology assistance/dependency:
    - ◆ Apnea monitors.
    - ◆ Tracheostomy tubes.
    - ◆ Continuous positive airway pressure (CPAP) and bilevel positive airway pressure (BiPAP).
    - ◆ Home mechanical ventilators.
    - ◆ Vascular access devices.
    - ◆ Dialysis.
    - ◆ Feeding tubes.
    - ◆ Intraventricular shunts.

- **Current treatment strategies for the special challenged or technology-assisted patient.**

nor a unified definition of what a "specially challenged" patient is. The number is large, however, as evidenced by the more than 74 million "hits" received in response to a recent Internet search for the term *specially challenged patient*.

Underreporting of abuse is also widespread. Many times, especially when the abused person lives at home with others, the victim is unable to report abuse to the authorities because the

Underreporting of abuse is widespread.

person's physical or mental conditions prohibit a call for help. Although this is not a total picture, it is known that more than 3 million children are victims of abuse annually, more than 560,000 cases of elder abuse are reported in the United States every year, and 3 to 4 million people are victims of spousal or partner abuse annually.

Finally, more than 8 million disabled patients are receiving health care from professional providers, and it is estimated that millions of others receive care from family members or volunteers. In sum, given these numbers, this is not a statement of "*if* you will have a specially challenged patient" but rather "*when* you will."

PATHOPHYSIOLOGY

A person may be receiving care at home for any of multiple reasons. Perhaps the patient's condition is not severe enough to warrant admission into a hospital or rehabilitation center. Perhaps the patient's status or condition is expected to improve over time, and he wants to be with his family. Some patients, however, have conditions that will not improve, but they want to live at home and, with the help of medical technology, they can do so with the greatest degree of normalcy possible.

Although the patient's primary care providers are usually knowledgeable about the equipment or technology being used, they may not be as well versed in what to do if that equipment fails or the patient's status begins to deteriorate.

Although it is impossible to discuss everything that you may encounter regarding special needs patients, this topic is intended to provide you with the knowledge and the mental processing required to meet the needs of abused patients, mentally retarded patients, and patients with disabilities. Tertiary care hospitals that care for such patients often maintain an on-call person for specialized conditions and/or equipment.

Abuse

Child abuse occurs when a child falls victim to abuse or neglect. In fact, child abuse has been the only major cause of infant and child death to increase in the past 30 years. It ranges from actual physical and emotional harm to neglect of the body's basic needs. The abuser is not necessarily the parent and can be a babysitter, foster parent, sibling, stepsibling, stepparent, or anyone else responsible for the child's care.

Generally, child abuse falls into one of three categories: physical abuse (which can include neglect), emotional abuse, and sexual abuse. *Physical abuse* occurs when improper or excessive action is taken that injures or causes harm. *Neglect* is the provision of inadequate attention or respect to someone who has a claim to that attention. *Emotional abuse* occurs when a child is regularly threatened, yelled at, humiliated, ignored, blamed, or otherwise emotionally mistreated. *Sexual abuse* occurs when a child is subject to an older child's or adult's advances of a sexual nature and can include both contact and non-contact events.

Elder abuse may occur in care centers and other medical institutions, but it can also occur at home. Any elderly person is especially at risk if he is cared for by someone who is under stress from other sources. Abuse of the elderly can occur in many forms and can include neglect, physical abuse, sexual abuse, financial abuse, and/or emotional and mental abuse. At highest risk are elderly patients who are bedridden, demented, incontinent, frail, or experiencing disturbed sleep patterns (▶ **Figure 59-1**).

Elder abuse in the form of neglect is similar to pediatric neglect: It is the care provider's withholding of attention or medical care to which the victim is entitled. This type of neglect could occur passively or actively, the difference being the intent of the care provider. In situations of *active neglect*, the care provider intentionally fails to meet the obligations to the elderly victim.

In *passive neglect*, the failure is said to occur unintentionally and is often the result of the care provider's feeling overwhelmed by the needed tasks. Regardless of the reason, this type of neglect could be manifested as failure to provide adequate nutrition or hydration, to provide medications or access to medical services when warranted, or to care for personal hygiene. The development of bedsores because the care provider is not turning the patient as needed to prevent the breakdown of the skin is also a form of passive neglect.

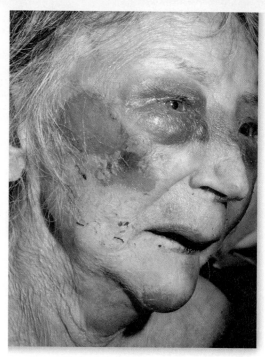

Figure 59-1 Physical abuse of an elderly person can have dire consequences because of the patient's frailty.

Physical abuse can involve the hitting, restraining, shaking, or shoving of an elderly patient. Because of elderly patients' frail status, the injuries sustained from these attacks can be significant.

Sexual abuse is said to occur when unwanted or unwarranted advances of a sexual nature (either through body contact or exposure) are made to which the older person does not or cannot consent.

Financial abuse consists of the care provider exploiting the material possessions, property, credit, or monetary assets of the elderly patient for his own personal gain.

With *emotional/mental abuse*, psychological distress or mental harm is inflicted on the elderly patient through verbal assaults, verbal insults, threats of physical harm, or simply ignoring the patient.

Mental Illnesses

Mental (or emotional) illnesses can present as unique challenges to the paramedic. The impairment that the patient demonstrates may range from being so mild that it is almost imperceptible to being significant enough that communicating with the patient is almost impossible. Generally, though, the term *mental retardation* encompasses disabilities that affect the nervous system and typically

TABLE 59-1 Causes of Mental Retardation

Down syndrome	This is a disorder in which the patient is born with an extra 21st chromosome. The disability usually results in characteristic facial features well as learning disabilities and multiple physical problems (heart, vision, intestinal, lung).
Fragile X syndrome	This disorder is the second most common inherited form of mental retardation. The result is the body's inability to produce a certain protein needed for normal brain growth and development. Patients with fragile X syndrome also have characteristic facial features and severe mental retardation. Over time, the person may also present with cardiac, behavioral, speech, and motor abnormalities.
Autism	Autism is a genetic-based developmental disorder of the brain, which results in mild to significant impairment of social interaction and communication skills. Although the cause is still being debated, it is usually suspected by the parents when the child fails to reach developmental milestones.
Fetal alcohol syndrome	This is caused by excessive alcohol consumption by the mother during pregnancy. It is occasionally confused with Down syndrome, as patients with both syndromes have similar facial features. A patient with this disorder often displays mental disabilities, hyperactivity, and delayed physical growth.
Phenylketonuria (PKU), hypothyroidism	These are both metabolic disorders that can affect how the body processes materials needed for functioning. In both these conditions, the abnormal metabolic activity of the body results in mental retardation and other cognitive and behavioral deficits.
Rett syndrome	This syndrome, which afflicts females almost exclusively, is characterized by a genetic mutation of the X chromosome. The child usually displays normal early development, but this is followed by progressive loss of purposeful motion, inability to speak, behavioral disorders, abnormal skeletal growth, and loss of motor skills previously acquired.

have a negative impact on intelligence level and how the person learns. These disabilities may also cause problems such as speech impediments, behavioral disorders, language difficulties, and some movement disorders. **Table 59-1** describes some of the more common causes of mental retardation.

Disabilities

The term *disabilities* is often used as an encompassing label that includes impairments, activity limitations, and participation restrictions. The medical model for "disabilities" views it as a problem of the patient that was caused by disease, trauma, inheritance, or other factors that necessitate sustained medical care for the individual. As such, trying to discuss all the disabilities known to medicine far exceeds the intent of this topic.

As an alternative, what will be discussed are the more common disabilities that can or may result in acute deterioration of the patient or leaves him dependent on medical technology—either way, the patient's deterioration or equipment malfunction necessitates the summoning of EMS to treat the patient. In these situations, the intent is not to diagnose the disability and provide curative care but rather to recognize the dysfunction caused by the disability and provide supportive care to the body system that is failing.

Paralysis refers to the complete loss of function in one or more groups of muscles. Paralysis is caused by damage or dysfunction of the nervous system (especially the spinal cord) or the brain. Common causes for paralysis include trauma to the head, spinal cord, or vertebral column. Strokes can also cause residual paralysis when the area of the brain that controls certain muscle groups is damaged.

Neuromuscular diseases can also result in paralysis that typically originates in the extremities and progressively causes weakness and paralysis to the muscles of the trunk and respiratory system. Common diagnoses include amyotrophic lateral sclerosis, Guillain-Barré syndrome, muscular dystrophy, poliomyelitis, myasthenia gravis, and multiple sclerosis.

Patients who are paralyzed are susceptible to multiple other problems as well. For example, if the paralysis involves the respiratory muscles, the patient may be ventilator dependent. Patients with paralysis also have frequent respiratory infections resulting from the inability to cough and clear out inhaled debris from the airway. They are also susceptible to urinary tract infections (totally paralyzed patients are routinely catheterized).

In addition, because they are wheelchair confined or bedridden, paralyzed patients may develop pressure necrosis (bedsores) over the bony areas of the body. If a feeding tube is inserted, the insertion site may become infected or the tube may become occluded. Secondary emergencies from this can include sepsis, dyspnea, chest pain, open soft tissue deterioration, unrecognized injury, and many other problems.

Obesity is a definite concern in the United States today. It is estimated that more than 40 percent of people in the United States are obese. In addition, obesity is the second leading cause of preventable death today, after smoking. Long-term body deterioration from obesity can result in coronary heart disease, type 2 diabetes, immobility, sleep apnea, and hypertension, to name a few problems—all of which can reduce the life span of the patient should no corrective measures be taken (see Table 59-2).

Obesity can occur for a number of reasons. Whereas the short explanation is that the patient is consuming more calories than he is burning (i.e., overeating with a sedentary lifestyle), obesity can be caused by physiologic problems as well. For example, a patient with hypothyroidism may have a lowered metabolic rate, which means he burns calories more slowly.

Some medications, such as central nervous system (CNS) depressants and anticonvulsant medications, can lower the metabolic rate and contribute to weight gain. Genetic factors have been cited as contributing to obesity in some people as well. It has also been noted that obese people tend to form relationships with each other, and their children are often obese as well (be it from genetics, predisposition, or lifestyle).

Traumatized patients are another type of specially challenged patient for whom

TABLE 59-2   Effects of Excess Weight on Organ Systems

Organ System	Disease State
Cardiovascular	Hypertension, coronary artery disease, congestive heart failure, cerebrovascular accident
Respiratory	Obstructive sleep apnea, asthma, chronic obstructive pulmonary disease
Endocrine and reproductive	Diabetes mellitus, infertility, birth defects, menstrual disorders
Gastrointestinal	Esophageal reflux, liver disease
Musculoskeletal	Osteoarthritis, gout, back injuries, immobility
Psychological	Depression, suicide

> **Head trauma can easily result in a multitude of residual disabilities.**

the paramedic may be called on to care. Head trauma (or more specifically, brain trauma) in patients can easily result in a multitude of residual disabilities. The disability may be mild, such as changes in speech pattern or mild cognitive changes, or can be so severe as to leave the patient unresponsive to external stimuli and dependent on ventilators for breathing; feeding tubes for nutrition; and care providers for day-to-day washing, turning, and bedding changes. Most previous head injury patients, though, fall somewhere between those two extremes.

Trauma to the brain can occur at any age and may result in permanent damage, as evidenced by changes in cognition, learning abilities, emotional abilities, and/or muscle weakness or paralysis.

Technology Assistance/ Dependency

Whereas some medical equipment is designed to enhance the quality of life and allow patient independence (e.g., feeding tubes or urinary catheters), other medical equipment found in the home setting actually sustains life (e.g., mechanical ventilators). As a paramedic, you must remain abreast of current home medical care and equipment, as it is common for EMS to be summoned to a patient whose home medical equipment has failed or is no longer able to support the patient's vital functions.

Apnea monitors are designed to constantly monitor the patient's breathing sta-

tus and then emit a warning signal should breathing cease. Some are also designed to monitor the heart rate, as changes in the heart rate may signal failure of the respiratory system. This type of equipment is commonly found in a home with an infant, especially a newborn who was born prematurely. These devices will emit a loud piercing sound to signal a problem and often will emit a series of beeps indicating how long the machine has been alerting.

Tracheostomy tubes (▶ Figure 59-2) are used when it becomes necessary to provide a new surgical opening for the airway in patients with certain medical and/or traumatic conditions. More specifically, a tracheostomy is a surgical opening through the anterior neck and into the trachea that serves as an alternative site for air entry and exit from the body (bypassing the mouth and nose). The site for this surgical opening is usually the inferior trachea, somewhere near the second through fourth tracheal ring anteriorly.

A tracheostomy may be used as a permanent opening and is then referred to as a *stoma*. This technique is commonly performed for patients who have either long-term upper airway problems or medical conditions that result in long-term dependence on mechanical ventilation.

Continuous positive airway pressure (CPAP)

and *bilevel positive airway pressure* (BiPAP) machines are both designed to provide a therapeutic back-pressure during exhalation via an airway circuit attached to a mask that covers the mouth and/or nose. Whereas the CPAP device provides a constant positive pressure during the entire ventilatory cycle, the BiPAP machine provides a higher pressure during inhalation and a lower pressure during exhalation.

The primary therapeutic goal of both devices is to keep the small bronchiole airways open during exhalation, which in turn improves both oxygenation and ventilation; it also lowers the work of breathing. These devices are commonly used on patients with sleep apnea or certain chronic lung diseases. Some CPAP and BiPAP machines also allow the administration of oxygen during use.

Home mechanical ventilators are designed to assist a patient who cannot breathe adequately on his own. The patient may have any one of several reasons to be dependent on a ventilator, but these causes typically center around either the brain's inability to initiate a spontaneous breath, a structural defect of the thorax or lungs that prohibits or greatly diminishes normal gas exchange, or a disease process that renders the respiratory muscles of the body useless, most commonly spinal cord injury.

Commonly, the responding paramedic will learn the exact reason for the ventilator dependency while ascertaining the

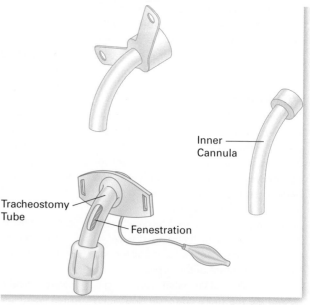

Inner Cannula

Tracheostomy Tube

Fenestration

Figure 59-2 A tracheostomy tube for older children and adults has an outer cannula and an inner cannula.

patient's medical history. Causes include (but are not limited to) a history of a debilitating stroke, brain damage following head trauma, long-term pulmonary problems (e.g., chronic obstructive pulmonary disease [COPD] or lung cancer), and neuromuscular diseases.

The two types of ventilators are negative pressure ventilators and positive pressure ventilators. *Negative pressure ventilators*, such as the "iron lung," encircle the patient's chest and generate a negative pressure around the thoracic cage. The negative pressure created by the devices draws out the rib cage, which, in turn, creates a negative intrathoracic pressure, thereby causing air to be drawn into the lungs.

The most commonly encountered mechanical ventilators, though, are *positive pressure ventilators*, which push air into the airway (i.e., positive pressure), much like the EMS provider who squeezes a bag-valve mask. Exhalation then ensues when the positive pressure stops, and the chest wall and lungs recoil.

Home ventilation units typically have two or three controls: one is for the ventilatory rate, one is for adjusting the size of each breath (i.e., tidal volume), and some units may have one control that adjusts the amount of oxygen that is provided during ventilation if so required by the patient. Tidal volume in most ventilators is adjustable, whereas the ventilatory rate and oxygen supply (if so equipped) may be either fixed or adjustable. The ventilator is attached to the patient by large-diameter tubing, referred to as the ventilator circuit.

Ventilators may also have several alarms that help the primary care provider identify whether the ventilator is functioning properly. In fact, EMS may be summoned to care for a patient when one of these alarms alerts a warning. Because of variances in the device, the particular ventilator your patient uses may or may not have the following alarms:

- **High-pressure alarm.** A high-pressure alarm is activated when the pressure needed to cause lung inflation exceeds the present value. This can be from increased airway resistance caused by increased secretions (mucus plugs) occluding the tracheostomy tube, kinking of the ventilator circuit, movement of the tracheostomy tube, bronchospasms, or the patient coughing during inspiration. The alarm can also be triggered by decreased lung

compliance. Causes of decreased lung compliance include the development of a pneumothorax, progressive pneumonia, acute pulmonary edema, or alveolar collapse (atelectasis).

- **Low-pressure alarm.** The low-pressure alarm is usually set to activate when the tidal volume falls 50 to 100 mL below the set tidal volume. This usually indicates a problem in the breathing circuit, such as a disconnected segment or a leak in the cuff of the tracheostomy tube.

- **Apnea alarm.** A patient on a ventilator may still have some respiratory effort, but it is inadequate to sustain life. As such, the home ventilator may not trigger a breath until the patient starts to breathe in. In these models, the apnea alarm sounds when the patient stops breathing. Causes are usually physiologic and include decreased mental status, overmedication, and respiratory muscle fatigue.

- **Low FiO_2.** A low fraction of inspired oxygen (FiO_2) alarm will occur when the oxygen source is disconnected or depleted.

Vascular access devices (VADs) are devices that are used when a patient is in need of ongoing intravenous medications. Usually VADs are placed in a surgically created pocket under the surface of the skin in patients who are in need of medication for longer than seven to ten days, but they may also be needed on a long-term basis as well (▶ Figure 59-3). The type and duration of use of the device is largely dependent on the medical needs and disease process for which the patient is being treated.

Annually, more than 500,000 devices of this nature are in use. They are typically placed in patients who have ongoing chemotherapy, peritoneal dialysis, hemodialysis, total parenteral nutrition (TPN), and antibiotic therapy needs.

As a paramedic, your system may allow you to administer medications and fluid via VADs. Know that these devices require specific training that is beyond the scope of this topic. Always follow local protocol

Ventilators may have alarms to help the primary care provider identify whether the ventilator is functioning properly.

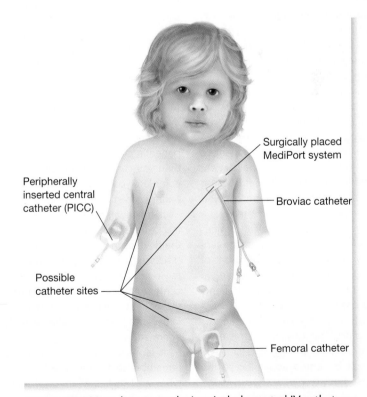

Figure 59-3 Vascular access devices include central IV catheters such as a PICC line, central venous lines such as the Broviac catheter, and implants ports such as the MediPort system.

Peripherally inserted central catheter (PICC)

Possible catheter sites

Surgically placed MediPort system

Broviac catheter

Femoral catheter

and use these access sites only if you are specifically trained and comfortable with the procedure. Do not initiate an IV in an arm that contains a vascular device (shunt).

Dialysis is a medical procedure designed to support the lost function of the kidneys, although total replacement of all renal functions is not possible. Dialysis removes the buildup of toxins that occurs when the kidneys can no longer filter out these toxins. *Hemodialysis* is the type of dialysis in which blood is extracted from the body and sent through a dialyzer. The *dialyzer* filters the blood from the body via a membrane that also uses a dialysate fluid to help cleanse the blood. Following the cleansing process, the blood is returned to the body.

The process takes anywhere from two to five hours for ongoing removal of blood for filtration, followed by the filtered blood being returned to the body. Dialysis typically occurs in a dialysis center and must be repeated two or three times per week.

Peritoneal dialysis is another type of dialysis that is done in the home or the extended care facility. With this type of dialysis (which the paramedic is more likely to encounter), dialysate fluid that contains glucose and minerals is instilled via gravity into a port that leads into the peritoneal cavity. The fluid then surrounds the intestines, where it interacts with the body to remove waste products. After a specific amount of time, the fluid is removed from the abdominal cavity and replaced with fresh fluid.

Because this form of dialysis is not as effective as hemodialysis, it must be repeated several times a day. However, owing to current technology, the procedure is relatively easy for the patient to perform and, thus, allows the patient greater freedom in daily activities because he is not bound to several long appointments a week at the dialysis center.

Feeding tubes are medical devices that provide nutrition to patients who cannot chew and/or swallow because of medical conditions or trauma resulting in paralysis or unconsciousness. Patients receiving their nourishment this way are said to be receiving *enteral feeding* or *tube feeding.* The device is typically a flexible tube that is long and small in diameter. It is named according to the site of insertion. If it is inserted through the nose and ends in the stomach, it is a *nasogastric tube,* or *NG-tube.* If the tube is inserted through the mouth and to the stomach, it is an *orogastric tube,* or *OG-tube.* Some feeding tubes are inserted through the skin into the stomach (G-tubes) or jejunum (J-tubes).

Intraventricular shunts are used mainly in pediatric patients who have medical illnesses or anatomical defects that result in either the overproduction of cerebrospinal fluid (CSF) in the brain, inadequate reabsorption of CSF, or irregular flow of CSF through the ventricles and/or meningeal layers. When excess CSF accumulates, the patient is said to have *hydrocephalus.*

Regardless of the reason for the hydrocephalus, because the skull is a fixed size and cannot expand to accommodate the extra fluid, the pressure within the skull (intracranial pressure [ICP]) builds, which can then result in compression of brain tissue. To alleviate the rising ICP, a *shunt* (a long, hollow, tubelike device) is surgically placed. It originates within a ventricle of the brain and extends to a blood vessel in the neck, heart, or abdomen to drain extra CSF and keep the ICP within an acceptable level. In some patients, responding paramedics may also find a reservoir on the side of the skull, placed beneath the scalp, which collects the excess CSF for laboratory testing purposes.

ASSESSMENT AND MANAGEMENT

Unless you are caring for the patient in some type of medical facility, specialized residential facility, or group home, if the patient is unresponsive it may be difficult to recognize or get information regarding many of the aforementioned conditions or types of medical equipment. If the patient's clinical status is mild, however, then you can usually obtain a history and complete your physical exam because the patient can still communicate with you.

If, however, during your assessment of the patient, you start to identify some of the developmental or cognitive problems discussed previously, or if the patient is relying on medical equipment and is non-communicative, you will need to rely on the patient's primary care provider (be it family or professional heath care) for your information.

It is important for the paramedic to remember that it is impossible to cover all types and makes of medical technology used in the home; therefore, the paramedic should always approach the patient or caregiver and ask the following questions to help determine the best course of action for ongoing assessment and care:

- Where would I get the best information regarding this piece of equipment?
- What does this device do for the patient?
- Can I replicate its function should the device fail? Remember that the most important support is to the airway or ventilation.
- Will this equipment have an effect on how I assess the patient or on the findings I may discover?
- Has this problem ever occurred previously, and if so, what fixed it?
- Has anyone attempted already to remediate the problem?
- Are there specific considerations I need to make when deciding how to best prepare the patient for movement and transport him?

You may also need to rely on the care provider to obtain the patient's medical history and information about any care that has been provided thus far relative to the current emergency. During your assessment of the patient with special challenges, incorporate the following treatment interventions as appropriate:

1. **Ensure scene safety.** Although not a patient care step per se, the paramedic must always ensure the safety of himself and his crew when responding to any call.

2. **Consider spinal immobilization.** The patient with special challenges may have fallen; therefore, immobilization may be warranted. Because the patient may have other skeletal abnormalities (e.g., kyphosis) that preclude normal immobilization techniques, be sure to use padding to align and secure the patient to the best of your ability.

3. **Assess the airway.** Carefully assess the airway to ensure that it is clear from any blood, vomitus, heavy secretions, or other fluids. Sometimes people with special challenges cannot chew food or swallow well, and the paramedic may find partially chewed food occluding the airway. If this is the case, progressively treat the airway occlusion until it is removed (suctioning, manual techniques, simple mechanical techniques, advanced mechanical

techniques). In obese patients, extra adipose tissue in the cheeks, lower jaw, and anterior neck places pressure on the tongue and airway structures, causing closure. Position these patients with a towel behind the shoulder blades to facilitate an open airway (if no cervical problems are suspected). If the patient has a stoma, use a French catheter to suction it out should it be occluded with mucus or secretions.

4. **Assess the breathing.** The critical question here is to ascertain whether the patient is breathing adequately. Assess for chest rise and fall, listen to alveolar breath sounds, and note the patient's speech patterns (if the patient is able to talk). A patient who has good alveolar breath sounds, has normal chest excursion, and is speaking in full sentences is still breathing adequately. If the patient is on a mechanical ventilator, use the same parameters (chest excursion and breath sounds) to ascertain whether it is still ventilating properly. If it is not, consider using your own mechanical ventilator if you are equipped with one, or use a bag-valve-mask (BVM) device to replace the ventilator. Exercise extreme caution to ensure that you are ventilating at an appropriate rate and depth. If the patient has a stoma, use a pediatric mask attached to the BVM and ventilate over the stoma. If a tracheostomy tube is placed in the stoma hole, attach the BVM directly to this (▶ **Figure 59-4**). You may need to seal the mouth and nose should the glottic opening still be patent.

5. **Assess central and peripheral circulation.** Assess the patient for adequate or inadequate peripheral perfusion following normal assessment techniques. Also assess for indications of hemorrhage if the patient is a victim of trauma or is relying on some medical equipment (e.g., urinary catheters or VADs) that has somehow dislodged, causing local trauma or bleeding. Treat the patient with a hemorrhage as you normally would, consider any patient with indications of poor peripheral perfusion to be unstable, position him appropriately, and keep him warm.

6. **Complete the secondary assessment.** After managing any lost function to the airway, breathing, and circulation in the specially challenged patient, complete a secondary assessment to note whether any other minor conditions are present (treating them appropriately as well). During the secondary assessment, note any signs of abuse and learn as much as you can about any medical technology on which the patient is reliant. Be careful when preparing the patient for movement to the ambulance, and make allowances for proper handling of the patient's medical equipment. Typi-

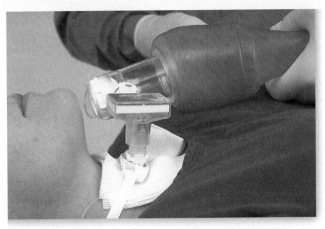

Figure 59-4 The paramedic can ventilate a patient with a tracheostomy by attaching the bag-valve device to the tracheostomy tube's 15/22 mm adapter.

cally, your on-scene time with specially challenged patients is longer than for nonchallenged patients because of the additional time needed for assessment and proper packaging for transport.

Overall, the care you render for specially challenged patients will depend on the condition(s) for which you were summoned. Most tertiary centers have a program to educate local EMS on special needs patients who are released to the community (e.g., VAD patients) and have consultative services for these patients. Always remember, though, to maintain an open and patent airway, ensure that breathing remains adequate, and make sure peripheral perfusion is intact. Consider summoning advanced life support (ALS) for a patient who is critically unstable or deteriorating. Become familiar with the medical technology on which the patient may be relying, and provide careful and expedient transport to the hospital.

TRANSITIONING • • • • • • • •

REVIEW ITEMS

1. You arrive on scene for a patient with an altered mental status. You note during your physical exam that the patient has a VAD placed beneath the skin in the upper left thoracic region. Knowing this, what can you conclude about the patient's medical history?

    a. The patient has a pulmonary dysfunction.

    b. The patient is suffering from cancer.

    c. The patient is likely terminal and probably has a do not resuscitate (DNR) order.

    d. The patient's medical condition warrants ongoing medication injections.

2. A two-year-old male patient has a history of hydrocephalus, and the parents state that the boy's mental status has been continually deteriorating over the past eight hours. What might be a cause for this?

    a. There is likely bleeding into the brain tissue.

    b. The shunt is probably blocked and the ICP is increasing.

c. Because of the medical history, the child's electrolytes are deranged.

d. The child may be suffering from ongoing child abuse.

3. A morbidly obese patient is found supine and unresponsive in his home. You hear loud sonorous airway sounds with each breath. What action should you take next?

   a. Position some folded towels between the shoulder blades.

   b. Provide endotracheal intubation with an appropriate-size ET tube.

   c. Initiate positive pressure ventilation at 12/minute with 100 percent oxygen.

   d. Suction out the airway with a rigid-tip catheter, then provide positive pressure ventilation.

4. Your patient has a history of a traumatic injury that has left him completely paralyzed. What type of medical equipment will he most likely be dependent on for survival?

   a. VAD   b. apnea monitor

   c. peritoneal dialysis   d. mechanical ventilator

5. A patient who uses a CPAP or BiPAP machine will likely have what type of medical history?

   a. sleep apnea   b. renal failure

   c. traumatic brain injury   d. neuromuscular disease

APPLIED PATHOPHYSIOLOGY

A patient has been diagnosed with a neuromuscular disease that has left him dependent on care providers for ongoing care. The patient is ventilator dependent, has a feeding tube inserted, and has a urinary catheter placed.

1. Given this history, what other clinical conditions is he at risk for developing that may result in the summoning of EMS?

2. Discuss the problems with airway and ventilation maintenance in a patient with morbid obesity who is found unresponsive and apneic.

3. Discuss how morbid obesity can also have a detrimental effect on the following body systems:

   a. Cardiovascular

   b. Pulmonary

   c. Musculoskeletal

   d. Psychological

CLINICAL DECISION MAKING

You are called for a "medical equipment alarm" at a residential address. On arrival you are met by an elderly female who seems very distressed. She explains that her husband came home from the hospital the previous day, after suffering a major stroke a month ago. He is now reliant on a mechanical ventilator for breathing through a tube placed in his neck. She tells you that the ventilator's alarm keeps sounding.

1. Based on this brief history, what would be at least two etiologies for the ventilator alarm to be sounding?

The primary assessment reveals the patient to be responsive to noxious stimuli with nonpurposeful motion. You note that the ventilator alarm is indicating "high airway pressure," and you note heavy secretions to the stoma placed in the anterior neck. The pulse oximeter reading is 93 percent, and the heart rate is 110 beats per minute.

2. Is this patient suffering from an airway disturbance or a ventilatory disturbance?

3. What action should you take to initially care for this patient?

After managing the situation described, you continue your assessment. You find that the pupils are midsize and responsive, the airway remains patent, peripheral pulses are present, capillary refill is <2 seconds, the skin is warm and slightly diaphoretic, the blood pressure is 138/86, the heart rate is now 88 beats per minute, and the pulse oximeter reads 96 percent. After placing the patient back on the ventilator, the ventilator resumes functioning without any alarms sounding.

4. How could you confirm clinically that the ventilator's operation is actually resulting in adequate ventilations for the patient?

5. What conditions are you still considering as the possible cause? Would you consider any other conditions as a possible cause?

6. Explain why this patient is at a greater risk for:

   a. Respiratory infections

   b. Sepsis

   c. Pressure ulcers

Standard EMS Operations

Competency Knowledge of operational roles and responsibilities to ensure patient, public, and personnel safety.

TOPIC

OPERATING AN AMBULANCE SAFELY

INTRODUCTION

Operating the ambulance and providing emergency care are essential roles of the paramedic. During each major phase of an ambulance call, the paramedic is responsible for safely performing the duties that will benefit those who require assistance. The major phases of an ambulance call include daily pre-run, dispatch, en route to the scene, at the scene, en route to the receiving facility, at the receiving facility, en route to the station, and post-run.

DAILY PRE-RUN

In an emergency, the paramedic must be properly prepared to respond. This includes having himself and his unit ready for whatever type of call is received. Preparations for the day are normally performed by the staff at the beginning of the shift. Typical pre-run activities include the following:

- **Preparing for the activities of the day.** It is important to take pride in yourself, your ambulance, and the services you provide to others. You should be prepared physically and mentally for the day ahead.
- **A briefing from the exiting crew** (if possible).
- **Inspection of the ambulance.** Make a thorough bumper-to-bumper inspection of the ambulance using the checklist provided by your service. If a problem is noted with your vehicle, know your service's policies for reporting and correcting it. Conduct routine maintenance on all ambulances. Some of the usual items inspected on a daily basis include interior and exterior of the vehicle, wheels, tires, windows, mirrors, doors, lights, oil, fluids, radio, horn, siren, and fuel.
- **Inspection of all equipment.** Each state mandates the equipment required to be carried by EMS response units. Use the checklist provided by your service to ensure that all equipment and supplies are present, and verify that everything is working properly (▶ **Figure 60-1**).
- **Notify dispatch when you are available to respond to an emergency call.**

TRANSITION *highlights*

- *Thorough review of the phases of an ambulance run:*
  - Pre-run.
  - Dispatch.
  - En route to the scene.
  - At the scene.
  - En route to the receiving facility.
  - At the receiving facility.
  - En route to the station.
  - Post-run.
- *Current guidelines for using aeromedical transport.*

DISPATCH

When an emergency arises, help is usually a phone call away. In most areas, an individual dials 911 to access emergency fire, police, and EMS personnel. The call is received by an emergency medical dispatcher, who attempts to ascertain the pertinent information about the nature of the emergency and determines which services will initially respond to the call. The information obtained from the caller may not be completely accurate. The responding unit should confirm the information and use it to prepare for the call.

> Make a thorough bumper-to-bumper inspection of the ambulance using the checklist provided by your service.

EN ROUTE TO THE SCENE

Emergency care cannot be provided to a patient if the responding unit does not arrive safely on the scene. Following the established safety procedures, obeying the laws, and driving

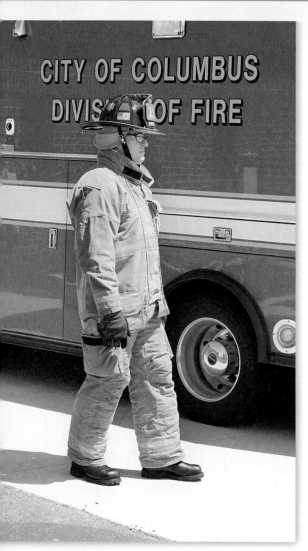

Figure 60-1 An ambulance carries full protective gear, including turnout gear, eye protection, helmet, and gloves. (© Ken Kerr)

safely will help you arrive ready to help those in need.

Call Preparation

- Advise dispatch that your unit is en route to the scene.
- Relax and prepare yourself mentally for the call and the drive.
- Based on the dispatched information, discuss with your partner what equipment may be needed and who will perform specific duties at the scene.
- Plan the safest route to the call. Use your maps and global positioning system (GPS) navigation before you leave. Avoid schools, railroad crossings, detours, construction sites, bridges, and

> **Know the capabilities and limitations of your vehicle.**

tunnels if possible. The time of day, day of the week, and weather conditions may influence your route.
- Limit use of escort vehicles or multiple-vehicle responses unless absolutely necessary and the driver cannot locate the patient or hospital. Remember that most motorists are expecting only one emergency vehicle. Second and third vehicles in an escort situation are more frequently involved in collisions.

Obey the Laws

- Know the state and local laws and regulations that apply when operating an ambulance. Emergency vehicle operators are frequently granted certain exemptions with regard to speed, parking, passage through traffic signals, and direction of travel as long as they do so with due regard for others.
- It is never acceptable for a paramedic to disobey the laws that govern his actions. Failure to follow the laws may result in tickets, lawsuits, loss of certification, or jail time.

Safe Driving

- Emergency vehicle operator training helps a paramedic develop the skills to safely operate an ambulance. Remember that emergency operations put both the providers in the ambulance and motorists around the ambulance at greater risk of injury.
- Seatbelts should be worn at all times by everyone inside the ambulance.
- Proper driving techniques, such as holding the steering wheel with both hands and checking your mirrors, should be followed. Good techniques help make good drivers.
- Follow your laws and protocols for use of emergency lights, sirens, and horns. Although a little time may be saved by using them, their use also increases the risk of incidents. Be aware of the effects these emergency devices can have on your patients, other drivers, and yourself.

- Know the capabilities and limitations of your vehicle. Each vehicle performs differently. You will need to become accustomed to how your ambulance accelerates and decelerates; the kind of space it requires for its fenders and bumpers; how it brakes; and how it corners.
- Weather conditions affect driving conditions, so adjust your driving accordingly. Allow for decreased visibility at night, in fog, and during rain, snow, and ice storms. Roads are most slippery as a rainstorm begins, and hydroplaning can occur at speeds as low as 35 miles per hour. Sleet, freezing rain, packed snow, and ice are slippery conditions that increase the possibility of skidding. Maintaining proper control of your vehicle in these conditions may be more difficult, so exercise caution.
- Drive defensively and always maintain a safe distance between your ambulance and other vehicles. Other drivers may be unpredictable, so be vigilant and anticipate the unexpected.
- Avoid backing up if possible. If you must back up, use a spotter to guide the backing process.

AT THE SCENE

Once at the scene, you will begin to assess the situation and provide emergency care to your patient. On scene, follow these guidelines:

- Notify dispatch of your arrival on scene (▶ **Figure 60-2**).
- Determine where and how to park the ambulance. Choose a safe location that will allow you to easily load the patient into the unit and depart from the scene.
- Perform a full scene size-up. Remember that you are responsible for the safety of those on the scene.
- Take all Standard Precautions that are necessary. As a general rule, paramedics should match the level of protection being worn by other responders at the scene. Remember that those responding to emergencies near a roadway must, by law, wear approved high-visibility apparel.
- Request additional resources if they are necessary, or cancel them if they are not.
- Assess your patient and provide the appropriate basic and advanced emergency care.

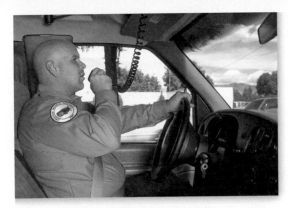

Figure 60-2 **Notify dispatch when you arrive at the scene.** (© Ken Kerr)

- Properly package the patient and transfer him to the waiting ambulance.
- Ensure that all hazards have been controlled and, if applicable, that care for the scene has been transferred to the appropriate agency.
- Ensure that you have all your equipment and have disposed properly of any wastes.

EN ROUTE TO THE RECEIVING FACILITY

The next phase of an emergency call is going to the receiving facility. Follow these guidelines:

- Notify dispatch that you are leaving the scene and are en route to the appropriate medical facility.
- Ensure that everyone in the vehicle is wearing safety belts properly.
- If you are the provider with the patient, continue to provide emergency care throughout transport. Keep the driver informed of the patient's condition.
- If you are driving to the receiving facility, make sure to drive safely and responsibly at all times. Do not use lights and siren en route to the hospital unless they are necessary based on the patient's clinical condition. Plan a safe route that minimizes the risks and discomfort to those in the ambulance.
- Notify the receiving medical facility that you are en route to the facility.

AT THE RECEIVING FACILITY

Once you arrive at the receiving facility, do the following:

- Notify dispatch of your arrival at the medical facility and park appropriately.
- Properly transfer the care of the patient by providing an oral report to the appropriate medical personnel at the receiving facility. Be sure to also transfer any of the patient's personal belongings.
- Assist emergency department personnel in moving the patient to a hospital bed and provide additional assistance as requested by the staff (▶ **Figure 60-3**).
- Complete a prehospital care report, and leave a copy at the emergency department.
- Prepare the ambulance to return to service as soon as possible. Clean the patient compartment, exchange equipment and supplies per protocol, prepare the cot, and ensure that all equipment is ready for the next call.
- Notify dispatch of your availability to take another emergency call.

EN ROUTE TO THE STATION

Once you return to the ambulance, you should notify dispatch that you are returning to the station or to the appropriate response area. Drive safely. It may be necessary to refuel at this time, based on protocol.

POST-RUN

After arriving back at the station, do the following:

- Notify dispatch of your arrival back at the station.
- Clean, sanitize, or disinfect all equipment appropriately, based on protocol.
- Replace any supplies that were used on the call that could not be exchanged previously.
- Change and replace any dirty linens or uniforms.
- Refuel and wash the ambulance.
- Complete any unfinished paperwork.

AIR MEDICAL TRANSPORT

In many cases, local and state guidelines define the criteria for use of air medical transport. Consider some of the potential disadvantages of using air transport, such as weather, response time, altitude limitations, aircraft size, terrain, cost, and patient condition before requesting a helicopter.

If it is necessary to use air medical transport, the following information should be provided by your department: whom to contact, the nature and location of the incident, the landing zone or helipad location, wind direction (if known), and any other potential hazards the

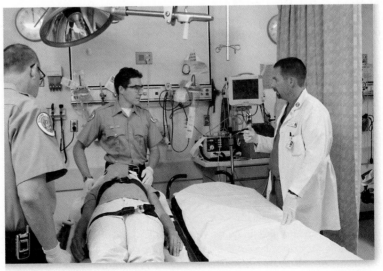

Figure 60-3 **It is essential that information exchange among providers be rapid, thorough, and accurate.**

service may encounter in response to your request.

In some instances, a landing zone may need to be set up. If so, follow these basic guidelines:

- Ensure that the landing area is clear from debris, traffic, wires, lines, and bystanders and rescue personnel.
- Landing zones should be a minimum of 60 × 60 feet during daytime operations and 100 × 100 feet at night. The terrain should have a slope not greater than 7 degrees. It is best to consult with your local flight service for their suggested minimum landing zone requirements.
- Mark the area with a highly visible device, such as tape during the day and flashing lights at night. Use flares only if fire is not a danger, and the area has been wet down.
- Assign one person to guide the pilot into the landing zone. He should wear proper protection and consider the wind direction.
- Approach and leave the helicopter only when the pilot indicates. In general, the aircraft should be shut down before personnel approach it. Be careful to crouch and avoid the aircraft's blades at all times.
- Follow the instructions of the crew in patient preparation and aircraft operation.
- Cooperate with the crew and transfer patient care to them appropriately. Be familiar with the cot used by local air ambulance providers in your area.

TRANSITIONING

REVIEW ITEMS

1. What factor should *not* affect the route you select to respond to an emergency call?
    a. time of day
    b. road construction
    c. color of the ambulance
    d. day of the week

2. Before leaving the receiving facility, you must _____.
    a. sterilize all equipment
    b. ensure proper patient transfer
    c. refill the fuel tank
    d. perform triage

3. Safe driving practices include _____.
    a. using lights and sirens when returning to the station
    b. using safety belts
    c. driving with one hand
    d. driving while asleep

4. Hydroplaning can occur _____.
    a. when the roads are dry
    b. only at high speeds
    c. at speeds as little as 35 miles per hour
    d. only if the steering wheel is let go

5. Which of the following should *not* be avoided when responding to a call?
    a. schools and school buses
    b. railroads and traffic jams
    c. multilane roadways and pedestrian-free areas
    d. bridges and tunnels

APPLIED KNOWLEDGE

1. Explain the importance of being well prepared to respond to an emergency.

2. Explain how different environmental factors may influence your response.

3. Why are good driving basics a necessity for ambulance operators?

4. List three circumstances that might influence the use of air medical services.

5. Discuss the importance of traffic laws while operating an ambulance in emergency mode.

CLINICAL DECISION MAKING

It is 5:00 AM, and you have just arrived at the station for your shift. After you clock in, the exiting crew members tell you that they had a very busy night. As you approach your unit, you see your partner checking the oil and ensuring that the vehicle is in proper working condition.

1. What do you do now?

2. Why is checking the equipment prior to answering any calls an essential part of your duties?

3. Is it necessary to check all supplies on the unit? Why or why not?

Dispatch advises you to respond to a call at a local nursing home with which you are familiar. You are advised that the female patient has a bloody nose. You and your partner respond appropriately to the call. After leaving the station, it begins to rain.

4. What concerns do you have as you proceed to the scene?

5. When you arrive at the nursing facility, what should you do?

After you ensure that the scene is safe and provide the initial emergency care to your patient, you determine no immediate life threats. The bleeding had stopped prior to your arrival, and the patient has no other complaints. The nursing facility has requested, however, that the

patient be treated and transported to the local hospital for physician evaluation.

6. What do you need to do before you leave the scene?

7. Will you use emergency lights and sirens en route to the hospital? Why or why not?

After arriving safely at the receiving facility, you and your partner transfer the patient and her belongings to the physician on duty. After completing your paperwork and cleaning the unit, you notify dispatch of your availability. Dispatch advises you to report back to the station.

8. What duties should you perform when you arrive back at the station?

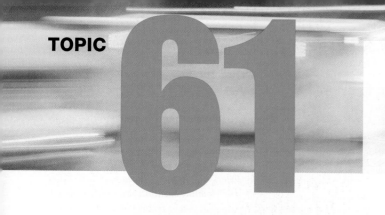

Standard EMS Operations

Competency Knowledge of operational roles and responsibilities to ensure patient, public, and personnel safety.

MULTIPLE-CASUALTY INCIDENTS AND INCIDENT MANAGEMENT

TRANSITION *highlights*

- *Review of what a multiple-casualty incident is.*
- *The NIMS framework.*
- *How the Incident Command System within NIMS is to be deployed during an MCI.*
- *The START triage format.*
- *The psychological stress that may arise in EMS secondary to an MCI.*

INTRODUCTION

A multiple-casualty incident (MCI) is any event that places a great demand on personnel or equipment. MCIs range from vehicle collisions with a few injured passengers to major disasters. Although most large-scale incidents require more time, resources, and support from other agencies, the principles for managing any MCI are fundamentally the same, regardless of the size of the emergency.

To manage any MCI effectively, the following must be accomplished:

- Enough help and resources, both personnel and equipment, must be obtained.
- Emergency vehicles must respond to and have access to the emergency scene.
- The appropriate emergency medical care must be provided to every patient.
- Patients requiring care must be transported to hospitals for treatment.
- Effective communication must be ensured.

- Follow-up care for both the patients and rescue personnel must be received.

The Department of Homeland Security developed and administers the National Incident Management System (NIMS). NIMS provides a framework to guide all levels of governmental, nongovernmental, and private agencies to work together to prevent, protect against, respond to, recover from, and mitigate the effects of incidents, regardless of cause, size, location, or complexity, in order to reduce the loss of life and property and harm to the environment.

NIMS is composed of five major components that are designed to work together:

- **Preparedness** involves a combination of assessment; planning; procedures and protocols; training and exercises; personnel qualifications, licensure, and certification; equipment certification; and evaluation and revision.
- **Communications and Information Management** utilizes the concepts of interoperability, reliability, scalability, and portability, as well as the resiliency and redundancy of communications and information systems.
- **Resource Management** defines mechanisms and establishes the process to identify requirements, order and acquire, mobilize, track and report, recover and demobilize, reimburse, and inventory resources.
- **Command and Management** is designed to provide a flexible structure based on three key organizational constructs: the Incident Command System, Multiagency Coordination Systems, and Public Information.
- **Ongoing Management and Maintenance** is facilitated through two components: the National Integration Center (NIC) and Supporting Technologies.

The Incident Command System (ICS) is a subset of the NIMS. It is based on successful business practices and decades of lessons learned in the organization and management of emergency incidents. The ICS is a flexible, cost-effective system that can be used to match the complexities and demands of a single or multiple incidents. It is applicable across all disciplines and is legally required to be used during some incidents, such as those involving hazardous materials. The ICS is structured to facilitate activities in five major functional areas:

- **Command.** Establishes and prioritizes objectives and has overall responsibility at the incident.
- **Operations.** Develops the tactical objectives and directs the use of tactical resources to carry out the plan.
- **Planning.** Prepares and documents the plan, collects and evaluates information, and maintains resource status and documentation for incident records.
- **Logistics.** Provides support, resources, and other services needed to meet the incident needs.
- **Finance/Administration.** Monitors costs related to the incident. Provides accounting, procurement, time recording, and cost analyses.
- **Intelligence and Investigation.** Sometimes added as a sixth area.

Every agency that responds to a disaster is required to be NIMS compliant. Various levels of incident management training are available to emergency personnel. The courses "FEMA IS-700: NIMS, An Introduction" and "ICS-100: Introduction to ICS," or their equivalents, are required for paramedics; however, particular organizations and positions might require additional training.

The initial training helps emergency responders understand the systems, use common terminology, communicate effectively with other agencies, identify the objectives to be accomplished during the incident, designate organizational resources, and manage the various spans of control and accountability throughout an incident.

Paramedics can better prepare themselves to respond to large-scale incidents by receiving additional training, participating in training activities, and using the principles of these systems in smaller-scaled incidents based on their protocols.

BRANCH UNITS

The incident commander (▶ Figure 61-1) may establish a number of branches to implement the plan effectively. The commander may assign a unit leader who will supervise the activities within the unit. Common units used for EMS personnel include triage, treatment, staging, transport, and communications. Many paramedics also participate in the care provided following the incident.

Triage

The triage unit sorts patients by criticality and assigns priorities for emergency care and transport. As a paramedic, you may be directed to assist in or may be completely responsible for accurate and efficient triage of the patients at an MCI. Triage is one of the first functions performed at the scene, and it directly affects all the other aspects of the operation.

There are typically two types of triage: primary and secondary. *Primary triage* occurs immediately on arrival of the first EMS crew. It is usually performed by the most knowledgeable and experienced EMS personnel first on the scene. Primary triage is used on the scene to rapidly categorize a patient's condition as one of the following:

- **Red/Highest Priority/Immediate/ Priority 1: Treatable Life- Threatening Illness or Injuries.** This category is assigned to patients with the most critical injuries who may be able to survive the incident with quick treatment and transport. Most of the treatable problems in this category correlate with the primary assessment. Patients in this category may have airway and breathing difficulties, uncontrolled or severe bleeding, decreased mental status, severe medical problems, shock, and/or severe burns.
- **Yellow/Second Priority/Delayed/ Priority 2: Serious But Not Life- Threatening Illness or Injuries.** This category is assigned to patients who are suffering severe injuries but still have a good chance of survival. The treatable problems in this category usually correlate with the findings identified during a rapid trauma assessment, such as burns without

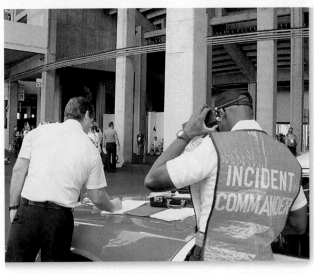

Figure 61-1 The incident commander directs the response and coordinates resources. Wearing reflective vests makes it easier to identify personnel.

airway problems, major or multiple bone or joint injuries, and back injuries.

- **Green/Lowest Priority/Minor/ Priority 3: "Walking Wounded."** This category is assigned to patients who are capable of walking. Patients in this category have injuries that will not reduce their chance of survival, such as fractures and soft tissue injuries without life-threatening bleeding.
- **Black/Deceased/Priority 4 (sometimes called Priority 0): Dead or Fatally Injured.** This category is assigned to patients who, despite the provision of emergency care, will not survive or who are already dead. Examples include patients with exposed brain matter, in cardiac arrest, or decapitated, and those who are incinerated.

Secondary triage is used for patient reevaluation after the patient is moved to the treatment area. Depending on the size of the incident, it may be necessary to retriage and reassign a patient to a different group based on the patient's presentation. Various techniques and systems are used to triage a patient, so it is necessary to be familiar with your local procedures and protocols. The Centers for Disease Control and Prevention (CDC) guidelines and START (Simple Triage and Rapid Transport) systems are two of the most commonly used.

> **Every agency that responds to a disaster is required to be NIMS compliant.**

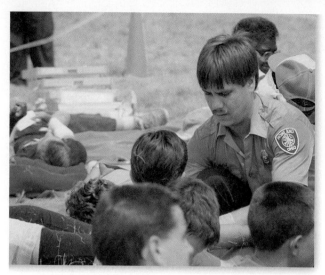

FIGURE 61-2 Patients are treated after triage, in order of priority.

START TRIAGE The START triage is performed primarily to initially categorize older children and adult patients for priority movement to the triage unit. It should not take more than 30 seconds per patient to complete. The assessment in START includes the following:

- **Respiratory status.** Any patient who is able to walk is considered low priority and is tagged "green." The paramedic should assess the respiratory status of those who cannot walk. If the patient is not breathing, the paramedic should open the patient's airway. If the patient remains apneic, tag him "black." If the patient's respiratory rate is greater than 30 per minute or inadequate, tag him "red." If it is less than 30 per minute, assess his perfusion status.
- **Perfusion status.** The paramedic should then assess the patient's radial pulse and capillary refill. If the patient has a radial pulse and his capillary refill is less than 2 seconds, the paramedic should then proceed to the mental status examination. If the patient's capillary refill is greater than 2 seconds or the radial pulse is absent, tag the patient "red."
- **Mental status.** The paramedic should ask the patient to squeeze his fingers. If the patient follows the command, tag him "yellow." If the patient is not alert, does not obey the commands, or is unresponsive, tag him "red."

After the patients are tagged appropriately, they can be identified, sorted, treated, and transported according to their criticality by rescue personnel at the incident.

Treatment

The treatment unit provides emergency care based on the priority assigned to the patient. Patients should be fully immobilized, if needed, and moved from the triage unit to the treatment unit in order of their priority (▶ **Figure 61-2**). The treatment area should be a safe distance from the incident and close to the area where the ambulances arrive. Larger-scaled incidents may require use of more than one treatment unit. A morgue should be established and used appropriately. Follow local protocol.

Staging

The staging unit holds ambulances, helicopters, and additional equipment until they are assigned to a particular task. The staging unit leader monitors, inventories, and directs the available ambulances to and from the treatment area. The staging unit leader should also provide the responding EMS personnel with maps to the appropriate receiving facilities.

Transport

The transport unit leader ensures that ambulances are accessible and that transportation does not occur without the direction of the incident commander. Patients should be transported based on their priority. The transport unit leader must consider the following when making decisions on where to transport each patient:

- Distribution of patients to each medical facility
- Surge capacity of each hospital or medical facility
- Need for transport to a specialty medical facility, such as a burn unit or pediatric emergency department
- The need for constant coordination and communication

The transport unit leader should radio the hospital and provide a brief patient report and estimated time of arrival. Ambulatory patients may be transported via bus with adequate personnel and supplies once the more critical patients have been transported. Deceased casualties should be transported to the morgue.

Communications

Emergency management is dependent on effective communication among all those involved. Without efficient communication, a paramedic should anticipate problems throughout the incident. Many communication problems, such as dead spots, frequency unavailability, and channel gridlock, are usually identified early but may still be encountered during an MCI. To reduce communication problems during an MCI, the details of a communication system should be established prior to an incident and should be incorporated into disaster drills. A communication plan should include the following:

- Incident-related policies and standards
- Systems and equipment to be used
- Training necessary to achieve integrated communications
- Responsibility assigned to those operating the system and equipment
- A reliable backup system

Follow-Through

After all the patients have been transported from an incident scene, the emergency personnel assist hospital personnel in follow-through care if necessary. If a paramedic's assistance is needed, the facility's incident manager will provide instructions. If the paramedic's assistance is not needed at the hospital, the paramedic should prepare to respond to other emergency calls.

PSYCHOLOGICAL STRESS

Psychological stress often affects the rescuers, as well as the patients, at the scene of an MCI. Personal safety, crying, anger, guilt, numbness, preoccupation with death, frustration, fatigue, and burnout are common concerns encountered by EMS personnel. Effective stress management should be considered prior to and incorporated into the relief efforts of any MCI. Stress management plans and activities should emphasize the following actions:

- Ensure that personnel are appropriately trained and aware of their specific tasks.
- Provide nourishing food and water.
- Ensure rest at regular intervals, maybe as often as once every one to two hours.

- Monitor personnel for signs of physical exhaustion, stress, or breakdown.
- Encourage rescue workers to talk to their colleagues about their experiences.

- Provide trained counselors to talk with personnel throughout and after the incident.
- Treat and transport immediately any rescuer who is injured or becomes ill during rescue operations.

TRANSITIONING

REVIEW ITEMS

1. Which of the following is *not* used when making decisions on where to take each patient involved in an MCI?
   a. the need for transport to a specialized facility
   b. the ability of each patient to pay for services from the receiving medical facility
   c. the distribution of patients to each medical facility
   d. the surge capacity of each hospital or medical facility

2. Which of the following activities is performed first at an MCI?
   a. triaging patients based on their presentations
   b. treating a patient's minor secondary injuries
   c. transporting all deceased patients to the morgue
   d. transporting all patients to a hospital as soon as you reach them regardless of the severity of their conditions

3. When using the START system, which of the following should be assessed first?

   a. mental status
   b. perfusion status
   c. respirations
   d. Glasgow Coma Scale

4. Which branch unit is responsible for holding the ambulances, helicopters, and additional equipment until they are assigned to a particular task?
   a. triage unit
   b. transport unit
   c. staging unit
   d. treatment unit

5. Which of the following NIMS component responsibilities includes ensuring that rescue personnel meet specific qualifications?
   a. Command and Management
   b. Preparedness
   c. Communications and Information Management
   d. Ongoing Management and Maintenance

APPLIED KNOWLEDGE

1. List and describe the branch units frequently used during an MCI.

2. Explain the process of triage.

3. What is the purpose of the incident management system?

4. How should START triage be used to assign priority to and properly tag a patient?

5. Discuss the importance of effective communications during an incident.

6. Discuss ways to help reduce responder stress throughout an incident.

7. Differentiate between primary and secondary triage.

CLINICAL DECISION MAKING

You and your partner are the first on the scene of a motor vehicle collision. Dispatch has advised you that, because of another major incident, you are the only unit available. Dispatch advises that backup will not be able to arrive on the scene for approximately 10 minutes. As you approach the scene, you note that three vehicles are involved, one of which is a motorcycle that appears to be missing a driver.

1. What concerns do you have as you approach the scene?

2. What information do you need to obtain?

After you determine that the scene is safe, you approach the vehicles. You are met by a patient who approaches you and states that he and his wife were inside vehicle 1. Their vehicle is an SUV with minor front-end damage. The driver, a 25-year-old man, states that they were on their way to the hospital because his wife is in labor when a man on a motorcycle passed them and hit the car ahead of them. The woman, who is 27 years old and obviously pregnant, states she is having contractions that are 10 minutes apart. She states says her abdomen is hurting but she has never been in labor before. Her husband denies any pain or complaints. Both patients are alert and oriented, deny any loss of consciousness, and state they were restrained.

3. As the most experienced provider on scene, what should you do now?

4. What should you instruct your partner to do?

After reassuring the patients in vehicle 1, you proceed to vehicle 2, as your partner begins to look in the nearby ditch for the driver of the motorcycle. Vehicle 2 is a minivan with extensive damage to the front passenger side. The driver of the vehicle is a 61-year-old woman who is alert and oriented. She is complaining of neck pain. She denies any loss of consciousness and says she was the only passenger in her vehicle.

Your partner states that he found the motorcycle driver, who was ejected into the ditch. The patient appears to be a teenage boy who is currently unresponsive, has a weak radial pulse, and has multiple abrasions and deformities to his upper and lower extremities.

5. Based on the scene size-up characteristics, what resources do you need?

6. What priority status would be assigned to each patient? Why?

7. What would your plan be for this incident?

8. Once additional units arrive, in what order would you have the patients transported? Why?

9. Despite your arrival first on the scene, explain why you and your partner will be the last to leave.

INDEX

Note: Page numbers followed by *f* represent figures and page numbers followed by *t* represent tables.